Respiratory Infections: Diagnosis and Treatment

Respiratory Infections: Diagnosis and Treatment

Editor: Mike Rudd

FOSTER ACADEMICS

www.fosteracademics.com

www.fosteracademics.com

FOSTER ACADEMICS

Cataloging-in-Publication Data

Respiratory infections : diagnosis and treatment / edited by Mike Rudd.
p. cm.
Includes bibliographical references and index.
ISBN 978-1-63242-800-4
1. Respiratory infections. 2. Respiratory infections--Diagnosis. 3. Respiratory infections--Treatment.
4. Respiratory organs--Diseases. I. Rudd, Mike.
RC740 .R47 2019
616.2--dc23

Foster Academics,
118-35 Queens Blvd., Suite 400,
Forest Hills, NY 11375, USA

ISBN 978-1-63242-800-4 (Hardback)

Printed and bound in China.

Contents

Preface

Respiratory infections include the infectious diseases of the respiratory tract. Such infections can be classified as lower respiratory tract infection or upper respiratory tract infection. The lower respiratory tract infections are more serious than the upper respiratory tract infections. Some respiratory tract infections are sinusitis, tonsillitis, pharyngitis, influenza, bronchitis and pneumonia. Human orthopneumovirus is a major cause of lower respiratory tract infections. It generally causes conditions like bronchiolitis and pneumonia. These can be diagnosed through physical examination, skin monitoring to check for hypoxemia, chest X-rays, blood tests, and lab test of respiratory secretions. This book explores all the important aspects of respiratory infections in the present day scenario. It includes some of the vital pieces of work being conducted across the world, on various topics related to the diagnosis and treatment of respiratory infections. This book is a resource guide for doctors as well as students.

This book unites the global concepts and researches in an organized manner for a comprehensive understanding of the subject. It is a ripe text for all researchers, students, scientists or anyone else who is interested in acquiring a better knowledge of this dynamic field.

I extend my sincere thanks to the contributors for such eloquent research chapters. Finally, I thank my family for being a source of support and help.

Editor

1

Respiratory Syncytial Virus Can Infect Basal Cells and Alter Human Airway Epithelial Differentiation

B. David Persson[1], Aron B. Jaffe[1], Rachel Fearns[2], Henry Danahay[3]*

1 Developmental and Molecular Pathways, Novartis Institutes for BioMedical Research, Cambridge, Massachusetts, United States of America, **2** Department of Microbiology, Boston University School of Medicine, Boston, Massachusetts, United States of America, **3** Respiratory Disease Area, Novartis Institutes for BioMedical Research, Horsham, United Kingdom

Abstract

Respiratory syncytial virus (RSV) is a major cause of morbidity and mortality worldwide, causing severe respiratory illness in infants and immune compromised patients. The ciliated cells of the human airway epithelium have been considered to be the exclusive target of RSV, although recent data have suggested that basal cells, the progenitors for the conducting airway epithelium, may also become infected *in vivo*. Using either mechanical or chemical injury models, we have demonstrated a robust RSV infection of $p63^+$ basal cells in air-liquid interface (ALI) cultures of human bronchial epithelial cells. In addition, proliferating basal cells in 2D culture were also susceptible to RSV infection. We therefore tested the hypothesis that RSV infection of this progenitor cell would influence the differentiation status of the airway epithelium. RSV infection of basal cells on the day of seeding (MOI≤0.0001), resulted in the formation of an epithelium that showed a profound loss of ciliated cells and gain of secretory cells as assessed by acetylated α-tubulin and MUC5AC/MUC5B immunostaining, respectively. The mechanism driving the switch in epithelial phenotype is in part driven by the induced type I and type III interferon response that we demonstrate is triggered early following RSV infection. Neutralization of this response attenuates the RSV-induced loss of ciliated cells. Together, these data show that through infection of proliferating airway basal cells, RSV has the potential to influence the cellular composition of the airway epithelium. The resulting phenotype might be expected to contribute towards both the severity of acute infection, as well as to the longer-term consequences of viral exacerbations in patients with pre-existing respiratory diseases.

Editor: Kevin Harrod, Lovelace Respiratory Research Institute, United States of America

Funding: This study was funded by Novartis Institutes for Biomedical Research. Authors B. D. Persson, A. B. Jaffe and H. Danahay are employees of Novartis Institutes for BioMedical Research. There are no patents, products in development or marketed products to declare. The funders had no role in study design, data collection and analysis, decision to publish, or preparation of the manuscript.

Competing Interests: This paper is financed by Novartis Institutes for Biomedical Research. The funder, Novartis Institutes for Biomedical Research provided support in the form of salaries for authors B. D. Persson, A. B. Jaffe and H. Danahay, but did not have any additional role in the study design, data collection and analysis, decision to publish, or preparation of the manuscript. The specific roles of these authors are articulated in the 'author contributions' section.

* Email: henry.danahay@novartis.com

Introduction

Human respiratory syncytial virus (RSV) infections are estimated to cause 64 million cases of respiratory disease worldwide leading to acute lower respiratory infections and 160,000 deaths annually [1,2]. RSV has seasonal epidemiology causing annual epidemics and virtually 100% of children are infected before the age of two. Neonates, young children, immune-compromised adults and the elderly are especially prone to severe infection, resulting in bronchiolitis associated with epithelial necrosis, sloughing of the airway epithelium, edema and increased secretion of mucus. RSV infection is also known to frequently exacerbate existing pulmonary conditions such as chronic obstructive pulmonary disease (COPD) and asthma [3,4,5]. Exposure to RSV does not provide life-long lasting immunity allowing for recurrent infections through life [6,7], and a greater understanding of the host response to this virus is expected to provide new insights into future therapy. To date, treatment of RSV disease is restricted to supportive care and prophylactic administration of palivizumab (Synagis), a monoclonal antibody directed to the fusion protein, for high-risk groups. No effective small molecule compounds or vaccines are currently available [8,9].

The major site of RSV infection in the human lung is the pseudostratified epithelium that lines the conducting airway. This epithelium is composed of apical multi-ciliated and secretory (goblet) cells with the $p63^+$ basal cell located directly beneath this layer. Elegant studies using well differentiated air-liquid interface (ALI) cultures of primary human bronchial epithelial cells (HBEC) have convincingly demonstrated that RSV has tropism for ciliated cells [10,11,12,13,14,15]. However, *in vivo* work using an infant baboon model and a pre-term lamb model have also described the potential for the airway basal cell to become infected by RSV. These studies propose that virus-induced damage to the surface epithelium enables access of RSV to an otherwise inaccessible, non-ciliated cell-type [16,17]. The identity of the infected, non-ciliated cell in these studies was not examined, but could potentially be a basal cell. Considering that respiratory diseases such as asthma and COPD can be associated with disrupted epithelial cell-cell junctions, impaired barrier function, and sloughing of the epithelium, basal cells might be reasonably expected to also be accessible to viruses such as RSV in patients with these pre-existing respiratory conditions [18,19,20,21,22]. The implications for infection of an airway basal cell are potentially widespread, especially in view of the key progenitor role it serves [23]. However, this remains a largely unexplored area, most likely because: 1) human airway basal cells in 'steady-state' ALI culture have been reported to not become infected by RSV, even after mechanical injury to the epithelium [11], and 2) human pathology studies largely implicate the ciliated cell as the major site of infection, and although infected non-ciliated cells have been described [24], basal cells have been considered to be resistant to RSV. It should however be considered that human pathology data are mostly restricted to pediatric cases [25,26,27]. To our knowledge, there are no pathology reports relating to RSV infection in adult patients with pre-existing conditions such as asthma or COPD, where epithelial barrier function can be chronically impaired. Furthermore, basal cells in a damaged epithelium will be required to be highly proliferative, that is in contrast to their slow turnover in the 'steady-state', healthy epithelium. The potential for RSV to infect basal cells in this highly proliferative state has not been explored. In view of the potential significance of an RSV infection of basal cells to human disease, recent *in vivo* data suggesting infection of basal cells together with outstanding questions regarding the identity of the infected non-ciliated cell, in human pathology studies, we have re-evaluated the basal cell tropism question in ALI cultures of HBEC.

Here we show that p63$^+$, primary human airway basal cells from multiple donors can be readily infected by different strains of RSV. We found that infection of basal cells occurred in both a 2D cell culture system, as well as in well-differentiated, polarized cultures grown at ALI. Mechanical injury (scratch wound) or chemical damage (low Ca^{2+} disruption of adherens junctions and desmosomes) both resulted in exposure of basal cells to RSV and a subsequent infection. The consequence of infection of the basal cell is that the resultant epithelium had a reduced density of ciliated cells and a greater proportion of mucin-containing goblet cells. This switch in epithelial phenotype might be reasonably expected to be a normal protective effect if appropriately regulated in a normal healthy individual, but could equally contribute towards airway occlusion and impaired mucociliary clearance in a patient with a pre-existing respiratory disease.

Furthermore, we have found that a number of interferons are able to phenocopy the effect of RSV on basal cell fate determination and have extended these observations to highlight that the endogenous production of the type III interferon IL-29 following RSV infection at least partially drives the loss of ciliated phenotype. To our knowledge, these are the first data to outline a mechanism by which RSV infection may contribute to airway epithelial remodeling and therefore the pathology of a number of respiratory diseases. Future therapies designed to regulate basal cell fate determination in the lung following injury or infection could represent novel approaches to the treatment of viral diseases in an adult host suffering from pre-existing conditions such as asthma, cystic fibrosis and COPD.

Results

RSV infects human airway basal cells

The experiments performed in these studies used well-differentiated cultures of the human airway epithelium that have been previously described by others [28,29,30]. This model utilizes p63$^+$ primary human airway basal cells cultured on a permeable support. The cells first proliferate and form a confluent epithelium (days 0–7), while submerged in growth medium, and then differentiate over days 8–21 while exposed to an air-liquid interface (ALI). This model has been widely used to study the regulation of airway epithelial growth and repair and to investigate RSV infection of the human airway [11,12,13,15]. When ALI cultures were exposed to recombinant RSV, engineered to express green fluorescent protein (RSV-A2-GFP) [31,32] (150,000 pfu/Transwell), we observed a widespread infection of ciliated cells (Figure 1A, B), consistent with published work [11,12,15]. Confocal microscopy failed to identify any GFP$^+$ infected cells in the basal region of the epithelium (Figure 1B), also consistent with previous reports [11,13,15]. To investigate whether an alteration in the integrity of the epithelial barrier would affect RSV tropism, we treated fully differentiated ALI cultures with a calcium-free medium using a protocol previously described to enable rhinovirus access to airway basal cells [33]. After a short exposure to calcium-free media, the supra-basal cell layer detached and could be easily removed, leaving a layer of predominantly p63$^+$ basal cells. RSV-A2-GFP was added to the remaining monolayer of p63$^+$ cells (150,000 pfu/Transwell) and at 16 hours post infection numerous dual positive GFP$^+$p63$^+$ cells were clearly evident across the insert (Figure 1C–D).

To test whether the infection of p63$^+$ basal cells with RSV was an artifact of treatment with Ca^{2+}-free media, we next mechanically injured the ALI cultures using the protocol described by Zhang et al. [11]. Intersecting thin scratches were made across the Transwell filter using a GUM stimulator, immediately after which 250,000 pfu of RV-A2-GFP was added. After a 30 minute exposure to RSV, the viral inoculum was removed and the cells cultured for a further 20 h. By 20 h after injury and infection, the scratch wound areas appeared to have covered over with epithelial cells (Figure 1E) and infected (GFP$^+$) cells were clearly visible within the wound area (Figure 1F). Confocal imaging of the wound area defined the infected cells as dual positive p63$^+$GFP$^+$, indicating infection of the airway basal cells (Figure 1G–I). To quantify the infection of basal cells within the scratch injury we outlined the approximate area of the injury in 12 imaged z-stacks (similar as indicated in Figure 1G–I), from 2 independent experiments, and counted the total number of p63$^+$ basal cells and GFP$^+$ infected cells. In total, of 214 p63$^+$ basal cells that were counted in the wound areas, 93 cells were RSV infected. In addition, we only found three infected cells within the marked scratch area that were neither p63$^+$ nor ciliated. In undamaged areas of the insert, an extensive infection of ciliated cells was observed. Together the data highlighted that RSV can infect basal cells if it is able to gain access to the sub-apical region of the epithelium.

An observation made in the two ALI injury/infection studies above, was that the p63 levels appeared to be reduced in the GFP$^+$ cells. To address whether RSV infection of basal cells could repress p63 protein expression, basal cells were seeded onto Transwell inserts and infected with RSV 3 h later. At 48 h after seeding (45 h post infection) cells were fixed and FACS sorted using the basal cell markers p63 and ITGA6 together with GFP as a marker of infected cells. We confirmed that 100% of infected cells were p63$^+$ITGA6$^+$ (Figure S1A–D) and that there was a significant reduction in the mean intensity of the p63 immunostaining (64.9$\pm$1.2% of uninfected control; $p<0.002$), consistent with observations made in the ALI studies.

Basal cell infection sustains the epithelial spread of RSV

Having demonstrated that RSV could infect basal cells both before and after the formation of a well-differentiated epithelium, we asked whether infected basal cells could sustain viral replication and enable the virus to spread in the context of a polarized epithelium, as observed in the infant baboon [16] and pre-term

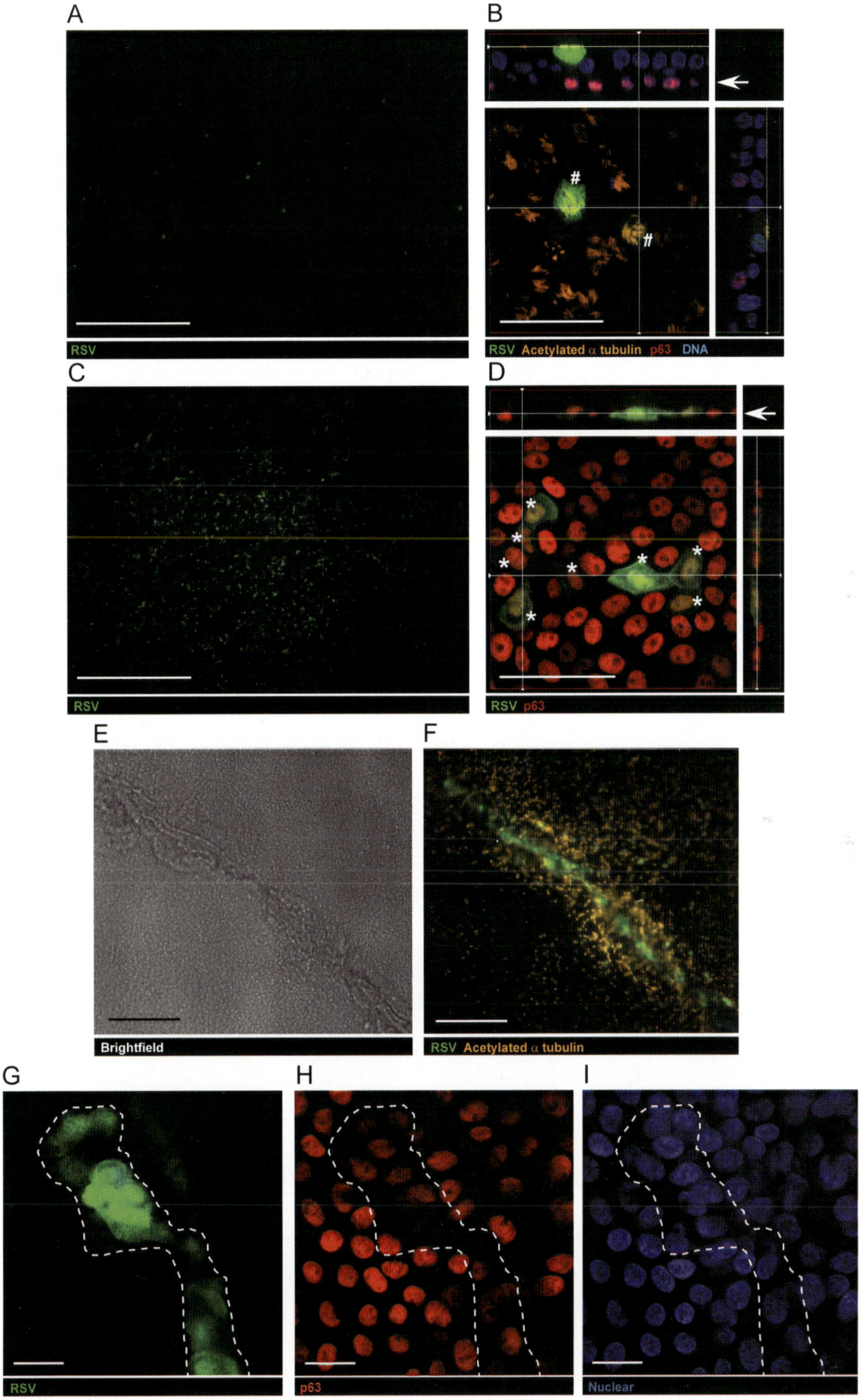
A
B
C
D
E
F
G
H
I
RSV
RSV Acetylated α tubulin p63 DNA
RSV
RSV p63
Brightfield
RSV Acetylated α tubulin
RSV
p63
Nuclear

Figure 1. RSV infection of both multi-ciliated and airway basal cells. Apical exposure of HBEC to RSV-A2-GFP led to the infection of multi-ciliated cells. GFP^+ (infected) cells were observed throughout the epithelium. These were identified as an acetylated α-tubulin$^+$, ciliated cell (#, orange) by confocal imaging (A–B). Under these conditions, the sub-apical $p63^+$ basal cells (red) did not become infected by RSV (B). Removal of the surface of the epithelium immediately before exposure to RSV resulted in numerous $p63^+GFP^+$ (*) cells 16 h later (C–D), consistent with infection of the airway basal cell. When well-differentiated cells were subjected to a mechanical scratch injury (E) followed by RSV infection multiple infected cells were clearly visible within the wound (F). A majority of the infected cells were determined as basal cells ($p63^+$) by confocal microscopy (G–I). Presented are representative images from three independent experiments in two different donors. White bar indicates 1,000 μm in A, C, 50 um in B, D, 500 μm in E–F and 20 μm in G–I.

lamb models [17]. To address this question we infected 100,000 basal cells before differentiation (3 h after seeding) with 100 pfu of RSV-A2-GFP, similarly to the experiment shown in Figure S1. Cells were cultured submerged in medium until day 7 and then exposed to ALI. Live cell images of the infected cultures were collected every 2–3 days over three weeks and GFP^+ cells were quantified to monitor viral infection. This analysis showed that RSV spread rapidly in the basal cell population until day 6 (line graph in Figure 2A, B), a time point where the uninfected control cultures were still predominantly $p63^+$ basal cells (data not shown). Viral titers in apical washes indicated that RSV was shed by the infected basal cells between days 3 and 6 post-seeding/infection (bar graph in Figure 2A). The numbers of GFP^+ cells then declined to approximately 20% of the maximum (Figure 2A), although viral titers in the media remained elevated. At day 13, coinciding with the time where ciliated cells first became apparent (Figure 2C), the numbers of GFP^+ cells began to increase, with infection of ciliated cells by day 20 (Figure 2D).

With evidence that an RSV infected basal cell could sustain viral replication, leading to spread of the infection throughout the course of epithelial formation and differentiation, we investigated how a range of viral doses could impact the epithelium. Basal cells infected with viral doses ranging from 1,000 pfu (MOI = 0.01) to 1 pfu (MOI = 0.00001) per insert formed a confluent monolayer with an intact barrier by 6 days post-seeding (equivalent to the behavior of uninfected cells), as judged by their ability to maintain a dry apical surface at ALI. Higher viral doses induced cell death and prevented the formation of a confluent cell monolayer so were not analyzed further (data not shown). Cells were examined at 21 days post infection to characterize their morphology and determine the extent of viral spread (Figure S2). At each of the viral doses examined, the infected cells were in an apical location (for example Figure 2D). However, the morphology of the infected cells and extent of viral spread was very different for the different viral doses (Figure S2A–D). Following infection with 1,000 pfu, numerous elongated, larger cells were apparent with evidence of syncytia (Figure S2A, E) and large, flat mono-nucleated cells (data not shown). The lower viral doses of 1 pfu and 10 pfu resulted in infected cells of a considerably smaller size (Figure S2C–D). The viral dose of 100 pfu generated RSV infected cells of small size as well as large flattened out cells (Figure S2B). Thus, even when inoculated at a low level, RSV was able to infect basal cells and spread in the basal cell population, resulting in widespread viral infection by the time of full differentiation.

RSV infection of basal cells results in loss of ciliated and gain of secretory cells

The data described above illustrate that in the presence of an ongoing RSV infection the airway epithelium was able to form a monolayer and differentiate. To determine whether RSV infection could influence the cellular composition of the epithelium, the cultures described above were assessed by quantitative immunofluorescence, using acetylated α-tubulin as a marker for ciliated cells and MUC5AC for secretory cells. At viral doses ≥10 pfu/Transwell (MOI: 0.0001), RSV infection resulted in a significant reduction in ciliated cells and an increase in $MUC5AC^+$ secretory cells by day 21 (Figure 3). At lower doses of RSV (<10 pfu/Transwell) the cellular composition of the epithelium was similar to that of the uninfected control and the infected (GFP^+) cells were exclusively ciliated cells (data not shown). This observation was verified in cells from three donors (Figure S3). In addition, to eliminate the possibility that the modified RSV-A2-GFP strain was not representative of wild-type RSV infection, we repeated the experiments using a clinical isolate designated RSV-A2-MOT092 (obtained from Dr. Edward Walsh, University of Rochester Medical School). For the clinical isolate we also had the possibility to stain for MUC5B in addition to MUC5AC and acetylated α-tubulin, as the GFP channel was not occupied by RSV-A2-GFP. For each experiment, one well was stained for RSV to verify viral infection (data not shown). RSV-A2-MOT0972 showed an identical epithelial phenotype with a loss of ciliated cells and an expansion of both $MUC5AC^+$ and $MUC5B^+$ secretory cells (Figure 3G). Together, these experiments illustrate that RSV infection of the progenitor basal cells induced a change in the phenotype of the resulting epithelium with an increased number of goblet cells and reduced number of ciliated cells.

Type III IFNs contribute to the RSV-induced change in epithelial phenotype

RSV infection of the airway epithelium has been demonstrated to induce the release of a number of secreted factors that likely regulate the host immune response, including: IL-1α, IL-1β, IL-4, IL-5, IL-6, IL-8, IL-10, IL-12, IL-13, IL-15, IL-17A, IL-18 and TNF-α [7,10,34,35,36,37,38,39,40]. RSV has also been shown to induce a type I (IFN-α and IFN-β) and type III (IFN-λ) interferon responses in multiple cell lines [10,12,36,39,41,42]. To assess the potential influence of the RSV-induced factors on the epithelial phenotype, we profiled their expression levels during differentiation. Basal cells were infected with 100 pfu of RSV-A2-GFP and expression levels of different soluble immune factors were determined by qRT-PCR at days 3, 7 and 14 days post-infection. Notably, RSV infection induced an early IL6, IFNβ and IFNλ (IL28A/B and IL29) response in the epithelium, which diminished over time (Figure 4A; note that due to the high similarity between IL28A and IL28B, our probes did not differentiate between the two). IFNγ and IL17A mRNAs were below the level of detection at each time point examined (data not shown) and there was no evidence for significant regulation of the other gene transcripts studied (Figure 4A). The RSV-induced changes in IFNλ mRNA levels correlated with a significant increase in levels of both IL-28A and IL-28B/IL-29 protein, which were detectable from day 7. The levels of these interferons declined over time and were undetectable at day 21 (Figure 4B). It was not possible to determine whether IL-28B was induced, as that interferon was grouped with IL-28A in the gene expression analysis and with IL-29 in the ELISA. The time for maximum concentrations of IL-28A, IL-28B and IL-29 correlated with the peak release of viral particles (bar graph in Figure 2A), consistent with the predicted anti-viral

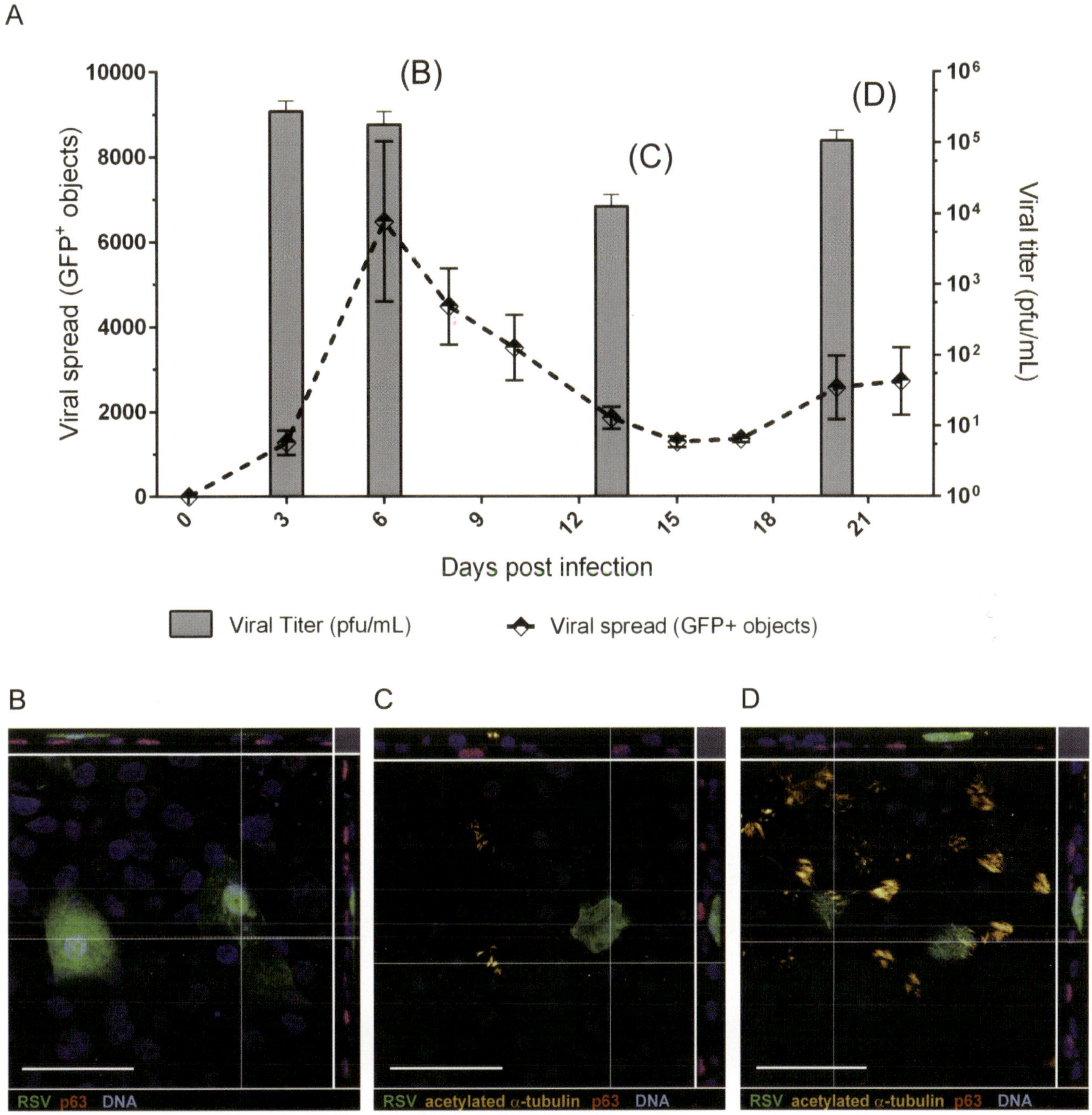

Figure 2. RSV infection of basal cells influences differentiation. The effects of RSV-A2-GFP infection of basal cells (100 pfu/insert, 3 h after seeding) were investigated over the duration of epithelial growth and differentiation. Infection of the epithelium was monitored by live cell imaging of GFP^+ objects every 2–3 days (A; dotted line) whilst viral release was determined by plaque assay at day 3, 6, 13 and 21 (A; filled bars). Mean data ± SEM from 3 independent studies are shown. Representative planar and transverse views by confocal microscopy showing RSV-A2-GFP infected cells at day 6 (B), infected non-ciliated cells at day 13 (C) and infected ciliated cells at day 20 (D). GFP was used to visualize RSV-infection (green), acetylated α-tubulin stain for cilia (orange) and p63 for basal cells (red). Scale bars indicate 50 μm.

response of the epithelium. Secreted IFN-β was below the level of detection at each time point examined (data not shown). We did not perform any further studies on IL6 as IL6 was not significantly up-regulated at 7 days post infection when the cells were brought to ALI to differentiate and was therefore unlikely to affect epithelial composition.

We next asked whether treatment with the RSV-induced cytokines could phenocopy the effect of RSV infection on the epithelial composition of air-liquid interface cultures. Concentrations of the different interferons were selected based on an initial pilot study that covered the range of 0.3 to 30 ng/mL for each. Based on this study, IL-28A, IL-28B and IL-29 were added at a concentration of 30 ng/mL with IFN-β being tested at 2.5 ng/mL as higher concentrations of IFN-β did not allow for a confluent cell layer to be formed. Cells were treated from days 0–21 in culture with fresh aliquots of mediator being added on every feeding.

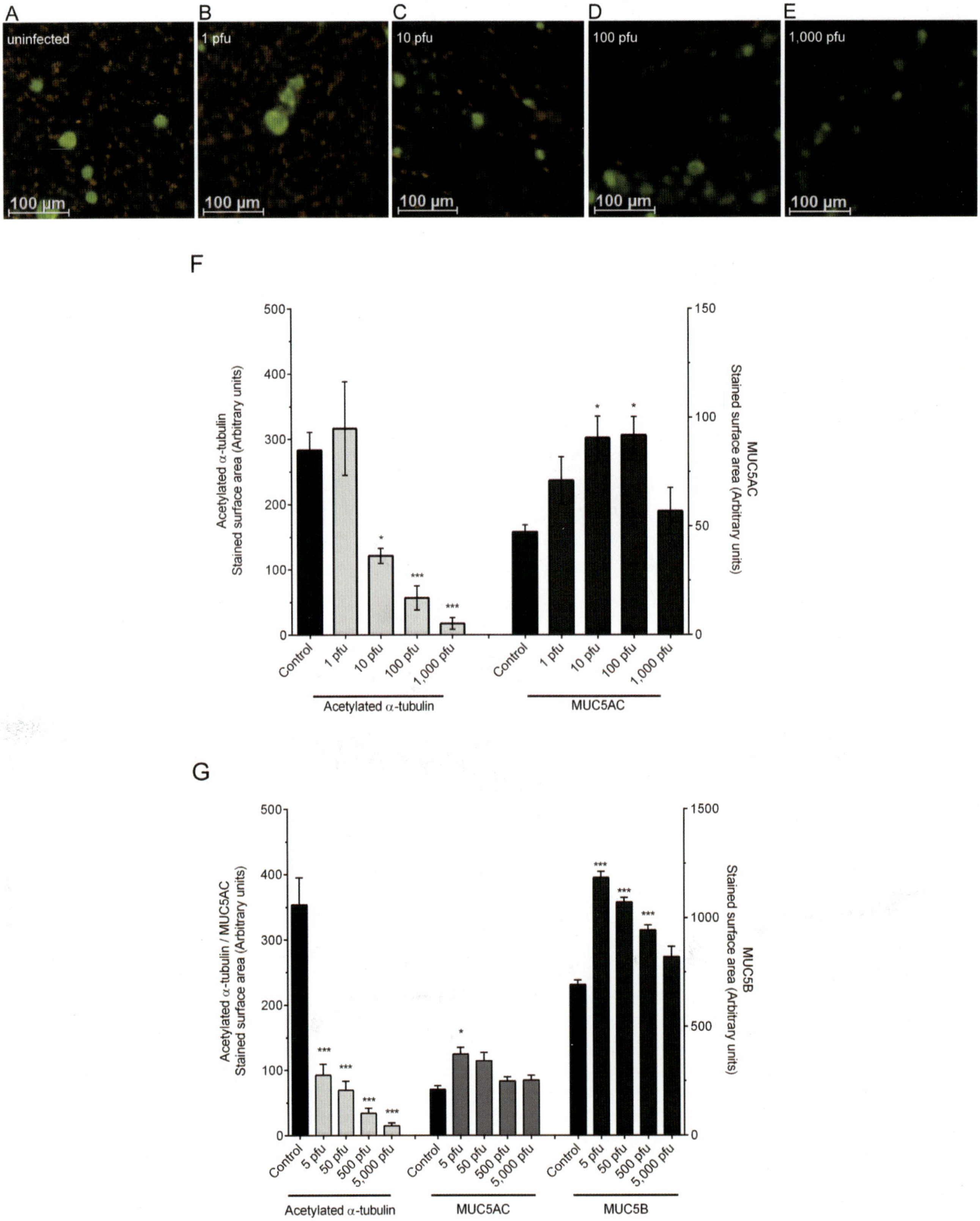

Figure 3. Epithelial composition following RSV infection. The effects of RSV-A2-GFP infection of basal cells on epithelial differentiation were assessed by quantitative immunofluorescence. Representative, images of HBEC cultures (21 days after seeding/infection) that were either uninfected (A) or infected with 1, 10, 100, or 1,000 pfu of RSV-A2-GFP (B–E, respectively). $MUC5AC^{+}$ goblet cells and acetylated a-$tubulin^{+}$ ciliated cells are pseudo-colored green and orange respectively. Staining for each of the cell types was quantified by image analysis (F). An alternative RSV strain, RSV-A2-MOT0972, was also assessed for effects on epithelial differentiation by quantitative immunofluoresence (G) as described above. For each study, mean data ± SEM from 6–9 inserts over three independent experiments are shown. Statistical significance was determined with a one-way ANOVA with post-hoc Dunnetts test compared to untreated control cells. * indicates $p<0.05$, **$p<0.01$ and ***$p<0.001$.

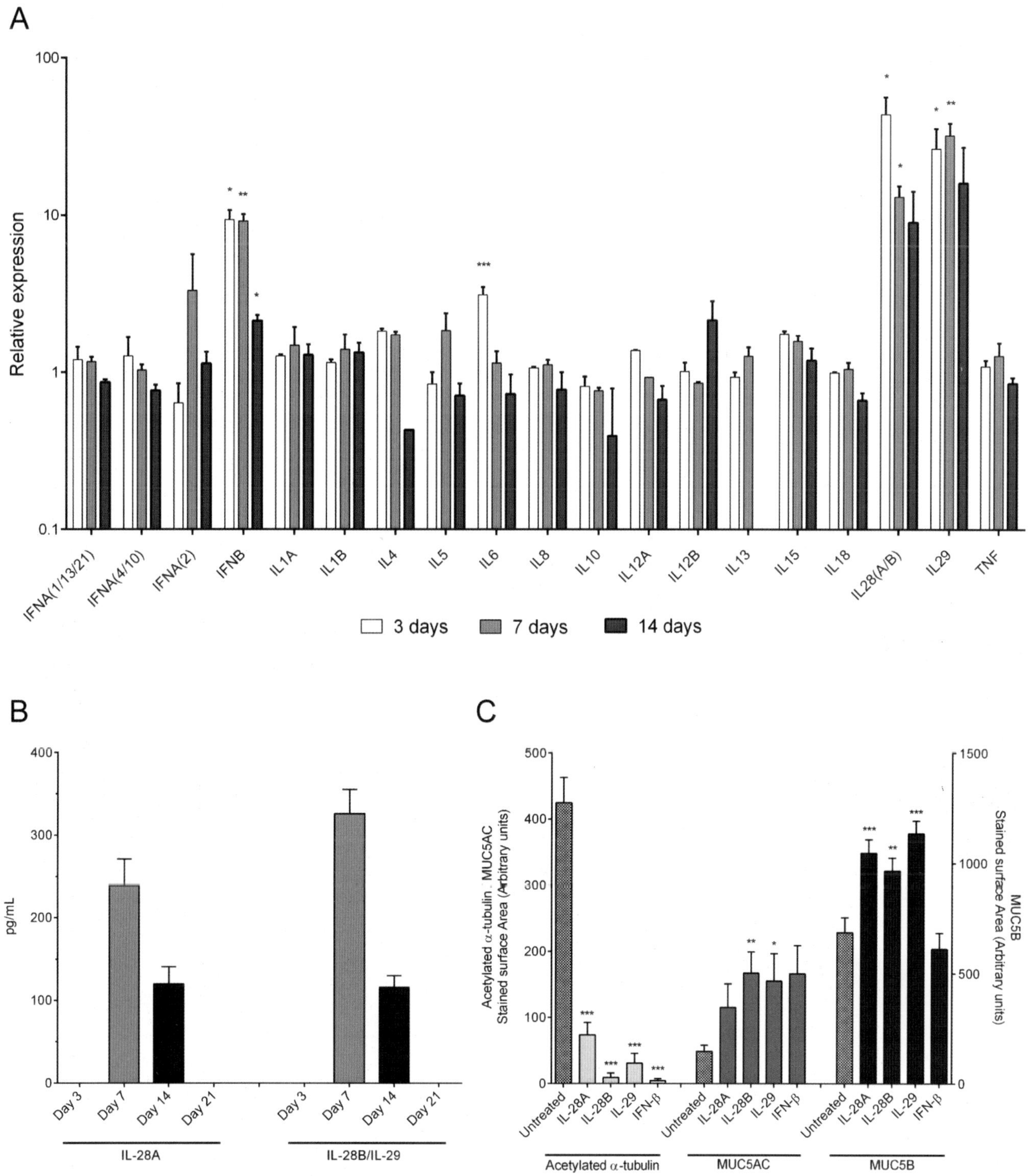

Figure 4. RSV infection induces an IFN-β and Type III interferon response in basal cells. The induction of an innate host response following RSV-A2-GFP infection of basal cells (100 pfu/insert, 3 h after seeding) was investigated over the duration of epithelial growth and differentiation. The expression of immune modulators was assessed at days 3, 7 and 14 after infection. qRT-PCR data are expressed relative to the time-matched, uninfected control (A). At day 3, 7, 14 and 21 media was collected and the levels of secreted IL-28A and IL-28B/IL-29 were determined by a sandwich ELISA (B). Quantitative immunofluorescence was used to assess the effects of IL-28A (30 ng/mL), IL-28B (30 ng/mL), IL-29 (30 ng/mL) or IFN-β (2.5 ng/mL) on epithelial differentiation (C). Mean data ± SEM from 9 inserts over 3 independent experiments are shown, except for panel B, in which 14 inserts over 5 independent experiments were analyzed. Statistical significance was determined with a one way ANOVA statistical test with post-hoc Dunnetts test compared to untreated control cells. *$p<0.05$, **$p<0.01$, and ***$p<0.001$.

Treatment with IL-28A, IL-28B, IL-29 or IFN-β resulted in an epithelial phenotype similar to that formed following RSV infection, with a significant loss in ciliated cells and expansion of MUC5AC and MUC5B secretory cells (Figure 4C). The epithelial remodeling caused by IL-28A, IL-28B, IL-29 and IFN-β indicated that the loss of ciliated cells observed during RSV infection could be driven by a type I and/or type III IFN response.

Finally, to address whether the RSV-induced production of IFN-β or the type III interferons are responsible for the observed change in epithelium, we neutralized the interferon response using antibodies directed against each of the induced ligands IL-28A, IL-28B, IL-29 and IFN-β, both as combination treatment and individually. All of the antibodies used for this experiment were verified to have neutralizing activity (Figure S4). One hundred pfu of RSV-A2-GFP was added to each well of HBECs 3 h post seeding and interferon neutralizing antibodies or isotype controls were included in the medium from day 0 to 21. The antibodies were replaced at each media exchange and at day 21 the cells were fixed and analyzed by quantitative immunofluorescence. Neutralization of the complete IFN response using a combination of all three antibodies caused a 3 to 4-fold increase in RSV spread (Figure 5A), demonstrating the importance of the innate immune response in limiting viral replication. Neutralization of IL-28B/IL-29 alone gave a similar increase in viral spread as combination treatment (Figure 5A), consistent with a key anti-viral role in limiting replication and spread. Next we assessed epithelial composition during interferon neutralization by quantitative immunofluorescence. We reasoned that if interferons had no effect in the epithelial composition, neutralization of the IFN ligands would result in reduced numbers of ciliated cells because of the increased degree of RSV infection under these conditions. However, neutralization of either all ligands together, or independently, resulted in similar numbers of ciliated cells compared to cells treated with an isotype control (Figure 5B). This result indicates that the interferons released as a consequence of RSV infection are at least in part responsible for causing the reduction in numbers of ciliated cells. The neutralization of the interferon response likewise had no effect on secretory cell numbers despite the increase in the number of infected cells. Taken together, these results show that RSV infection elicited an innate immune response of IFN-β and type III interferons at the transcriptional level together with detectable secretion of the type III interferons. Neutralization of the type III interferon response enhanced the viral infection but also at least partially protected the epithelium from loss of ciliated or gain of secretory cells.

Discussion

In this study we present data demonstrating that: 1) following epithelial injury, RSV could infect $p63^+$ airway basal cells, and 2) RSV infection of proliferating basal cells profoundly influenced the subsequent cellular composition of the epithelium. The airway basal cell is the key progenitor of the human conducting airway epithelium and the regulation of epithelial turnover, repair and subsequent differentiation are essential to maintain barrier function and protect the lung from inhaled pathogens and allergens. The present study provides the first evidence that RSV infection of primary human airway basal cells can divert epithelial differentiation towards a phenotype that has increased numbers of goblet cells and reduced numbers of ciliated cells. This phenotype was replicated using two different viral strains (Figure 3) in three different donors (Figure S4). These *in vitro* findings share a striking resemblance to those frequently observed in the human host with RSV infection, where patients have fewer ciliated cells and an increased number of secretory cells [43,44].

The relevance of the airway basal cell as an RSV-sensitive cell - type is somewhat controversial. Several studies have demonstrated that the ciliated cell is susceptible to infection by RSV *in vitro* [11,12,15] as well as in humans *in vivo* [24,26]. Indeed, the well-differentiated ALI HBEC system we have used also demonstrates a clear infection of the ciliated cell when RSV is added to the apical surface in the normal, steady-state system (Figure 1B). However, in a number of respiratory diseases the airway epithelium can be damaged and barrier function impaired. Potentially, this could expose the basal cell to pathogens and induce basal cell proliferation. Indeed, the Gern group recently demonstrated that impairing the barrier properties of the human airway epithelium in vitro, enabled infection of the otherwise inaccessible basal cell with rhinovirus [33]. In the case of RSV, there is some evidence to suggest that basal cells might become infected under certain conditions. Pathology studies have described RSV infected cells that do not have cilia, although their identity was not investigated further [24]. In addition, there are reports based on two animal models, infant baboons and pre-term lambs, which describe infection of airway basal cells [16,17] although the identity of the infected cell-type was not confirmed using cell-specific markers. Based on these findings, we considered that a re-evaluation of basal cell tropism for RSV and potential consequences of infection should be undertaken.

The overt RSV infection of $p63^+$ basal cells that we have observed in ALI cultures of HBEC is in contrast to the report of Zhang et al [11]. However, it should be noted that in that study, even though it was stated that no basal cells were infected after a scratch injury, infected cells were observed in and around the wound area, although their identity was not described [11]. Our data clearly show that irrespective of the method of epithelial injury, mechanical or chemical, RSV infected $p63^+$ basal cells were observed within hours of a brief exposure to virus. It is difficult to reconcile the differences in observations between the published scratch wound model and our own other than that we used cells at 2–4 weeks following the establishment of ALI as compared with 4–6 weeks. In both cases, cultures were well differentiated (evidenced by the presence of ciliated cells) although to our knowledge, any putative differences in basal cell populations at these times have not been described. Of note, the magnitude of $p63^+$ cell infection in the present study was extensive and far from being isolated to an occasional, rare cell type (Figure 1C–I) further supporting the concept that exposure of basal cells to RSV in a susceptible airway could result in significant infection.

Having established that basal cells within the mature ALI cultures could become infected with RSV following mechanical or chemical damage, we demonstrated that freshly seeded basal cells were also susceptible to infection (Figure 2, S1). Freshly seeded basal cells are highly proliferative as the cells attempt to 'repair' the epithelium. As such, a distinction should be made between the behavior of these dividing cells and the relatively quiescent basal cell in the healthy, fully developed epithelium. The lack of basal cell infection observed by Zhang et al [11] may relate to this difference in proliferative status of the cells. However, this would still not account for the differences in susceptibility to RSV infection following scratch injury between this work and the present study.

Using live cell imaging to follow the infected epithelium over time, it was clear that the initial infection of the basal cells was sustained and resulted in viral propagation that persisted until at least 21 days in culture (Figure 2, S2). As described above, even very low viral doses were capable of initiating a sustained infection

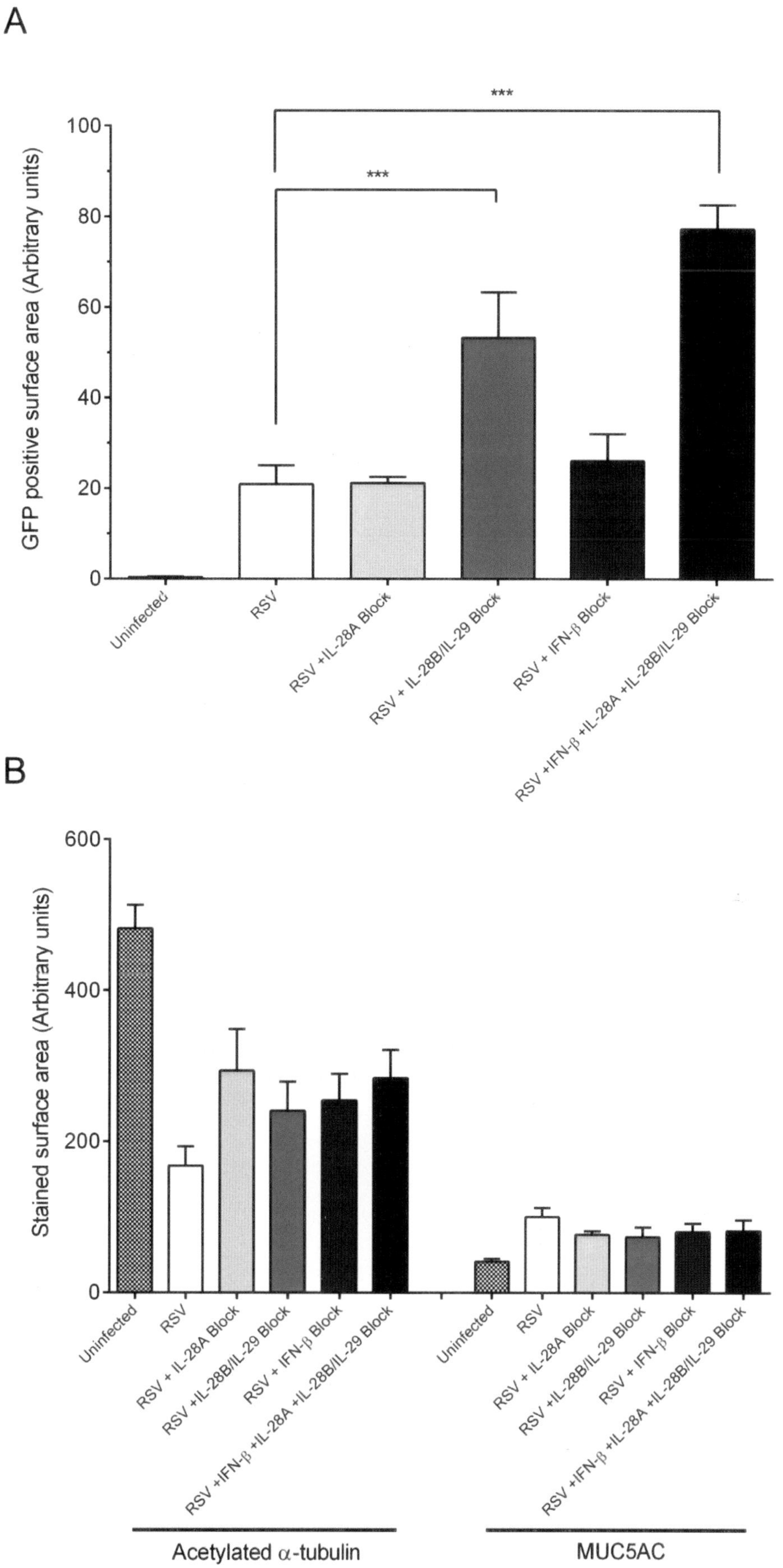
A
***
***
100
80
60
40
20
0
GFP positive surface area (Arbitrary units)
Uninfected
RSV
RSV +IL-28A Block
RSV + IL-28B/IL-29 Block
RSV + IFN-β Block
RSV +IFN-β +IL-28A +IL-28B/IL-29 Block
B
600
400
200
0
Stained surface area (Arbitrary units)
Uninfected
RSV
RSV + IL-28A Block
RSV +IL-28B/IL-29 Block
RSV + IFN-β Block
RSV +IFN-β +IL-28A +IL-28B/IL-29 Block
Uninfected
RSV
RSV + IL-28A Block
RSV +IL-28B/IL-29 Block
RSV + IFN-β Block
RSV +IFN-β +IL-28A +IL-28B/IL-29 Block
Acetylated α-tubulin
MUC5AC

Figure 5. Neutralization of the IFN response during RSV-A2-GFP infection. The effects of neutralization of IL-28A, IL-28B/IL-29 and IFN-β following RSV infection were assessed. GFP^+ surface area was used to assess the degree of RSV infection (A) and quantitative immunofluorescence was used to determine the balance of acetylated α-tubulin$^+$ and MUC5AC$^+$ cells. Mean data ± SEM are shown from 10–14 inserts over 4–6 independent experiments, respectively. Statistical significance was determined with a one way ANOVA statistical test with post-hoc Dunnetts test compared to untreated control cells, ***$p<0.001$.

that continued to generate infectious viral particles throughout the entire period of epithelial growth and differentiation. Between days 0–6 and then again from day 17 onwards, the numbers of infected cells in the epithelium increased. However, despite sustained infectious virus release, the numbers of infected cells declined from days 6–15. The failure to continue to infect the epithelium during days 6–15 is consistent with the work of Zhang et al [11], who showed a loss of susceptibility to RSV infection over this same period of culture. This may have been due to the concurrent induction of a protective interferon response (Figure 5B, 6A) that in some way limited spread and/or susceptibility of the epithelial cells to RSV. Accessibility of RSV to the basal cell may also account for the loss of susceptibility to infection at this time as confocal imaging of HBEC revealed a multilayered epithelium by day 6 in culture, with the p63$^+$ basal cell being covered by a p63$^-$ cell type (Figure 2B). Of note, the increase in infected cells from day 17 would coincide with the appearance of ciliated cells in the epithelium from day 13.

Interestingly, the initial viral dose did not necessarily relate to the final extent of infection. RSV doses of 1, 10 and 100 pfu showed an inverse correlation with the degree of infection by day 21 (Figure S2). A possible explanation for this is that low viral doses enabled a relatively normal epithelium to be formed with a relatively high proportion of ciliated cells for RSV to infect at later time points. It is remarkable that the degree of RSV infection appeared to reach a plateau at 20 days, even with a high number of uninfected ciliated cells present. This could imply that ciliated cells are infected relatively inefficiently by RSV (Figure 2) or that sub-populations exist with different viral susceptibilities. Support for this comes from the fact that even inoculation of well-differentiated HBEC cultures containing numerous ciliated cells, with high doses of RSV, or after an extended period of time, resulted in infection of only a fraction of this cell population (Figure 1A–B and Figure 2). Together, our data suggest that exposed basal cells were readily infected by RSV even when very low viral doses were used suggesting that RSV infection of the basal cells could be an underappreciated feature of RSV pathogenesis.

The data presented in Figure 3 provides strong evidence that RSV infection of airway basal cells resulted in a well-differentiated epithelium, but one that lacked ciliated cells and had increased numbers of secretory cells leading to a goblet cell hyperplasia and a hypersecretory phenotype [45]. The observed attenuation of p63 expression in infected basal cells may be consistent with an RSV-dependent switch in basal cell fate. A loss of p63 expression is essential to the commitment of undifferentiated dividing cells to undergo maturation [46]. It is also possible that RSV infection of emerging ciliated cells early in the course of differentiation led to a depletion in this cell type. In the context of human infection, such a change in epithelial phenotype may be a beneficial host response to limit viral spread by both limiting the numbers of ciliated cells and creating a localized mucus gel. Conversely, infection of the epithelial progenitor could drive an excessive switch in phenotype that may contribute to disease morbidity. At the higher viral doses, RSV resulted in some enlarged infected cells in the apical region of the epithelium, that was most pronounced at 1,000 pfu (Figure S2). These enlarged cells were negative for ciliated or secretory cell markers, were not apoptotic, but were often positive for cytokeratins 5 and/or 8 (data not shown). Similar enlarged multinucleated cells have been observed previously both in HBEC ALI cultures infected with RSV [15] and in post mortem biopsies from young children who succumbed to respiratory disease [24].

In view of the influence that soluble mediators such as IL-1β, IL-9 and IL-13 [47,48,49] can impart on airway epithelial formation, we considered the possibility that soluble factors induced by RSV infection might be modifying the epithelial phenotype. A number of secreted factors have been demonstrated to be released following infection with RSV, including: IL-1α, IL-1β, IL-4, IL-5, IL-6, IL-8, IL-10, IL-12, IL-13, IL-15, IL-17A, IL-18, TNF-α, IFN-α, IFN-β and IFN-λ [7,10,34,35,36,37,38,39,40]. Of these, only IL-6, IFN-β and the Type III interferons were expressed by the HBEC during the course of RSV infection (Figure 5A). It was surprising that IL-13, a widely recognized driver of goblet cell formation in the airways [49], was not induced by RSV infection in the present model system. Published studies have shown IL-13 to be induced following RSV infection [14,50,51,52]. The lack of effect in the present study may relate to the timing of infection (early basal cell infection versus infection of a mature epithelium) and/or the 5,000-fold lower viral dose we used. Of note, differences in innate immune responses between basal cells and a well-differentiated epithelium after RSV infection have been previously reported [13].

The RSV-induced expression of IFN-β and the type III interferons at the transcriptional level (Figure 4A) translated through to the secretion of detectable levels of IL-28A, IL-28B and IL-29 (Figure 4B). Even with the delay between mRNA and protein levels of IL-28A, IL-28B and IL-29 the concentrations peaked at a time point that correlated very well with high viral release, consistent with interferons playing an anti-viral role in RSV pathology. The induction of IFN-α/β by RSV has previously been reported in ALI HBEC [12], but a type III interferon response has so far only been described in nasal epithelial cells [41]. We were unable to detect significant levels of secreted IFN-β, consistent with the findings by Villenave et al. [15]. Neutralization of the endogenous IL-28B and IL-29 that was produced following RSV infection significantly increased the numbers of infected cells, supporting the anti-viral role for these mediators in the human airway epithelium. IL-28A and IFN-β neutralization did not affect the magnitude of the viral infection suggesting that these mediators have a less relevant, or even absent, role in the anti-viral response of the epithelium to RSV. That IL-28A neutralizing antibodies had no effect on viral spread was surprising as IL-28A is reported to share a common receptor and signaling pathway with IL-28B and IL-29 [53]. Pilot studies using A549 cells did confirm the neutralizing capacity of the anti-IL-28 antibody and selected dose (Figure S4), however it is possible that this failed to translate through to efficacy in a different cell type and in a study with an extended duration of exposure (24 h vs. 21 days). Alternatively, there may be a divergence of the signaling pathways between IL-28A and IL-28B/IL-29 in the HBEC cultures. With the interferon response maintained throughout the period of epithelial differentiation we addressed whether these mediators could influence the differentiation process. Exogenous addition of the IFN-β and the type III interferons had the capability to phenocopy the effect of

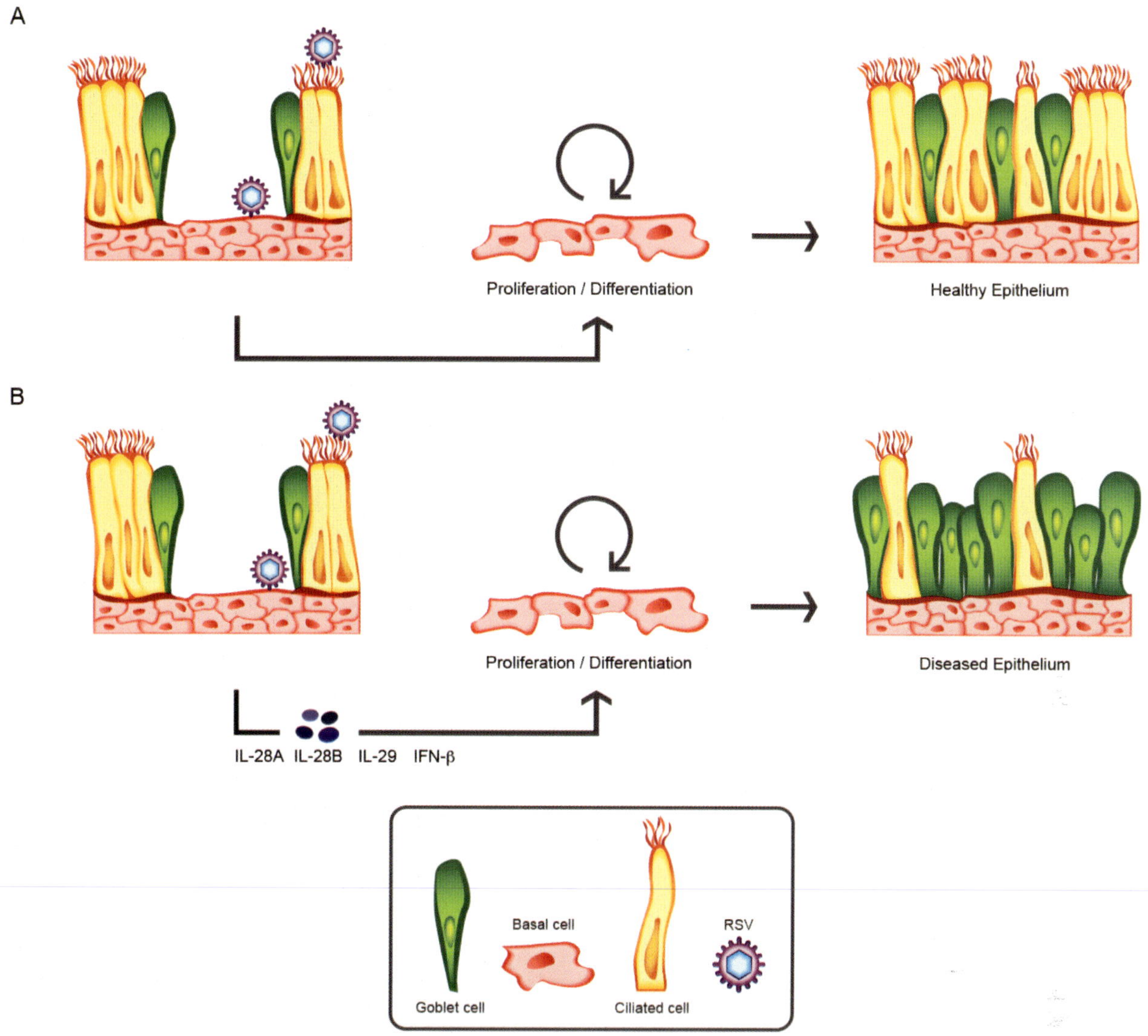

Figure 6. Proposed model for the impact of RSV infection of the airway basal cell. The multi-potent airway basal cell plays a central role in epithelial repair following injury, resulting in an epithelium composed of both ciliated and goblet cells (A). In patients with an impaired epithelial barrier, resulting from either the natural history of an RSV infection (epithelial sloughing) or because of a pre-existing respiratory disease, the airway basal cell can now become exposed to inhaled RSV particles (B). Infection of the basal cells by RSV results in the release of IL-28A, IL-28B, IL-29 and IFN-β that influences basal cell differentiation towards a hypersecretory phenotype i.e. gain of goblet cells and loss of ciliated cells that has the potential to contribute towards a disease exacerbation.

RSV infection on the epithelial composition (Figure 4C). Remarkably, despite the significantly enhanced viral infection of the IL-28B/IL-29 neutralized epithelium, the numbers of ciliated and secretory cells were unchanged from the IL-28B/IL-29 intact control. Based on the earlier dose-response data (Figure 3), it would have been predicted that the increased infection should have further reduced ciliated cell number and boost secretory cells. These data are therefore consistent with RSV-induced levels of endogenous IL-28B and IL-29 contributing towards both the loss of ciliated and gain of secretory cells.

Together, these data highlight that RSV infection of basal cells could have a significant, long-term impact on the biology of the airway epithelium (Figure 6). According to this model infection of the basal cells enables rapid and efficient RSV replication and spread of the infection. The infected epithelium mounts an early interferon response that plays a central role in the anti-viral response of the epithelium. However, in addition to the anti-viral effect of the endogenous production of IL-28B/IL-29, these mediatorscan also repress ciliated cell formation and increase secretory cell numbers. The impact is to push epithelial differentiation away from a 'normal' ciliated phenotype (Figure 6A) and towards a 'disease-like' pro-secretory function (Figure 6B). If this were to happen in infection of an individual, this change in epithelial phenotype may contribute to the excessive mucus production and occlusion of small airways that can occur following RSV infection. The balance between secretory and ciliated cells in the lung is critical to maintain a normal lung function. A degree of epithelial plasticity is beneficial to the healthy lung, allowing it to respond to injury by increasing the production of the protective mucus gel and in the case of RSV, reducing the number of susceptible ciliated cells. In diseases such as cystic fibrosis, COPD and asthma however, where epithelial barrier function can be compromised and the balance is already skewed towards the goblet cell, RSV infection of the basal cell might be predicted to further amplify that phenotype. Excessive mucus together with a reduced ciliated cell population can lead to direct airway occlusion, mucostasis and an increased risk of further infection or even bacterial colonization. As such, we would propose that infection of the basal cell by RSV may be a significant contributor to exacerbations of respiratory diseases and should be further investigated in human pathology. Strategies to regulate either the initial infection or response of airway basal cells may provide novel approaches for generating broad acting therapeutics under healthy or exacerbated conditions important for viral lung disease.

Methods

Cells and viruses

Human bronchial epithelial cells (HBEC) were purchased from Lonza and expanded in Bronchial Epithelial cell Growth Medium (BEGM) supplemented with the recommended additives (Singlequots, Lonza) until 80% confluent (P0 cells). Once confluent the cells were aliquoted and frozen down as 'P1' cells. For each experiment P1 cells were expanded to 80% confluence and seeded onto a 12-well Transwell permeable support (0.4 μM, Corning, NY) in BEGM media diluted 1:1 in DMEM (Lonza, Invitrogen) and supplemented with BEGM singlequots devoid of triiodothyronine (T3) and retinoic acid (differentiation media). All trans-retinoic acid (Sigma, 50 nM in ethanol) was added back fresh for each media exchange. Cells were infected by either RSV-A2-GFP [31,32], or a clinical isolate designated RSV-A2-MOT0972 (Obtained from Edward Walsh, University of Rochester Medical School) at various multiplicity of infection (MOI), as indicated in the text. Six days post-seeding the media was removed from the apical side and cells were cultured at ALI for an additional 14 days. Media was replaced three times a week with 1 mL on the basal side and for week one, 400 μL was added on the apical side.

RSV quantification

RSV-A2-GFP was grown in HEp-2 cells and purified by centrifugation through sucrose. Briefly, cells were infected with RSV at an MOI of 0.05. Ninety-six hours post-infection the cells were scraped into the media, which was collected and vortexed to release cell-associated viral particles. Cell debris was pelleted by centrifugation and the supernatant was loaded onto a 20% sucrose cushion in PBS and purified by centrifugation at 11,500 g. Pelleted virus was re-suspended in PBS containing 25% sucrose and flash frozen in liquid nitrogen. Aliquots of the virus were stored at −80°C. To quantify released virus from infected HBEC, 500 μL of warm DMEM was added to the apical side for 60 min and then collected. Aliquots were flash frozen in liquid nitrogen. All viral titers were determined by a conventional plaque assay. Ten-fold dilutions of cell supernatant were used to infect HEp-2 cells before overlaying with OptiMEM (Invitrogen) containing: 2% FCS (Invitrogen), 0.8% Methylcellulose (Sigma) and 1x Penicillin/Streptomycin (Invitrogen). Five days post-infection the cells were fixed with 80% cold methanol for 2 h, rinsed with ddH_2O and blocked with 5% dried milk in PBS. RSV infected cells were stained by RSV-F antibody (Serotec MCA490) followed by horseradish peroxidase conjugated secondary antibody (Abcam). Plaques were visualized by 4CN peroxidase substrate (KPL).

Epithelial denuding

Well-differentiated HBECs (at 21 days after seeding onto Transwell inserts) were rinsed three times in warm PBS (Invitrogen) to remove mucus. Once cleaned, warm S-MEM media (Invitrogen) was added for 20 min at 37°C (1 mL on the basal side and 500 μL on the apical side). Once separated the suprabasal layer was removed from the basal cell layer by vigorously pipetting up and down. The basal cell layer was washed several times using warm PBS until a single layer of cells could be observed. At this point cells were infected using 100,000 pfu of RSV-A2-GFP.

Scratch injury

100,000 cells were seeded onto a Transwell insert and grown to form a pseudostratified epithelium over 21 days as previously described [11]. Once fully differentiated the cells were washed once from the apical side using warm PBS followed by addition of 500 μL PBS. A GUM stimulator (generic dental tool) was used to carefully scratch several thin scratches that intersected each other. Once scratched 250,000 PFU of RSV-A2-GFP was added in 250 μL of warm HBEC growth media for 30 min at 37°C. After 30 min the apical media was removed, cells incubated at 37°C for 20 h followed by fixation using 4% paraformaldehyde.

Flow cytometry

100,000 cells were seeded onto a Transwell insert infected 3 h later with RSV-A2-GFP at an MOI of 0.1. Uninfected control cells were incubated with the respective volume of PBS. After 20 h cells where harvested and fixed by 2% paraformaldehyde for 10 min at RT, centrifuged for 5 min at 1,500 rcf and washed once in PBS. Fixed cells were permabilized by PBS+0.5% Triton X-100 for 15 min at RT, followed by washing once in PBS. Fixed and permabilized cells were stained for p63 (Abcam ab124762) and ITGA6 (Millipore MAB1378) at a dilution of 1:200 for 45 min, washed once, and incubated with an Alexaflour 568 and Alexaflour 647 conjugated secondary antibody (Invitrogen) at 1:1000 for 30 min. Flow cytometry was performed in PBS using a Fortessa cytometer.

Immunohistochemistry, live cell imaging and cell imaging analysis

Cells were fixed by 4% paraformaldehyde for 3 h at 4°C and blocked using 10% horse serum in immunofluorescence buffer containing: 130 mM NaCl, 13 mM Na_2HPO_4, 3.5 mM NaH_2PO_4, 0.2% Triton X-100 and 0.05% Tween-20 at pH 7.5. All imaging was performed using a Carl Zeiss spinning disk confocal microscope using antibodies against: acetylated α-tubulin (Sigma T6793) to stain ciliated cells, MUC5B (Santa Cruz sc-20119) and MUC5AC (Thermo Scientific MS145P) for secretory cells and p63 (Abcam ab124762) for basal cells. For staining RSV-A2-MOT0972 infected cells a goat anti-RSV antibody was used (Pierce PA1–7240). All Alexa-conjugated secondary antibodies were obtained from Invitrogen. To quantify epithelial composition quantitative immunofluorescence was performed by collecting 130 overlapping images at 10x magnification, for each 1 cm^2 Transwell insert, in Axiovision 4.8 (Carl Zeiss). This enabled almost the entire surface area of the insert to be captured and used for quantification removing any potential for operator bias. RSV-A2-GFP fluorescence was imaged using the same acquisition protocol. Converted images were analyzed by ImageJ [54] by measuring stained surface area over a pre-defined threshold, using the analyze particles routine. Data was normalized to uninfected control. For confocal microscopy, sections of the inserts were punched out using a 4 mm biopsy punch and mounted on a cover slide using ProLong Gold antifade reagent with DAPI (Invitrogen).

Quantitative PCR

Total RNA was harvested and isolated by using the RNeasy kit from Qiagen, according to the manufacturer's instructions (Qiagen). cDNA was generated by using the TaqMan reverse transcription reagents (Applied Biosystems) according to the manufacturer's instructions. All FAM probes were purchased from ABI (Invitrogen) as 20x Master mixes and designed for maximum gene coverage (Table S1). Gene expression reactions were performed with TaqMan 2x PCR Master Mix (Applied Biosystems) in a ViiA7 Real time PCR cycler (Applied Biosystems). All the data is expressed as expression relative to the untreated control.

ELISA

Basal supernatants were collected at day 3, 7, 14 and 21 post-infection. Uninfected samples were collected at the same time points. Collected supernatant was aliquoted and frozen until assayed for IL-28A or IL-28B/IL-29 production using a sandwich ELISA (R & D Systems). ELISA was performed according to the manufacturer's instructions. IFN content was compared to a 7-point 2-fold dilution standard curve from 8,000 pg/mL or 4,000 pg/mL.

IFN treatment

Soluble interferons were used at 30 ng/mL for IL-28A (R&D Systems), IL-28B (R&D Systems) and IL-29 (Gibco). For IFN-β (pbl Interferon Source) 2.5 ng/mL was used. Mediator was present in both apical and basal media for week one, and in the basal media once brought to ALI at day 6. Media was replaced three times a week and fresh mediator added. The experiment was terminated after 21 days by fixation using in 4% paraformaldehyde. Fixed cells were stained for epithelial composition using antibodies specific to acetylated α-tubulin, MUC5AC and MUC5B.

Blocking of IFN response

We used antibodies against IL-28A (R&D Systems at 1 μg/mL), IL-28B/IL-29 (R&D Systems 12.5 μg/mL) and IFN-β (R&D Systems at 2 μg/mL) to neutralize the induced IFN response. Concentrations used had been verified to neutralize an induced IFN response in A549 cells to at least 50% (Figure S4). All treatments were performed as combination treatment or individual with matched isotype control. One week after seeding the media was removed from the apical side and cells were allowed to differentiate. Mediator was present in both apical and basal media for week one. The antibody treatment continued for the full 21 days. At day 21 cells were fixed by 4% paraformaldehyde and stained for epithelial composition using antibodies specific to MUC5AC and acetylated α-tubulin.

Analysis of results

Data are presented as mean ± SEM unless otherwise stated. All statistical analyses were performed in GraphPad 6 (GraphPad software Inc., San Diego, CA) using analysis of variance (ANOVA) followed by a Dunnett's multiple comparison test. Significance was assumed when $p<0.05$.

Supporting Information

Figure S1 Flow cytometry analysis of RSV-A2-GFP infected basal cells. RSV infection of HBEC cells at 3 h post seeding allowed for an extensive infection of basal cells. At 45 h post infection cells were harvested, fixed and stained for the basal cell markers p63 and ITGA6. Close to 100% of the cells on the inserts were basal cells as indicated by positive p63 and ITGA6 stain (A–B). In addition, infected cells showed a significant reduction in p63 levels but not ITGA6 (C–D). Presented are representative flow cytometry data from three independent donors.

Figure S2 RSV-A2-GFP infection 21 days post infection. The effect of RSV-A2-GFP infection of basal cells (1–1,000 pfu/Transwell, D to A respectively, 3 h after seeding) was investigated over the duration of epithelial growth and differentiation by fluorescence imaging. Lower viral doses (C–D) exclusively generated infected cells with a condensed-morphology that gradually disappeared as the viral dose increased (A–D). The highest viral dose studied (1,000 pfu) resulted in the formation of an epithelium with large patches of infection (A, GFP^+ cells) that were confirmed as syncytia by confocal imaging (E). Representative images from three independent experiments are shown, RSV infected cells are colored green.

Figure S3 RSV induced epithelium phenotype was independent of donor. HBEC cells from three different donors were investigated to rule out any for donor variability in the loss of cilia phenotype. Cells were infected at a Transwell insert 3 h after seeding using a range of RSV-A2-GFP from 1–1000 pfu/Transwell. After 21 days in culture the cells were stained for cilia using acetylated α-tubulin. Cells from all donors were cultured and imaged in parallel and three inserts from each donor was examined. Data is presented as the average ± SD, from 2 independent experiments and a total of 4–6 inserts per viral dose.

Figure S4 Validation of neutralizing activity of anti-interferon antibodies. Antibodies intended to neutralize IL-28A, IL-28B, IL-29 and IFN-β were all verified to neutralize a stimulated response in A549 cells. A549 cells were seeded into a 12 well plate (1.2×10^5 cells/well) and stimulated for 2 h using 10 ng/mL of IL-28A (R & D Systems), IL-28B (R & D Systems) or IFN-β (pbl bioscience). The increasing concentrations of neutralizing antibodies added were based on the manufacturer's neutralization data. After 24 h of treatment total RNA was collected using Buffer AVL from the RNAeasy kit (Qiagen) and RNA purified according to the manufacturer's instructions. qRT-PCR was performed using 40 ng of total cDNA analyzing ISG15 for IL-28A/IL-28B/IL-29 stimulation (A–B) and CXCL10 for IFN-β stimulation (C). The concentration of antibody that resulted in a >50% pathway inhibition was used in the experiments presented in Figure 6.

Table S1 qRT-PCR primer used and accession number. All primers and probes where ordered from Invitrogen with the ordering number listed below.

Acknowledgments

We would specifically like to thank Lina Cabal Romero for providing the illustration for Figure 6. In addition we are grateful for the clinical isolated provided by Dr. Ed Walsh at the University of Rochester, Medical School. We appreciate all the help with the experiments for figures 4 and 5 provided by Stephanie Petit, and the input from Frank Martin on the flow cytometry experiments. Special thanks to all members of the Danahay and

Jaffe labs as well as the entire Regenerative Medicine Hub for helpful comments though the course of this work.

Author Contributions

Conceived and designed the experiments: BDP ABJ HD. Performed the experiments: BDP. Analyzed the data: BDP HD. Contributed reagents/materials/analysis tools: ABJ HD. Wrote the paper: BDP ABJ RF HD.

References

1. Nair H, Nokes DJ, Gessner BD, Dherani M, Madhi SA, et al. (2010) Global burden of acute lower respiratory infections due to respiratory syncytial virus in young children: a systematic review and meta-analysis. Lancet 375: 1545–1555.
2. (2013) The 10 leading causes of death in the world, 2000 and 2011. World Health Organization.
3. Ramaswamy M, Groskreutz DJ, Look DC (2009) Recognizing the importance of respiratory syncytial virus in chronic obstructive pulmonary disease. COPD 6: 64–75.
4. Westerly BD, Peebles RS Jr (2010) Respiratory syncytial virus infections in the adult asthmatic–mechanisms of host susceptibility and viral subversion. Immunol Allergy Clin North Am 30: 523–539, vi–vii.
5. Collins PL, Crowe JEJ (2007) Respiratory syncytial virus and metapneumovirus; D. M. Knipe PMH, D. E. Griffin, R. A. Lamb, M. A. Martin, B. Roizman, and S. E. Straus, editor. Philadelphia, PA: Lippincott Williams & Wilkins. 1601–1646 p.
6. Collins PL, Graham BS (2008) Viral and host factors in human respiratory syncytial virus pathogenesis. J Virol 82: 2040–2055.
7. Gonzalez PA, Bueno SM, Carreno LJ, Riedel CA, Kalergis AM (2012) Respiratory syncytial virus infection and immunity. Rev Med Virol 22: 230–244.
8. Delgado MF, Coviello S, Monsalvo AC, Melendi GA, Hernandez JZ, et al. (2009) Lack of antibody affinity maturation due to poor Toll-like receptor stimulation leads to enhanced respiratory syncytial virus disease. Nat Med 15: 34–41.
9. Maggon K, Barik S (2004) New drugs and treatment for respiratory syncytial virus. Rev Med Virol 14: 149–168.
10. Villenave R, Shields MD, Power UF (2013) Respiratory syncytial virus interaction with human airway epithelium. Trends Microbiol.
11. Zhang L, Peeples ME, Boucher RC, Collins PL, Pickles RJ (2002) Respiratory syncytial virus infection of human airway epithelial cells is polarized, specific to ciliated cells, and without obvious cytopathology. J Virol 76: 5654–5666.
12. Zhang L, Collins PL, Lamb RA, Pickles RJ (2011) Comparison of differing cytopathic effects in human airway epithelium of parainfluenza virus 5 (W3A), parainfluenza virus type 3, and respiratory syncytial virus. Virology 421: 67–77.
13. Smith CM, Kulkarni H, Radhakrishnan P, Rutman A, Bankart MJ, et al. (2013) Ciliary dyskinesia is an early feature of respiratory syncytial virus infection. Eur Respir J.
14. Mata M, Sarrion I, Armengot M, Carda C, Martinez I, et al. (2012) Respiratory syncytial virus inhibits ciliagenesis in differentiated normal human bronchial epithelial cells: effectiveness of N-acetylcysteine. PLoS One 7: e48037.
15. Villenave R, Thavagnanam S, Sarlang S, Parker J, Douglas I, et al. (2012) In vitro modeling of respiratory syncytial virus infection of pediatric bronchial epithelium, the primary target of infection in vivo. Proc Natl Acad Sci U S A 109: 5040–5045.
16. Papin JF, Wolf RF, Kosanke SD, Jenkins JD, Moore SN, et al. (2013) Infant Baboons Infected with Respiratory Syncytial Virus Develop Clinical and Pathologic Changes that Parallel Those of Human Infants. Am J Physiol Lung Cell Mol Physiol.
17. Meyerholz DK, Grubor B, Fach SJ, Sacco RE, Lehmkuhl HD, et al. (2004) Reduced clearance of respiratory syncytial virus infection in a preterm lamb model. Microbes Infect 6: 1312–1319.
18. Chung KF (2001) Cytokines in chronic obstructive pulmonary disease. Eur Respir J Suppl 34: 50s–59s.
19. Sethi S, Mahler DA, Marcus P, Owen CA, Yawn B, et al. (2012) Inflammation in COPD: implications for management. Am J Med 125: 1162–1170.
20. Holgate ST, Roberts G, Arshad HS, Howarth PH, Davies DE (2009) The role of the airway epithelium and its interaction with environmental factors in asthma pathogenesis. Proc Am Thorac Soc 6: 655–659.
21. Swindle EJ, Collins JE, Davies DE (2009) Breakdown in epithelial barrier function in patients with asthma: identification of novel therapeutic approaches. J Allergy Clin Immunol 124: 23–34; quiz 35–26.
22. Xiao C, Puddicombe SM, Field S, Haywood J, Broughton-Head V, et al. (2011) Defective epithelial barrier function in asthma. J Allergy Clin Immunol 128: 549–556 e541–512.
23. Rock JR, Randell SH, Hogan BL (2010) Airway basal stem cells: a perspective on their roles in epithelial homeostasis and remodeling. Dis Model Mech 3: 545–556.
24. Johnson JE, Gonzales RA, Olson SJ, Wright PF, Graham BS (2007) The histopathology of fatal untreated human respiratory syncytial virus infection. Mod Pathol 20: 108–119.
25. Ebbert JO, Limper AH (2005) Respiratory syncytial virus pneumonitis in immunocompromised adults: clinical features and outcome. Respiration 72: 263–269.
26. Power OTaUF (2011) Cellular and Molecular Characteristics of RSV-Induced Disease in Humans, Human Respiratory Syncytial Virus Infection. In: Resch DB, editor.
27. Levenson RM, Kantor OS (1987) Fatal pneumonia in an adult due to respiratory syncytial virus. Arch Intern Med 147: 791–792.
28. Fulcher ML, Randell SH (2013) Human nasal and tracheo-bronchial respiratory epithelial cell culture. Methods Mol Biol 945: 109–121.
29. Ross AJ, Dailey LA, Brighton LE, Devlin RB (2007) Transcriptional profiling of mucociliary differentiation in human airway epithelial cells. Am J Respir Cell Mol Biol 37: 169–185.
30. Gray TE, Guzman K, Davis CW, Abdullah LH, Nettesheim P (1996) Mucociliary differentiation of serially passaged normal human tracheobronchial epithelial cells. Am J Respir Cell Mol Biol 14: 104–112.
31. Hallak LK, Collins PL, Knudson W, Peeples ME (2000) Iduronic acid-containing glycosaminoglycans on target cells are required for efficient respiratory syncytial virus infection. Virology 271: 264–275.
32. Hallak LK, Spillmann D, Collins PL, Peeples ME (2000) Glycosaminoglycan sulfation requirements for respiratory syncytial virus infection. J Virol 74: 10508–10513.
33. Jakiela B, Brockman-Schneider R, Amineva S, Lee WM, Gern JE (2008) Basal cells of differentiated bronchial epithelium are more susceptible to rhinovirus infection. Am J Respir Cell Mol Biol 38: 517–523.
34. Lotz MT, Peebles RS Jr (2012) Mechanisms of respiratory syncytial virus modulation of airway immune responses. Curr Allergy Asthma Rep 12: 380–387.
35. Bueno SM, Gonzalez PA, Pacheco R, Leiva ED, Cautivo KM, et al. (2008) Host immunity during RSV pathogenesis. Int Immunopharmacol 8: 1320–1329.
36. Oshansky CM, Zhang W, Moore E, Tripp RA (2009) The host response and molecular pathogenesis associated with respiratory syncytial virus infection. Future Microbiol 4: 279–297.
37. Garofalo RP, Hintz KH, Hill V, Ogra PL, Welliver RC, Sr. (2004) Production of interferon gamma in respiratory syncytial virus infection of humans is not associated with interleukins 12 and 18. J Med Virol 73: 289–294.
38. van Benten IJ, van Drunen CM, Koopman LP, KleinJan A, van Middelkoop BC, et al. (2003) RSV-induced bronchiolitis but not upper respiratory tract infection is accompanied by an increased nasal IL-18 response. J Med Virol 71: 290–297.
39. Spann KM, Tran KC, Chi B, Rabin RL, Collins PL (2004) Suppression of the induction of alpha, beta, and lambda interferons by the NS1 and NS2 proteins of human respiratory syncytial virus in human epithelial cells and macrophages [corrected]. J Virol 78: 4363–4369.
40. Zdrenghea MT, Telcian AG, Laza-Stanca V, Bellettato CM, Edwards MR, et al. (2012) RSV infection modulates IL-15 production and MICA levels in respiratory epithelial cells. Eur Respir J 39: 712–720.
41. Okabayashi T, Kojima T, Masaki T, Yokota S, Imaizumi T, et al. (2011) Type-III interferon, not type-I, is the predominant interferon induced by respiratory viruses in nasal epithelial cells. Virus Res 160: 360–366.
42. Harris J, Werling D (2003) Binding and entry of respiratory syncytial virus into host cells and initiation of the innate immune response. Cell Microbiol 5: 671–680.
43. Black CP (2003) Systematic review of the biology and medical management of respiratory syncytial virus infection. Respir Care 48: 209–231; discussion 231–203.
44. Wong JY, Rutman A, O'Callaghan C (2005) Recovery of the ciliated epithelium following acute bronchiolitis in infancy. Thorax 60: 582–587.
45. Openshaw PJ, Tregoning JS (2005) Immune responses and disease enhancement during respiratory syncytial virus infection. Clin Microbiol Rev 18: 541–555.
46. Yang A, Schweitzer R, Sun D, Kaghad M, Walker N, et al. (1999) p63 is essential for regenerative proliferation in limb, craniofacial and epithelial development. Nature 398: 714–718.
47. Lai H, Rogers DF (2010) New pharmacotherapy for airway mucus hypersecretion in asthma and COPD: targeting intracellular signaling pathways. J Aerosol Med Pulm Drug Deliv 23: 219–231.
48. Vermeer PD, Harson R, Einwalter LA, Moninger T, Zabner J (2003) Interleukin-9 induces goblet cell hyperplasia during repair of human airway epithelia. Am J Respir Cell Mol Biol 28: 286–295.
49. Laoukili J, Perret E, Willems T, Minty A, Parthoens E, et al. (2001) IL-13 alters mucociliary differentiation and ciliary beating of human respiratory epithelial cells. J Clin Invest 108: 1817–1824.
50. Moore ML, Chi MH, Luongo C, Lukacs NW, Polosukhin VV, et al. (2009) A chimeric A2 strain of respiratory syncytial virus (RSV) with the fusion protein of RSV strain line 19 exhibits enhanced viral load, mucus, and airway dysfunction. J Virol 83: 4185–4194.
51. Castilow EM, Meyerholz DK, Varga SM (2008) IL-13 is required for eosinophil entry into the lung during respiratory syncytial virus vaccine-enhanced disease. J Immunol 180: 2376–2384.

2

Entry Properties and Entry Inhibitors of a Human H7N9 Influenza Virus

Youhui Si[9], Jianguo Li[9], Yuqiang Niu[9], Xiuying Liu, Lili Ren, Li Guo, Min Cheng, Hongli Zhou, Jianwei Wang*, Qi Jin*, Wei Yang*

Ministry of Health Key Laboratory of Systems Biology of Pathogens, Institute of Pathogen Biology, Chinese Academy of Medical Sciences & Peking Union Medical College, Beijing, China

Abstract

The recently identified human infections with a novel avian influenza H7N9 virus in China raise important questions regarding possible risk to humans. However, the entry properties and tropism of this H7N9 virus were poorly understood. Moreover, neuraminidase inhibitor resistant H7N9 isolates were recently observed in two patients and correlated with poor clinical outcomes. In this study, we aimed to elucidate the entry properties of H7N9 virus, design and evaluate inhibitors for H7N9 virus entry. We optimized and developed an H7N9-pseudotyped particle system (H7N9pp) that could be neutralized by anti-H7 antibodies and closely mimicked the entry process of the H7N9 virus. Avian, human and mouse-derived cultured cells showed high, moderate and low permissiveness to H7N9pp, respectively. Based on influenza virus membrane fusion mechanisms, a potent anti-H7N9 peptide (P155-185-chol) corresponding to the C-terminal ectodomain of the H7N9 hemagglutinin protein was successfully identified. P155-185-chol demonstrated H7N9pp-specific inhibition of infection with IC_{50} of 0.19 μM. Importantly, P155-185-chol showed significant suppression of A/Anhui/1/2013 H7N9 live virus propagation in MDCK cells and additive effects with NA inhibitors Oseltamivir and Zanamivir. These findings expand our knowledge of the entry properties of the novel H7N9 viruses, and they highlight the potential for developing a new class of inhibitors targeting viral entry for use in the next pandemic.

Editor: Tony Wang, SRI International, United States of America

Funding: This work was supported by grants from National Science and Technology Major Project of China (2012ZX10002007-003), National Basic Research Program of China (2011CB504800), National Natural Science Foundation of China (81271831 and 81301442) and an intramural grant from the Institute of Pathogen Biology (2013IPB103). The funders had no role in study design, data collection and analysis, decision to publish, or preparation of the manuscript.

Competing Interests: The authors have declared that no competing interests exist.

* Email: wyang@ipb.pumc.edu.cn (WY); zdsys@vip.sina.com (QJ); wangjw28@163.com (JW)

[9] These authors contributed equally to this work.

Introduction

The emergence of a severe human illness caused by a novel avian influenza H7N9 virus has recently been reported in China [1]. Although H7 viruses have occasionally been found to infect humans (H7N2 [2], H7N3 [3] and H7N7 [4,5]), no human infections with H7N9 viruses have been reported previously [6]. As of August 12 2013, a total of 135 laboratory-confirmed patients were officially reported in mainland China, and 44 (32.6%) of them had died [7]. A large portion of the infected people had a history of poultry exposure [1,8], even though H7N9 viruses are considered epidemic and low-pathogenic in poultry. Sequence analyses have shown that H7N9 viruses have several molecular signatures of adaptation to grow in mammalian species, including the ability to bind to mammalian cell receptors and to grow at temperatures close to the normal mammalian body temperature [9]. Moreover, the H7N9 virus contains an internal gene cassette from an H9N2 virus [10], which has the ability to infect and move rapidly between numerous avian and mammalian hosts [11]. Thus far, H7N9 has not been found to be transmissible from human to human but should be closely watched in the future.

The neuraminidase (NA) inhibitors are currently available for the treatment of H7N9 virus infection. However, the antiviral resistant H7N9 isolates with NA R292K mutant were recently observed in two patients and correlated with poor clinical outcome. It is with high possibility that the H7N9 virus will be reemerging in the next flu season. Therefore, discovering novel antiviral targets and drug candidates are urgently anticipated for this high lethal viral disease. The entry of influenza virus into host cells establishes the first step of the whole viral life cycle and represents a promising target for novel antiviral drug development. This study was aimed to elucidate the entry characteristics of H7N9 virus, design and evaluate inhibitors for H7N9 virus entry.

Materials and Methods

Cells, plasmids, peptides and reagents

The MDCK, A549, NCI-H1650, 293T, Hela, Vero E6, CHO and NIH3T3 cells were purchased from The American Type Culture Collection (ATCC, Manassas, VA, USA). The Huh7.5.1 cells were provided by Dr Francis V. Chisari (Scripps Research Institute, La Jolla, CA, USA), and the chick embryo fibroblast

(CEF) cells were derived from specific-pathogen-free fertilized eggs purchased from Vital River Laboratory Animal Technology Co., Ltd. Fibroblasts were prepared from 12-day old embryos under a specific procedure for the chicken embryo collection approved by the Ethics Committee of the Institute of Pathogen Biology. All the cells were maintained in DMEM medium (Invitrogen, Carlsbad, CA, USA) supplemented with 10% fetal bovine serum (Gibco, Carlsbad, CA, USA), 1% nonessential amino acids (Gibco, Carlsbad, CA, USA), and 1% penicillin and streptomycin (Gibco, Carlsbad, CA, USA) at 37°C under 5% CO_2.

pCAGGS.MCS-based expression plasmids carrying codon-optimized NA or HA genes for influenza A virus A/Brisbane/59/2007 (H1N1), A/California/04/2009 (H1N1), A/Brisbane/10/2007 (H3N2), A/Anhui/1/2005 (H5N1) and A/Anhui/1/2013 (H7N9) were constructed by inserting synthesized sequences into KpnI/SacI restriction sites of pCAGGS [12] (addgene).

Peptides for P155-185, $B7^{NP}$, GBVA10-9 and Scrambled controls were synthesized by standard Fmoc-solid phase methods at Scilight Biotechnology LLC (Beijing, China). The cholesterol moiety was attached to P155-185 via a reaction between the thiol group of an extra cysteine residue and added C-terminally to P155-185 as well as a bromoacetyl derivative of cholesterol (P155-185-Chol).

Chloroquine diphosphate and Zanamivir hydrate were purchased from Tokyo Chemical Industry Co., Ltd (Tokyo, Japan). Bafilomycin A1 and dynasore hydrate were obtained from Sigma-Aldrich (St Louis, MO, USA). Oseltamivir carboxylate was from Hoffmann-La Roche, Ltd (Basel, Switzerland).

Production and optimization of HA-mediated pseudovirions (HANApp)

Lentiviral pseudotyped particles were produced in 293T cells (70% confluence) and co-transfected with pNL-4.3-Luc-R^-E^-, pCAGGS-HA and pCAGGS-NA constructs using a standard PEI-based transfection protocol [13,14,15]. Following transfection, the 293T cells were washed once with phosphate-buffered saline and maintained in Opti-MEM I Reduced Serum Medium (Gibco, Carlsbad, CA, USA). For optimizing the infectivity of the produced pseudotyped particles, viral supernatants were generated in 6-well plates as described above. To determine the optimal transfection quantities of pCAGGS-HA and pCAGGS-NA plasmids, one plasmid amount was maintained at 0.5 µg, while the other was varied at 0.1 µg, 0.25 µg, 0.5 µg, 1 µg or 1.5 µg. The culture supernatants were collected at different times post-transfection (24 h, 36 h, 48 h) and incubated with a series of concentrations (0, 2, 4, 6, 8, 10 µg/ml) of TPCK-treated trypsin (Sigma-Aldrich, St. Louis, MO, USA) for 1 h at 37°C. The final culture supernatants were filtered through a 0.45 µm filter (Millipore, Billerica, MA), and aliquots were stored at -70°C until use.

Pseudotyped particle neutralization assay

H7N9pp was mixed with serially diluted neutralized monoclonal antibodies against H1, H3, H5 or H7, which was provided by Dr Li Guo, [12,16] for 1 h at 37°C followed by incubation with MDCK cells cultured in a 96-well plate (1×10^4 cells per well) for 3 h before changing the media. Isotype IgG was included as a control. Infectivity was evaluated at 48 h post-infection by a luciferase assay.

HANApp entry assay

The pseudotyped viral supernatants prepared above were incubated with cells in 96-well plates for 3 h at 37°C before changing the media. Infectivity was evaluated at 48 h post-infection by a luciferase assay (Promega, Madison, WI, USA) and normalized to that of MDCK cells. To test the antiviral activity of the indicated synthetic peptides, HANApp was treated with serially diluted peptides for 0.5 h at 37°C, and then incubated with MDCK cells in 96-well plates for 3 h at 37°C before changing the media. To determine the effects of the chemicals on virus infection, MDCK cells were seeded into 96-well plates and treated with serially diluted chemicals for 1 h at 37°C followed by infection with HANApp. The dynasore treated group was conducted in Opti-MEM I Reduced Serum Medium, while the other groups were in complete growth medium. Infectivity was evaluated at 48 h post-infection by a luciferase assay.

Superinfection assay

293T cells were transfected in 96-well plates (70% confluence) with various amounts of pCAGGS-N9 (0 µg, 0.0375 µg, 0.075 µg and 0.15 µg) using a standard PEI-based transfection protocol. Twenty-four hours post-transfection, N9-expressing cells were infected with HANApp as described above [13]. Vesicular stomatitis virus G protein-pseudotyped particles (VSVGpp) were included as a control. For the NA inhibitor treatments, 293T cells were transfected in 96-well plates (70% confluence) with 0.15 µg pCAGGS-N9 using PEI. Four hours post-transfection, the cells were washed with pre-warmed PBS, and 100 µl of fresh media containing the indicated concentrations of Zanamivir hydrate were added to each plate followed by infection with H7N9pp as described above. Infectivity was evaluated at 30 h post-infection by a luciferase assay.

H7N9 influenza virus infection

The A/Anhui/1/2013 (H7N9) viruses were provided by the CDC, China. The viruses were isolated and passaged in 9-day-old specific pathogen-free chicken embryos. All the experiments with H7N9 viruses were performed in approved enhanced biosafety level 3 (BSL-3) containment laboratories. The H7N9 influenza virus was treated with 2 µM P155-185, P155-185-Chol or scrambled peptide for 0.5 h at 37°C, followed by incubation with MDCK cells cultured in 24-well plates (4×10^5 cells per well) at 0.1 MOI. The inoculum was removed at 2 h post-infection, and the cells were washed twice with DMEM prior to the addition of Opti-MEM I Reduced Serum Medium containing 1 µg/ml TPCK-trypsin with or without 100 nM Zanamivir hydrate (ZA) or 200 nM Oseltamivir carboxylate (OS). Treatment of H7N9 influenza virus with 5 µM chloroquine diphosphate, 2.5 nM bafilomycin A1 or 10 µM dynasore hydrate was also performed as described above. H7N9 influenza virus RNA copies were quantified at 24 h post-infection by qRT-PCR according to the WHO protocol for the detection of Avian Influenza A (H7N9) Virus. The cytopathic effects were visually inspected under an inverted microscope at 48 h post-infection.

Statistical analyses

The data are expressed as the means ± SEM, and all the experiments were repeated at least three times. The data were analyzed with unpaired two-tailed *t* tests with SPSS 16 and GraphPad Prism 5 software.

Results

Production of the H7-pseudotyped particle system

Hemagglutinin (HA) sequence alignments of influenza A virus A/Brisbane/59/2007 (H1N1), A/California/04/2009 (H1N1), A/Brisbane/10/2007 (H3N2), A/Anhui/1/2005 (H5N1) and

A/Anhui/1/2013 (H7N9) were analyzed. The HA cleavage site sequence of H7N9 is P-K-G-R, which is consistent with low pathogenic avian influenza H7 [17]. Western blot analysis also showed that, in contrast to H5N1, the H7N9 HA0 protein cannot be effectively cleaved into functional HA1 and HA2 subunits by intracellular proteases (Fig. 1A). Because HA0 cleavage is a prerequisite for viral entry, we treated the HA pseudotyped particles (HANApp) with a series of concentrations of TPCK trypsin to improve the infectivity of HANApp. As shown in Fig. 1B, in the absence of TPCK-treated trypsin, the H7N9pp was completely non-infectious. However, after incubation with 2 μg/ml TPCK-treated trypsin, H7N9pp could efficiently infect the cells, whereas the proteolysis mode and entry of H5N1pp was quite different from the other tested viruses.

To further optimize the H7N9pp system, we systematically tested the effects of various HA/NA ratios and virus harvest times on the infectivity of H7N9pp. As shown in Fig. 1C, the 293T culture supernatants collected from 24 h post-transfection with 1.5 μg pNL-4.3-Luc-R-E-, 0.5 μg pCAGGS-HA and 0.5 μg pCAGGS-NA constructs exhibits high infectivity with lowest background. To determine whether the produced H7N9pp could mimic the influenza virus entry process, an antibody-mediated neutralization assay was performed. As shown in Fig. 1D, H7N9pp entry was specifically inhibited by an antibody against H7 but not antibodies against H1, H3 or H5 [12]. These findings suggest that H7N9pp-mediated infection has similar properties to H7N9 and thus can be used as an alternative research model for the early events of H7N9 infection.

Hemagglutinin-mediated entry tropism of H7N9

Recent studies have demonstrated that the novel H7N9 virus can bind to both avian (α2,3-linked sialic acid) and human (α2,6-linked sialic acid) receptors [18,19]. It remained unknown whether the unique characteristics of H7N9 receptor binding could affect host tropism with regards to viral entry. Therefore, the entry efficiencies of various HANApp were compared using multiple species and tissue-derived cells (Fig. 2A). The infection efficiencies of each H7N9pp were measured and normalized to that of MDCK cells. Among the 10 examined cell types, chicken embryonic fibroblasts (CEF) and human 293T cells were highly susceptible to H7N9pp. Cells derived from human lung (A549 and NCI-H1650), human hepatoma (Huh7.5.1), African green monkey kidney (Vero E6) and Madin-Darby canine kidney (MDCK) supported moderate H7N9pp infections. However, cells of mouse kidney (NIH3T3), hamster ovary (CHO) and human cervical carcinoma (Hela) were nearly non-permissive to H7-mediated infection.

Neuraminidase N9 limits H7-mediated infection

It has been reported that NA is essential for virus release from host cells [20], and the expression of NA alone can inhibit influenza virus superinfection by removing the SA receptor from the cell surface [13]. To investigate whether H7N9 neuraminidase N9 could inhibit H7N9pp infection, 293T cells expressing various amounts of N9 were infected with H7N9pp, and infectivity was evaluated at 30 h post-infection (Fig. 2B). H7N9pp entry was specifically inhibited in a N9 dosage-dependent manner, whereas the entry of VSVGpp and H5N1pp were unaffected. This N9-mediated H7N9pp superinfection exclusion was partially blocked by the treatment of Zanamivir, a NA inhibitor (Fig. 2C). These results suggest that N9 neuraminidase may play an important role in regulating H7N9 superinfection, and wild type N9 is sensitive to NA inhibitors.

Inhibition of H7N9 virus by peptides and chemicals

To screen for drug candidates against this novel H7N9 virus, we assessed the antiviral potential of several peptides and chemicals using the H7N9pp system *in vitro*. The amino acid sequences of related synthetic peptides are listed in Fig. 3A. As shown in Fig. 3C, P155-185-chol corresponding to the C-terminal ectodomain of the H7 protein (Fig. 3B) showed significant inhibitory effects against H7N9pp infection but not H5N1pp infection, suggesting that the antiviral activity of P155-185-chol was specific to H7. The IC_{50} value of P155-185-chol to H7N9pp was approximately 0.19 μM. However, the unconjugated P155-185 peptide had no inhibitory effects on either H7N9pp or H5N1pp infection. In addition, we tested several previously reported antiviral peptides for H7N9pp inhibition. $B7^{NP}$, a peptide derived from the fibroblast growth factor 4 signal sequence [21,22], exhibits broad-spectrum antiviral activity against influenza viruses *in vitro*. It was demonstrated that the peptide specifically binds to the viral hemagglutinin protein to inhibit the attachment to the cellular receptor, preventing infection. GBVA10-9, a peptide derived from GB virus A [23], may influence virus entry by affecting the integrity of host cell and virus membranes. It has been reported that the effect of GBVA10-9 on HCV entry is genotype independent. Both peptides also showed inhibitory effects against both H7N9pp and H5N1pp infections in a concentration-dependent manner at low micromolar levels (Fig. 3C).

To further investigate whether P155-185-chol was effective against live H7N9 virus propagation *in vitro* when treated alone or in combination with well-characterized NA inhibitors, the A/Anhui/1/2013 (H7N9) virus infection model in MDCK cells was used. Intracellular viral RNA copies, expression of influenza nucleoprotein (NP) and cytopathic effects were measured. As shown in Fig. 3D, 3E and 3F, A/Anhui/1/2013 (H7N9) virus replication in MDCK cells was effectively inhibited by single drug treatments of P155-185-chol (2 μM), ZA (100 nM) and OS (200 nM), respectively. Surprisingly, when P155-185-chol was used in combination with ZA or OS, A/Anhui/1/2013 (H7N9) virus replication was nearly completely blocked (3D, 3E and 3F).

A number of cellular events are involved in influenza virus entry. Thus, we next determined whether H7-mediated infection was sensitive to several specific inhibitors. Dynasore [24] (a specific inhibitor of dynamin), bafilomycin A1[25,26] (a highly specific inhibitor of vacuolar type H+-ATPase) and chloroquine [27,28] (a 9-aminoquinolone with well-known anti-malarial effects) have been previously reported to inhibit the growth of influenza virus in cell culture. As shown in Fig. 4A, dynasore also showed inhibitory effects on the entry of H7N9pp into MDCK cells. The IC_{50} value of dynasore was 3.84 μM in the absence of fetal bovine serum or 16.89 μM in the presence of 10% fetal bovine serum. Bafilomycin A1 was a powerful inhibitor of H7N9pp infection at 2.5 nM. Concentrations of bafilomycin A1 as low as 10 nM almost completely prevented H7N9pp infection in MDCK cells (Fig. 4B). Similarly, live H7N9 virus exhibited a corresponding reduction upon bafilomycin A1 treatment under the same condition. However, the inhibitory effects of 10 μM dynasore on H7N9 virus were not significant (Fig. 4C). Chloroquine had no effects on H7N9pp entry but conferred a weak inhibition against H7N9 virus at 5 μM. Cytotoxicity assays demonstrated that all of the indicated concentrations of peptides and chemicals did not produce cytotoxicity in MDCK cells (Fig. 4A, 4B and 3C).

Discussion

The human infection with H7 subtypes of influenza viruses mainly resulted in conjunctivitis and mild upper respiratory

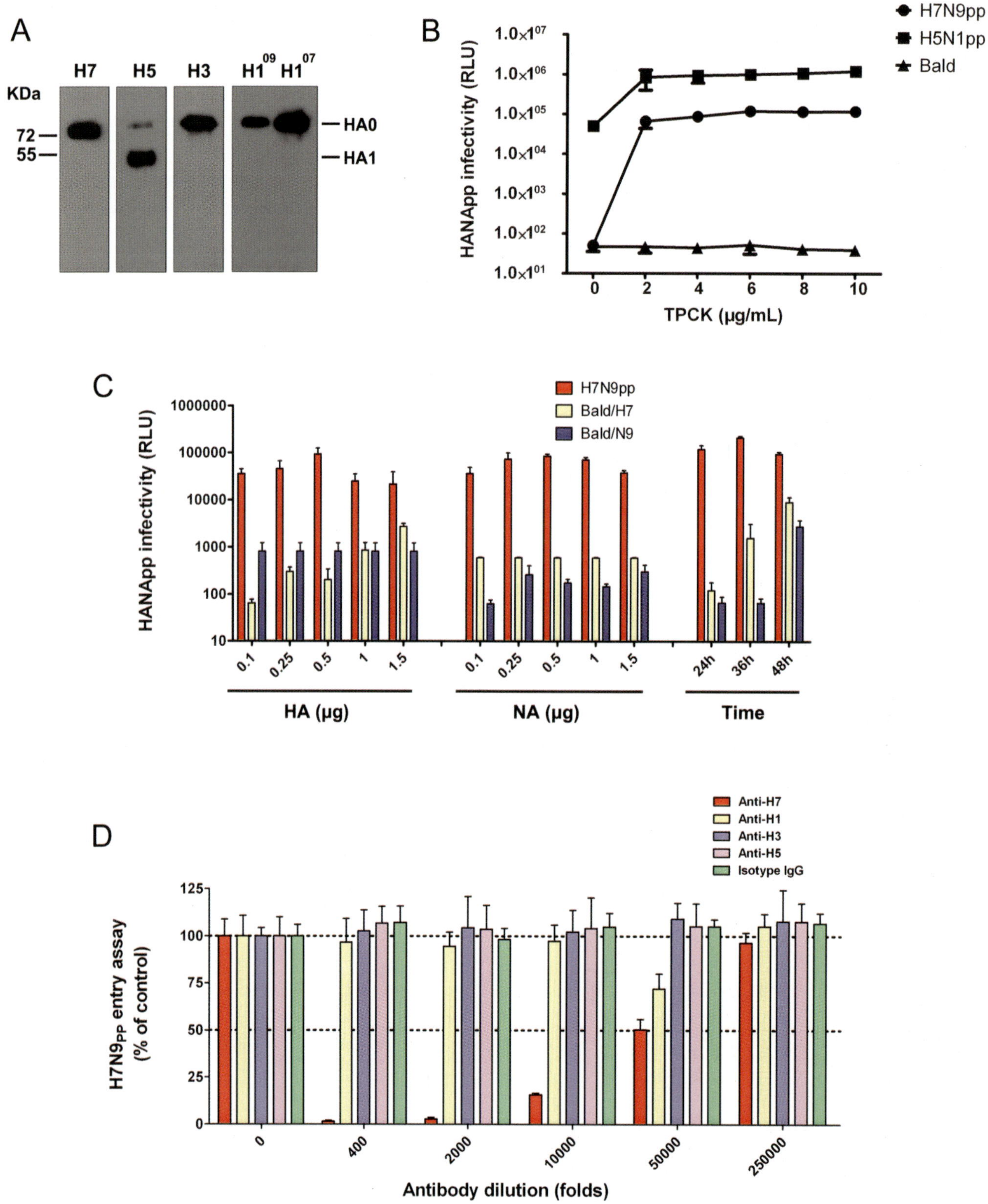

Figure 1. Production and characterization of the H7-pseudotyped particle system. (A) Western blot analysis was performed using lysates from 293T cells transfected with the recombinant pCAGGS plasmids expressing H7 (A/Anhui/1/2013), H5 (A/Anhui/1/2005), H3 (A/Brisbane/10/2007), $H1^{09}$ (A/California/04/2009) and $H1^{07}$ (A/Brisbane/59/2007). Specific bands corresponding to HA0 and HA1 are indicated on the right. **(B)** TPCK-treated trypsin treatment is required for H7N9pp infection. The infectivities of H7N9pp and H5N1pp were determined after treatment with different concentrations of TPCK-treated trypsin (0, 2, 4, 6, 8, 10 μg/ml). Bald virus refers to culture supernatants collected from 293T cells co-transfected with 1.5 μg pNL-4.3-Luc-R^-E^- and 0.5 μg pCAGGS-H7 in the absence of pCAGGS-N9 and was used as a control. **(C)** Optimization of H7N9pp packaging. 293T cells were co-transfected with pNL-4.3-Luc-R^-E^-, pCAGGS-HA and pCAGGS-NA constructs. pCAGGS-HA was maintained at 0.5 μg, while

pCAGGS-NA was varied at 0.1 μg, 0.25 μg, 0.5 μg, 1 μg or 1.5 μg, and the reverse was also performed. The infectivity of 293T culture supernatants collected from different times (24 h, 36 h, 48 h) post-transfection with 1.5 μg pNL-4.3-Luc-R⁻E⁻, 0.5 μg pCAGGS-HA and 0.5 μg pCAGGS-NA constructs was determined as described above. Bald/H7 refers to culture supernatants collected from 293T cells co-transfected with 1.5 μg pNL-4.3-Luc-R⁻E⁻ and the indicated amount of pCAGGS-HA (In 'NA(ug)', Bald/H7 refers to culture supernatants collected from 293T cells co-transfected with 1.5 μg pNL-4.3-Luc-R-E- and 0.5 μg pCAGGS-HA). Bald/N9 refers to culture supernatants collected from 293T cells co-transfected with 1.5 μg pNL-4.3-Luc-R⁻E⁻ and the indicated amount of pCAGGS-NA (In 'HA(ug)', Bald/N9 refers to culture supernatants collected from 293T cells co-transfected with 1.5 μg pNL-4.3-Luc-R-E- and 0.5 μg pCAGGS-NA). Both Bald/H7 and Bald/N9 were included as negative controls. **(D)** Antibody neutralization assays. H7N9pp was incubated with serially diluted monoclonal antibodies against H1, H3, H5 or H7 for 1 h at 37°C before inoculation onto MDCK cells. The cells were lysed, and luciferase activity was determined at 48 h post-infection. Viral entry in the absence of antibody (0 Ab) was set at 100%. Isotype IgG was included as a negative control.

symptoms. However, the recently H7N9 outbreak in China caused high lethal rate. HA is synthesized as a precursor HA0, which is subsequently cleaved into HA1 and HA2 for its full function [29,30]. It has been demonstrated that the cellular proteolytic conversion of HA0 to HA1 and HA2 is an essential step for viral entry and multiplication within the infected host and thus is associated with pathogenicity of influenza viruses [31,32]. In the present study, H7N9 possess an HA cleavage site with a monobasic motif susceptible to only several trypsin-like proteases limited in a few cell types. These suggested that the existence of a multi-basic cleavage site is not essential for the high pathogenicity of avian influenza virus in humans.

To facilitate H7N9 study, we developed an H7N9-pseudotyped particle system bearing virus HA and NA glycoproteins. The produced H7N9pp was neutralized specifically by an antibody against H7 but not antibodies against H1, H3 or H5. In addition,

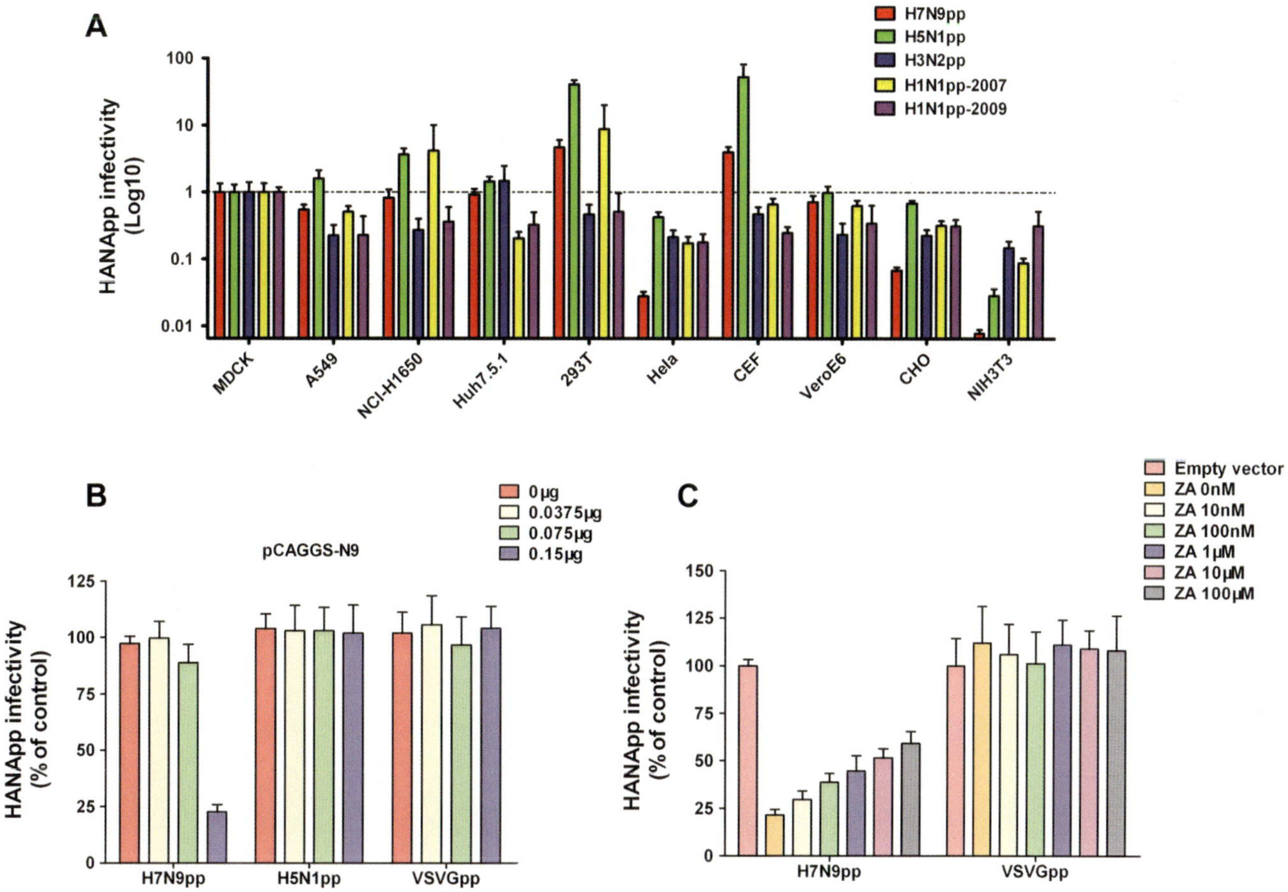

Figure 2. Cell permissiveness to H7N9pp and N9-mediated H7N9pp superinfection exclusion. (A) Different subtypes of HANApp with equal amounts of p24 antigen were incubated with various cells derived from different species and tissues, and the transduction efficiencies were measured and normalized to that of MDCK cells. **(B)** N9 expression specifically inhibits H7N9pp infection. 293T cells were transfected with various amounts of pCAGGS-N9 (0 μg, 0.0375 μg, 0.075 μg and 0.15 μg) and then infected with equal amounts of H7N9pp at 24 h post-transfection. Pseudovirus infection was determined by a luciferase activity assay and normalized to that of cells transfected with vector alone. VSVGpp was included as negative control. **(C)** N9-mediated H7N9pp inhibition can be partially blocked with NA inhibitor Zanamivir (ZA). N9-expressing 293T cells were treated with the indicated concentrations of ZA and then infected with H7N9pp. Pseudovirus infection was determined by a luciferase activity assay and normalized to that of cells transfected with vector alone. VSVGpp was included as a negative control.

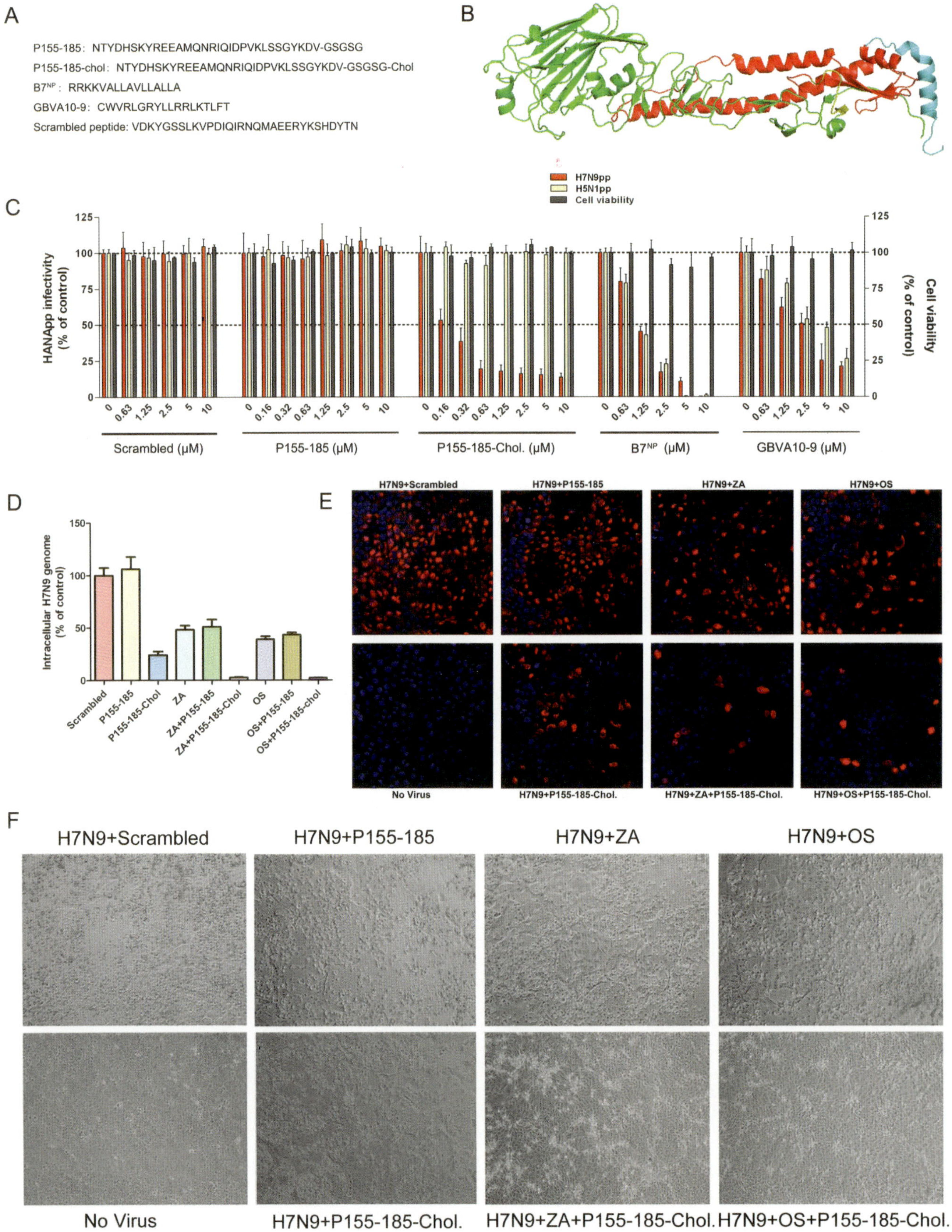

Figure 3. Inhibition of H7N9 virus by peptides. (A) Amino acid sequences of the indicated synthetic peptides. **(B)** Location of P155-185. Structure of HA. HA1, green; HA2, red; fusion peptide, yellow; P155-185, cyan. **(C)** Characterization of the antiviral activity of the synthetic peptides. Viral entry without peptide treatment was set at 100%. A scrambled peptide was included as a negative control. Cytotoxicity of the peptides to MDCK

cells was measured by a MTT assay. **(D)** The inhibitory effect of P155-185-chol against H7N9 influenza virus in combination with neuraminidase inhibitors. P155-185-chol 2 μM; P155-185 2 μM; scrambled peptide 2 μM; ZA, 100 nM Zanamivir hydrate; OS, 200 nM Oseltamivir carboxylate. **(E)** The same experiments as panel D were performed. H7N9-infected MDCK cells were fixed at 36 h after the indicated treatments and processed for immunostaining and observed under confocal microscope. Fixed cell monolayers were immunostained with an anti-influenza A nucleoprotein (NP) murine monoclonal antibody (MAB8251; Millipore) and Alexa 594 conjugated secondary antibody (red). Nuclei were stained with DAPI (blue). **(F)** The same experiments as panel D were performed. The cytopathic effect of H7N9-infected MDCK cells in the presence or absence of the indicated treatments was visually inspected under an inverted microscope at 48 h post-infection.

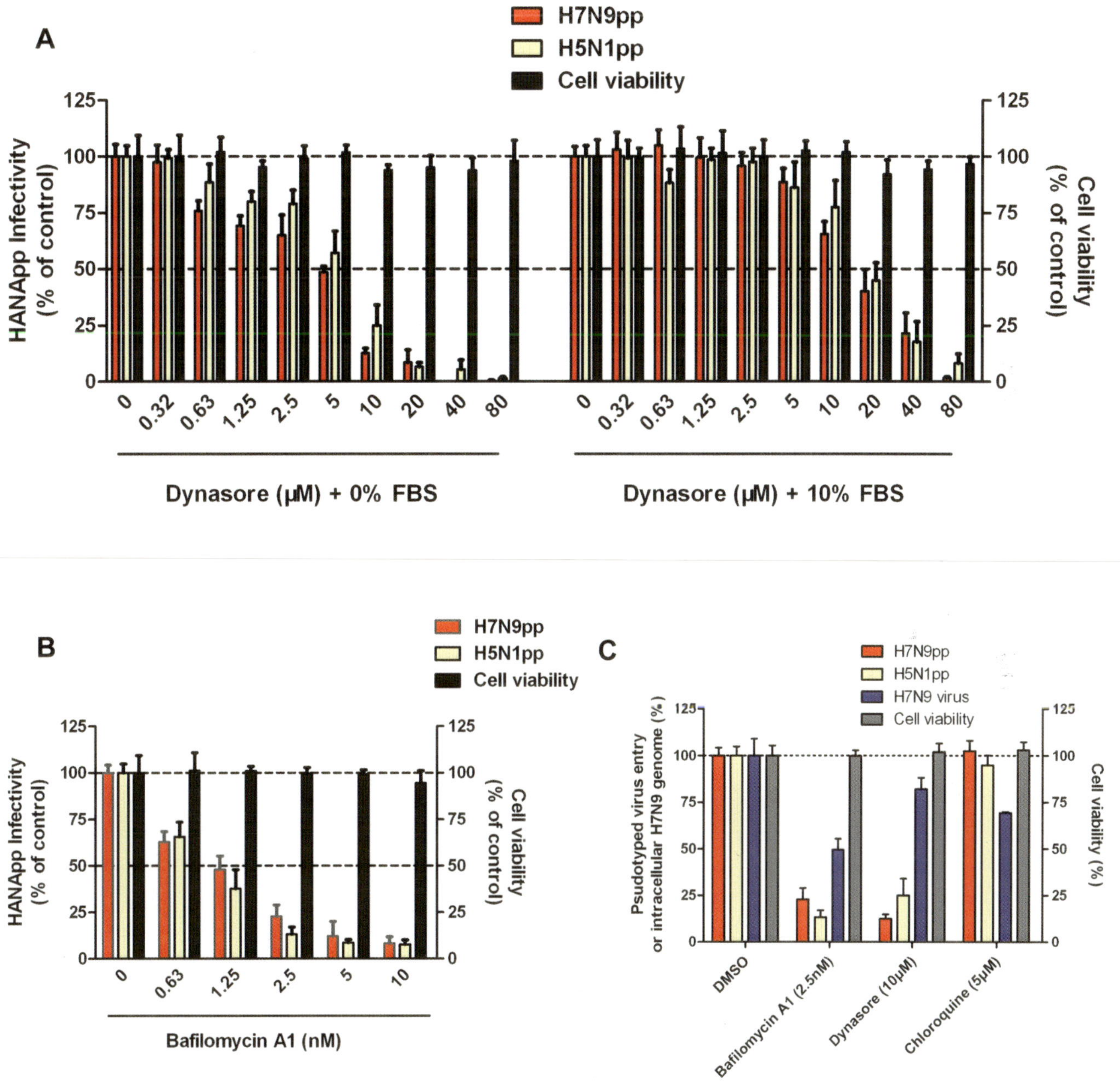

Figure 4. Inhibition of H7N9 virus by chemicals. (A) Inhibition of HA-mediated infection by dynasore. Dynasore's concentrations range from 0 to 80 μM in the absence (left) or presence (right) of 10% fetal bovine serum (FBS). MDCK cells were kept at 37°C in Opti-MEM I Reduced Serum Medium with or without 10% FBS at all times. Dynasore was added 1 h prior to HANApp infection. Pseudovirus infection was determined by a luciferase activity assay 48 h post-infection. Viral entry in the 0 μM treatment control group was set at 100%. **(B)** The inhibitory effect of bafilomycin A1. MDCK cells were pretreated with bafilomycin A1 (concentration range 0 nM to 10 nM) for 1 h at 37°C followed by infection with HANApp. Pseudovirus infection was determined by a luciferase activity assay at 48 h post-infection. Viral entry in the 0 nM treatment control group was set at 100%. **(C)** Antiviral effects of bafilomycin A1, dynasore and chloroquine. Viral entry in the DMSO treated control group was set at 100%. The cytotoxicity of the chemicals at indicated concentrations for MDCK cells was also measured by a MTT assay.

H7N9pp infection was also sensitive to bafilomycin A1 and dynasore as well as other influenza A viruses. These findings suggest that H7N9pp could mimic the influenza virus entry process. Recent studies have demonstrated that the novel H7N9 virus can bind to both avian-type (α2,3-linked SA) and human-type (α2,6-linked SA) receptors. These presented us questions about whether the changed Receptor-Binding ability of the novel H7N9 viruses can affect tropism and pathogenesis of these viruses in mammals. However, the HA-mediated entry assay indicated that the tropism of H7N9 was quite similar to avian H5N1 rather than human pandemic influenza. Until now, information is still limited about the transmission and pathogenicity associated with this novel avian influenza H7N9 virus.

Currently, the NA inhibitors Oseltamivir and Zanamivir are the front-line therapeutic options against this novel H7N9 influenza virus, which contains an S31N mutation in its M2 protein and thus confers resistance to the M2 ion channel blockers [1]. However, recent studies have reported that H7N9 isolates with the R292K mutation are resistant to Zanamivir, Peramivir and Oseltamivir [33]. Two of 14 patients infected with the novel H7N9 influenza virus possessing an R292K NA mutation had a poor clinical outcome [34]. Therefore, discovering novel antiviral targets and drug candidates is urgently expected. HA-mediated virus-host membrane fusion is a prerequisite for the viral life cycle and is a promising antiviral target. Based on the HA-dependent membrane fusion model [35,36], we designed a cholesterol-conjugated peptide, named P155-185-chol, which is derived from the amino acid 155-185 region of H7N9 HA2. P155-185-chol demonstrated H7N9pp-specific inhibition of infection and exhibited significant inhibitory effects against H7N9 virus.

In summary, our study demonstrated that the established H7N9-pseudotyped particle system can largely mimic the entry properties of the H7N9 virus, thus providing a relatively safe experimental system for studying the entry of H7N9 virus and for high-throughput screening of entry inhibitors, such as small molecules, peptides or antibodies. A potent anti-H7N9 peptide (P155-185-chol) was successfully identified in this study. When used in combination with neuraminidase inhibitors (Oseltamivir, Zanamivir), P155-185-chol showed additive and significant inhibitory effects against H7N9. By virtue of its distinct mechanisms of inhibition, P155-185-chol may be further optimized to improve its activity, highlighting a potential therapeutic candidate for H7N9 infections that can be used in combination with other anti-flu drugs.

Author Contributions

Conceived and designed the experiments: WY QJ JW. Performed the experiments: YS JL YN LR LG HZ. Analyzed the data: YS JL YN. Contributed reagents/materials/analysis tools: XL MC. Contributed to the writing of the manuscript: WY YS.

References

1. Gao R, Cao B, Hu Y, Feng Z, Wang D, et al. (2013) Human infection with a novel avian-origin influenza A (H7N9) virus. N Engl J Med 368: 1888–1897.
2. Trock SC, Huntley JP (2010) Surveillance and control of avian influenza in the New York live bird markets. Avian Dis 54: 340–344.
3. Pasick J, Berhane Y, Hooper-McGrevy K (2009) Avian influenza: the Canadian experience. Rev Sci Tech 28: 349–358.
4. Fouchier RA, Schneeberger PM, Rozendaal FW, Broekman JM, Kemink SA, et al. (2004) Avian influenza A virus (H7N7) associated with human conjunctivitis and a fatal case of acute respiratory distress syndrome. Proc Natl Acad Sci U S A 101: 1356–1361.
5. Koopmans M, Wilbrink B, Conyn M, Natrop G, van der Nat H, et al. (2004) Transmission of H7N7 avian influenza A virus to human beings during a large outbreak in commercial poultry farms in the Netherlands. Lancet 363: 587–593.
6. World Health Organization website. Available: http://www.who.int/influenza/human_animal_interface/faq_H7N9/en/. Accessed 2014 Feb 14.
7. World Health Organization website. Available: http://www.who.int/influenza/human_animal_interface/influenza_h7n9/09_ReportWebH7N9Number.pdf?ua=1. Accessed 2013 Aug 17.
8. Chen Y, Liang W, Yang S, Wu N, Gao H, et al. (2013) Human infections with the emerging avian influenza A H7N9 virus from wet market poultry: clinical analysis and characterisation of viral genome. Lancet.
9. Watanabe T, Kiso M, Fukuyama S, Nakajima N, Imai M, et al. (2013) Characterization of H7N9 influenza A viruses isolated from humans. Nature.
10. Kageyama T, Fujisaki S, Takashita E, Xu H, Yamada S, et al. (2013) Genetic analysis of novel avian A(H7N9) influenza viruses isolated from patients in China, February to April 2013. Euro Surveill 18: 20453.
11. Dong G, Luo J, Zhang H, Wang C, Duan M, et al. (2011) Phylogenetic diversity and genotypical complexity of H9N2 influenza A viruses revealed by genomic sequence analysis. PLoS One 6: e17212.
12. Zhao R, Cui S, Guo L, Wu C, Gonzalez R, et al. (2011) Identification of a highly conserved H1 subtype-specific epitope with diagnostic potential in the hemagglutinin protein of influenza A virus. PLoS One 6: e23374.
13. Huang IC, Li W, Sui J, Marasco W, Choe H, et al. (2008) Influenza A virus neuraminidase limits viral superinfection. J Virol 82: 4834–4843.
14. Li R, Song D, Zhu Z, Xu H, Liu S (2012) An induced pocket for the binding of potent fusion inhibitor CL-385319 with H5N1 influenza virus hemagglutinin. PLoS One 7: e41956.
15. Guo Y, Rumschlag-Booms E, Wang J, Xiao H, Yu J, et al. (2009) Analysis of hemagglutinin-mediated entry tropism of H5N1 avian influenza. Virol J 6: 39.
16. Oh HL, Akerstrom S, Shen S, Bereczky S, Karlberg H, et al. (2010) An antibody against a novel and conserved epitope in the hemagglutinin 1 subunit neutralizes numerous H5N1 influenza viruses. J Virol 84: 8275–8286.
17. Kido H, Okumura Y, Takahashi E, Pan HY, Wang S, et al. (2008) Host envelope glycoprotein processing proteases are indispensable for entry into human cells by seasonal and highly pathogenic avian influenza viruses. J Mol Genet Med 3: 167–175.
18. Xiong X, Martin SR, Haire LF, Wharton SA, Daniels RS, et al. (2013) Receptor binding by an H7N9 influenza virus from humans. Nature.
19. Ramos I, Krammer F, Hai R, Aguilera D, Bernal-Rubio D, et al. (2013) H7N9 influenza viruses interact preferentially with alpha2,3-linked sialic acids and bind weakly to alpha2,6-linked sialic acids. J Gen Virol.
20. Moscona A (2005) Neuraminidase inhibitors for influenza. N Engl J Med 353: 1363–1373.
21. Jones JC, Turpin EA, Bultmann H, Brandt CR, Schultz-Cherry S (2006) Inhibition of influenza virus infection by a novel antiviral peptide that targets viral attachment to cells. J Virol 80: 11960–11967.
22. Jones JC, Settles EW, Brandt CR, Schultz-Cherry S (2011) Identification of the minimal active sequence of an anti-influenza virus peptide. Antimicrob Agents Chemother 55: 1810–1813.
23. Liu X, Huang Y, Cheng M, Pan L, Si Y, et al. (2013) Screening and rational design of hepatitis C virus entry inhibitory peptides derived from GB virus A NS5A. J Virol 87: 1649–1657.
24. de Vries E, Tscherne DM, Wienholts MJ, Cobos-Jimenez V, Scholte F, et al. (2011) Dissection of the influenza A virus endocytic routes reveals macropinocytosis as an alternative entry pathway. PLoS Pathog 7: e1001329.
25. Wang H, Jiang C (2009) Influenza A virus H5N1 entry into host cells is through clathrin-dependent endocytosis. Sci China C Life Sci 52: 464–469.
26. Ochiai H, Sakai S, Hirabayashi T, Shimizu Y, Terasawa K (1995) Inhibitory effect of bafilomycin A1, a specific inhibitor of vacuolar-type proton pump, on the growth of influenza A and B viruses in MDCK cells. Antiviral Res 27: 425–430.
27. Di Trani L, Savarino A, Campitelli L, Norelli S, Puzelli S, et al. (2007) Different pH requirements are associated with divergent inhibitory effects of chloroquine on human and avian influenza A viruses. Virol J 4: 39.
28. Ooi EE, Chew JS, Loh JP, Chua RC (2006) In vitro inhibition of human influenza A virus replication by chloroquine. Virol J 3: 39.
29. Garten W, Klenk HD (1999) Understanding influenza virus pathogenicity. Trends Microbiol 7: 99–100.
30. Stieneke-Grober A, Vey M, Angliker H, Shaw E, Thomas G, et al. (1992) Influenza virus hemagglutinin with multibasic cleavage site is activated by furin, a subtilisin-like endoprotease. EMBO J 11: 2407–2414.
31. Horimoto T, Kawaoka Y (1994) Reverse genetics provides direct evidence for a correlation of hemagglutinin cleavability and virulence of an avian influenza A virus. J Virol 68: 3120–3128.
32. Senne DA, Panigrahy B, Kawaoka Y, Pearson JE, Suss J, et al. (1996) Survey of the hemagglutinin (HA) cleavage site sequence of H5 and H7 avian influenza viruses: amino acid sequence at the HA cleavage site as a marker of pathogenicity potential. Avian Dis 40: 425–437.
33. Yen HL, McKimm-Breschkin JL, Choy KT, Wong DD, Cheung PP, et al. (2013) Resistance to neuraminidase inhibitors conferred by an R292K mutation in a human influenza virus H7N9 isolate can be masked by a mixed R/K viral population. MBio 4.

34. Hu Y, Lu S, Song Z, Wang W, Hao P, et al. (2013) Association between adverse clinical outcome in human disease caused by novel influenza A H7N9 virus and sustained viral shedding and emergence of antiviral resistance. Lancet.
35. Park HE, Gruenke JA, White JM (2003) Leash in the groove mechanism of membrane fusion. Nat Struct Biol 10: 1048–1053.
36. Lee KK, Pessi A, Gui L, Santoprete A, Talekar A, et al. (2011) Capturing a fusion intermediate of influenza hemagglutinin with a cholesterol-conjugated peptide, a new antiviral strategy for influenza virus. J Biol Chem 286: 42141–42149.

3

Proteomics-Identified Bvg-Activated Autotransporters Protect against *Bordetella pertussis* in a Mouse Model

Daan de Gouw[1,2], Marien I. de Jonge[1,2], Peter W. M. Hermans[1,2¤], Hans J. C. T. Wessels[3], Aldert Zomer[1,2], Alinda Berends[1,2], Catherine Pratt[5], Guy A. Berbers[4], Frits R. Mooi[1,2,4], Dimitri A. Diavatopoulos[1,2*]

1 Laboratory of Pediatric Infectious Diseases, Department of Pediatrics, Radboud University Medical Centre, Nijmegen, The Netherlands, **2** Laboratory of Medical Immunology, Department of Laboratory Medicine, Radboud University Medical Centre, Nijmegen, The Netherlands, **3** Nijmegen Centre for Mitochondrial Disorders, Department of Laboratory Medicine, Radboud Proteomics Centre, Radboud University Medical Centre, Nijmegen, The Netherlands, **4** Netherlands Centre for Infectious Disease Control, National Institute for Public Health and the Environment (RIVM), Bilthoven, The Netherlands, **5** Public Health England, Centre for Emergency Preparedness and Response, Porton Down, Salisbury, United Kingdom

Abstract

Pertussis is a highly infectious respiratory disease of humans caused by the bacterium *Bordetella pertussis.* Despite high vaccination coverage, pertussis has re-emerged globally. Causes for the re-emergence of pertussis include limited duration of protection conferred by acellular pertussis vaccines (aP) and pathogen adaptation. Pathogen adaptations involve antigenic divergence with vaccine strains, the emergence of strains which show enhanced *in vitro* expression of a number of virulence-associated genes and of strains that do not express pertactin, an important aP component. Clearly, the identification of more effective *B. pertussis* vaccine antigens is of utmost importance. To identify novel antigens, we used proteomics to identify *B. pertussis* proteins regulated by the master virulence regulatory system BvgAS *in vitro.* Five candidates proteins were selected and it was confirmed that they were also expressed in the lungs of naïve mice seven days after infection. The five proteins were expressed in recombinant form, adjuvanted with alum and used to immunize mice as stand-alone antigens. Subsequent respiratory challenge showed that immunization with the autotransporters Vag8 and SphB1 significantly reduced bacterial load in the lungs. Whilst these antigens induced strong opsonizing antibody responses, we found that none of the tested alum-adjuvanted vaccines - including a three-component aP - reduced bacterial load in the nasopharynx, suggesting that alternative immunological responses may be required for efficient bacterial clearance from the nasopharynx.

Editor: Eliane Namie Miyaji, Instituto Butantan, Brazil

Funding: D.d.G. is supported by Grant 125020001 from the Netherlands Organization of Scientific Research (ZonMw). The funders had no role in study design, data collection and analysis, decision to publish, or preparation of the manuscript.

Competing Interests: The authors have declared that no competing interests exist.

* Email: dimitri.diavatopoulos@radboudumc.nl

¤ Current address: Crucell – Johnson and Johnson, Leiden, The Netherlands

Introduction

Pertussis (or whooping cough) is a highly contagious, acute respiratory disease of humans caused by the Gram-negative bacterium *Bordetella pertussis*. Although pertussis-related mortality has dropped significantly after the introduction of childhood vaccination, pertussis has resurged in many industrialized countries, with particularly large outbreaks occurring in 2010 and 2012 in Australia, the USA, the UK, the Netherlands, and several other countries [1–4]. This increase in pertussis incidence is seen mainly in (vaccinated) adolescents and adults, providing a reservoir for transmission of pertussis to unvaccinated or partially vaccinated newborns, who are at greatest risk of developing severe pertussis [5–7].

Although current pertussis vaccines are effective in limiting the development of severe clinical symptoms, they are much less effective in preventing colonization of the upper respiratory tract and consequently do not adequately reduce circulation in the population [8]. Moreover, vaccine-induced protection wanes rapidly leaving vaccinated individuals susceptible to develop disease after 5–7 years [9]. The apparent inability of current vaccines to significantly reduce the circulation of *B. pertussis* may have facilitated pathogen adaptation. Pathogen adaptation has resulted in antigenic divergence between vaccine strains and circulating strains and the emergence of strains, designate P3 strains, which show enhanced *in vitro* expression of a number of virulence-associated genes [10,11]. Most recently, strains belonging to the P3 lineage have emerged which do not produce pertactin (Prn), a component of most aPs. Prn-deficient strains have reached frequencies of up to 55% in some countries [12–15]. Efforts to improve the immunogenicity of pertussis vaccines have thus far focused on skewing immunity towards more effective bacterial clearance, for instance through the use of novel adjuvants [16,17]. However, the emergence of Prn-deficient strains also highlights a need to identify novel protective antigens, which may be included in improved aPs.

The expression of nearly all pertussis virulence factors, including the antigens present in aPs, is positively regulated by the two-component sensory transduction system BvgAS (reviewed in [18]). Bvg-activated proteins are generally associated with virulence and modulation or evasion of host immunity [19] and play an important, or even essential role, during infection. These proteins therefore represent potential vaccine targets. *In vitro*, low temperature and increasing concentration of nicotinic acid or sulfate are known to suppress the Bvg-system, resulting in the transition from virulent (Bvg^+) through intermediate (Bvg^i) to nonvirulent (Bvg^-) bacteria [20]. In this study, we analyzed the Bvg^+, Bvg^i, and Bvg^- phase-dependent protein content of two clinical isolates derived from the P1 and P3 lineages which dominated globally *before* and *after* the 1990s, respectively [11,21]. Conserved *in vivo* expressed candidates were then evaluated for their ability to confer protection against respiratory infection in mice.

Results

Proteomic analysis and vaccine antigen selection

The regulation of the Bvg-system is dependent on environmental signals, including free sulfate [20]. In this study, we compared the proteome of two currently circulating *B. pertussis* lineages under *in vitro* Bvg^+ (low sulfate), Bvg^i (medium sulfate), and Bvg^- (high sulfate) conditions. *B. pertussis* strains B1917 and B1920 were used as representatives for the P3 and P1 lineages, respectively [21]. Bacterial cultures were grown in four replicates under different Bvg conditions, fractionated into cytosolic and membrane protein fractions and analyzed by mass spectrometry. This approach identified a total of 940 proteins in B1917 and 952 proteins in B1920, with 91% overlap between these strains (see Text S1 and Figure 1A), representing ~28% of the predicted 3449 protein-coding ORFs in the *B. pertussis* genome [22]. The IDEAL-Q algorithm [23] was used to identify proteins that were ≥2.5 fold higher expressed under Bvg^+ or Bvg^i conditions compared to the Bvg^- condition, which yielded 159 and 104 Bvg-activated proteins in B1917 and B1920, respectively (Table S1).

Since P3 and P1 strains both circulate in the population [21], novel antigens should target both lineages. We therefore first selected proteins that were Bvg-activated in both strains, resulting in 51 potential candidates (Figure 1A). Aggregation based on function and predicted subcellular localization showed that these 51 candidates were significantly enriched for proteins involved in cellular processes (n = 6, 15%), outer membrane proteins (n = 6, 20%) and extracellular proteins (n = 10, 44%; Figure 1B and C). Subsequent selection based on Bvg-dependent *in vitro* transcription levels [10], presence in the core genome of *B. pertussis* [25] and predicted surface-exposed localization [26] yielded 15 vaccine candidates (Figure 1A). Of these 15 proteins, eight represent known *B. pertussis* protective antigens (Figure 1A), thus validating our strategy to identify virulence factors, some of which have proven immunogenic properties. Of the remaining candidates, the autotransporters SphB1 and Vag8, the TonB-dependent receptor for iron transport BfrD, the zinc protease BP2497, and the outer membrane porin protein Q (OmpQ), were selected for further examination (Figure 1A). Although the outer membrane ligand binding protein BipA and FhaC are also promising vaccine candidates based on these criteria, their vaccine potential was not assessed due to limited resources.

The list of vaccine candidates was supplemented with proteins that were highly abundant under all Bvg conditions, as these may also represent attractive targets for the host immune response. Based on protein abundance estimation by emPAI [27] (Table S2), the two most abundant proteins, outer membrane proteins A and P (OmpA, OmpP), were also selected for further analysis.

Recombinant protein production and vaccination

To analyze the protective potential of the selected vaccine candidates, recombinant His-tagged fusion proteins were expressed, purified, and refolded. BfrD and OmpQ could not be produced due to low expression and protein degradation. The five remaining proteins were adjuvanted with alum (5 µg for each antigen, 1 µg for SphB1 due to low protein yield) and administered to BALB/c mice (six mice per group) as stand-alone antigens by subcutaneous injection at day 0 and 14. In parallel, groups of mice were vaccinated with a 3-component aP or with PBS and/or alum. Three weeks after the final vaccination, mice were challenged by intranasal infection with *B. pertussis* strain B1917. B1917 was chosen as the challenge strain, as it belongs to the predominant P3 lineage, which has spread worldwide [11,24]. Importantly, the amino acid sequences of the tested antigens are highly conserved in all sequenced *B. pertussis* strains [24].

aP-vaccinated mice showed the strongest (>220-fold) reduction in bacterial load in the lungs at both 3 and 7 days after infection. Of the novel vaccine candidates, rOmpA did not confer any protection. Although vaccination with rOmpP and rBP2497 resulted in a small but significant reduction of bacterial numbers in the lungs at day 3 (1.7 and 1.8-fold, respectively), these differences were not observed at day 7, suggesting that these proteins have only limited vaccine potential (Figure 2A and B). In contrast, vaccination with either rSphB1 or rVag8 resulted in a nearly 10-fold reduction in bacterial load in the lungs at day 3 and a more pronounced 26 and 68-fold reduction at day 7, respectively (Figure 2A and B). Of note, although alum-vaccination induced a significant 7.3-fold reduction in bacterial load in the upper respiratory tract (URT) at day 7 compared to the PBS group, none of the vaccines, including aP, was able to reduce bacterial load in the URT (Figure 2C and D).

Antibody responses to vaccine antigens

To determine the potential role of antibodies in vaccine-mediated opsonization, ELISA was performed using sera from vaccinated mice. Figure 3 suggests that all vaccine candidates induced production of antigen-specific IgG. The absence of pre-existing antigen-specific antibodies was confirmed using pre-immune serum. To assess binding to native epitopes on the bacterial surface, flow cytometry was used to measure binding of antibodies in serum and nasal lavage to the challenge strain B1917 grown under Bvg^+ and Bvg^- conditions. Serum antibodies from rVag8, rSphB1, and aP-vaccinated mice opsonized Bvg^+ bacteria at significant levels. Although opsonization levels were reduced for Bvg^- bacteria, rVag8 and aP-vaccinated mice sera still bound significantly to Bvg^- bacteria (Figure 4A), which is most likely due to residual expression of these proteins under Bvg^- conditions (Table S2). For nasal lavage samples, binding to Bvg^+ bacteria was only detected for rVag8 and aP-treated animals (Figure 4B).

Finally, whole-cell ELISA was performed for each antigen. Analysis of the subtype distribution of opsonizing IgG1, IgG2a, and IgG2b antibodies showed that IgG1 was the dominant subtype for each antigen (Figure 4C, D en E).

In vivo expression of vaccine antigens

To determine whether the selected vaccine candidates were expressed during infection, naïve adult BALB/c mice were infected intranasally with B1917 or B1920. Seven days after infection, gene expression was analyzed on bacteria isolated from

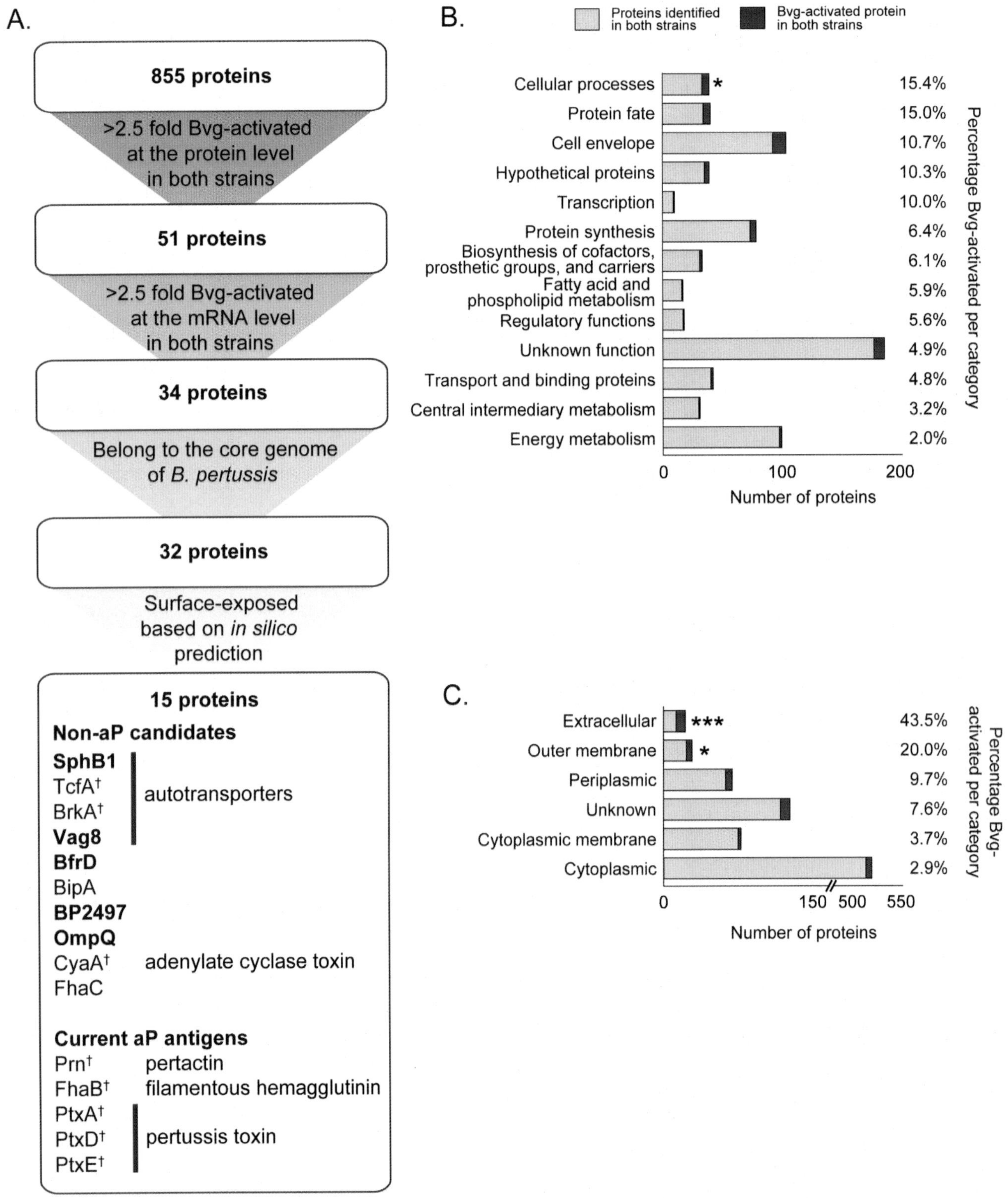

Figure 1. Vaccine antigen selection and functional clustering of Bvg-activated proteins. A) Putative protein antigens were selected based on ≥2.5-fold Bvg-activation at both protein (this work) and mRNA level [10], presence in the core genome of *B. pertussis* [25], and PSORTb v3.0 predicted surface accessibility (outer membrane or extracellular) [26]. This resulted in the identification of 15 putative vaccine candidates. † known *B. pertussis* protective antigens. Proteins in bold were selected for further examination. The proteins in bold The 855 and 51 proteins that were respectively identified and Bvg-activated at the protein level in both strains, were grouped by functional categories (**B**) and PSORTb-predicated subcellular localization (**C**). The relative frequency of Bvg-activated proteins compared to the total number of annotated proteins identified in both strains for each functional class are listed on the right-hand side. Asterisks indicate statistically significant enrichment of Bvg-activated proteins in a certain class as determined by Fisher's exact test. *$p<0.05$, ***$p<0.0005$.

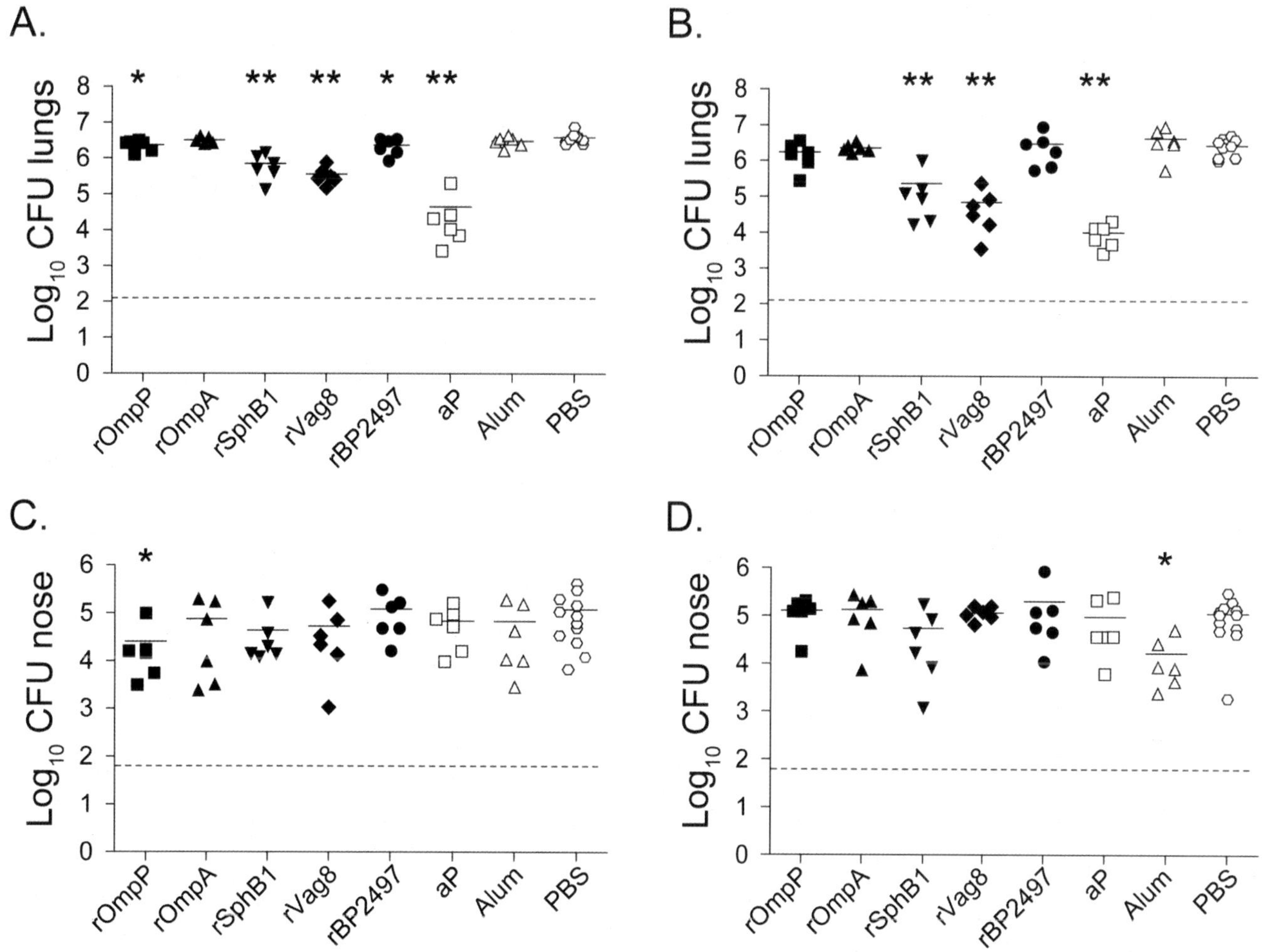

Figure 2. Effect of immunization with novel vaccine candidates on infection with *B. pertussis* in the lower and upper respiratory tract. Naïve adult female BALB/c mice were subcutaneously immunized as described in the text and infected intranasally with 2×10^7 CFU of *B. pertussis* strain B1917. The bacterial load in the lungs and nose was quantified three (**A&C**) and seven (**B&D**) days after challenge. Each symbol represents one mouse. Horizontal lines represents the mean. Dashed lines indicate the lower limit of detection. *$p<0.05$, **$p<0.005$ relative to PBS mice; 2-tailed Mann-Whitney *U* test.

the lungs for the five vaccine candidate genes as well as for *ptxA*, *prn*, *fhaB*, and *fim3*, which encode all currently used aP antigens except for Fim2. The expression of these genes was compared to the *kpsT* gene, which encodes a protein involved in capsule biosynthesis that has previously been identified as a Bvg$^-$ gene [28]. Transcriptional analysis showed that all vaccine candidates and aP antigens were highly expressed in the lungs of mice in relation to *kpsT* (Figure 5).

Discussion

The increase in pertussis outbreaks and the many adaptations observed in *B. pertussis* populations, including the down-regulation of Prn, indicates that more potent pertussis vaccines are warranted. Here, using an integrated 'omics' approach, we identified OmpP, OmpA, SphB1, Vag8, and BP2497 as *in vivo* expressed vaccine candidates. Stand-alone immunization with the autotransporters SphB1 and Vag8 induced significant protection against lower respiratory tract (LRT) infection, at a level which was only 10- and 3-fold lower compared to the reference 3-component aP vaccine (containing Ptx, Prn, and FHA), respectively. Thus far, four *B. pertussis* autotransporters have shown to confer protection in the mouse model, Prn [29], TcfA [30], SphB1, and Vag8, suggesting that these proteins represent an attractive class of protective antigens.

Since aluminum adjuvants typically induce a strong T helper type 2 (Th2) response and high levels of antibodies [31], we primarily focused on the contribution of antibodies to protection. Although all five selected vaccine candidates induced significant levels of specific serum IgGs (predominantly IgG1), only rSphB1 and rVag8 conferred significant protection. A potential explanation for this result may be that only antibodies to rSphB1 and rVag8 opsonized *B. pertussis* (Figure 4). The inability of antibodies specific for rOmpP, rOmpA, and rBP2497 to successfully opsonize bacteria may be due to incorrect folding of the recombinant proteins, which is essential to induce bactericidal antibodies particularly to integral outer membrane proteins like OmpP and OmpA [32].

At present, the exact mechanisms of protection induced by SphB1 and Vag8 remain unknown. Antibodies to these proteins may facilitate phagocytosis and subsequent killing, or result in the deposition of complement factors on the bacterial surface. Alternatively, antibodies may neutralize the biological activity of these antigens. For instance, antibodies against Vag8 may enhance

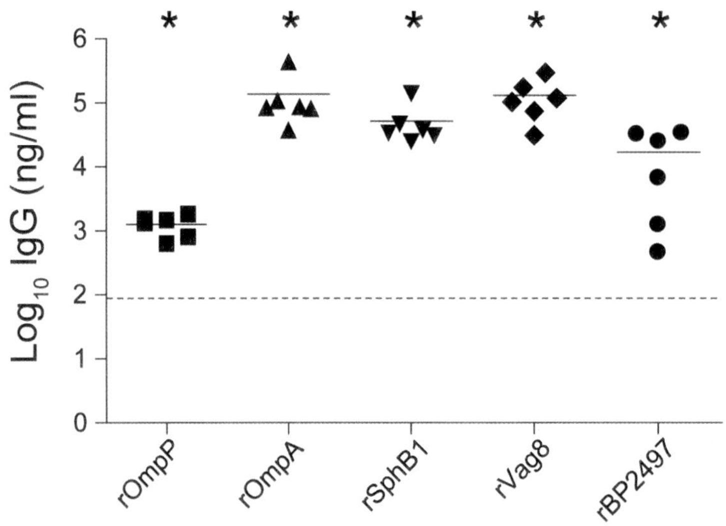

Figure 3. Detection of antigen-specific IgG in the serum of immunized mice. Post-immune serum (day 28) was used to determine the amount of total IgG specific for each recombinant antigens using ELISA as described in the text. Each symbol represents one mouse and the geometric mean is represented by a line. Dashed lines indicate the lower limit of detection (93 ng/ml). *$p<0.05$; 1-tailed Wilcoxon Signed Rank Test.

the susceptibility of *B. pertussis* to complement-mediated killing [33]. Interestingly, SphB1 induced similar protection levels compared as Vag8 (Figure 2), despite much lower opsonization levels (Figure 4). This could be a direct consequence of the lower absolute expression levels of *sphB1* during infection compared to *vag8* (Figure 5). Alternatively, the lower level of opsonizing antibodies may still be sufficient to effectively neutralize the biological activity of SphB1 on the bacterial surface. SphB1 is a serine protease which plays an essential role in the maturation of the adhesin and immune-modulating factor FHA [34]. Previous studies have shown that deletion of the *sphB1* gene dramatically attenuated the ability of *B. pertussis* to infect mice [35] and enhanced phagocytosis [36]. Taken together with our observation that *sphB1* is not expressed at high levels during infection, this gene represents a very attractive target because even low concentrations of neutralizing antibodies may be sufficient for protection.

Although we found that SphB1 and Vag8 were both expressed during infection in naïve mice, antibodies against these (recombinant) antigens were undetectable in convalescent pertussis patients (data not shown). Although it is possible that these proteins have poor intrinsic immunogenicity in humans during natural infection, another explanation may be that vaccinated individuals who are subsequently infected with *B. pertussis* preferentially respond to only a limited number of immunodominant vaccine antigens, also known as original antigenic sin [37].

Finally, an important observation was that none of the vaccine formulations, including aP, was able to reduce bacterial colonization of the URT. As colonization of the URT is probably essential for transmission, this may explain epidemiological studies which show that high circulation of *B. pertussis* occurs despite widespread aP vaccination [38]. Similarly, recent observations in the baboon model have shown that aP-vaccinated baboons are protected against disease but remain susceptible to colonization and are able to transmit the disease [8]. These data suggest that the immunological mechanisms which are required for effective clearance from the lungs (e.g. antibodies [39]) are distinct from those in the URT, an observation which has also been made for other respiratory bacterial pathogens, including *Streptococcus pneumonia* [40–42]. Cellular immunity in particular may represent an important component for effective clearance of the URT [43] and in order to prevent both disease *and* colonization, a combined antibody and cellular response may be required [8,17,44–47].

Materials and Methods

Ethics statement

Animal experiments were approved by the Radboudumc Committee for Animal Ethics and conducted in accordance with the relevant Dutch legislation. Bacterial strains were collected by regional Medical Microbiology Laboratories from patients suspected of whooping cough and sent to the National Institute for Public Health and the Environment (RIVM) in the context of routine surveillance (as required by law). The strains are sent to the RIVM for confirmation of clinical diagnosis, species determination and subtyping. Strictly anonymized patient information is included, which is limited to age, sex and postal code. For this type of surveillance ethical evaluation or patient consent are not required. The strains have been used in previous studies [48].

Bacterial strains and growth conditions

Culture samples of *B. pertussis* strains grown under Bvg^+, Bvg^i, and Bvg^- conditions in chemically defined THIJS medium [49] from a previous study [10] were used for proteomic analysis (four replicates). For modulation of the BvgASR regulatory system, magnesium sulfate was added to cultures at a final concentration of 5 and 50 mM to induce Bvg^i and Bvg^- conditions respectively. In the absence of additional sulfate, the concentration of free sulfate was determined to be 0.02 mM, thereby inducing Bvg^+ conditions. Correct modulation of the Bvg system by sulfate was confirmed in previous work [10]. Bacteria harvested at mid-log (OD_{620} of 0.5–0.6) were used for protein isolation.

For recombinant protein expression, *Escherichia coli* OverExpress C41(DE3) (Lucigen, USA) was grown in Luria Bertani medium (LB) containing appropriate antibiotics (ampicillin, kanamycin and/or chloramphenicol at a concentration of 50 µg/ml) at 37°C.

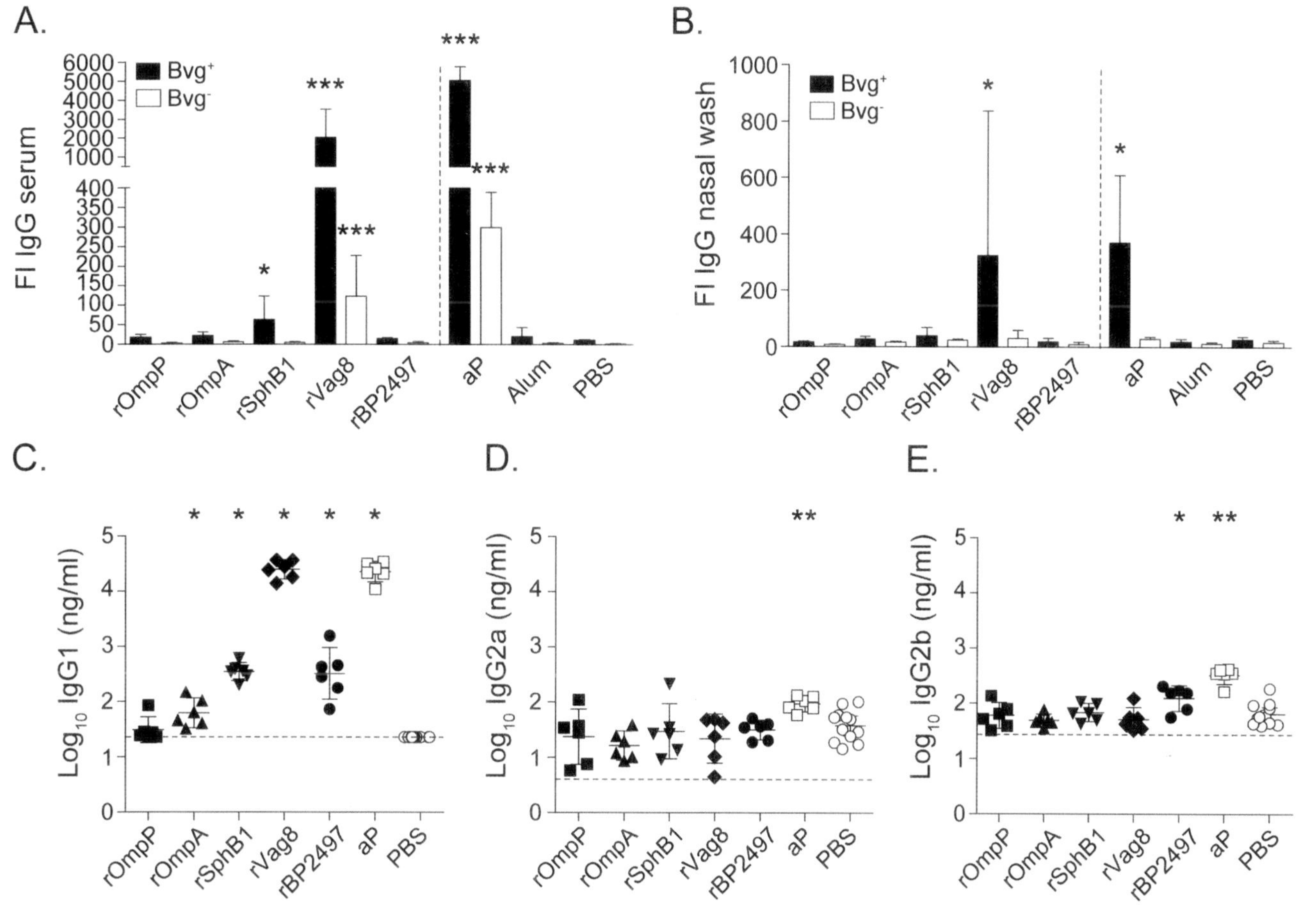

Figure 4. Antibody-mediated opsonization of *B. pertussis*. The binding of serum (**A**) and nasal lavage (**B**) IgG antibodies to Bvg^+ or Bvg^- grown *B. pertussis* B1917 was determined using flow cytometry. Bars represent the geometric mean ±95% confidence interval (CI) of 6 individual mice. **p*<0.05, ****p*<0.0005 relative to PBS group; Kruskal-Wallis test followed by a Dunns *post-hoc* test (α = 5%). To determine the distribution of IgG subtypes, whole-cell ELISA was performed with the post-immunization serum samples to detect pertussis-specific IgG1 (**C**), IgG2a (**D**), and IgG2b (**E**). Each symbol represents one mouse and the geometric mean is represented by a line. Dashed lines indicate the lower limit of detection (23, 4, and 27 ng/ml for IgG1, IgG2a, and IgG2b, respectively). For IgG1, a 1-tailed Wilcoxon Signed Rank Test was performed because IgG1 levels of the PBS mice were below the detection limit. IgG2a and IgG2b levels were statistically compared to the PBS mice using a 2-tailed Mann-Whitney *U*-test. **p*<0.05, ***p*<0.005.

Proteomics analysis

Bacterial pellets from 5 ml of mid-log culture were lysed by sonication. Cytosolic and membrane protein fractions were then isolated using the ReadyPrep Protein Extraction Kit Membrane I (Bio-Rad Laboratories, Hercules, CA, USA), according to the manufacturers protocol. The obtained soluble and insoluble fractions, containing the cytosolic and membrane (-associated) proteins respectively, were precipitated using the ReadyPrep 2-D clean-up Kit (Bio-Rad Laboratories). Protein pellets were then dissolved in 8 M urea in 10 mM Tris-HCl pH 8.0 and subjected to in-solution digestion and C18 reversed phase nano flow LC-MS/MS analysis as described in Text S1.

Recombinant antigen production

The DNA sequences of the selected vaccine antigens lacking their N-terminal signal sequences and/or other targeting domains to allow cytosolic expression, were codon optimized for expression in *E. coli*, synthesized by GenScript (USA), and cloned into pET28-TEVsite vector (modified from pET28a vector, Novagen, Denmark) to generate N-terminally His_6-tagged proteins (Table S3). *E. coli* OverExpress C41(DE3) (Lucigen, USA) was cultured to an OD_{600} = 0.6–0.7 at 37°C, after which recombinant protein expression was induced through the addition of 1 mM Isopropyl β-D-1-thiogalactopyranoside (IPTG) for 3 hours. For cell lysis, bacteria were sonicated in Bacterial Protein Extraction Reagent (B-PER, Thermo Scientific). Recombinant proteins in inclusion bodies were dissolved in 20 mM sodium phosphate, 500 mM NaCl, 4 M urea and 20 mM imidazole and purified on a AKTA FPLC system using affinity chromatography on a HisTrap FF crude 1 ml column prepacked with Ni Sepharose 6 Fast Flow (GE Healthcare, Sweden) as described [50]. Protein concentrations were determined using the 2-D Quant Kit (GE Healthcare, USA). Recombinant proteins were refolded by rapid 50-fold dilution in refolding buffer (for rBP2315 and rBP2497 according to [51] and for rBP0840 and rBP0943 according to [52]) Refolding of rBP0216 was performed in 10 mM Benzamidine, 1 mM EDTA, 100 mM NaCL, 1 M urea, and 50 mM diethanolamine (pH9.5).

Vaccination

Individual groups of six naïve female, 6–8 week old BALB/c mice (Charles River) were immunized subcutaneously on day 0 and 14 with 5 µg of recombinant protein (1 µg for rBP0216 due to

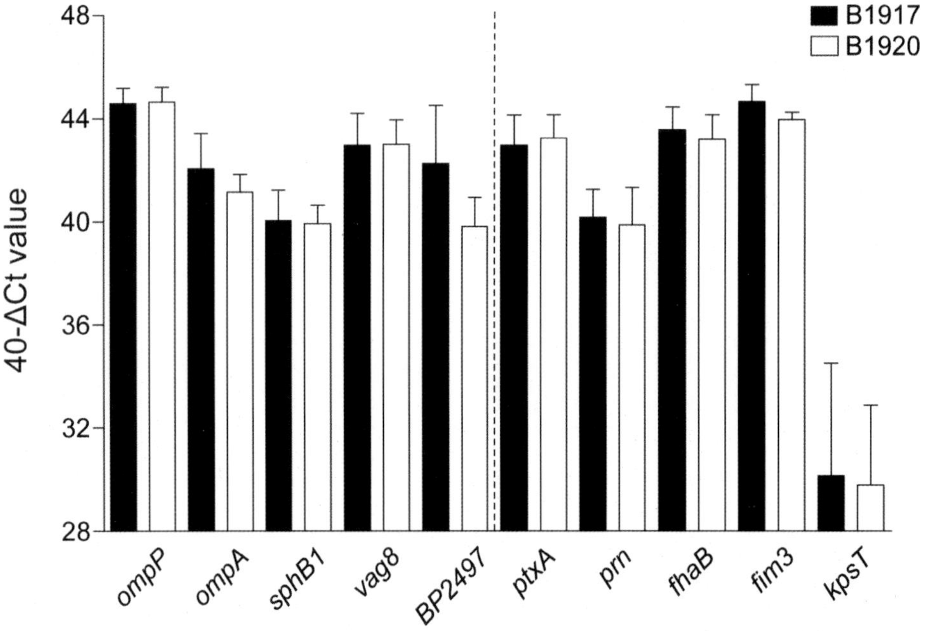

Figure 5. *In vivo* expression of vaccine-candidate genes. Naïve adult female BALB/c mice (n = 4) were infected intranasally with *B. pertussis* strain B1917 or B1920. After 7 days, bacteria were collected through broncho-alveolar lavage and used for *in vivo* transcriptional analysis using antigen-specific primers as described in the text. The transcription data is expressed as 40-ΔCt value, which is a measure of expression relative to the *recA* household gene (ΔCt = Ct *target* – Ct *recA*). The number 40 represents the number of PCR cycles. A 40-ΔCt value of 40 indicates that the gene is expressed at equal levels as *recA*, while higher values correspond to higher expression.

low protein yield) mixed 1:1 in 1.3% alum adjuvant (Alhydrogel; Sigma). As a control, mice were immunized with PBS and Alhydrogel, or with PBS alone. Since the PBS group was the most used group for statistical comparisons, 12 mice were included in this group to enhance the statistical power. In order to compare efficacy to current aPs, one group of mice was immunized with 1/50th of the human dose (equals 1.16 µg of *B. pertussis* protein) of the commercial hexavalent 3-component acellular pertussis vaccine *Infanrix* (GSK, Belgium). On day 35, mice were challenged by intranasal (i.n.) infection with 2×10^7 colony forming units (CFU) of *B. pertussis* strain B1917 in 40 µL. Bacterial load in the nasopharynx and lungs was determined on day 38 and 42 (3 and 7 days after challenge) as described previously [50]. Including the 7 day time-point allowed comparison to aP vaccination, which in mice typically leads to clearance of the pathogen from the lungs within 7 days [17]. Furthermore, the 3 day time point allowed us to determine whether the selected antigens are able to induce early protection against infection. Serum samples were collected on days 0, 28, 38, and 42.

In vivo transcriptional analysis

Groups of 4 female, naïve 6–8 week old BALB/c mice (Charles River) were infected i.n. with *B. pertussis* strain B1917 or B1920 as described above. After 7 days (at the peak of infection), bacteria were collected from the lungs through a bronchoalveolar lavage (BAL) with PBS and stabilized with RNA Protect Bacteria Reagent (Qiagen). Total RNA was extracted using the RNeasy Mini kit (Qiagen) and contaminating genomic DNA was removed by DNase treatment (DNAfree, Ambion). Bacterial RNA was enriched and amplified using the MICROBEnrich (Ambion) and SensationPlus FFPE Amplification (Affymetrix) kits, respectively. Enriched RNA was reverse-transcribed using the SuperScript One-Cycle cDNA Kit (Invitrogen) and used for quantitative real-time PCR analysis (primer sequences available on request). To determine relative expression levels, ΔCt values were calculated by subtracting the Ct value of the *recA* (BP2546) household gene from the Ct value of the target gene [53]. The transcription data are expressed as 40-ΔCt value, with 40 representing the number of PCR cycles as detection limit. A 40-ΔCt value of 40 indicates that the gene is expressed at equal levels as *recA*, while higher values correspond to increased expression.

Antibody analysis

Protein ELISA. IgG titers against the recombinant antigens in mouse and human sera were determined by sandwich enzyme-linked immunosorbent assay (ELISA) analysis, essentially as described previously [50].

Whole-cell ELISA. The binding of IgG subtypes to whole bacteria was measured using a whole-cell ELISA method adapted from Abdillahi and Poolman [54]. Briefly, ELISA plates were coated with Bvg$^+$ mid-log culture of the challenge strain B1917, washed with PBS containing 0.05% Tween 20 (PBST), blocked with 1% BSA/PBS, and incubated with mouse serum. Bound IgG1, IgG2a, and IgG2b was detected using anti-mouse secondary antibodies (BD Pharmingin and Southern Biotech) and appropriate substrates. The optical density was measured on an ELISA plate reader (Tecan Infinite F50) and antibody subtype concentrations were determined by comparison to standard curves with known concentrations of each IgG subtype.

Opsonization. 1% BSA/PBS was used for all dilutions. 10^6 CFU of Bvg$^+$ and Bvg$^-$ B1917 (challenge strain) were incubated with serum or nasal lavage (NL) samples from vaccinated mice for 30 min at 4°C. Bacteria were fixed in 2% paraformaldehyde and surface-bound IgG was detected using anti-mouse IgG-Fc-FITC-conjugated antibodies (Sigma-Aldrich) on a BD LSRII flow cytometer (BD Biosciences). The amount of surface-bound antibodies was expressed in arbitrary units as a fluorescence index (FI), calculated by multiplying the geometric mean fluorescence intensity by the percentage of FITC-positive bacteria [55]. Data were analyzed using FlowJo version 7.6.5.

Statistical analyses

A 2-tailed Mann-Whitney *U* test was used for comparison of bacterial load in NL and lung homogenate between PBS-vaccinated mice and recombinant antigen-vaccinated mice. A Kruskal-Wallis test followed by a Dunns *post-hoc* test ($\alpha = 5\%$) was used for comparison of antibody-mediated opsonization by serum and NL samples between PBS-vaccinated mice and recombinant antigen-vaccinated mice. A 1-tailed Wilcoxon Signed Rank Test was used to determine whether ELISA measured IgG levels were significantly above the detection limit. All statistical analyses were performed using the GraphPad Prism software program, version 5.0, where $p<0.05$ was considered significant.

Supporting Information

Table S1 Proteomics data of statistically significant Bvg-regulated proteins identified in the cytosolic and membrane fraction of *B. pertussis* strains B1917 (P3) and B1920 (P1).

Table S2 Protein abundance of all proteins identified in the cytosolic and membrane fraction of *B. pertussis* strains B1917 (P3) and B1920 (P1).

Table S3 Constructing His-fusions of the selected candidate antigens.

Text S1 Supplemental Methods.

Acknowledgments

We thank Maurice van Dael en Jolein Gloerich (Radboud Proteomics Centre, Radboud University Medical Centre, Nijmegen, the Netherlands) for technical assistance regarding proteomics experiments and Fred van Opzeeland, Elles Simonetti, and Saskia van Selm (Laboratory of Pediatric Infectious Diseases, Department of Pediatrics, Radboud University Medical Centre, Nijmegen, The Netherlands; Laboratory of Medical Immunology, Department of Laboratory Medicine, Radboud University Medical Centre, Nijmegen, The Netherlands) for assistance with the animal experiments.

Author Contributions

Conceived and designed the experiments: DdG MdJ PH FM DD. Performed the experiments: DdG AB CP. Analyzed the data: DdG HW AZ. Contributed reagents/materials/analysis tools: HW AZ GB. Contributed to the writing of the manuscript: DdG FM DD.

References

1. Boulton J (2013) The UK pertussis epidemic: implications for immunisation. Br J Nurs 22: 1046–1050.
2. Campbell P, McIntyre P, Quinn H, Hueston L, Gilbert GL, et al. (2012) Increased population prevalence of low pertussis toxin antibody levels in young children preceding a record pertussis epidemic in Australia. PLoS One 7: e35874.
3. van der Maas NA, Mooi FR, de Greeff SC, Berbers GA, Spaendonck MA, et al. (2013) Pertussis in the Netherlands, is the current vaccination strategy sufficient to reduce disease burden in young infants? Vaccine 31: 4541–4547.
4. Witt MA, Katz PH, Witt DJ (2012) Unexpectedly limited durability of immunity following acellular pertussis vaccination in preadolescents in a North American outbreak. Clin Infect Dis 54: 1730–1735.
5. Bisgard KM, Pascual FB, Ehresmann KR, Miller CA, Cianfrini C, et al. (2004) Infant pertussis: who was the source? Pediatr Infect Dis J 23: 985–989.
6. de Greeff SC, Mooi FR, Westerhof A, Verbakel JM, Peeters MF, et al. (2010) Pertussis disease burden in the household: how to protect young infants. Clin Infect Dis 50: 1339–1345.
7. Kowalzik F, Barbosa AP, Fernandes VR, Carvalho PR, Avila-Aguero ML, et al. (2007) Prospective multinational study of pertussis infection in hospitalized infants and their household contacts. Pediatr Infect Dis J 26: 238–242.
8. Warfel JM, Zimmerman LI, Merkel TJ (2013) Acellular pertussis vaccines protect against disease but fail to prevent infection and transmission in a nonhuman primate model. Proc Natl Acad Sci U S A.
9. Mooi FR, Van Der Maas NA, De Melker HE (2013) Pertussis resurgence: waning immunity and pathogen adaptation - two sides of the same coin. Epidemiol Infect: 1–10.
10. de Gouw D, Hermans PW, Bootsma HJ, Zomer A, Heuvelman K, et al. (2014) Differentially expressed genes in *Bordetella pertussis* strains belonging to a lineage which recently spread globally. PLoS One 9: e84523.
11. Mooi FR, van Loo IH, van Gent M, He Q, Bart MJ, et al. (2009) *Bordetella pertussis* strains with increased toxin production associated with pertussis resurgence. Emerg Infect Dis 15: 1206–1213.
12. Barkoff AM, Mertsola J, Guillot S, Guiso N, Berbers G, et al. (2012) Appearance of *Bordetella pertussis* strains not expressing the vaccine antigen pertactin in Finland. Clin Vaccine Immunol 19: 1703–1704.
13. Lam C, Octavia S, Ricafort L, Sintchenko V, Gilbert GL, et al. (2014) Rapid increase in pertactin-deficient *Bordetella pertussis* isolates, Australia. Emerg Infect Dis 20: 626–633.
14. Otsuka N, Han HJ, Toyoizumi-Ajisaka H, Nakamura Y, Arakawa Y, et al. (2012) Prevalence and genetic characterization of pertactin-deficient *Bordetella pertussis* in Japan. PLoS One 7: e31985.
15. Pawloski LC, Queenan AM, Cassiday PK, Lynch AS, Harrison M, et al. (2013) Prevalence and molecular characterization of pertactin-deficient *Bordetella pertussis* in the US. Clin Vaccine Immunol.
16. Polewicz M, Gracia A, Garlapati S, van Kessel J, Strom S, et al. (2013) Novel vaccine formulations against pertussis offer earlier onset of immunity and provide protection in the presence of maternal antibodies. Vaccine 31: 3148–3155.
17. Ross PJ, Sutton CE, Higgins S, Allen AC, Walsh K, et al. (2013) Relative contribution of Th1 and Th17 cells in adaptive immunity to *Bordetella pertussis*: towards the rational design of an improved acellular pertussis vaccine. PLoS Pathog 9: e1003264.
18. Decker KB, James TD, Stibitz S, Hinton DM (2012) The *Bordetella pertussis* model of exquisite gene control by the global transcription factor BvgA. Microbiology 158: 1665–1676.
19. de Gouw D, Diavatopoulos DA, Bootsma HJ, Hermans PW, Mooi FR (2011) Pertussis: a matter of immune modulation. FEMS Microbiol Rev 35: 441–474.
20. Melton AR, Weiss AA (1993) Characterization of environmental regulators of *Bordetella pertussis*. Infect Immun 61: 807–815.
21. Bart MJ, van Gent M, van der Heide HG, Boekhorst J, Hermans P, et al. (2010) Comparative genomics of prevaccination and modern *Bordetella pertussis* strains. BMC Genomics 11: 627.
22. Parkhill J, Sebaihia M, Preston A, Murphy LD, Thomson N, et al. (2003) Comparative analysis of the genome sequences of *Bordetella pertussis*, *Bordetella parapertussis* and *Bordetella bronchiseptica*. Nat Genet 35: 32–40.
23. Tsou CC, Tsai CF, Tsui YH, Sudhir PR, Wang YT, et al. (2010) IDEAL-Q, an automated tool for label-free quantitation analysis using an efficient peptide alignment approach and spectral data validation. Mol Cell Proteomics 9: 131–144.
24. Bart MJ, Harris SR, Advani A, Arakawa Y, Bottero D, et al. (2014) Global population structure and evolution of *Bordetella pertussis* and their relationship with vaccination. MBio 5: e01074.
25. King AJ, van Gorkom T, Pennings JL, van der Heide HG, He Q, et al. (2008) Comparative genomic profiling of Dutch clinical *Bordetella pertussis* isolates using DNA microarrays: identification of genes absent from epidemic strains. BMC Genomics 9: 311.
26. Yu NY, Wagner JR, Laird MR, Melli G, Rey S, et al. (2010) PSORTb 3.0: improved protein subcellular localization prediction with refined localization subcategories and predictive capabilities for all prokaryotes. Bioinformatics 26: 1608–1615.
27. Ishihama Y, Oda Y, Tabata T, Sato T, Nagasu T, et al. (2005) Exponentially modified protein abundance index (emPAI) for estimation of absolute protein amount in proteomics by the number of sequenced peptides per protein. Mol Cell Proteomics 4: 1265–1272.
28. Neo Y, Li R, Howe J, Hoo R, Pant A, et al. (2010) Evidence for an intact polysaccharide capsule in *Bordetella pertussis*. Microbes Infect 12: 238–245.
29. Roberts M, Tite JP, Fairweather NF, Dougan G, Charles IG (1992) Recombinant P.69/pertactin: immunogenicity and protection of mice against *Bordetella pertussis* infection. Vaccine 10: 43–48.
30. Sukumar N, Love CF, Conover MS, Kock ND, Dubey P, et al. (2009) Active and passive immunizations with *Bordetella* colonization factor A protect mice

against respiratory challenge with *Bordetella bronchiseptica*. Infect Immun 77: 885–895.

31. Stevens TL, Bossie A, Sanders VM, Fernandez-Botran R, Coffman RL, et al. (1988) Regulation of antibody isotype secretion by subsets of antigen-specific helper T cells. Nature 334: 255–258.
32. Nurminen M, Butcher S, Idanpaan-Heikkila I, Wahlstrom E, Muttilainen S, et al. (1992) The class 1 outer membrane protein of *Neisseria meningitidis* produced in *Bacillus subtilis* can give rise to protective immunity. Mol Microbiol 6: 2499–2506.
33. Marr N, Shah NR, Lee R, Kim EJ, Fernandez RC (2011) *Bordetella pertussis* autotransporter Vag8 binds human C1 esterase inhibitor and confers serum resistance. PLoS One 6: e20585.
34. Mazar J, Cotter PA (2006) Topology and maturation of filamentous haemagglutinin suggest a new model for two-partner secretion. Mol Microbiol 62: 641–654.
35. Coutte L, Willery E, Antoine R, Drobecq H, Locht C, et al. (2003) Surface anchoring of bacterial subtilisin important for maturation function. Mol Microbiol 49: 529–539.
36. Mobberley-Schuman PS, Weiss AA (2005) Influence of CR3 (CD11b/CD18) expression on phagocytosis of *Bordetella pertussis* by human neutrophils. Infect Immun 73: 7317–7323.
37. Kim JH, Skountzou I, Compans R, Jacob J (2009) Original antigenic sin responses to influenza viruses. J Immunol 183: 3294–3301.
38. de Greeff SC, de Melker HE, van Gageldonk PG, Schellekens JF, van der Klis FR, et al. (2010) Seroprevalence of pertussis in The Netherlands: evidence for increased circulation of *Bordetella pertussis*. PLoS One 5: e14183.
39. Kirimanjeswara GS, Mann PB, Harvill ET (2003) Role of antibodies in immunity to *Bordetella infections*. Infect Immun 71: 1719–1724.
40. Malley R, Trzcinski K, Srivastava A, Thompson CM, Anderson PW, et al. (2005) CD4+ T cells mediate antibody-independent acquired immunity to pneumococcal colonization. Proc Natl Acad Sci U S A 102: 4848–4853.
41. Trzcinski K, Thompson CM, Srivastava A, Basset A, Malley R, et al. (2008) Protection against nasopharyngeal colonization by *Streptococcus pneumoniae* is mediated by antigen-specific CD4+ T cells. Infect Immun 76: 2678–2684.
42. Zhang Z, Clarke TB, Weiser JN (2009) Cellular effectors mediating Th17-dependent clearance of pneumococcal colonization in mice. J Clin Invest 119: 1899–1909.
43. Lu YJ, Gross J, Bogaert D, Finn A, Bagrade L, et al. (2008) Interleukin-17A mediates acquired immunity to pneumococcal colonization. PLoS Pathog 4: e1000159.
44. Dunne A, Ross PJ, Pospisilova E, Masin J, Meaney A, et al. (2010) Inflammasome activation by adenylate cyclase toxin directs Th17 responses and protection against *Bordetella pertussis*. J Immunol 185: 1711–1719.
45. Fedele G, Spensieri F, Palazzo R, Nasso M, Cheung GY, et al. (2010) *Bordetella pertussis* commits human dendritic cells to promote a Th1/Th17 response through the activity of adenylate cyclase toxin and MAPK-pathways. PLoS One 5: e8734.
46. Higgins SC, Jarnicki AG, Lavelle EC, Mills KH (2006) TLR4 mediates vaccine-induced protective cellular immunity to *Bordetella pertussis*: role of IL-17-producing T cells. J Immunol 177: 7980–7989.
47. Warfel JM, Merkel TJ (2013) *Bordetella pertussis* infection induces a mucosal IL-17 response and long-lived Th17 and Th1 immune memory cells in nonhuman primates. Mucosal Immunol 6: 787–796.
48. van Gent M, Bart MJ, van der Heide HG, Heuvelman KJ, Mooi FR (2012) Small mutations in *Bordetella pertussis* are associated with selective sweeps. PLoS One 7: e46407.
49. Thalen M, van den IJ, Jiskoot W, Zomer B, Roholl P, et al. (1999) Rational medium design for *Bordetella pertussis*: basic metabolism. J Biotechnol 75: 147–159.
50. Cron LE, Stol K, Burghout P, van Selm S, Simonetti ER, et al. (2011) Two DHH subfamily 1 proteins contribute to pneumococcal virulence and confer protection against pneumococcal disease. Infect Immun 79: 3697–3710.
51. Hijnen M, van Gageldonk PG, Berbers GA, van Woerkom T, Mooi FR (2005) The *Bordetella pertussis* virulence factor P.69 pertactin retains its immunological properties after overproduction in *Escherichia coli*. Protein Expr Purif 41: 106–112.
52. McConnell MJ, Pachon J (2011) Expression, purification, and refolding of biologically active *Acinetobacter baumannii* OmpA from *Escherichia coli* inclusion bodies. Protein Expression and Purification 77: 98–103.
53. Livak KJ, Schmittgen TD (2001) Analysis of relative gene expression data using real-time quantitative PCR and the 2(-Delta Delta C(T)) Method. Methods 25: 402–408.
54. Abdillahi H, Poolman JT (1988) Typing of group-B *Neisseria meningitidis* with monoclonal antibodies in the whole-cell ELISA. J Med Microbiol 26: 177–180.
55. Hyams C, Camberlein E, Cohen JM, Bax K, Brown JS (2010) The *Streptococcus pneumoniae* capsule inhibits complement activity and neutrophil phagocytosis by multiple mechanisms. Infect Immun 78: 704–715.

4

High Rate of A(H1N1)pdm09 Infections among Rural Thai Villagers, 2009–2010

Benjawan Khuntirat[1], In-Kyu Yoon[1], Malinee Chittaganpitch[2], Whitney S. Krueger[3], Krongkaew Supawat[2], Patrick J. Blair[4], Shannon D. Putnam[5], Robert V. Gibbons[1], Darunee Buddhari[1], Pathom Sawanpanyalert[2], Gary L. Heil[3], John A. Friary[3], Gregory C. Gray[3*¤]

1 Department of Virology, Armed Forces Research Institute of Medical Sciences, Bangkok, Thailand, **2** National Institute of Health, Ministry of Public Health, Nonthaburi, Thailand, **3** College of Public Health and Health Professions and Emerging Pathogens Institute, University of Florida, Gainesville, Florida, United States of America, **4** Naval Medical Research Center - Asia, Singapore, Singapore, **5** Naval Health Research Center, San Diego, California, United States of America

Abstract

Background: Pandemic influenza A(H1N1)pdm09 emerged in Thailand in 2009. A prospective longitudinal adult cohort and household transmission study of influenza-like illness (ILI) was ongoing in rural Thailand at the time of emergence. Symptomatic and subclinical A(H1N1)pdm09 infection rates in the cohort and among household members were evaluated.

Methods: A cohort of 800 Thai adults underwent active community-based surveillance for ILI from 2008–2010. Acute respiratory samples from ILI episodes were tested for A(H1N1)pdm09 by qRT-PCR; acute and 60-day convalescent blood samples were tested by A(H1N1)pdm09 hemagglutination inhibition assay (HI). Enrollment, 12-month and 24-month follow-up blood samples were tested for A(H1N1)pdm09 seroconversion by HI. Household members of influenza A-infected cohort subjects with ILI were enrolled in household transmission investigations in which day 0 and 60 blood samples and acute respiratory samples were tested by either qRT-PCR or HI for A(H1N1)pdm09. Seroconversion between annual blood samples without A(H1N1)pdm09-positive ILI was considered as subclinical infection.

Results: The 2-yr cumulative incidence of A(H1N1)pdm09 infection in the cohort in 2009/2010 was 10.8% (84/781) with an annual incidence of 1.2% in 2009 and 9.7% in 2010; 83.3% of infections were subclinical (50% in 2009 and 85.9% in 2010). The 2-yr cumulative incidence was lowest (5%) in adults born ≤1957. The A(H1N1)pdm09 secondary attack rate among household contacts was 47.2% (17/36); 47.1% of these infections were subclinical. The highest A(H1N1)pdm09 secondary attack rate among household contacts (70.6%, 12/17) occurred among children born between 1990 and 2003.

Conclusion: Subclinical A(H1N1)pdm09 infections in Thai adults occurred frequently and accounted for a greater proportion of all A(H1N1)pdm09 infections than previously estimated. The role of subclinical infections in A(H1N1)pdm09 transmission has important implications in formulating strategies to predict and prevent the spread of A(H1N1)pdm09 and other influenza virus strains.

Editor: Steven Riley, Imperial College London, United Kingdom

Funding: This work was supported by the US Armed Forces Health Surveillance Center - Global Emerging Infections Surveillance and Response System (multiple grants to GCG, PJB, SDP, and IKY) and National Institute of Allergy and Infectious Diseases (R01 AI068803 to GCG). The funders had no role in study design, data collection and analysis, decision to publish, or preparation of the manuscript.

Competing Interests: The authors have declared that no competing interests exist.

* Email: gcgray2@gmail.com

¤ Current address: Duke University School of Medicine, Duke Infectious Diseases, and Duke Global Health Institute, Durham, North Carolina, United States of America

Introduction

Pandemic influenza A(H1N1)pdm09 emerged in North America in March 2009 and rapidly spread to other parts of the world, eventually replacing previous seasonal H1N1 virus strains. Several studies from different countries established a pattern of higher A(H1N1)pdm09 infection rates in school-age children relative to young adults, with older adults having the lowest infection rates [1–6]. These studies were primarily community-based serological surveys that relied on non-prospective cohort designs and convenience sampling rather than sampling of prospective longitudinal cohorts. Household transmission studies were also conducted during the 2009 pandemic to characterize A(H1N1)pdm09 transmission in confined settings. Several household studies reported a wide range (8% to 45%) of secondary attack rates [7–10]. These studies were mainly conducted during the early stages of the pandemic (April to August 2009) based on household investigations usually triggered by sentinel A(H1N1)pdm09 cases. In addition, some studies reported subclinical A(H1N1)pdm09 infection rates of 9% to 50% of all A(H1N1)pdm09 infections in adults [1,7,11–13], and 9% to 25% among household members [7–10]. Estimating the proportion of subclinical infections is relevant because these infections may contribute to virus transmission [14].

In Thailand, like other tropical countries, influenza activity tends to occur in a biphasic seasonal pattern (June to August and January to March) with sporadic infection throughout the year [15]. Between May 2009 and November 2010, three waves of the influenza pandemic influenza A(H1N1)pdm09 were clearly documented in Thailand (Figure 1). During this 18-month period, it was estimated that nearly one half of the Thai population may have been infected by the pandemic influenza A(H1N1)pdm09 [16].

At the time of pandemic onset in 2009, a prospective longitudinal cohort study was ongoing in Kamphaeng Phet, Thailand in which 800 adults (age range 20–85 years) were undergoing active surveillance for influenza-like illness (ILI) from 2008 to 2010. The study also included a household transmission component triggered by confirmed influenza virus (IFV) infections in the cohort [17–18]. This provided a unique opportunity to investigate the epidemiology and transmission of A(H1N1)pdm09, yielding information about A(H1N1)pdm09 infection rates in adults and their household members in a community setting, and providing estimates of subclinical infection rates and risk factors.

Materials and Methods

Ethics Statement

The study was approved by the institutional review boards of the Thai Ministry of Public Health (MOPH), Walter Reed Army Institute of Research (WRAIR), Naval Medical Research Unit No. 2 (NAMRU-2), US Army Medical Research and Materiel Command, University of Iowa, and University of Florida. Written informed consent was obtained from all study subjects (or their parents if applicable) and assent was obtained from children older than seven years.

Although the study was designed to focus chiefly upon studying subclinical avian influenza infections, reviewing IRBs approved the study to include all influenza A infections.

Prospective Longitudinal Cohort

Approximately 800 adult subjects living in Kamphaeng Phet province (KPP), Thailand, a rural province located about 350 km north of Bangkok, were enrolled in a prospective longitudinal cohort study. Details of study methods have been previously published [17–18]. Briefly, cohort subjects were enrolled from April to October 2008. Clinical and demographic questionnaires were administered, blood samples were obtained, and digital thermometers were provided at enrollment. Active surveillance for influenza-like illness (ILI) was conducted through weekly home visits by study staff. Weekly questionnaires were administered to detect any changes in clinical status. Subjects were also encouraged to contact study staff if they developed any febrile episodes. If the subject met the ILI case definition (measured temperature ≥38°C with sore throat or cough for ≥4 hours), an acute blood sample and acute respiratory samples (one nasal and one throat swab) were collected. At day 60 after the acute visit, a convalescent blood sample was collected. Semi-quantitative real-time reverse transcriptase polymerase chain reaction (qRT-PCR) was performed on respiratory samples to detect influenza A or B. Serological testing of the paired acute/convalescent blood samples was performed by hemagglutination inhibition assay (HI) against IFV.

Annual follow-up visits at 12 and 24 months after enrollment were performed in 2009 and 2010 during which clinical questionnaires were administered and blood samples were obtained. The questionnaires assessed changes in demographic or health status during the preceding year. Serological testing of the enrollment and annual follow-up blood samples was conducted by influenza HI to monitor for changes in influenza antibody titers over time. An IFV infection was considered to be subclinical if IFV

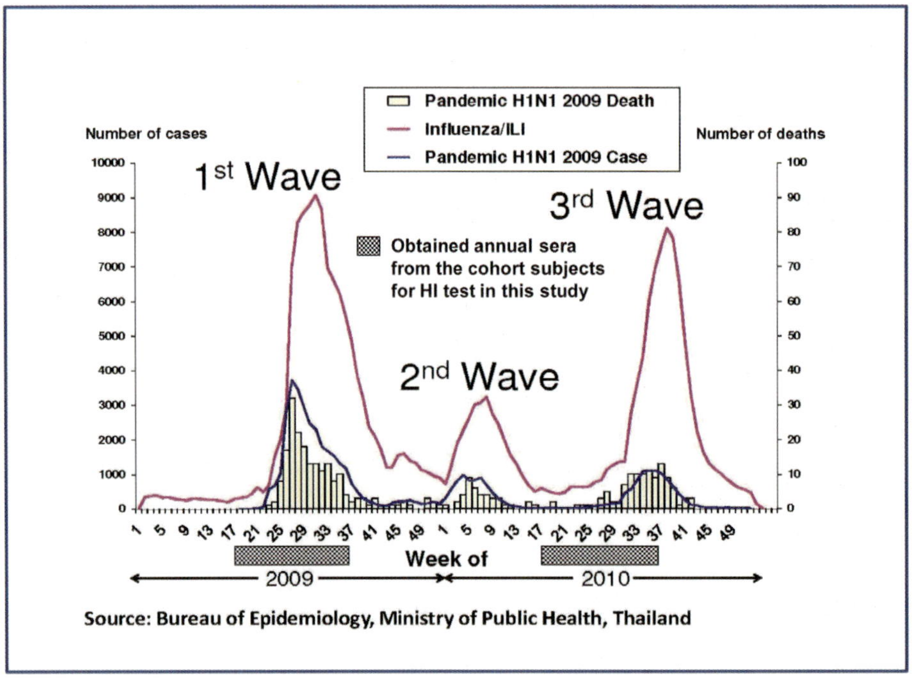

Figure 1. Three waves of the pandemic influenza A(H1N11)pdm09 in Thailand. Source: Bureau of Epidemiology, Ministry of Public Health, Thailand.

HI seroconversion occurred between annual blood samples without an IFV-positive ILI detected during the intervening surveillance period.

Household Transmission Investigations

When a cohort subject developed an ILI in which an acute respiratory sample tested positive for influenza A by qRT-PCR, that cohort subject's household members ≥6 months old were enrolled in a household transmission investigation. A blood sample was collected at enrollment (day 0) from each household member (i.e., contact subject). If a contact subject developed ILI during the following 60 days, acute respiratory samples (one nasal and one throat swab) were additionally collected from that contact subject for qRT-PCR for influenza A and B. A questionnaire was administered to each contact subject to assess the degree of contact with the cohort subject and identify any illnesses during the preceding 7 days. Weekly follow-up visits were conducted with the contact subjects for 60 days after initiation of the household investigation. At day 60, a convalescent blood sample was collected from each contact subject.

Laboratory Methods

Blood samples were transported at room temperature and respiratory swabs were transported in Micro Test M4RT Viral Transport Media (Remel, Inc., Lenexa, KS, USA) at 4°C within the same day to the field laboratory at Kamphaeng Phet-AFRIMS Virology Research Unit (KAVRU) in KPP, Thailand, where qRT-PCR for IFV was performed. Serological testing by HI was performed at the University of Florida Global Pathogens Laboratory in Gainesville, Florida, USA.

Hemagglutination Inhibition (HI) assay. Enrollment and annual follow-up serum samples were tested using the World Health Organization (WHO) or US Centers for Disease Control and Prevention (CDC) HI protocol as previously described [17,19] against 2 human viruses: A/Brisbane/59/2007(H1N1), and A/Mexico/4108/2009(H1N1); and 2 swine viruses: A/SW/Gent/7625/99(H1N2) and A/SW/Lutol/3/2000(H1N1). Acute and convalescent serum samples collected from ILI episodes were tested against A/Mexico/4108/2009(H1N1). IFV strains were grown in fertilized eggs. Sera were pretreated with receptor-destroying enzyme and hemabsorbed with either guinea pig or turkey erythrocytes. Titer results were reported as the reciprocal of the highest dilution of serum that inhibited virus-induced hemagglutination of 0.65% (guinea pig) or 0.50% (turkey) solution of erythrocytes as previously described [17]. An HI titer of ≥1:40 was considered as positive. Seroconversion between paired samples was considered to be 4-fold or greater rise in HI titer.

Semi-quantitative real-time qRT-PCR. The procedures have been previously described [18]. Briefly, RNA was extracted from 140 µl of each nasal and throat swab using QIAamp viral RNA extraction kit (Qiagen Inc., Valencia, CA, USA) and screened via a qRT-PCR protocol developed by the US CDC. The protocol was designed to first screen for influenza A, and then through separate reactions, to rapidly determine influenza subtype. The human RNase P gene primer set was also used as an internal positive control for human RNA in each specimen.

Infection with A(H1N1)pdm09 was considered to have occurred if (a) a respiratory sample was positive for A(H1N1)pdm09 by qRT-PCR, or (b) a 4-fold or greater increase in HI titer (seroconversion) against A(H1N1)pdm09 occurred between paired annual sera or paired ILI sera, with a second titer of at least 1:40. If paired sera were not available, a single high titer of at least 1:40 was considered to indicate recent infection.

Statistical Methods

Risk factors for bivariate associations with HI results were initially examined using binary logistic regression and proportional odds modeling [20]. An exact method was used for sparse data, and the score test was used to evaluate the proportional odds assumption. Covariates with p values <0.25 were considered for inclusion in multivariate models. Final multivariate models were designed using manual backwards elimination. Analyses were performed using SAS v9.2 (SAS Institute Inc., Cary, NC, USA).

Results

Between April and October 2008, field staff enrolled a total of 800 adults (100 from each of 8 sites). Details of participant demographics at enrollment have been previously described [17]. The median age of the 800 participants was 49.6 years. Only 1.6% of the cohort reported ever receiving a human influenza vaccine and 11.4% reported ever being exposed to swine. Over the 24-month follow-up period, 49 subjects withdrew their participation and 45 replacement enrollments were added. A total of 768 participants (96%) completed the 12-month annual follow-up and 784 participants (98%) completed the 24-month annual follow-up visit. Overall, 747 participants (93%) remained enrolled for the entire study duration by completing enrollment and both 12- and 24-month follow-up visits.

Prospective Longitudinal Cohort

Seroprevalence of elevated HI antibodies against A(H1N1)pdm09 increased from 1.7% and 1.3% in 2008 and 2009, respectively, to 10.3% in 2010 (Table 1). Based on serological results from 2009, cohort subjects born ≤1957 were more likely to have elevated A(H1N1)pdm09 antibodies compared to those born after 1957 (Table 1); however, in 2010, cohort subjects born after 1957 were more likely to have positive HI titer against A(H1N1)pdm09. The birth year of 1957 was chosen as the cut-point since it has been shown that immunity to A(H1N1)pdm09 virus could be acquired as a result of previous exposure to a 1918-like A(H1N1) virus circulating during the period 1918–1957 [1]. The seroconversion rate in those born after 1957 was ≥12%, more than double the rate in those born <1957 (Table 1). None of the subjects who seroconverted to A(H1N1)pdm09 were seropositive (i.e., A(H1N1)pdm09 HI titer ≥1:40) in their 2009 sera.

From January 2009 to December 2010, 53 cohort subjects met the case definition for ILI; 10 of these subjects were confirmed to have A(H1N1)pdm09 infection by qRT-PCR. Most (70%, 7/10) of these subjects were born after 1957. Prior to ILI occurrence, none of the 10 subjects had pre-existing A(H1N1)pdm09 antibody. Only 3 of these subjects had A(H1N1)pdm09 seroconversion in the paired ILI sera. Among the remaining 7 subjects with A(H1N1)pdm09-positive qRT-PCR, 5 were seronegative in both of the paired ILI sera and 2 did not have sufficient paired sera for HI testing.

When comparing A(H1N1)pdm09 seroconversions from the enrollment and annual follow-up blood samples and the qRT-PCR data from ILI acute respiratory samples, 5 subjects had A(H1N1)pdm09 infection by both qRT-PCR and HI, 5 by qRT-PCR only, and 74 by HI alone. Among these 84 cohort subjects with A(H1N1)pdm09 infection, only 14 subjects reported ILI [10 were A(H1N1)pdm09-positive by qRT-PCR; 4 were negative by qRT-PCR]. Most (83.3%, 70/84) of the A(H1N1)pdm09 infections among the cohort subjects were subclinical. The proportion of subclinical infections among cohort subjects born after 1957 was higher than those born ≤1957 (Table 1).

Table 1. Evidence of A(H1N1)pdm09 infection among cohort subjects, Kamphaeng Phet, Thailand.

Category	Birth Year			Total (%)
	≤1957 (%)	1958–1968 (%)	≥1969 (%)	
Seroprevalence[a]				
(HI titer ≥1:40)				
Enrollment (2008)	4/280 (1.4)	4/207 (1.9)	3/159 (1.9)	11/646 (1.7)
12-month (2009)	7/338 (2.1)	2/243 (0.8)	2/186 (1.1)	11/767 (1.4)
24-month (2010)	21/339 (6.2)	34/252 (13.5)	26/199 (13.1)	81/790 (10.3)
Seroconversion[b]	17/337 (5.0)	31/249 (12.4)	25/195 (12.8)	73/781 (9.3)
A(H1N1)pdm09 infection[c]	21 (2.7)	34 (4.4)	29 (3.7)	84 (10.8)
Subclinical infection[d]	15 (17.9)	31 (36.9)	24 (28.6)	70 (83.3)

[a]HI testing not conducted in some subjects due to insufficient serum volume.
[b]≥4-fold increase in HI titer of 2009/2010 sera.
[c]Positive respiratory sample for A(H1N1)pdm09 by qRT-PCR or ≥4-fold increase in HI titer of paired annual sera/paired ILI sera.
[d]≥4-fold increase in HI titer of paired annual sera/paired ILI sera without positive respiratory sample for A(H1N1)pdm09 by qRT-PCR.

Using binary logistic regression analysis, several covariates were associated with an increased risk for seroconversion against A/Mexico/4108/2009(H1N1) (Table 2). Cohort subjects born after 1957 were more likely to have seroconversion than those born ≤ 1957 (unadjusted OR = 2.7, 95% CI = 1.4–5.0 for subjects born between 1958 and 1968; unadjusted OR = 2.8, 95% CI = 1.5–5.3 for subjects born after 1968). Indoor water use was associated with an increased risk for seroconversion (unadjusted OR = 2.1, 95% CI = 1.2–3.9). Cohort subjects living in Phran Kratai district were more likely to have seroconversion than those living in Mueng district (unadjusted OR = 2.7, 95% CI = 1.7–4.4). Elevated titers against A/SW/Gent/7625/99(H1N2) and A/SW/Lutol/3/2000(H1N1) were also associated with A(H1N1)pdm09 seroconversion (unadjusted OR = 6.4, 95% CI = 3.8–10.7; unadjusted OR = 8.2, 95% CI = 3.6–18.6, respectively). There was a trend for elevated antibody against seasonal A/Brisbane/59/2007(H1N1) to be associated with an increased risk of seroconversion against pandemic A/Mexico/4108/2009(H1N1) (unadjusted OR = 1.7, 95% CI = 0.9–2.9).

Household Transmission Investigations

Thirty-six contact subjects (age range 1–70 years) living in the same household as the 10 cohort subjects with A(H1N1)pdm09-positive qRT-PCR were enrolled. Paired day 0 and 60 sera from these contact subjects were evaluated by HI against A(H1N1)pdm09 [A/Mexico/4108/2009(H1N1)]; three contact subjects missed their day 60 blood draw. Of the 36 contact subjects, 6 had ILI of which all were A(H1N1)pdm09-positive by qRT-PCR (Table 3). Five of these 6 contact subjects had HI seroconversion against A(H1N1)pdm09, and one was seronegative at both day 0 and 60. Of the 30 contact subjects without ILI, 8 had seroconversion against A(H1N1)pdm09, and 3 had elevated antibody against A(H1N1)pdm09. Of the 8 contact subjects with seroconversion, 3 reported having a respiratory illness within 7 days prior to enrollment. None of the 3 seropositive contact subjects reported having a respiratory illness within 7 days prior to enrollment. Therefore, the A(H1N1)pdm09 infection rate among household members was 47.2% (17/36) and the proportion with subclinical infection was 47.1% (8/17) (Table 4). The majority (88.2%, 15/17) of A(H1N1)pdm09 infections among contact subjects was in those individuals born after 1957. The highest infection rate (70.6%, 12/17) was in school-age children (born between 1990 and 2003) as shown in Table 4.

Discussion

Our report is one of the few combined prospective longitudinal cohort and household transmission studies conducted during the A(H1N1)pdm09 pandemic that describes the epidemiology of A(H1N1)pdm09 in a tropical region. The proportion of A(H1N1)pdm09 infections in our cohort that were subclinical was very high (83.3%). This proportion was higher than some prior estimates (approximately 50%) from a few comparable studies [11–13]. This may be due to differences in our study design. For example, the age range of our cohort population was between 20–85 years (mean age = 49.6 years), whereas the age range in the study by Aho et al. [11] and Khaokham et al. [13] was 20–28 years (mean age = 21 years) and 19–58 years (median age = 24.7 years), respectively. In addition, the proportion of adults older than 60 years in our study (23%) was greater than in the community cohort study by Chen et al. [12] (7%). Our age composition was, however, unlikely to be the only factor in these differences since the rate of subclinical infections in our cohort was high even among those born after 1957. An additional possibility is that active surveillance in our cohort was conducted before and during the course of the pandemic from April 2008 to December 2010. Aho et al. [11], Chen et al. [12], and Khaokham et al. [13] conducted their studies during the early stages of the pandemic (i.e., November 2009, June to October 2009, and September to October 2009, respectively). The rate of subclinical A(H1N1)pdm09 infection in the current study is consistent with that from a recently published multi-year prospective household-based cohort study in Vietnam conducted from 2007 to 2010 [21]. That study reported 84.4% of A(H1N1)pdm09-infected subjects did not have ILI. Subclinical A(H1N1)pdm09 infection may contribute to a substantial fraction of virus transmission as suggested by a simulation study [14]. The household transmission investigations in our study also revealed a high subclinical A(H1N1)pdm09 infection rate among household contacts (47.1%) which was higher than the range (9% to 25%) reported by previous household transmission studies conducted during the early pandemic phase from April to August 2009 [7–10]. To confirm infections among household contacts, Suess et al. [10] used only qRT-PCR, while Jackson et al. [8] performed only

Table 2. Risk factors for ≥4-fold increase in hemagglutination inhibition (HI) titer against A/Mexico/4108/2009(H1N1) from 2009 to 2010 among cohort subjects, Kamphaeng Phet, Thailand; odds ratios calculated by binary logistic regression.

Variables	Total N	A/Mexico/4108/2009(H1N1)		
		≥4-fold increase N (%)	Unadjusted OR (95% CI)	Adjusted OR (95% CI)
Birth Year				
>1968	195	25 (34.2)	2.8 (1.5–5.3)	2.2 (1.1–4.3)
1958–1968	249	31 (42.5)	2.7 (1.4–5)	2.5 (1.3–4.8)
≤1957	337	17 (23.3)		Reference
Gender				
Male	318	29 (39.7)	1 (0.6–1.6)	-
Female	463	44 (60.3)		
Indoor Water				
Yes	528	59 (80.8)	2.1 (1.2–3.9)	-
No	253	14 (19.2)		
Geographical Region				
Phran Kratai District	298	44 (60.3)	2.7 (1.7–4.4)	2.6 (1.5–4.5)
Mueng District	483	29 (39.7)		Reference
Swine Exposure				
Yes	87	7 (9.6)	0.8 (0.4–1.9)	-
No	694	66 (90.4)		
Developed a respiratory illness in the last 12 months[a]				
Yes	423	44 (60.3)	1.3 (0.8–2.2)	-
No	357	29 (39.7)		
A/Brisbane/59/2007(H1N1)				
Positive	143	19 (26)	1.7 (1.0–2.9)	-
Negative	638	54 (74)		
A/SW/Gent/7625/99(H1N2)				
Positive	211	48 (65.8)	6.4 (3.8–10.7)	5.8 (3.4–10.0)
Negative	570	25 (34.2)		Reference
A/SW/Lutol/3/2000(H1N1)				
Positive	26	11 (15.1)	8.2 (3.6–18.6)	3.7 (1.5–9.6)
Negative	755	62 (84.9)		Reference

Abbreviation: OR, odds ratio; CI, confidence interval.
[a]Covariate has some missing values.

serological testing. On the other hand, Cowling et al. [7] and Papenburg et al. [9] included both qRT-PCR and serological testing for A(H1N1)pdm09 infection.

Cohort subjects born ≤1957 (age ≥52 years) were less likely to have A(H1N1)pdm09 seroconversion, comparable to the findings from other studies [12]. Multivariate analyses suggested that adults born after 1957 were more susceptible to A(H1N1)pdm09 infection (adjusted OR = 2.1, 95% CI, 1.1–4.2 for subjects born after 1968; adjusted OR = 2.4, 95% CI, 1.2–4.6 for those born between 1958 and 1968). These findings support the hypothesis that older adults may have acquired partial immunity to A(H1N1)pdm09 from previous exposure to a 1918-like A(H1N1) virus circulating between 1918 and 1957 [1], or from a lifetime of exposure to influenza A resulting in broad heterotypic immunity [22–26]. Cross-reactive antibody to the A(H1N1)pdm09 virus has also been demonstrated in archival serum samples from adult recipients of trivalent inactivated influenza vaccines during 2007–2009 seasons [23]. However, only 4 of 84 cohort subjects with A(H1N1)pdm09 infection reported ever receiving human influenza vaccines. Hence, we posit that a high prevalence of cross-reacting antibody to the A(H1N1)pdm09 virus seems unlikely. Local geographical area was also associated with A(H1N1)pdm09 infections. Subjects living in Phran Kratai district had higher adjusted odd ratios for A(H1N1)pdm09 infection (adjust OR = 2.6; 95% CI, 1.5–4.5) compared with those living in Mueng district. Since Phran Kratai district has approximately 3 times more pigs per person than does Mueng district (KPP Livestock Office data), cohort subjects living in Phran Kratai district may have had antibodies to swine viruses which were cross-reactive with A(H1N1)pdm09. This is supported by the fact that elevated antibodies against the two swine viruses, A/SW/Gent/7625(H1N2) and A/SW/Lutol3/2000(H1N1), were associated

Table 3. Description of contact subjects living with A(H1N1)pdm09-infected cohort subjects, Kamphaeng Phet, Thailand.

Year of Infection	ID of Cohort Subject with A(H1N1)pdm09 Infection	Number of Enrolled Contacts/Total Household Members	Number of Contact Subjects with:				
			ILI	A(H1N1)pdm09-positive by qRT-PCR	Hemagglutination Inhibition (HI) Titer against A/Mexico/4108/2009(H1N1)		
					Seroconversion[a]	Positive[b]	Negative
2009	T20133AIS	6[c]/6	1	1	0	0	6
	T50492AIS	1/6	0	0	0	1	0
	T20159AIS	9/9	5	5	6	0	3
2010	T70655AIS	3/3	0	0	0	1	2
	T40378AIS	2/2	0	0	2	0	0
	T40379AIS	2[c]/2	0	0	0	0	2
	T50448AIS	6/6	0	0	3	0	3
	T80750AIS	2/2	0	0	1	1	0
	T20119AIS	2/2	0	0	1	0	1
	T20129AIS	3[c]/5	0	0	0	0	3
Total	**N = 10**	**36/43**	**6**	**6**	**13**	**3**	**20**

[a]≥4-fold increase in HI titer from day 0 to day 60 sera.
[b]Single positive HI titer ≥1:40.
[c]Missing convalescent sample for one subject.

Table 4. Age distribution of contact subjects with laboratory-confirmed A(H1N1)pdm09 infection, Kamphaeng Phet, Thailand.

Birth Year	Number of Enrolled Contact Subjects	Number of A(H1N1)pdm09-positive by qRT-PCR[a]	Number of A(H1N1)pdm09-positive by Seroconversion or Single Positive HI Titer	Number of Symptomatic[b] A(H1N1)pdm09 Infection	Number of Subclinical[c] A(H1N1)pdm09 Infection
≤1957	5	0	2	0	2
1958–1968	2	1	2	2	0
1969–1989	9	1	1	1	0
1990–2003	16	3 (1)	9	4	6
≥2004	4	1	2	2	0
Total	**36**	**6 (1)**	**16**	**9**	**8**

[a]Number in parenthesis refers to sample determined to be positive by qRT-PCR without documented seroconversion or single positive HI titer.
[b]Symptomatic infections include those having positive respiratory sample for A(H1N1)pdm09 by qRT-PCR or ≥4-fold increase in HI titer of paired ILI sera or single positive HI titer with ILI or respiratory illness within 7 days prior to study enrollment.
[c]Subclinical infections include those having ≥4-fold increase in HI titer of paired ILI sera or single positive HI titer without ILI or respiratory illness within 7 days prior to study enrollment.

with A(H1N1)pdm09 seroconversion among the cohort subjects (Table 2). A similar finding was reported by Kyriakis et al. [27] that pigs infected or vaccinated with European swine influenza viruses had cross-reactive antibodies against A(H1N1)pdm09. It is of note that swine exposure was not associated with the A(H1N1)pdm09 infection (Table 2).

The cumulative incidence of A(H1N1)pdm09 infection by qRT-PCR and HI seroconversion in the cohort from January 2009 to December 2010 was 10.8% with an annual incidence of 1.2% and 9.7% in 2009 and 2010, respectively. Previous studies estimated the incidence of A(H1N1)pdm09 infection among adults to range from 6% to 13% during the early pandemic (May to September 2009) [2–4,6,12] and from 3% to 41% during November 2009 to May 2010 [28–31]. These wide ranges are likely a result of varying study designs, study periods, laboratory methods, and sample sources.

The A(H1N1)pdm09 secondary attack rate (SAR) among household members of cohort subjects was 47.2% (50% in 2009, 45% in 2010). Previous A(H1N1)pdm09 household transmission studies conducted during the early pandemic (April to August 2009) reported a wide range (4% to 45%) of SARs [8–10,32–35]. Most of these studies used only clinical symptoms (ILI) [32–33] or serology [8] to identify secondary A(H1N1)pdm09 cases, or performed qRT-PCR only for clinically suspected secondary cases [10,34–35]. In contrast, the study by Papenburg et al. [9] sought secondary A(H1N1)pdm09 cases among all consented household members (symptomatic or not) performing laboratory diagnostic testing to include serology and qRT-PCR. That study reported a SAR of 45% for laboratory-confirmed A(H1N1)pdm09 similar to the SAR in our study. It is well accepted that influenza can present with a broad range of symptoms and severities, including atypical and subclinical infections. Thus, underestimation of IFV infection by 25–50% may occur depending on the surveillance system and diagnostic criteria [36–40]. As demonstrated in previous studies [9,41] and substantiated by our work, serological evaluation in combination with molecular analysis (qRT-PCR) can improve the sensitivity of case detection.

Our study had some limitations. Only adults over 20 years of age were enrolled in the cohort. Since children are at high risk of A(H1N1)pdm09 infection [42], our sampling method may have excluded a substantial portion of individuals at-risk. However, children were indeed included in the household transmission investigations in which school-aged subjects were found to have the highest A(H1N1)pdm09 infection rate. The small sample size in the household transmission component of our study limited what conclusions could be made. Nevertheless, the A(H1N1)pdm09 secondary attack rate among household members in our study was similar to those demonstrated in previous studies. Other limitations are related to the serological assay. It is possible that HI seropositivity against A(H1N1)pdm09 may have been due to cross-reactive IFV strains. Furthermore, the HI cut-off of 1:40 was chosen in order to be comparable with other studies; however, different cut-offs would change our findings.

Our study was unique in evaluating the 2009 influenza pandemic in several ways. First, it combined a prospective longitudinal cohort study undergoing active ILI surveillance with a household transmission component. Second, it was already fully operational at the outset of the pandemic. Third, it continued operating for the full duration of the pandemic. Keeping these aspects of the study in mind, our results demonstrate that subclinical A(H1N1)pdm09 infection occurred frequently among Thai adults in this rural population. The role of these subclinical infections in A(H1N1)pdm09 transmission has important implications in formulating strategies to predict and control the spread of A(H1N1)pdm09 and other IFV strains. For instance, if a large portion of viral infections are subclinical, hospital-based surveillance will not well-represent a population's influenza ecology. Hence, public health officials should consider these large numbers of subclinical infections in developing future influenza surveillance and control programs. The effort to capture subclinical data need not be as extensive and expensive as this cohort study. For example, subclinical infection data might be collected through modest household transmission studies, where secondary attack rates (clinical and subclinical) among persons in the same household as index cases may be used as a surrogate for general population data.

Acknowledgments

This study was made possible through collaborations between the Global Pathogens Laboratory, University of Florida Emerging Pathogens Institute, USA (formerly the Center for Emerging Infectious Diseases, University of Iowa, College of Public Health, USA); United States Army Medical Component-Armed Forces Research Institute of Medical Sciences (USAMC-AFRIMS), Bangkok, Thailand; and the National Institute of Health, Ministry of Public Health, Bangkok, Thailand.

We thank John Paul Burks, Ben Anderson, Clint McDaniel, and Danielle Peters (University of Florida Global Pathogens Laboratory); Dr. Alexander Klimov (Influenza Division, Centers for Disease Control and Prevention, Atlanta, Georgia), Dr. Richard Webby (St Jude Children's Research Hospital, Memphis, Tennessee), Dr. Dennis Senne (National Veterinary Services Laboratories, Ames, Iowa), Dr. Chris Olsen (School of Veterinary Medicine, University of Wisconsin-Madison, Madison, Wisconsin, USA), and Dr. Malik Peiris (Chair, Department of Microbiology, University of Hong Kong, Hong Kong, China) for sharing their viruses and antisera; and the staff at the Kamphaeng Phet-AFRIMS Virology Research Unit (KAVRU), especially Ms. Rungkarn Hangsuwan, for their administrative, laboratory, and logistic support.

Author Contributions

Conceived and designed the experiments: IKY PJB SDP RVG GCG . Performed the experiments: BK IKY MC KS DB PS GLH. Analyzed the data: BK IKY WSK JAF. Wrote the paper: BK IKY WSK GCG.

References

1. Bandaranayake D, Huang QS, Bissielo A, Wood T, Mackereth G, et al. (2010) Risk factors and immunity in a nationally representative population following the 2009 influenza A(H1N1) pandemic. PLoS One 5: e13211.
2. Gilbert GL, Cretikos MA, Hueston L, Doukas G, O'Toole B, et al. (2010) Influenza A (H1N1) 2009 antibodies in residents of New South Wales, Australia, after the first pandemic wave in the 2009 southern hemisphere winter. PLoS One 5: e12562.
3. Grills N, Piers LS, Barr I, Vaughan LM, Lester R, et al. (2010) A lower than expected adult Victorian community attack rate for pandemic (H1N1) 2009. Aust N Z J Public Health 34: 228–231.
4. McVernon J, Laurie K, Nolan T, Owen R, Irving D, et al. (2010) Seroprevalence of 2009 pandemic influenza A(H1N1) virus in Australian blood donors, October - December 2009. Euro Surveill 15: pii = 19678.
5. Miller E, Hoschler K, Hardelid P, Stanford E, Andrews N, et al. (2010) Incidence of 2009 pandemic influenza A H1N1 infection in England: a cross-sectional serological study. Lancet 375: 1100–1108.
6. Tandale BV, Pawar SD, Gurav YK, Chadha MS, Koratkar SS, et al. (2010) Seroepidemiology of pandemic influenza A (H1N1) 2009 virus infections in Pune, India. BMC Infect Dis 10: 255.
7. Cowling BJ, Chan KH, Fang VJ, Lau LL, So HC, et al. (2010) Comparative epidemiology of pandemic and seasonal influenza A in households. N Engl J Med 362: 2175–2184.
8. Jackson ML, France AM, Hancock K, Lu X, Veguilla V, et al. (2011) Serologically confirmed household transmission of 2009 pandemic influenza A (H1N1) virus during the first pandemic wave–New York City, April-May 2009. Clin Infect Dis 53: 455–462.
9. Papenburg J, Baz M, Hamelin MÈ, Rhéaume C, Carbonneau J, et al. (2010) Household transmission of the 2009 pandemic A/H1N1 influenza virus: elevated laboratory-confirmed secondary attack rates and evidence of asymptomatic infections. Clin Infect Dis 51: 1033–1041.
10. Suess T, Buchholz U, Dupke S, Grunow R, an der Heiden M, et al. (2010) Shedding and transmission of novel influenza virus A/H1N1 infection in households–Germany, 2009. Am J Epidemiol 171: 1157–1164.
11. Aho M, Lyytikäinen O, Nyholm JE, Kuitunen T, Rönkkö E, et al. (2010) Outbreak of 2009 pandemic influenza A(H1N1) in a Finnish garrison–a serological survey. Euro Surveill 15: pii = 19709.
12. Chen MI, Lee VJ, Lim WY, Barr IG, Lin RT, et al. (2010) 2009 influenza A(H1N1) seroconversion rates and risk factors among distinct adult cohorts in Singapore. JAMA 303: 1383–1391.
13. Khaokham CB, Selent M, Loustalot FV, Zarecki SM, Harrington D, et al. (2013) Seroepidemiologic investigation of an outbreak of pandemic influenza A H1N1 2009 aboard a US Navy vessel–San Diego, 2009. Influenza Other Respir Viruses 7: 791–798.
14. Hsu SB, Hsieh YH (2008) On the role of asymptomatic infection in transmission dynamics of infectious diseases. Bull Math Biol 70: 134–155.
15. Simmerman JM, Chittaganpitch M, Levy J, Chantra S, Maloney S, et al. (2009) Incidence, seasonality and mortality associated with influenza pneumonia in Thailand: 2005–2008. PLoS One 4: e7776.
16. Iamsirithaworn S, AKarasewi P, Yingyong T, Suthachana S, Pittayawonganon C, et al. (2011) Three waves of the 2009 H1N1 influenza pandemic in Thailand. Siriraj Med J 63: 64–67.
17. Khuntirat BP, Yoon IK, Blair PJ, Krueger WS, Chittaganpitch M, et al. (2011) Evidence for subclinical avian influenza virus infections among rural Thai villagers. Clin Infect Dis 53: e107–116.
18. Krueger WS, Khuntirat B, Yoon IK, Blair PJ, Chittaganpitch M, et al. (2013) Prospective Study of Avian Influenza Virus Infections among Rural Thai Villagers. PLoS One 8: e72196.
19. Kayali G, Setterquist SF, Capuano AW, Myers KP, Gill JS, et al. (2008) Testing human sera for antibodies against avian influenza viruses: horse RBC hemagglutination inhibition vs. microneutralization assays. J Clin Virol 43: 73–78.
20. Capuano AW, Dawson JD, Gray GC. (2007) Maximizing Power in Seroepidemiological Studies Through Use of The Proportional Odds Model. Influenza Other Respi Viruses 1: 87–93.
21. Horby P, Mai le Q, Fox A, Thai PQ, Thi Thu Yen N, et al. (2012) The epidemiology of interpandemic and pandemic influenza in Vietnam, 2007–2010: the Ha Nam household cohort study I. Am J Epidemiol 175: 1062–1074.
22. Greenberg SB, Couch RB, Kasel JA (1974) An outbreak of an influenza type A variant in a closed population: The effect of homologous and heterologous antibody on infection and illness. Am J Epidemiol 100: 209–215.
23. Hancock K, Veguilla V, Lu X, Zhong W, Butler EN, et al. (2009) Cross-reactive antibody responses to the 2009 pandemic H1N1 influenza virus. N Engl J Med 361: 1945–1952.
24. Larson HE, Tyrrell DA, Bowker CH, Potter CW, Schild GC (1978) Immunity to challenge in volunteers vaccinated with an inactivated current or earlier strain of influenza A(H3N2). J Hyg (Lond) 80: 243–248.
25. Pereira MS, Chakraverty P, Schild GC, Coleman MT, Dowdle WR (1972) Prevalence of antibody to current influenza viruses and effect of vaccination on antibody response. Br Med J 4: 701–703.
26. Potter CW, Jennings R, Phair JP, Clarke A, Stuart-Harris CH. (1977) Dose-response relationship after immunization of volunteers with a new, surface-antigen-adsorbed influenza virus vaccine. J Infect Dis 135: 423–431.
27. Kyriakis CS, Olsen CW, Carman S, Brown IH, Brookes SM, et al. (2010) Serologic cross-reactivity with pandemic (H1N1) 2009 virus in pigs, Europe. Emerg Infect Dis 16: 96–99.
28. Achonu C, Rosella L, Gubbay JB, Deeks S, Rebbapragada A, et al. (2011) Seroprevalence of pandemic influenza H1N1 in Ontario from January 2009-May 2010. PLoS One 6: e26427.
29. Cox CM, Goodin K, Fisher E, Dawood FS, Hamilton JJ, et al. (2011) Prevalence of 2009 pandemic influenza A (H1N1) virus antibodies, Tampa Bay Florida - November-December, 2009. PLoS One 6: e29301.
30. Lerdsamran H, Pittayawonganon C, Pooruk P, Mungaomklang A, Iamsirithaworn S, et al. (2011) Serological response to the 2009 pandemic influenza A (H1N1) virus for disease diagnosis and estimating the infection rate in Thai population. PLoS One 6: e16164.
31. Zhang X, He J, Li L, Zhu X, Ke C, et al. (2011) Serologic survey of the pandemic H1N1 2009 virus in Guangdong Province, China: a cross sectional study. PLoS One 6: e23034.
32. Cauchemez S, Donnelly CA, Reed C, Ghani AC, Fraser C, et al. (2009) Household transmission of 2009 pandemic influenza A (H1N1) virus in the United States. N Engl J Med 361: 2619–2627.
33. France AM, Jackson M, Schrag S, Lynch M, Zimmerman C, et al. (2010) Household transmission of 2009 influenza A (H1N1) virus after a school-based outbreak in New York City, April-May 2009. J Infect Dis 201: 984–992.
34. Morgan OW, Parks S, Shim T, Blevins PA, Lucas PM, et al. (2010) Household transmission of pandemic (H1N1) 2009, San Antonio, Texas, USA, April-May 2009. Emerg Infect Dis 16: 631–637.
35. Odaira F, Takahashi H, Toyokawa T, Tsuchihashi Y, Kodama T, et al. (2009) Assessment of secondary attack rate and effectiveness of antiviral prophylaxis among household contacts in an influenza A(H1N1)v outbreak in Kobe, Japan, May-June 2009. Euro Surveill 14: pii = 19320.
36. Babcock HM, Merz LR, Dubberke ER, Fraser VJ (2008) Case-control study of clinical features of influenza in hospitalized patients. Infect Control Hosp Epidemiol 29: 921–926.
37. Boivin G, Hardy I, Tellier G, Maziade J (2000) Predicting influenza infections during epidemics with use of a clinical case definition. Clin Infect Dis 31: 1166–1169.
38. Call SA, Vollenweider MA, Hornung CA, Simel DL, McKinney WP (2005) Does this patient have influenza? JAMA 293: 987–997.
39. Harper SA, Bradley JS, Englund JA, File TM, Gravenstein S, et al. (2009) Seasonal influenza in adults and children–diagnosis, treatment, chemoprophylaxis, and institutional outbreak management: clinical practice guidelines of the Infectious Diseases Society of America. Clin Infect Dis 48: 1003–1032.
40. Ong AK, Chen MI, Lin L, Tan AS, Nwe NW, et al. (2009) Improving the clinical diagnosis of influenza–a comparative analysis of new influenza A (H1N1) cases. PLoS One 4: e8453.
41. Zambon M, Hays J, Webster A, Newman R, Keene O (2001) Diagnosis of influenza in the community: relationship of clinical diagnosis to confirmed virological, serologic, or molecular detection of influenza. Arch Intern Med 161: 2116–2122.
42. Riley S, Kwok KO, Wu KM, Ning DY, Cowling BJ, et al. (2011) Epidemiological characteristics of 2009 (H1N1) pandemic influenza based on paired sera from a longitudinal community cohort study. PLoS Med 8: e1000442.

5

High Basal Expression of Interferon-Stimulated Genes in Human Bronchial Epithelial (BEAS-2B) Cells Contributes to Influenza A Virus Resistance

Lai-Giea Seng, Janet Daly, Kin-Chow Chang, Suresh V. Kuchipudi*

School of Veterinary Medicine and Science, University of Nottingham, Sutton Bonington Campus, Leicestershire, United Kingdom

Abstract

Respiratory epithelial cells play a key role in influenza A virus (IAV) pathogenesis and host innate response. Transformed human respiratory cell lines are widely used in the study of IAV−host interactions due to their relative convenience, and inherent difficulties in working with primary cells. Transformed cells, however, may have altered susceptibility to virus infection. Proper characterization of different respiratory cell types in their responses to IAV infection is therefore needed to ensure that the cell line chosen will provide results that are of relevance *in vivo*. We compared replication kinetics of human H1N1 (A/USSR/77) IAVs in normal primary human bronchial epithelial (NHBE) and two commonly used respiratory epithelial cell lines namely BEAS-2B and A549 cells. We found that IAV replication was distinctly poor in BEAS-2B cells in comparison with NHBE, A549 and Madin-Darby canine kidney (MDCK) cells. IAV resistance in BEAS-2B cells was accompanied by an activated antiviral state with high basal expression of interferon (IFN) regulatory factor-7 (*IRF-7*), stimulator of IFN genes (*STING*) and IFN stimulated genes (ISGs). Treatment of BEAS-2B cells with a pan-Janus-activated-kinase (JAK) inhibitor decreased IRF-7 and ISG expression and resulted in increased IAV replication. Therefore, the use of highly resistant BEAS-2B cells in IAV infection may not reflect the cytopathogenicity of IAV in human epithelial cells *in vivo*.

Editor: Michael Nevels, University of Regensburg, Germany

Funding: This project is funded by a Ministry of Higher Education, Government of Malaysia PhD scholarship awarded to LS. The funders had no role in study design, data collection and analysis, decision to publish, or preparation of the manuscript.

Competing Interests: The authors have declared that no competing interests exist.

* Email: suresh.kuchipudi@nottingham.ac.uk

Introduction

Influenza A viruses (IAVs) infect a wide spectrum of avian and mammalian hosts with a range of clinical manifestations from mild or in-apparent infection to severe fatal disease. The dangerous features of IAVs are their highly infectious nature, broad host range, and their inherent nature to frequently mutate and/or reassort from mixed infections, resulting in emergence of new strains. Despite ongoing vaccination programmes, influenza is still one of the leading causes of human deaths, with 3–5 million cases of severe illness and up to 500,000 deaths each year (http://www.who.int/mediacentre/factsheets/fs211/en/). IAVs have been shown to readily overcome vaccine specificity and develop resistance against the few available antiviral drugs such as neuraminidase inhibitors [1].

While seasonal influenza virus infection typically causes contagious respiratory disease in humans with relatively low mortality rate, infections with some of the highly pathogenic avian influenza (HPAI) viruses of the H5N1 subtype could cause up to 60% mortality [2]. The unusual severity of HPAI H5N1 virus infections in humans has been attributed to hyperacute dysregulation of pro-inflammatory cytokines and chemokines often referred to as a 'cytokine storm' [3,4]. It has previously been shown that pigs are inherently more resistant to HPAI H5N1 virus infection than humans, with reduced infectious virus production and pro-inflammatory response [5]. It is increasingly clear that host responses critically contribute to the disparate clinical outcomes of IAV infection.

Respiratory epithelial cells are the primary early targets of IAVs and are key players in the host innate immune responses to IAV infection. The first step in IAV infection is the attachment of viral haemagglutinin (HA) to host cell sialic acid (SA) receptors [6]. Avian influenza viruses show preferential binding to SA receptors linked to galactose with an alpha 2–3 linkage (SAα 2,3 Gal) whereas classical human influenza viruses preferentially bind to alpha 2,6 linked SA receptors (SAα 2,6 Gal) [7,8]. Human respiratory epithelial cells express both alpha 2,3 and alpha 2,6 receptors [9] and are permissive to a range of avian and mammalian influenza virus replication. Hence, respiratory epithelial cells are important in the study of influenza virus−host interactions.

As alternatives to primary normal human bronchial epithelial (NHBE) cells, immortalised human respiratory cell lines are often used as they are easily accessible, cost-effective and can be propagated almost indefinitely. For example, adenovirus-12 SV40 transformed human bronchial epithelial cells (BEAS-2B) and adenocarcinomic human alveolar basal epithelial cells (A549) are two of the most common cell lines used in the study of IAV−host interactions [10–12] and in infections with other respiratory viruses such as human respiratory syncytial virus [13,14].

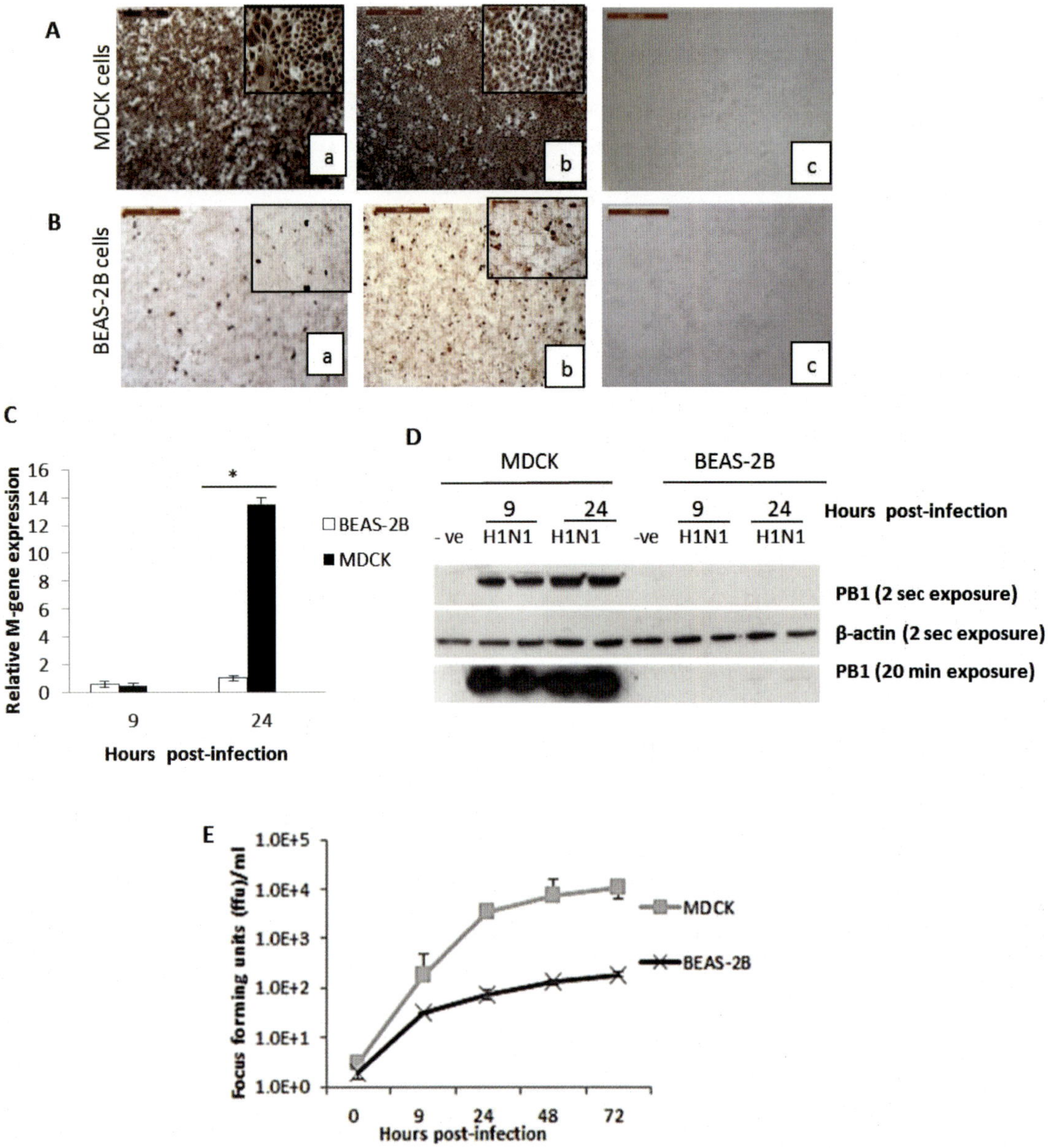

Figure 1. BEAS-2B cells were considerably less permissive to influenza virus replication than MDCK cells. (A) MDCK and BEAS-2B cells were infected with USSR H1N1 or H2N3 influenza viruses at 1.0 MOI (based on MDCK cells), and viral NP expression was determined at 6 h post-infection (hpi). All MDCK cells were positive for viral NP at 6 hpi with (Aa) human H1N1 and (Ab) avian H2N3 viruses. (B) In contrast, few corresponding virus positive BEAS-2B cells were found (Ba and Bb). Mock infected MDCK (Ac) and BEAS-2B (Bc) cells showed no staining. MDCK cells and BEAS-2B cells were infected with H1N1 virus (dose equivalent to MOI 1.0 as per MDCK titration) to determine cellular expression of viral M gene RNA, normalized to 18Sr RNA (C), PB1 protein expression at 9 and 24 hpi (D), and infectious virus output at 9, 24, 48 and 72 hpi (D). In BEAS-2B cells, (C) viral M gene expression was much lower than MDCK cells, (D) little or no PB1 protein was detected (only detected faint bands for PB1 after prolonged exposure for 20 min) and (E) less infectious progeny virus was produced over 72 h of infection. ** ($p<0.01$).

Many immortalized cell lines such as Madin-Darby canine kidney (MDCK), Vero and baby hamster kidney (BHK21) cells are readily permissive to influenza virus replication and are also widely used for *in vitro* virus infection studies. However, IAV replication kinetics can vary depending on the virus strain and the type of cell line. For example, MDCK cells support more rapid growth of influenza viruses than Vero cells [15]. However little is known about the differences in IAV replication between primary human respiratory epithelial cells and cell lines. It has been shown that antiviral response pathways are dysregulated in cancer cells due to immortal transformation [16–18]. Therefore, there may be differences in antiviral mechanisms between primary cells and transformed cells that could result in differences in virus replication and cellular responses to virus infection.

Consequently, it is likely that IAV replication kinetics and cellular responses to virus infection could be different between primary and immortalized respiratory cells. Proper characterization, in particular of viral growth, in different respiratory cell types is therefore needed to allow rational selection of the most appropriate cells for addressing specific influenza research questions.

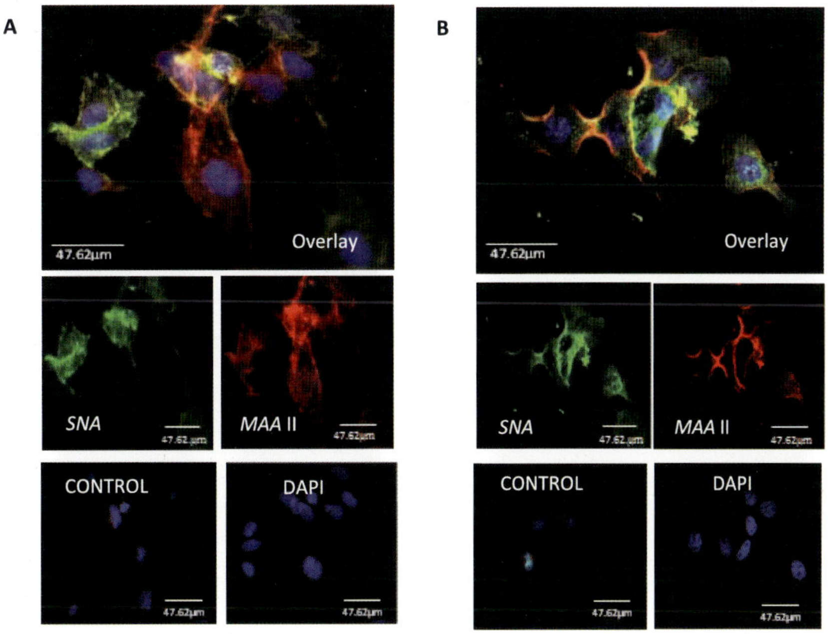

Figure 2. Similar distribution of human and avian influenza virus receptors on BEAS-2B and MDCK cells. Human (SAα2,6-Gal [green]) and avian (SAα2,3-Gal [red]) virus receptors were detected on (A) BEAS-2B and (B) MDCK cells by lectins *SNA* and *MAA* II, respectively. Co-expression of both receptors was found in BEAS-2B and MDCK cells. Negative controls were performed without lectin incubation.

In order to characterize differences in virus replication between human primary and transformed respiratory epithelial cells, we compared virus replication and cellular responses to human H1N1 IAV infections in NHBE, BEAS-2B and A549 cells. We found that BEAS-2B cells are highly resistant to avian and human IAV infections in comparison with NHBE and A549 cells.

Materials and Methods

Cells and viruses

BEAS-2B (Sigma Aldrich) and NHBE (Lonza) cells were cultured in bronchial epithelial growth medium (BEGM, Lonza) at 37°C in an atmosphere of 5% CO_2. A549 cells (ATCC CCL-185) and MDCK cells were cultured in Dulbecco's Modified Eagle's Medium (DMEM) supplemented with 100 units/ml penicillin and 100 µg/ml streptomycin (Invitrogen), 10% fetal bovine serum (FBS) and 0.3 g/l L-glutamine. A549 cells were switched to BEGM 48 h before virus challenge.

A low pathogenicity avian influenza (LPAI) H2N3 virus (A/mallard duck/England/7277/06) and a moderately pathogenic human influenza H1N1 (A/USSR/77) virus were used. All viruses were grown by allantoic inoculation of 10-day-old embryonated hens' eggs. Viruses were titrated in MDCK cells using an immunocytochemical focus assay [19].

Virus infection of cells

At 80% confluence, cells were rinsed twice with phosphate buffered saline (PBS) and infected with H1N1 or H2N3 IAVs at multiplicity of infection (MOI) of 1.0, based on virus titration values on MDCK cells, in infection medium comprising 2% Ultroser G (Pall Biosepra, Portsmouth, UK), 500 ng/ml TPCK trypsin (Sigma-Aldrich Ltd.) and antibiotics in Ham's F12. At 2 h incubation, cells were rinsed twice with PBS and fresh infection medium added. Cells were further incubated for 4, 6 or 22 h. Cells infected for 6 h were fixed in acetone: methanol (1:1) for 10 min and were subjected to immunocytochemical staining using a murine monoclonal antibody to influenza nucleoprotein (NP) as previously described [5]. At 10 and 24 h post infection, culture supernatants were collected for infectious virus titration on MDCK cells as previously described [19]. Total RNA was extracted using RNeasy plus kit (Qiagen) following the manufacturer's instructions.

Influenza receptor detection

Influenza virus receptors on cultured cells were characterized using FITC-labelled *Sambucus nigra agglutinin* (*SNA*) (Vector Labs) for SAα 2,6 Gal, and biotinylated *Maackia amurensis* agglutinin II (*MAA* II) (Vector Labs) for SAα 2,3 Gal in a previously described lectin-cytochemical method [20].

Influenza PB1 protein expression

Infected cells were lysed using RIPA lysis buffer (Santa Cruz) and cellular proteins were separated on a Tris-glycine gel and blotted onto polyvinylidene difluoride (PVDF) membrane. Viral polymerase basic 1(PB1) protein expression was detected by western blot analysis using a goat polyclonal primary anti-PB1 antibody (Santa Cruz), followed by donkey anti-goat IgG-horseradish peroxidase (IgG-HRP) (Santa Cruz), and subsequently visualized by standard enhanced chemiluminescence reaction ECL detection kit (Amersham Life Science Ltd).

Viral and host gene expression

Quantification of expression of viral and host genes based on cDNA converted from total RNA (Superscript III first strand cDNA synthesis kit, Invitrogen) was performed on a LightCycler-96 (Roche, Mannheim, Germany) using the SYBR green or TaqMan method. Primers and probe used for detecting influenza matrix (M) gene expression were as previously described [21]. Primers for the expression analysis of *IL-6, IFNβ, and Mx1* were as described in Nelli et al. (2012) [22]. Predesigned primers

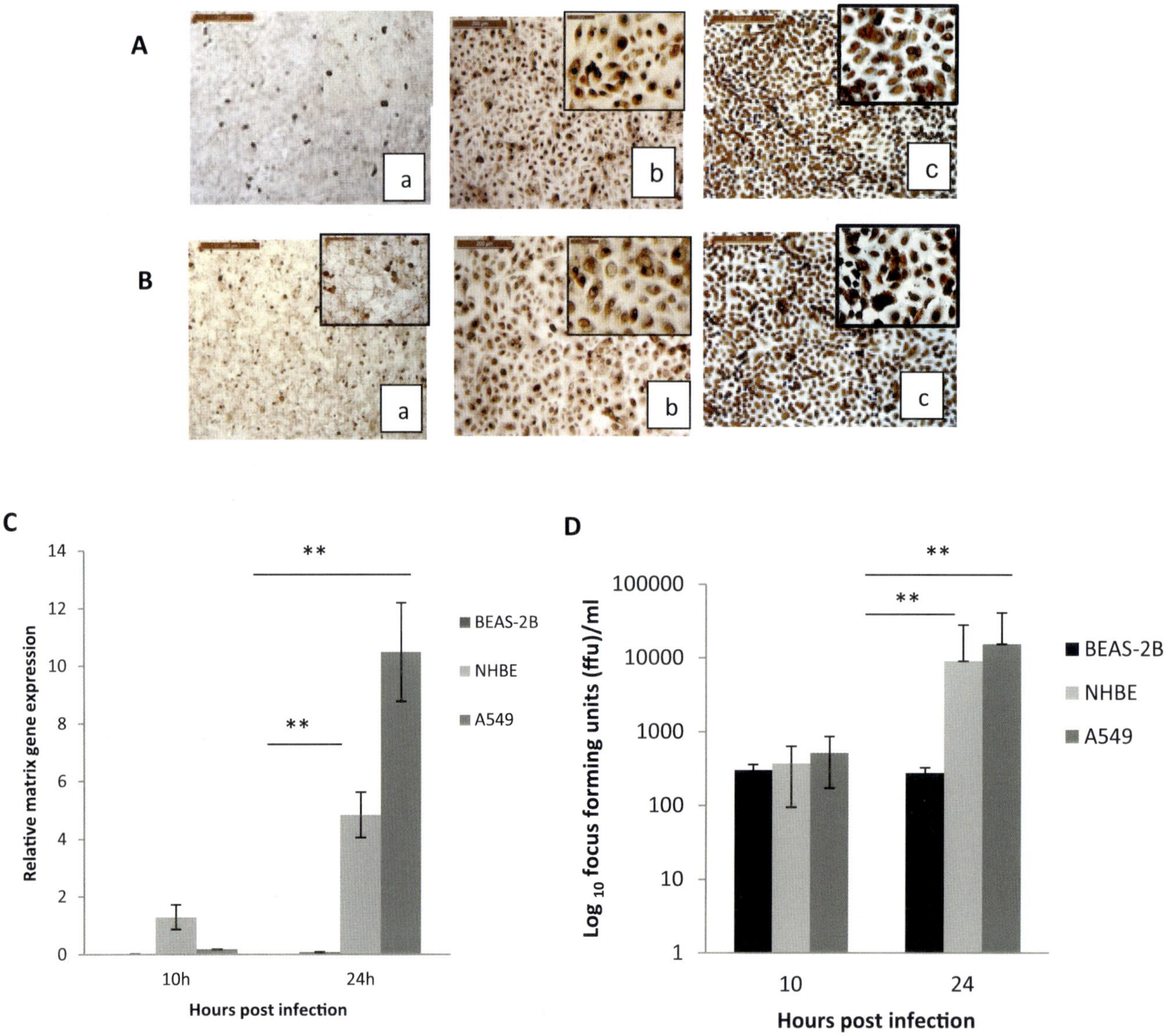

Figure 3. BEAS-2B cells were more resistant than human primary NHBE cells and human A549 cells to human H1N1 (A) and avian H2N3 (B) influenza virus. Cells were infected with the respective virus at a dose that was equivalent to 1.0 MOI in MDCK cells. For both viruses, few BEAS-2B cells (a), most NHBE cells (b), and virtually all A549 cells (c) were positive for viral NP at 6 h of infection. At 24 h of infection with human H1N1 virus (C and D), M gene expression (C) and infectious virus production (D) from BEAS-2B cells were significantly less than corresponding NHBE and A549 cells, with A549 cells showing the highest M gene expression (C) and infectious virus production (D). **$p<0.01$.

(KiCqStart SYBR Green Primers) for expression analysis of *ISG15*, *STING*, *IRF-7* and *IRF-3* were purchased from Sigma Aldrich. Other primer sequences are as follows: interferon beta (*IFN-β*) sense: 5′- ACCTCCGAAACTGAAGATCTCCTA-3′, antisense: 5′- TGCTGGTTGAAGAATGCTTGA-3′; *ISG15* sense: 5′- AGATCACCCAGAAGATCG-3′, antisense: 5′-TG-TTATTCCTCACCAGGATG-3′; *STING* sense: 5′-CTATTTC-TACTACTCCCTCCC-3′antisense: 5′- CGCAGATATCCGA-TGTAATATG-3′; *Mx1* sense: 5′- TTCTGGGTCGGAGGC-TACAG-3′, antisense: 5′- TGGATGGCGGCGTTCT-3′; *IRF-7* sense: 5′- TCTTCTTCCAAGAGCTGG-3′, antisense: 5′- CT-ATCCAGGGAAGACACAC-3′; *IL-6* sense: 5′- GGTA-CATCCTCGACGGCATCT-3′, antisense: 5′- GTGCCTCTT-TGCTGCTTTCAC-3′. Data were normalized to 18S rRNA expression using a relative standard curve method [23].

JAK inhibition

BEAS-2B cells were treated with 2.5 or 5.0 μM concentration of pyridine 6 (P6) [2-(1,1-dimethylethyl)-9-fluoro-3,6-dihydro-7H-benz[h]-imidaz[4,5-f]isoquinolin-7-one, Calbiochem], a pan-Janus-activated-kinase (JAK) inhibitor [24]. JAK inhibitor P6 was dissolved in DMSO. Following pre-treatment of cells with different concentrations of P6 or corresponding amounts of DMSO as controls for 24 h, medium was removed and cells were rinsed with PBS before infecting with H1N1 influenza virus at MOI of 1.0, based on viral titration values on MDCK cells. Cells were immunostained for viral NP at 6 h of infection. At 24 h infection, ISG expression, influenza viral M gene was quantified from total RNA, and progeny virus output in culture media was determined by immunocytochemical focus assays on MDCK cells.

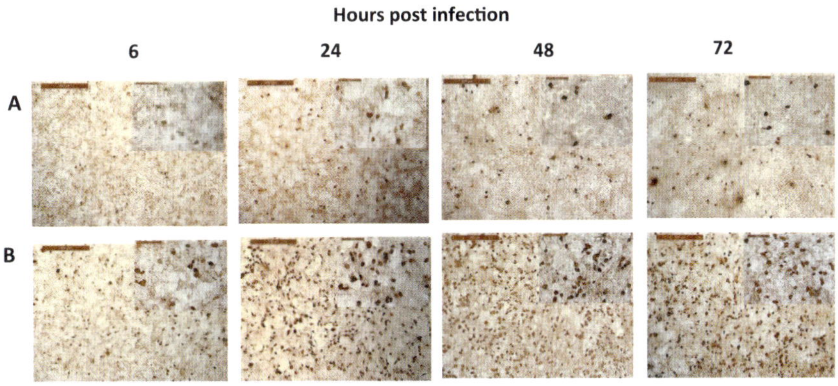

Figure 4. BEAS-2B cells showed greater accumulation of avian H2N3 virus than human H1N1 virus in prolonged cultures. At 6h of infection with H1N1 (A) and H2N3 (B) virus (at MOI 1.0 based on MDCK cells titration), there was little difference in virus accumulation as determined by viral NP detection. However, over 72h of H2N3 virus infection, there was progressive increase in NP intensity and number of infected cells (B). Such increases were barely detected in H1N1 virus infected BEAS-2B cells (A).

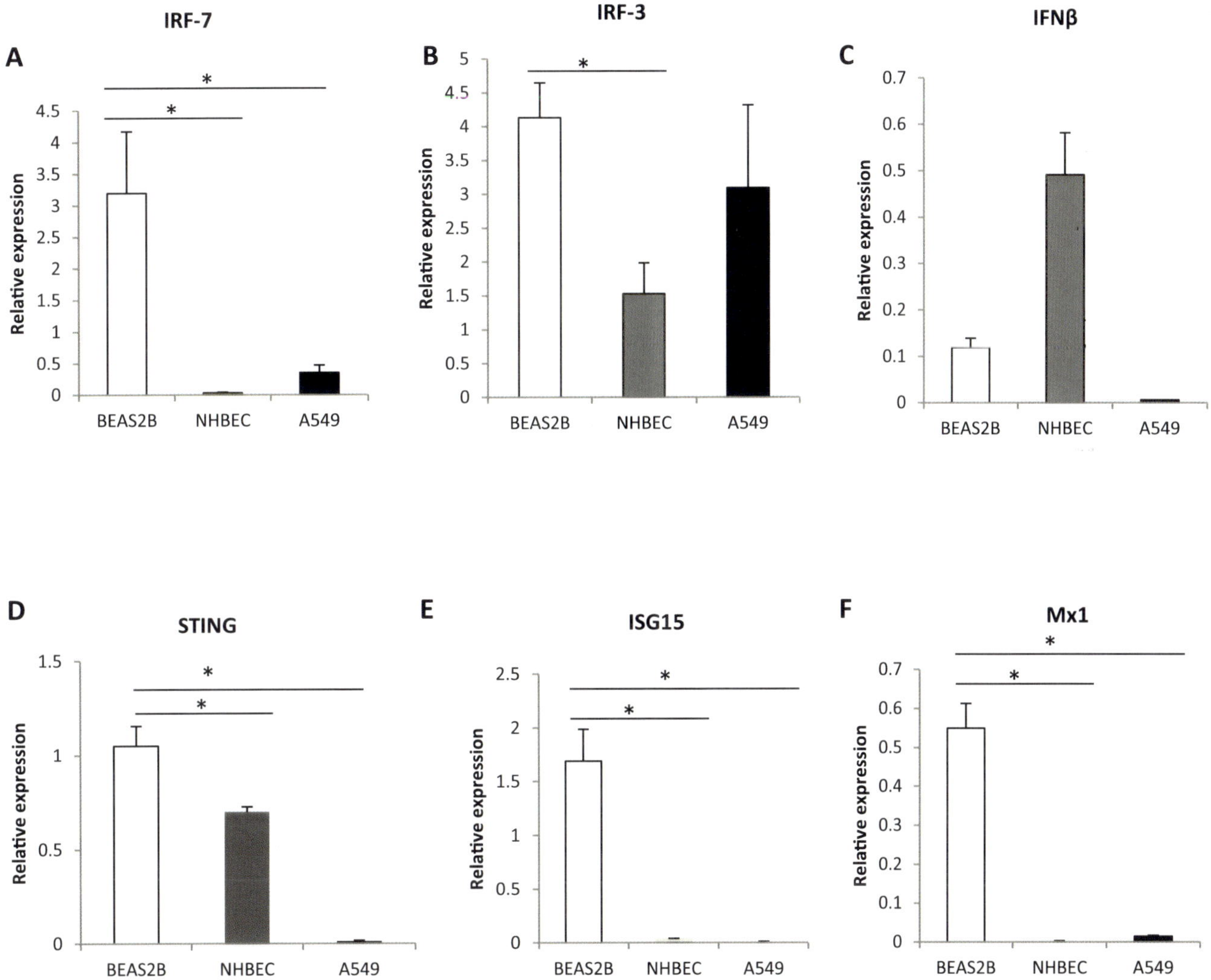

Figure 5. Resistance of BEAS-2B to influenza virus infection associated with high basal expression of *IRF-7* and several ISGs. The basal expression of a selection of genes associated with antiviral function was determined in the three human epithelial cell types (BEAS-2B, NHBE and A549 cells). In BEAS-2B cells, (A) basal *IRF-7* expression was significantly higher than the other two cell types ($p<0.05$). Basal basal expression of (D) *STING* (E) *ISG15* and (F) *Mx1* in BEAS-2B cells was also significantly higher ($p<0.05$) than in NHBE and A549 cells. Data normalized to 18S rRNA expression. Data points represent mean of 3 biological replicates. Error bar = SEM, *$p<0.05$.

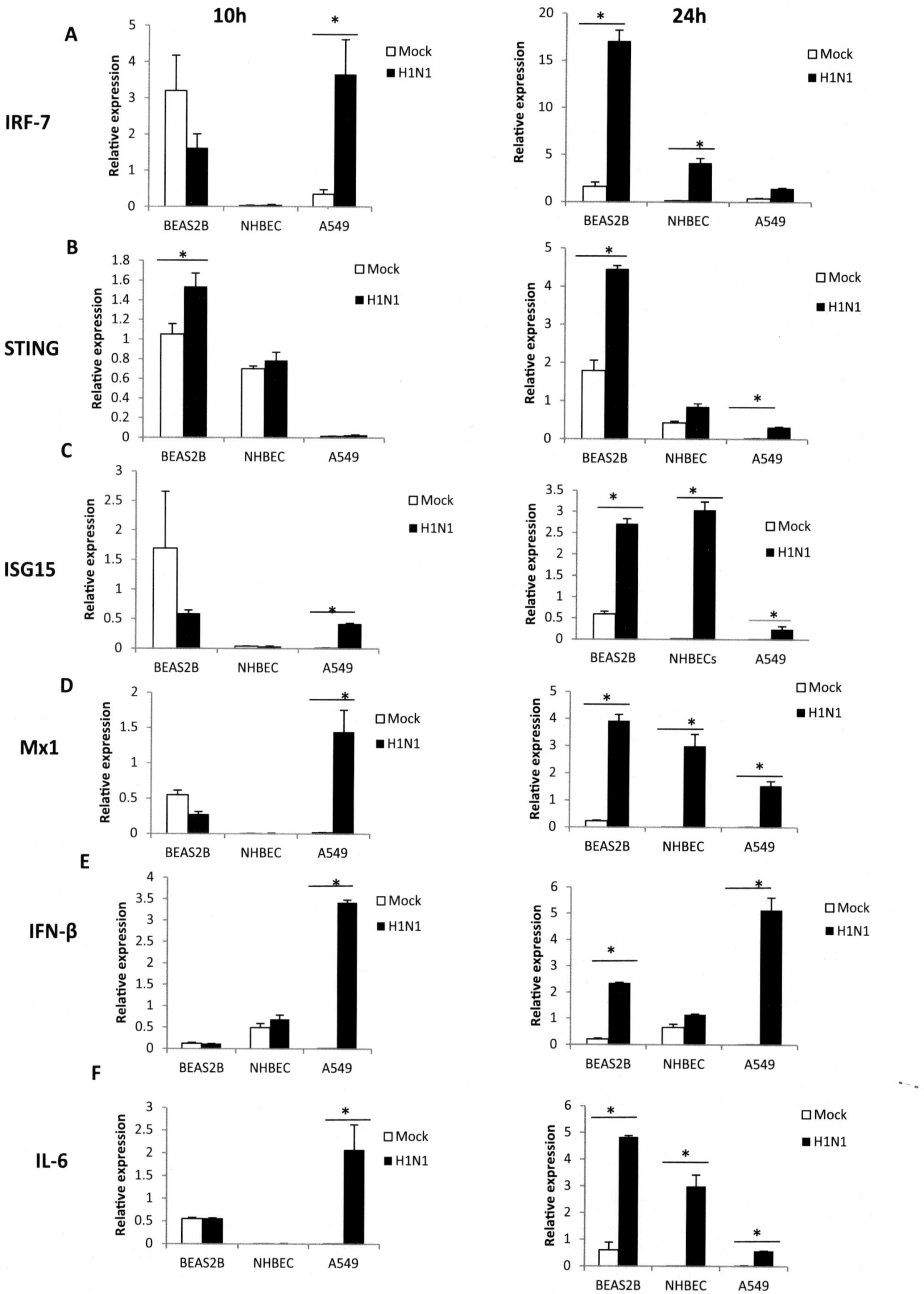
10h
24h
A
IRF-7
B
STING
C
ISG15
D
Mx1
E
IFN-β
F
IL-6
Relative expression
Mock
H1N1
BEAS2B
NHBEC
NHBECs
A549
*

Figure 6. BEAS-2B cells displayed strong induction of *IRF-7* and several ISGs at 24 h of H1N1 virus infection. Human epithelial BEAS-2B, NHBE and A549 cells were infected with human H1N1 virus at 1.0 MOI (based on MDCK cells). At 10 h of infection, expression pattern of antiviral genes (A) *IRF-7*, (B) *STING* (C) *ISG15*, (D) *Mx1*, (E) *IFN-β* and (F) *IL-6* was unremarkable in BEAS-2B and NHBE cells; however *IRF-7*, *ISG15*, *Mx1*, *IFN-β* and *IL-6* expression were up-regulated in A549 cells. Notably, all genes analyzed in BEAS-2B cells were significantly up-regulated by 24 h of infection; BEAS-2B cells expressed the highest *IRF-7*, *STING*, *Mx1* and *IL-6* RNA amongst the three cell types. Data normalized to 18S rRNA expression. Data points represent mean of 3 biological replicates. Error bar = SEM, $^*p<0.05$.

Statistical analysis

Statistical analyses for quantitative reverse transcriptionPCR (qRT-PCR) data were carried out using Relative Expression Software Tool (REST, Qiagen) [25]. Statistical analysis of infectious virus titration data was performed by a two-sample *t* test using Minitab software version 16 (16.2.2.).

Results

BEAS-2B cells were highly resistant to influenza virus infection relative to MDCK cells

BEAS-2B and MDCK cells were infected with USSR H1N1 and LPAI H2N3 IAVs at MOI of 1.0, based on viral titration values on MDCK cells. MDCK cells infected for 6 h with human H1N1 (Figure 1Aa) or avian H2N3 (Figure 1Ab) IAVs showed 100% detection of viral NP. In sharp contrast, less than 5% of BEAS-2B cells were positive for viral NP (Figure 1B).

To evaluate the kinetics of virus replication, cellular expression of viral M gene RNA, viral PB1 protein and infectious virus production were compared between H1N1 virus-infected MDCK and BEAS-2B cells. At 24 h infection, M gene expression was significantly higher ($p<0.05$) in MDCK cells than in BEAS-2B cells, which showed little increase in M gene expression with time (Figure 1C).

Protein expression of viral PB1 protein was barely detectable in H1N1 virus infected BEAS-2B cells whereas corresponding MDCK cells consistently showed much higher levels of PB1 (Figure 1D). Similarly, BEAS-2B cells released significantly less ($p<0.05$) infectious virus than MDCK cells at 9, 24, 48 and 72 h of infection (Figure 1E).

BEAS-2B and MDCK cells showed similar distribution of human and avian influenza virus receptors

To determine if the cellular distribution of virus receptors on BEAS-2B and MDCK cells could account for the difference in viral replication between the two cell types, SA-linkage specific lectin cytochemistry was performed. Similar co-expression of both human (SAα2,6-Gal [green]) and avian (SAα2,3-Gal [red]) type influenza virus receptors was found in BEAS-2B (Figure 2A) and MDCK cells (Figure 2B), suggesting that there was no qualitative difference in virus receptors between the two cell types.

BEAS-2B cells were more resistant than human primary NHBE cells and human A549 cells to human H1N1 and avian H2N3 influenza viruses

To compare the susceptibility of BEAS-2B cells with primary NHBE and A549 cells, the three cell types were infected with USSR H1N1 or avian H2N3 viruses at MOI of 1.0 (based on MDCK cells). Viral NP at 6 h of infection with H1N1 virus (Figure 3A) and H2N3 virus (Figure 3B) showed that few BEAS-2B cells, most NHBE cells and virtually all A549 cells were positive for viral NP. We then quantified viral M gene RNA expression and progeny virus release in all three cell type at 10 and 24 h of H1N1 virus infection. M gene expression (Figure 3C) and infectious virus production (Figure 3D) from BEAS-2B cells were significantly less than corresponding NHBE and A549 cells at 24 h of H1N1 virus infection ($p<0.05$), with A549 cells showing the highest M gene expression (Figure 3C) and infectious virus production (Figure 3D).

BEAS-2B cells displayed differential accumulation of human H1N1 and avian H2N3 viruses in extended cultures

As BEAS-2B cells were more resistant to influenza virus infection (Figures 1 and 3), they were infected with human H1N1 and avian H2N3 viruses (at 1.0 MOI based on MDCK cells) over an extended period of 72 h (Figure 4). At 6 h of infection, there was little difference in virus accumulation as determined by viral NP detection. However over 72 h of H2N3 virus infection, there was progressive increase in NP intensity and number of infected cells (Figure 4B). Such changes were barely detected in H1N1 virus infected BEAS-2B cells (Figure 4A). Thus, virus accumulation in resistant BEAS-2B cells varied according to virus subtype.

BEAS-2B cells showed high basal expression of *IRF-7* and several ISGs

To gain insight into the relative resistance of BEAS-2B cells to H1N1 influenza virus infection, the basal expression of a selection of genes associated with antiviral function was determined in the three human epithelial cell types (BEAS-2B, NHBE and A549 cells) (Figure 5). In BEAS-2B cells, basal *IRF-7* expression was significantly higher than the other two cell types ($p<0.05$) (Figure 5A). Notably, basal expression of *STING* (Figure 5D), *ISG15* (Figure 5E) and *Mx1* (Figure 5F) in BEAS-2B cells was also significantly higher ($p<0.05$) than in NHBE and A549 cells.

BEAS-2B cells displayed strong induction of *IRF-7* and ISGs at 24 h of H1N1 virus infection

To evaluate the antiviral response to influenza virus, the three human epithelial cell types were infected with the human H1N1 virus at 1.0 MOI (based on MDCK cells). In BEAS-2B cells at 10 h of infection, *IRF-7* (Figure 6A), *ISG15* (Figure 6C) and *Mx1* (Figure 6D) expression were significantly down-regulated ($p<0.05$) while *STING* expression (Figure 6B) was significantly up-regulated ($p<0.05$); expression of *IFN-β* and *IL-6* was unchanged (Figure 6 E–F). NHBE cells showed no significant change in antiviral gene response, and in *IFN-β* and *IL-6* expression at 10 h infection (Figure 6E–F). In corresponding A549 cells, all antiviral genes (except *STING*), *IFN-β* and *IL-6* were significantly up-regulated ($p<0.05$) (Figure 6A–F). By 24 h of infection, however, expression of all four anti-viral genes and *IFN-β* and *IL-6* was clearly up-regulated ($p<0.05$) in all three cell types; BEAS-2B cells displayed the highest expression of *IRF-7*, *STING*, *Mx1* and *IL-6*.

JAK-STAT pathway inhibition increased susceptibility of BEAS-2B cells to influenza virus infection

To assess the role of high basal and strong induced expression of ISGs at 24 h of influenza virus infection, BEAS-2B cells were treated with pyridine 6 (P6), a pan-JAK inhibitor known to shut down ISG expression [24]. P6-treated BEAS-2B cells showed

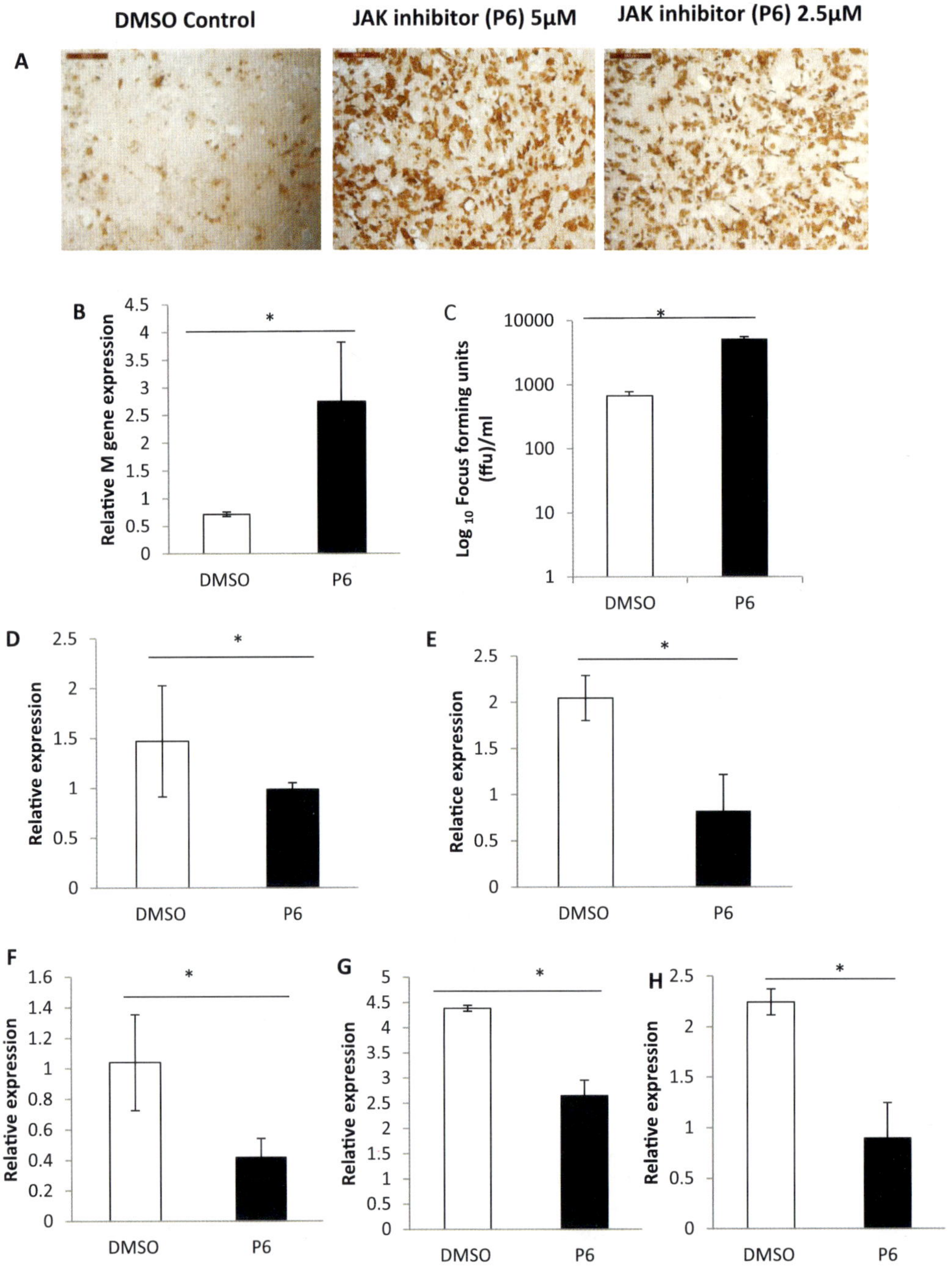

Figure 7. Pan-JAK inhibitor P6 decreased ISG expression and increased susceptibility of BEAS-2B cells to H1N1 influenza virus infection. (A) BEAS-2B cells treated with P6 inhibitor showed enhanced susceptibility to H1N1 influenza virus infection as evident by greater viral NP expression in P6 treated cells compared with DMSO control. BEAS-2B cells were pre-treated with P6 at a final concentration of 2.5 or 5 µM for 24 h and infected with H1N1 influenza virus at 1.0 MOI (based on MDCK cells). At 6 h post-infection cells were immunostained for viral NP. (B) P6 treated (2.5 µM) BEAS-2B cells showed higher influenza M gene RNA expression and (C) produced higher levels of infectious progeny virus at 24 h of H1N1 influenza virus infection. Increased influenza virus replication in P6 treated BEAS-2B cells corresponded to decreased expression of (D) *IRF-7* (E) IL-6 (F) *ISG15* (G) *STING* (H) *Mx1* compared with the controls. Total RNA extracted at 24 h infection from P6 or DMSO pre-treated cells was used for gene expression analysis re normalized to 18S rRNA expression. Culture supernatants collected at 24 h virus infection from P6 or DMSO pre-treated cells were subjected to infectious virus titration on MDCK cells using an immunocytochemical focus assay. Data points represent mean of 3 biological replicates with error bars showing standard deviation, $^*p<0.05$.

increased susceptibility to H1N1 virus infection as seen by greater number viral NP positive cells at 6 h of infection compared with DMSO controls (Figure 7A). BEAS-2B cells treated with P6 (2.5 µM) showed significantly higher ($p<0.05$) M gene RNA (Figure 7B) and produced significantly ($p<0.05$) higher levels of infectious progeny virus at 24 h of virus infection (Figure 7C). As expected the expression of anti-viral genes namely IRF-7, *IL-6*,

ISG15, *STING* and *Mx1* was significantly reduced in P6 treated BEAS-2B cells.

Discussion

In this study, BEAS-2B cells were shown to be significantly resistant to avian H2N3 and human H1N1 IAV infection compared with MDCK, NHBE and A549 cells. Influenza virus PB1 protein is an essential subunit of influenza virus RNA polymerase and plays a key role in influenza virus replication [26]. Poor replication of influenza viruses in BEAS-2B cells was associated with little PB1 protein expression in contrast to corresponding abundance of PB1 in MDCK cells. Viral HA binding to host SA receptors initiates IAV replication and the specific SA receptor distribution pattern of cells determines IAV susceptibility [20]. We found similar patterns of co-expression of avian and mammalian type influenza receptors in BEAS-2B and MDCK cells, which indicated that the resistance of BEAS-2B cells was not due to the absence of specific virus receptors.

Comparison of the kinetics of IAV replication showed that BEAS-2B cells were also highly resistant to IAV replication compared with the NHBE and A549 cells. In contrast to our findings, an earlier study found similar viral PB1 gene expression between BEAS-2B and A549 cells [27]. The reason for this difference is not clear, however the previous finding used different influenza virus strains, i.e. A/Udorn/72 (H3N2) and A/WSN/33 (H1N1), and the results were based on qRT-PCR quantification of PB1 gene expression rather than PB1 protein expression and infectious virus release. Thus it is possible that the choice of virus strains or a difference in the methodology may be responsible for the different observations.

Influenza virus replication in cell cultures can be different depending on the origin of influenza viruses. For example, human, avian and swine influenza viruses showed different replication kinetics in NHBE cells with human IAVs growing to higher titres [28]. In contrast, we found that BEAS-2B cells were relatively more resistant to human H1N1 than avian H2N3 influenza virus infection. These findings suggest that BEAS-2B cells do not reflect the natural host restriction pattern of NHBE cells to IAV infection.

In order to establish the molecular basis for the IAV resistance in BEAS-2B cells, we evaluated the regulation of antiviral pathways before and after H1N1 virus infection. We found significantly higher basal expression of *IRF-7* in BEAS-2B cells compared with NHBE and A549 cells. *IRF-7* plays a key role in mediating host resistance against influenza virus replication. For example, *IRF-7* knockdown resulted in enhanced PR8 influenza virus production in A549 cells and MDCK cells [29]. This study also found high basal expression of key antiviral genes namely *STING*, *ISG15* and *Mx1* in BEAS-2B cells relative to NHBE and A549 cells. *ISG15* is one of the most highly induced IFN-induced proteins and inhibits replication of a wide range of viruses including IAVs [30]. High basal expression of Mx is also a key marker of virus resistance in cells. For example, vesicular stomatitis virus (VSV) resistant human pancreatic ductal adenocarcinoma (PDA) cell lines displayed high basal expression of ISGs *MxA* and 2′,5′-oligoadenylate synthetase (*OAS*) in comparison with VSV susceptible PDA cells [31]. *STING* plays an important role in host defence against a range of intra-cellular pathogens and acts as a cytosolic DNA sensor [32]. The collective evidence suggests that resistance of BEAS-2B cells to IAV infection is mediated by high basal expression of antiviral genes and their subsequent strong induction (by 24 h) in response to infection. Furthermore, high basal expression of cytosolic DNA sensor *STING* in BEAS-2B cells raises the possibility that these cells could also be resistant to DNA viruses. Hence, it is prudent to determine the susceptibility of BEAS-2B cells to other viruses to assess its usefulness as an *in vitro* model for the study of virus cytopathogenesis.

Distinct profiles of antiviral gene responses following IAV infection were also noticed among the three respiratory epithelial cells (BEAS-2B, NHBE and A549 cells). In particular, the regulation of antiviral genes at 10 h of virus infection was highly variable among the cell types. Notably, A549 cells showed significantly higher expression of *IFN-β* and *IL-6* expression than BEAS-2B and NHBE cells at 10 h of infection. This could be due to higher levels of IAV replication in A549 cells compared with other cells. IL-6 is a vital innate immune cytokine in the protection against severe influenza A infection [33]. *IL-6* induction was highest in A549 cells at 10 h of infection, while it was highest at 24 h of infection in BEAS-2B and NHBE cells. While we do not know the significance of the distinct cytokine expression profiles among the three cells, clearly there were inherent differences in IAV cytopathogenesis in these cells. It is well recognised that inhibition of JAK/STAT signalling results in reduced ISG expression [31]. We showed that JAK/STAT inhibition by P6 treatment reversed the antiviral state of BEAS-2B cells as evident by the lower mRNA level of ISGs. Enhanced susceptibility of P6 treated BEAS-2B cells to IAV infection is evident from increased viral M gene RNA detection and increased production of infectious progeny virus.

In conclusion, comparison of IAV replication in three human respiratory epithelial cell types along with MDCK cells showed BEAS-2B cells to be highly resistant to avian H2N3 and human H1N1 IAV infection. Resistance of BEAS-2B cells to H1N1 virus was mediated by high basal expression of antiviral genes namely *IRF-7*, *STING*, *ISG15* and *Mx1*. JAK/STAT inhibition by P6 treatment reversed the antiviral state of BEAS-2B cells and resulted in increased H1N1 virus replication. Studies continue to make inferences on IAV pathogenesis based on results of infected BEAS-2B cells [27,34,35]. However, it is clear from our data that IAV replication and host response in BEAS-2B cells are different from primary NHBE cells. Our findings warrant evaluation of BEAS-2B cells for suitability for use with other human respiratory viruses. This study highlights the importance of using appropriate cell culture models that closely reflect viral pathogenesis in a given host species to make valid inferences.

Acknowledgments

We are grateful to Dr Ian Brown and Dr Sharon Brookes of Animal Health and Veterinary Laboratory Agency, Weybridge, UK for their help during the course of the work and kind supply of the influenza A viruses.

Author Contributions

Conceived and designed the experiments: KCC SVK. Performed the experiments: LS SVK. Analyzed the data: LS SVK JD KCC. Wrote the paper: LS SVK KCC JD.

References

1. Samson M, Pizzorno A, Abed Y, Boivin G (2013) Influenza virus resistance to neuraminidase inhibitors. Antiviral Research 98: 174–185.
2. Nelli RK, Dunham SP, Kuchipudi SV, White GA, Baquero BP, et al. (2012) Mammalian Innate Resistance to Highly Pathogenic Avian Influenza H5N1 Virus Infection is Mediated through Reduced Pro-inflammation and Infectious Virus Release. J Virol.
3. Wang H, Ma S (2008) The cytokine storm and factors determining the sequence and severity of organ dysfunction in multiple organ dysfunction syndrome. The American Journal of Emergency Medicine 26: 711–715.

4. Thitithanyanont A, Engering A, Uiprasertkul M, Ekchariyawat P, Wiboon-ut S, et al. (2010) Antiviral immune responses in H5N1-infected human lung tissue and possible mechanisms underlying the hyperproduction of interferon-inducible protein IP-10. Biochemical and Biophysical Research Communications 398: 752–758.
5. Nelli RK, Dunham SP, Kuchipudi SV, White GA, Baquero BP, et al. (2012) Mammalian Innate Resistance to Highly Pathogenic Avian Influenza H5N1 Virus Infection is Mediated through Reduced Pro-inflammation and Infectious Virus Release. Journal of Virology.
6. Matrosovich M, Stech J, Klenk H (2009) Influenza receptors, polymerase and host range. Rev Sci Tech 28: 203–217.
7. Nelli R, Kuchipudi S, White G, Perez B, Dunham S, et al. (2010) Comparative distribution of human and avian type sialic acid influenza receptors in the pig. BMC Veterinary Research 6: 1–9.
8. Gagneux P, Cheriyan M, Hurtado-Ziola N, van der Linden ECMB, Anderson D, et al. (2003) Human-specific Regulation of α2–6-linked Sialic Acids. Journal of Biological Chemistry 278: 48245–48250.
9. Shinya K, Ebina M, Yamada S, Ono M, Kasai N, et al. (2006) Avian flu: influenza virus receptors in the human airway. Nature 440: 435–436.
10. Guillot L, Le Goffic R, Bloch S, Escriou N, Akira S, et al. (2005) Involvement of Toll-like Receptor 3 in the Immune Response of Lung Epithelial Cells to Double-stranded RNA and Influenza A Virus. Journal of Biological Chemistry 280: 5571–5580.
11. Perwitasari O, Torrecilhas AC, Yan X, Johnson S, White C, et al. (2013) Targeting Cell Division Cycle 25 Homolog B To Regulate Influenza Virus Replication. Journal of Virology 87: 13775–13784.
12. Chakrabarti A, Vipat V, Mukherjee S, Singh R, Pawar S, et al. (2010) Host gene expression profiling in influenza A virus-infected lung epithelial (A549) cells: a comparative analysis between highly pathogenic and modified H5N1 viruses. Virol J 7: 219.
13. Satkunanathan S, Kumar N, Bajorek M, Purbhoo MA, Culley FJ (2014) Respiratory Syncytial Virus Infection, TLR3 Ligands, and Proinflammatory Cytokines Induce CD161 Ligand LLT1 Expression on the Respiratory Epithelium. J Virol 88: 2366–2373.
14. Munday DC, Emmott E, Surtees R, Lardeau C-H, Wu W, et al. (2010) Quantitative Proteomic Analysis of A549 Cells Infected with Human Respiratory Syncytial Virus. Molecular & Cellular Proteomics 9: 2438–2459.
15. Youil R, Su Q, Toner TJ, Szymkowiak C, Kwan WS, et al. (2004) Comparative study of influenza virus replication in Vero and MDCK cell lines. J Virol Methods 120: 23–31.
16. van den Elsen PJ, Holling TM, van der Stoep N, Boss JM (2003) DNA methylation and expression of major histocompatibility complex class I and class II transactivator genes in human developmental tumor cells and in T cell malignancies. Clin Immunol 109: 46–52.
17. Fernandez M, Porosnicu M, Markovic D, Barber GN (2002) Genetically Engineered Vesicular Stomatitis Virus in Gene Therapy: Application for Treatment of Malignant Disease. Journal of Virology 76: 895–904.
18. Stojdl DF, Lichty B, Knowles S, Marius R, Atkins H, et al. (2000) Exploiting tumor-specific defects in the interferon pathway with a previously unknown oncolytic virus. Nat Med 6: 821–825.
19. Kuchipudi SV, Dunham SP, Nelli R, White GA, Coward VJ, et al. (2012) Rapid death of duck cells infected with influenza: a potential mechanism for host resistance to H5N1. Immunol Cell Biol 90: 116–123.
20. Kuchipudi S, Nelli R, White G, Bain M, Chang K, et al. (2009) Differences in influenza virus receptors in chickens and ducks: implications for interspecies transmission. J Mol Gen Med 3: 143–151.
21. Spackman E, Senne DA, Myers TJ, Bulaga LL, Garber LP, et al. (2002) Development of a Real-Time Reverse Transcriptase PCR Assay for Type A Influenza Virus and the Avian H5 and H7 Hemagglutinin Subtypes. Journal of Clinical Microbiology 40: 3256–3260.
22. Nelli RK, Dunham SP, Kuchipudi SV, White GA, Baquero-Perez B, et al. (2012) Mammalian innate resistance to highly pathogenic avian influenza H5N1 virus infection is mediated through reduced proinflammation and infectious virus release. J Virol 86: 9201–9210.
23. Kuchipudi S, Tellabati M, Nelli R, White G, Perez B, et al. (2012) 18S rRNA is a reliable normalisation gene for real time PCR based on influenza virus infected cells. Virology Journal 9: 230.
24. Pedranzini L, Dechow T, Berishaj M, Comenzo R, Zhou P, et al. (2006) Pyridone 6, A Pan-Janus–Activated Kinase Inhibitor, Induces Growth Inhibition of Multiple Myeloma Cells. Cancer Res 66: 9714–9721.
25. Pfaffl MW, Horgan GW, Dempfle L (2002) Relative expression software tool (REST) for group-wise comparison and statistical analysis of relative expression results in real-time PCR. Nucleic Acids Res 30: e36.
26. Toyoda T (1996) [Molecular dissection of the influenza virus RNA polymerase]. Uirusu 46: 131–143.
27. Buggele WA, Johnson KE, Horvath CM (2012) Influenza A virus infection of human respiratory cells induces primary microRNA expression. J Biol Chem 287: 31027–31040.
28. Ilyushina NA, Ikizler MR, Kawaoka Y, Rudenko LG, Treanor JJ, et al. (2012) Comparative study of influenza virus replication in MDCK cells and in primary cells derived from adenoids and airway epithelium. J Virol 86: 11725–11734.
29. Hamamoto I, Takaku H, Tashiro M, Yamamoto N (2013) High yield production of influenza virus in Madin Darby canine kidney (MDCK) cells with stable knockdown of IRF7. PLoS One 8: e59892.
30. Zhao C, Collins MN, Hsiang T-Y, Krug RM (2013) Interferon-induced ISG15 pathway: an ongoing virus host battle. Trends Microbiol 21: 181–186.
31. Moerdyk-Schauwecker M, Shah NR, Murphy AM, Hastie E, Mukherjee P, et al. (2013) Resistance of pancreatic cancer cells to oncolytic vesicular stomatitis virus: Role of type I interferon signaling. Virology 436: 221–234.
32. Nakhaei P, Hiscott J, Lin R (2010) STING-ing the Antiviral Pathway. J Mol Cell Biol 2: 110–112.
33. Dienz O, Rud JG, Eaton SM, Lanthier PA, Burg E, et al. (2012) Essential role of IL-6 in protection against H1N1 influenza virus by promoting neutrophil survival in the lung. Mucosal Immunol 5: 258–266.
34. Le Goffic R, Pothlichet J, Vitour D, Fujita T, Meurs E, et al. (2007) Cutting Edge: Influenza A virus activates TLR3-dependent inflammatory and RIG-I-dependent antiviral responses in human lung epithelial cells. J Immunol 178: 3368–3372.
35. Guillot L, Le Goffic R, Bloch S, Escriou N, Akira S, et al. (2005) Involvement of toll-like receptor 3 in the immune response of lung epithelial cells to double-stranded RNA and influenza A virus. J Biol Chem 280: 5571–5580.

6

Utilisation and Off-Label Prescriptions of Respiratory Drugs in Children

Sven Schmiedl[1,2]*, Rainald Fischer[3], Luisa Ibáñez[4,5], Joan Fortuny[6], Olaf H. Klungel[7], Robert Reynolds[8], Roman Gerlach[9], Martin Tauscher[9], Petra Thürmann[1,2], Joerg Hasford[10], Marietta Rottenkolber[10]

1 Department of Clinical Pharmacology, School of Medicine, Faculty of Health, Witten/Herdecke University, Witten, Germany, **2** Philipp Klee-Institute for Clinical Pharmacology, HELIOS Clinic Wuppertal, Wuppertal, Germany, **3** Pneumologische Praxis München-Pasing, Munich, Germany, **4** Fundació Institut Català de Farmacologia, Hospital Universitari Vall d'Hebron, Barcelona, Spain, **5** Departament de Farmacologia, Terapèutica i Toxicologia, Universitat Autònoma de Barcelona, Barcelona, Spain, **6** Novartis Farmaceutica S.A., Barcelona, Spain, **7** Utrecht Institute for Pharmaceutical Sciences, Division Pharmacoepidemiology and Clinical Pharmacology, Utrecht University, Utrecht, the Netherlands, **8** Epidemiology, Pfizer, New York, New York, United States of America, **9** National Association of Statutory Health Insurance Physicians of Bavaria, Munich, Germany, **10** Institute for Medical Information Sciences, Biometry, and Epidemiology, Ludwig-Maximilians-Universitaet, Munich, Germany

Abstract

Respiratory drugs are widely used in children to treat labeled and non-labeled indications but only some data are available quantifying comprehensively off-label usage. Thus, we aim to analyse drug utilisation and off-label prescribing of respiratory drugs focusing on age- and indication-related off-label use. Patients aged ≤18 years documented in the Bavarian Association of Statutory Health Insurance Physicians database (approx. 2 million children) between 2004 and 2008 were included in our study. Annual period prevalence rates (PPRs) per 10,000 children and the proportion of age- and indication-related off-label prescriptions were calculated and stratified by age and gender. Within the study period, highest PPRs were found for the fixed combination of clenbuterol/ambroxol (between 374–575 per 10,000 children) and the inhaled short acting beta-2-agonist salbutamol (between 378–527 per 10,000 children). Highest relative PPR increase was found for oral salbutamol (approx. 39-fold) whereas the most distinct decrease was found for oral long-acting beta-2-agonist clenbuterol (−97%). Compound classes most frequently involved in off-label prescribing were inhaled bronchodilative compounds (91,402; 37.3%) and oral beta-2-agonists (26,850; 22.5%). The highest absolute number of off-label prescriptions were found for inhaled salbutamol (n = 67,084; 42.0%) and oral clenbuterol/ambroxol (fixed combination, n = 18,897; 20.7%). Off-label prescribing due to indication was of much greater relevance than age-related off-label use. Most frequently, bronchodilative compounds were used off-label to treat respiratory tract infections. Highest off-label prescription rates were found in the youngest patients without relevant gender-related differences. Off-label prescribing of respiratory drugs is common especially in young children. Bronchodilative drugs were most frequently used off-label for treating acute bronchitis or upper respiratory tract infections underlining the essential need for a more rational prescribing in this area.

Editor: Imti Choonara, Nottingham University, United Kingdom

Funding: The PROTECT project has received support from the Innovative Medicines Initiative Joint Undertaking (www.imi.europa.eu) under Grant Agreement n° 115004, resources of which are composed of financial contribution from the European Union's Seventh Framework Programme (FP7/2007–2013) and EFPIA companies' in kind contribution. In addition, as a special form of the IMI JU grant, Utrecht University received a direct financial contribution from Pfizer. The funders had no role in study design, data collection and analysis, decision to publish, or preparation of the manuscript.

Competing Interests: RF, LI, OK, RG, MT, JH, and MR have no conflicts of interest. PT and SS report personal lecture fees from Rottapharm Madaus (Cologne, Germany). RR is employed by Pfizer belonging to EFPIA (European Federation of Pharmaceutical Industries and Association) member companies in the IMI J Ua n d costs related to their part in the research were carried by the respective company as in-kind contribution under the IMI JU scheme. JF is employed by Novartis Farmaceutica S.A., Barcelona, Spain belonging to EFPIA (European Federation of Pharmaceutical Industries and Association) member companies in the IMI JU and costs related to their part in the research were carried by the respective company as in-kind contribution under the IMI JU scheme.

* Email: sven.schmiedl@helios-kliniken.de

Introduction

Respiratory drugs are frequently prescribed to paediatric patients for a wide range of airway diseases but most of these drugs are only approved for asthma and COPD from a particular age onwards [1,2]. In young children, diagnosing asthma is difficult due to general limitations (e.g. ability to follow instructions for lung function measurements) which might contribute to a low fraction of patients with lung function testing and an under-diagnosis of asthma [3]. In addition, respiratory drugs are frequently used for symptomatic improvement of airway diseases (e.g. acute respiratory infections) or are prescribed as a diagnostic instrument to confirm a diagnosis of asthma [1,2]. All these reasons contribute to a high fraction of children receiving respiratory medication as off-label treatment [1,2], a factor which has been reported as a risk for adverse drug reactions [4–6].

Whereas some data are available about anti-asthmatic drug utilisation in children [7,8], the extent of off-label usage for these compounds has been quantified only in few studies [1,2,9]. Furthermore, generalizability of off-label results is limited due to e.g. national drug market characteristics and differing age groups of patients included in these studies [1,9]. In addition, some other aspects as for example time trends in off-label prescriptions or gender-related aspects have not been analysed in detail in these studies.

Thus, we aimed to analyse drug utilisation and indication- and age-related off-label use for respiratory drugs in children.

Methods

Database and study population

This study was performed using the Bavarian Association of Statutory Health Insurance Physicians database which covers approximately 2 million insured children aged ≤18 years (85% of the Bavarian paediatric population) excluding those with a private insurance [10]. All diagnoses of general practitioners and specialists were documented and a prescription was recorded in the database only if it was prescribed and filled at the pharmacy. Diagnoses and drugs were coded according to the International Classification of Diseases codes (ICD-10-GM) and the Anatomical Therapeutic Chemical (ATC-) classification, respectively [11,12]. Every child (≤18 years) receiving at least one prescription of respiratory drugs as stated in table 1 between 2004 and 2008 were included in the study. Analyses were restricted to drugs with an annual period prevalence rate (PPR) for the year 2008 of at least 0.1 per 10,000 children. All analyses were done using completely anonymised data only. The German law and the professional code of conduct for physicians do not ask for an ethical review for research with anonymised data.

Off-label analysis

For compounds stated in table 1, off-label analysis based on patient's age and indication was performed. The lower approved age and the approved indication were collected using the official summary of product characteristics (SPC) [13,14] and the Pharmaceutical Index for Germany [15] for the years 2004 and 2008 (beginning and end of the study period, table 1). If more than one age restriction existed for different devices or different years within the study period, we used the lowest age restriction for the respective ATC code. To analyse off-label prescriptions by indication, the widest definition was used if more than one definition for indications existed (table 1).

Statistical analysis

Annual period prevalence rates (PPRs) were calculated using the number of children with at least one prescription of interest during the year of interest (numerator) divided by the total number of children living in Bavaria at the end of the year (December, 31; denominator), based on the data of the Bavarian State Office for Statistics and Data Processing [16]. Under the assumption of equal age- and gender-distribution of children in the statutory and private health insurance, we used a correction factor (0.85) considering the statutory health insurance coverage of 85% of the total Bavarian population. Annual PPRs were calculated and stratifications by age (one-year age groups) and gender were performed.

Off-label prescriptions were analysed as proportion and stratifications by type of off-label prescriptions ('age', 'indication', and 'age&indication'), patient's age (one-year age groups) and gender were performed. All analyses were performed using IBM SPSS Statistics Version 20.0 and GNU R Version 3.0.1 (http://www.r-project.org/).

Results

Drug utilization

Within the study period, highest annual PPRs were found for the fixed combination of oral clenbuterol/ambroxol (between 374–575 per 10,000 children) and the inhaled short acting beta-2-agonist salbutamol (between 378–527 per 10,000 children). By comparing PPRs of 2004 and 2008, the highest absolute PPR increase was found for inhaled salbutamol (+149 per 10,000 children) whereas for clenbuterol/ambroxol, the most pronounced decrease was found (−113 per 10,000 children). Regarding relative PPR changes, highest increases were found for oral salbutamol (approx. 39-fold) and the fixed combination beclomethasone (approx. 2.5-fold) whereas the most distinct decrease was found for oral clenbuterol (−97%) and inhaled terbutaline (−77%, figure 1).

For 2008, age-related PPR patterns were similar for both genders but for most compounds, PPRs were higher for boys compared to girls. In children aged <6 years old, inhaled salbutamol and the fixed combination oral clenbuterol/ambroxol were the most frequently prescribed compounds whereas in adolescents (15–18 years), highest PPRs were found for salbutamol and budesonide (Table S1, S2).

Off-label prescriptions

The extent of off-label prescriptions related to the three types of off-label prescriptions 'age', 'indication' or 'age&indication' is shown in table 2 for the year 2008. The highest absolute number of off-label prescriptions including these three types of off-label prescribing were found for inhaled bronchodilative drugs (i.e. short-acting beta-2-agonist (SABA), long-acting beta-2-agonist (LABA), short-acting muscarinic antagonist (SAMA), and long-acting muscarinic antagonist (LAMA), including fixed combinations) with n = 91,402 (37.3% of all inhaled bronchodilative drugs) followed by oral beta-2-agonists (including fixed combinations) with n = 26,850 (22.5%). Regarding single compounds, inhaled salbutamol (n = 67,084; 42.0%) and oral clenbuterol/ambroxol (fixed combination, n = 18,897; 20.7%) were most frequently prescribed off-label. In most of these patients, off-label prescriptions due to "indication only" were present (inhaled bronchodilative drugs: 90,443 [99.0% of all off-label prescriptions], inhaled salbutamol 67,084 [100%], oral beta-2-agonists (including fixed combinations): 26,812 [99.9%], and oral clenbuterol/ambroxol (fixed combination): 18,897 [100%]; table 2).

By analyzing off-label indications in detail (combined analysis of off-label prescriptions due to 'indication' and 'age&indication'; table 3), we found that inhaled salbutamol was most frequently used off-label for treating acute bronchitis (n = 29,989, 44.7% of all off-label prescriptions due to 'indication' and 'age&indication') and acute upper respiratory infections (n = 23,827, 35.5% [multiple counting of off-label indications]). Similarly, oral clenbuterol/ambroxol (fixed combination) was most frequently prescribed off-label for treating acute upper respiratory infections (n = 9,131, 48.3%). For the compound classes most frequently used off-label (i.e. inhaled bronchodilative drugs and oral beta-2-agonists [including fixed combinations]), acute bronchitis and/or acute upper respiratory tract infections were the most common off-label indications (Table S3).

Regarding age, we observed the highest proportion of off-label prescriptions in youngest children aged under 6 years. For some compounds (e.g. formoterol) we found highest off-label prescriptions in youngest children and adolescents (u-shape; Table S4). We did not observe relevant differences in off label prescriptions between male and female children (Table S4). Focussing on

Table 1. Age restrictions and indications for selected respiratory drug classes.

Compound class	Compound	ATC-code*	Age restriction	Approved indication(s)
Inhaled SABA	Salbutamol	R03AC02	None	Asthma, chronic obstructive bronchitis, pulmonary emphysema with reversible obstruction, prophylaxis of allergic asthma and exercise-induced asthma
	Fenoterol	R03AC04	≥4 years	Asthma, chronic obstructive bronchitis, pulmonary emphysema with reversible obstruction, prophylaxis of allergic asthma and exercise-induced asthma
	Terbutaline	R03AC03	≥5 years	Asthma, chronic obstructive bronchitis, pulmonary emphysema with reversible obstruction
Inhaled SABA combination	Ipratropium/Fenoterol (fixed combination)	R03AK03	None	Asthma, COPD
	Reproterol/CGA (fixed combination)	R03AK05	None	Asthma
Inhaled LABA	Salmeterol	R03AC12	≥4 years	Asthma, COPD
	Formoterol	R03AC13	≥6 years	Asthma, COPD
Inhaled LABA/ICS	Salmeterol/Fluticasone (fixed combination)	R03AK06	≥4 years	Asthma, COPD
	Formoterol/Beclomethasone (fixed combination)	R03AK27	≥6 years	Asthma
	Formoterol/Budesonide (fixed combination)	R03AK28	≥6 years	Asthma, COPD
Inhaled SAMA	Ipratropium	R03BB01	None	Asthma, COPD
Inhaled LAMA	Tiotropium	R03BB04	≥18 years	COPD
ICS	Budesonide	R03BA02	None	Respiratory diseases (inclusive asthma and COPD) requiring ICS
	Beclomethasone	R03BA01	None	Respiratory diseases (inclusive asthma and COPD) requiring ICS
	Fluticasone	R03BA05	≥4 years	Asthma, COPD
	Ciclesonide	R03BA08	≥12 years	Asthma
Oral B2A	Salbutamol	R03CC02	None	Obstructive respiratory diseases, asthma, COPD, pulmonary emphysema
	Terbutaline	R03CC03	None	Obstructive respiratory diseases, asthma, COPD, pulmonary emphysema
	Tulobuterol	R03CC11	≥1year	Obstructive respiratory diseases, asthma, COPD, pulmonary emphysema
	Clenbuterol	R03CC13	None	Asthma, asthmatic bronchitis, chronic bronchitis, pulmonary emphysema
Oral B2A combinations	Clenbuterol/Ambroxol	R03CC63	None	Acute and chronic bronchitis, pulmonary emphysema, asthma
Others	Theophylline	R03DA04	≥1year	Asthma, COPD
	Montelukast	R03DC03	≥1 year	Asthma, prophylaxis of exercise-induced asthma
	Cromoglicic acid	R03BC01	≥2 years	Asthma

SABA: Short-acting beta-2-agonist, CGA: Cromoglicic acid, LABA: Long-acting beta-2-agonist, ICS: Inhaled corticosteroid, SAMA: Short-acting muscarinic antagonist, LAMA: Long-acting muscarinic antagonist, B2A: Beta-2-agonist. (*German version available at http://www.dimdi.de/static/de/amg/atcddd/index.htm).

changes over time (2004 versus 2008), the increase in the absolute number of off-label prescriptions was highest for inhaled (n = 21,841; +48.3%) and oral salbutamol (n = 5,422; +4,444.3%) whereas the highest decrease was found for CGA (n = −10,195; −75.8%) and oral clenbuterol/ambroxol (n = −6,196; −24.7%). In contrast, we found only small changes (less than 10%) in the proportion of off-label prescriptions for most compounds comparing 2004 and 2008 indicating that observed changes in absolute numbers of off-label prescriptions are mainly attributable to changes in absolute numbers of total prescriptions (Table S5).

Discussion

By analysing prescription patterns of respiratory drugs, we found highest PPRs for the fixed combination of clenbuterol/ambroxol and inhaled salbutamol. In our study, highest absolute numbers of off-label prescriptions were found for bronchodilative compounds including the most frequently prescribed drugs (i.e. inhaled salbutamol and the fixed combination of oral clenbuterol/ambroxol). For most compounds, off-label prescribing was mainly due to indication for treating respiratory tract infections.

Drug utilisation

Similar to our results, there are several studies reporting SABA and ICS as most prevalent respiratory drugs used in children [7,8,17]. Nevertheless, there is some inter-country variation as reported by Bianchi et al. [7]. Whereas SABA is the most prescribed anti-asthmatic drug class in e.g. Denmark and the USA, in Italy inhaled corticosteroids is the most frequently prescribed drug class. Despite similar results, a comparison of these studies with our results is limited due to some methodological aspects (e.g. differences in age groups and source of prescription data). Furthermore, national specialities in drug markets (i.e.

national drug approval for "older" compounds) and historically grown, specific national prescription behaviour might have contributed to some differences. In Germany, for example, a fixed combination of clenbuterol/ambroxol has been widely used whereas in other countries, no comparable fixed combination drug is available.

There are few studies reporting trends in asthma medication prescriptions [1,17]. Whereas Elkout et al. reported the fraction of patients aged less than 19 years of age treated with a particular drug class [17], Baiardi et al. presented the number of prescriptions for eleven compounds representing 90% of R03 (according to ATC) prescriptions given to children aged between 0 and 14 years of age [1]. Despite these methodological differences compared to our study reporting PPR, some issues are worth to be mentioned. Baiardi et al. [1] reported a stable number of inhaled salbutamol prescriptions whereas in our study, we found an increase in inhaled and oral salbutamol prescriptions which might correspond to a decreased prescriptions for the fixed combination of oral (long-acting beta-2-agonist) clenbuterol/ambroxol and oral terbutaline.

Off-label prescriptions

In our study, highest absolute numbers of off-label prescriptions were found for inhaled salbutamol and the fixed combination of oral clenbuterol/ambroxol. In most cases, off-label prescriptions were made to treat acute respiratory tract infections. In general, we found that a much higher proportion of off-label prescriptions were due to indication than due to age. This has also been reported by Baiardi et al. [1] whereas Sen et al. [9] did not report comprehensively age-related off-label usage and did primarily focus on indication-related off-label use.

Comparing our results for indication related off-label prescriptions with other studies, we found similar proportions for most compounds (Table S6). Nevertheless, some methodological issues will limit transferability of results. In addition to the issues mentioned already for the analyses conducted by Baiardi et al. [1], Sen et al. [9] did use general practice databases whereas in our study, prescriptions made by specialists are included too. Furthermore, we used the widest definition stated in the SPC for a specific compound whereas Baiardi et al. [1] did use more restrictive definitions of indications leading to a higher rates of off-label prescriptions for some compounds (Table S6). Since Zuidgeest et al. [2] did not report compound specific off-label rates, we abstained from presenting and discussing these results in detail.

As described by Baiardi et al. [1], respiratory tract infections and bronchiolitis were frequent off-label diagnoses in our study, too. Apart from formal implications of using drugs outside the approved indications, these results may underline a somewhat irrational prescribing which has been criticized before [18,19]. According to guidelines, systematic reviews, and meta-analyses, neither beta-2-agonists nor inhaled corticosteroids should be routinely recommended as treatment options for these indications due to lacking efficacy [20–23]. Of course in some patients, bronchodilators may lead to a transient clinical improvement but this should be weighed against potential adverse effects and the fact that most children will not benefit [20]. Nevertheless, as shown by de Brasi et al. [19] and Ochoa Sangrador et al. [24],

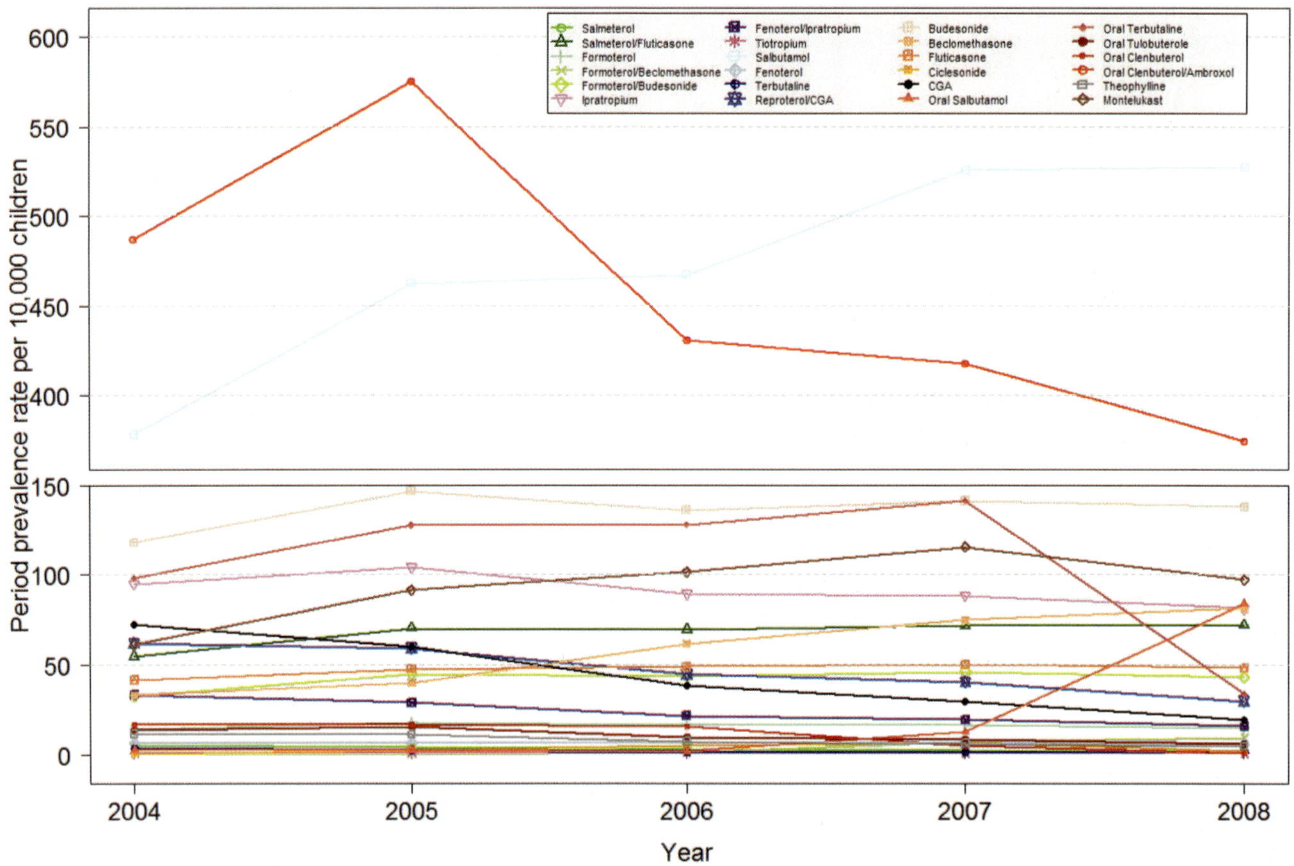

Figure 1. Annual period prevalence rates per 10,000 children (≤18 years) between 2004 and 2008.

Table 2. Number and proportion of off-label prescriptions stratified by off-label type (year 2008).

Compound class	Compound	All prescriptions (n)	Off-label overall (n,%)	Off-label due to age only (n)	Off-label due to indication only (n)	Off-label due to age and indication (n)
Inhaled SABA	**Salbutamol**	159,655	67,084 (42.0%)	0	67,084	0
	Fenoterol	1,452	383 (26.4%)	6	367	10
	Terbutaline	184	34 (18.5%)	0	33	1
Inhaled SABA combination	**Fenoterol/Ipratropium (fixed combination)**	3,998	1,722 (43.1%)	0	1,722	0
	Reproterol/CGA (fixed combination)	8,729	2,538 (29.1%)	0	2,538	0
Inhaled SABA (incl. combination) Total		174,018	71,761 (41.2%)	6	71,744	11
Inhaled LABA	**Salmeterol**	522	86 (16.5%)	9	75	2
	Formoterol	4,931	839 (17.0%)	88	730	21
Inhaled LABA/ICS	**Salmeterol/Fluticasone (fixed combination)**	27,600	4,278 (15.5%)	368	3,734	176
	Formoterol/Beclomethasone (fixed combination)	2,515	848 (33.7%)	11	827	10
	Formoterol/Budesonide (fixed combination)	13,833	2,584 (18.7%)	113	2,412	59
Inhaled LABA (incl. combination) Total		49,401	8,635 (17.5%)	589	7,778	268
SAMA	**Ipratropium**	21,822	10,910 (50.0%)	0	10,910	0
LAMA	**Tiotropium**	97	96 (99.0%)	9	11	76
Muscarinic antagonists (SAMA & LAMA) Total		21,919	11,006 (50.2%)	9	10,921	76
Inhaled bronchodilative drugs (SABA, LABA, SAMA, LAMA [incl. combination]) Total		**245,338**	**91,402 (37.3%)**	**604**	**90,443**	**355**
ICS	**Budesonide**	42,067	3,166 (7.5%)	0	3,166	0
	Beclomethasone	24,185	1,922 (7.9%)	0	1,922	0
	Fluticasone	17,097	5,360 (31.4%)	1,917	2,370	1,073
	Ciclesonide	326	110 (33.7%)	35	60	15
ICS total		83,675	10,558 (12.6%)	1,952	7,518	1,088
Oral B2A	**Salbutamol**	19,475	5,544 (28.5%)	0	5,544	0
	Terbutaline	6,940	2,012 (29.0%)	0	2,012	0
	Tulobuterol	1,201	330 (27.5%)	32	292	6
	Clenbuterol	113	67 (59.3%)	0	67	0
Oral B2A combination	**Clenbuterol/Ambroxol (fixed combination)**	91,385	18,897 (20.7%)	0	18,897	0
Oral B2A (incl. combination) total		119,114	26,850 (22.5%)	32	26,812	6
Others	**Theophylline**	1,184	451 (38.1%)	7	419	25
	Montelukast	33,501	12,826 (38.3%)	304	11,831	691
	Cromoglicic acid	5,087	3,247 (63.8%)	110	2,724	413
Others Total		39,772	16,524 (41.5%)	421	14,974	1,129
All drugs Total		**487,899**	**145,334 (29.8%)**	**3,009**	**139,747**	**2,578**

SABA: Short-acting beta-2-agonist, CGA: Cromoglicic acid, LABA: Long-acting beta-2-agonist, ICS: Inhaled corticosteroid, SAMA: Short-acting muscarinic antagonist, LAMA: Long-acting muscarinic antagonist, B2A: Beta-2-agonist.

Table 3. Number and proportion of the three most frequent off-label indications for drugs with at least 5,000 prescriptions (year 2008, multiple counting of off-label indications per prescription).

Compound class	Compound	All prescriptions (n)	Off-label due to 'indication' or 'age&indication' (n,% of all prescriptions)	Three most frequent off-label indications* (n, % of all off-label prescriptions due to 'indication' and 'age&indication')
Inhaled SABA	**Salbutamol**	159,655	67,084 (42.0%)	Acute bronchitis: 29,989 (44.7%), Acute upper respiratory infections: 23,827 (35.5%), Other diseases of upper respiratory tract: 13,267 (19.8%)
Inhaled SABA combination	**Reproterol/CGA (fixed combination)**	8,729	2,538 (29.1%)	Other disease of upper respiratory tract: 999 (39.4%), Acute upper respiratory tract infections: 402 (15.8%), Bronchitis nec: 259 (10.2%)
Inhaled LABA/ICS	**Salmeterol/Fluticasone (fixed combination)**	27,600	3,910 (14.2%)	Other diseases of upper respiratory tract: 1,066 (27.3%), Acute bronchitis: 751 (19.2%), Acute upper respiratory infections: 679 (17.4%)
	Formoterol/Budesonide (fixed combination)	13,833	2,471 (17.9%)	Other diseases of upper respiratory tract: 621 (25.1%), Acute upper respiratory infections: 456 (18.5%), Bronchitis nec: 428 (17.3%)
Inhaled SAMA	**Ipratropium**	21,822	10,910 (50.0%)	Acute bronchitis: 5,779 (53.0%), Acute upper respiratory infections: 4,124 (37.8%), Bronchitis nec: 2,033 (18.6%)
ICS	**Fluticasone**	17,097	3,443 (20.1%)	Acute bronchitis: 1,096 (31.8%), Acute upper respiratory infections: 977 (28.4%), Other diseases of upper respiratory tract: 847 (24.6%)
Oral B2A	**Oral Salbutamol**	19,475	5,544 (28.5%)	Acute upper respiratory infections: 2,431 (43.8%), Bronchitis nec: 2,020 (36.4%), Other diseases of upper respiratory tract: 1,001 (18.1%)
	Oral Terbutaline	6,940	2,012 (29.0%)	Acute upper respiratory infections: 880 (43.7%), Bronchitis nec: 773 (38.4%), Other diseases of upper respiratory tract: 348 (17.3%)
Oral B2A combination	**Oral Clenbuterol/ Ambroxol (fixed combination)**	91,385	18,897 (20.7%)	Acute upper respiratory infections: 9,131 (48.3%), Other diseases of upper respiratory tract: 2,767 (14.6%), Other respiratory diseases: 2,228 (11.8%)
Others	**Montelukast**	33,501	12,522 (37.4%)	Acute bronchitis: 3,868 (30.9%), Acute upper respiratory infections: 3,850 (30.7%), Other diseases of upper respiratory tract: 3,014 (24.1%)
	Cromoglicic acid	5,087	3,137 (61.7%)	Acute upper respiratory infections: 1,151 (36.7%), Acute bronchitis: 1,101 (35.1%), Other diseases of upper respiratory tract: 789 (25.2%)

SABA: Short-acting beta-2-agonist, CGA: Cromoglicic acid, LABA: Long-acting beta-2-agonist, ICS: Inhaled corticosteroid, SAMA: Short-acting muscarinic antagonist, B2A: Beta-2-agonist, nec: not elsewhere classified.
*Exclusive missing indications.

there is a relevant overuse of both compounds which has been attributed to e.g. physicians' recognition of disease severity, personal reassurance, and parental pressure [19]. On the other hand, by developing and implementing clinical guidelines, a more rational prescribing leading to less overtreatment seems reachable [25,26].

Limitations and Strengths

As for all observational studies, there are few limitations worth to be mentioned. First, as in most claims data analyses, we were not able to include clinical data (e.g. lung function parameter) and thus, we did focus on drug prescription instead of analysing patients in detail comparing on- and off-label users (as already done [27]). Second, we did analyse off-label treatment based on a compound- and not on a device-level using widest restrictions (age and/or indication) if different age restrictions or indications were mentioned in the respective summary of product characteristics. This approach will lead to an underestimation of off-label prescriptions for some compounds (e.g. formoterol, fixed combination of salmeterol/fluticasone) whereas for the majority of drugs or drug classes, all available devices have the same age restriction and labeled indication. Third, there are some uncertainties in matching specific ICD-codes needed for analyzing databases and indications stated in the SPC in particular when general terms have been used in the SPC. This might have influenced the number of calculated off-label prescriptions. Nevertheless, most of the terms used for defining off-label usage are comparable to other publications [1]. Fourth, within on-label prescriptions we did not discriminate between different compound classes regarding their efficiency. For example, asthma is a labeled indication for ipratropium but the role of anticholinergic compounds has been critically discussed in particular for asthmatic children [28]. Furthermore, inhaled SABA is the recommended reliever treatment whereas inhaled anticholinergics are considered only as alternative treatments according to the guidelines [29]. Fifth, since we use a statutory health insurance database, children with a private health insurance were not included. Hence, a bias due to socioeconomic status can not be excluded in our study. But one has to keep in mind that the database used covers with 85% the majority of the children in Bavaria.

Besides a few limitations, there are also some strengths of our study. First of all, we did use a large database with a good population coverage (85%) covering 2.0 million children. Second, not only data from general practitioners but also from specialists were included in our study. Third, since we did analyse a time period and did not only perform a cross-sectional analysis, we are able to quantify time trends in off-label prescriptions, which (to the best our knowledge) has not been performed before for children receiving respiratory medication.

Conclusion

In our study analysing respiratory drugs, we found highest PPRs for inhaled salbutamol and the fixed combination of oral clenbuterol/ambroxol. Off-label prescribing of respiratory drugs is common especially in young children. Bronchodilative drugs were most frequently used off-label for treating acute bronchitis or upper respiratory tract infections underlining the essential need for a more rational prescribing in this area.

Supporting Information

Table S1 Period prevalence rates for boys stratified by age for the year 2008. SABA: Short-acting beta-2-agonist, CGA: Cromoglicic Acid, LABA: Long-acting beta-2-agonist, ICS: Inhaled corticosteroid, SAMA: Short-acting muscarinic antagonist, LAMA: Long-acting muscarinic antagonist, B2A: Beta-2-agonist.

Table S2 Period prevalence rates for girls stratified by age for the year 2008. SABA: Short-acting beta-2-agonist, CGA: Cromoglicic Acid, LABA: Long-acting beta-2-agonist, ICS: Inhaled corticosteroid, SAMA: Short-acting muscarinic antagonist, LAMA: Long-acting muscarinic antagonist, B2A: Beta-2-agonist.

Table S3 Number and proportion of off-label indications (year 2008, multiple counting of off-label indications per prescription). SABA: Short-acting beta-2-agonist, CGA: Cromoglicic Acid, LABA: Long acting beta-2-agonist, ICS: Inhaled corticosteroid, SAMA: Short-acting muscarinic antagonist, LAMA: Long-acting muscarinic antagonist, B2A: Beta-2-agonist, nec: not elsewhere classified, n.a.: not applicable (i.e. labeled diagnoses).

Table S4 Number and proportion of off-label prescriptions stratified by off-label type, gender, and age group (year 2008). SABA: Short-acting beta-2-agonist, CGA: Cromoglicic Acid, LABA: Long-acting beta-2-agonist, ICS: Inhaled corticosteroid, SAMA: Short-acting muscarinic antagonist, LAMA: Long-acting muscarinic antagonist, B2A: Beta-2-agonist.

Table S5 Number and proportion of off-label prescriptions for the years 2004 to 2008. SABA: Short-acting beta-2-agonist, CGA: Cromoglicic Acid, LABA: Long-acting beta-2-agonist, ICS: Inhaled corticosteroid, SAMA: Short-acting muscarinic antagonist, LAMA: Long-acting muscarinic antagonist, B2A: Beta-2-agonist, n.a.: not applicable.

Table S6 Comparison of the proportion of off-label usage due to indication in several European countries. SABA: Short-acting beta-2-agonist, LABA: Long-acting beta-2-agonist, ICS: Inhaled corticosteroid, SAMA: Short-acting muscarinic antagonist.

Acknowledgment

The research leading to these results was conducted as part of the PROTECT consortium (Pharmacoepidemiological Research on Outcomes of Therapeutics by a European ConsorTium, www.imi-protect.eu) which is a public-private partnership coordinated by the European Medicines Agency. The views expressed in this article are the personal views of the authors and may not be understood or quoted as being made on behalf of or reflecting the position of the European Medicines Agency or one of its committees or working parties.

Author Contributions

Conceived and designed the experiments: SS RF LI JF OK RR RG MT PT JH MR. Analyzed the data: MR SS RF RG MT PT JH. Wrote the paper: SS MR RF LI JF OK RR RG MT PT JH.

References

1. Baiardi P, Ceci A, Felisi M, Cantarutti L, Girotto S, et al. (2010) In-label and off-label use of respiratory drugs in the Italian paediatric population. Acta Paediatr 99: 544–549.
2. Zuidgeest MG, van Dijk L, Smit HA, van der Wouden JC, Brunekreef B, et al. (2008) Prescription of respiratory medication without an asthma diagnosis in children: a population based study. BMC Health Serv Res 8: 16.
3. Bianchi M, Clavenna A, Sequi M, Bortolotti A, Fortino I, et al. (2012) Spirometry testing in a population of Italian children: age and gender differences. Respir Med 106: 1383–1388.
4. Conroy S (2011) Association between licence status and medication errors. Arch Dis Child 96: 305–306.
5. Neubert A, Dormann H, Weiss J, Egger T, Criegee-Rieck M, et al. (2004) The impact of unlicensed and off-label drug use on adverse drug reactions in paediatric patients. Drug Saf 27: 1059–1067.
6. Ufer M, Kimland E, Bergman U (2004) Adverse drug reactions and off-label prescribing for paediatric outpatients: a one-year survey of spontaneous reports in Sweden. Pharmacoepidemiol Drug Saf 13: 147–152.
7. Bianchi M, Clavenna A, Bonati M (2010) Inter-country variations in anti-asthmatic drug prescriptions for children. Systematic review of studies published during the 2000–2009 period. Eur J Clin Pharmacol 66: 929–936.
8. Zuidgeest MG, Koster ES, Maitland-van der Zee AH, Smit HA, Brunekreef B, et al. (2010) Asthma therapy during the first 8 years of life: a PIAMA cohort study. J Asthma 47: 209–213.
9. Sen EF, Verhamme KM, Neubert A, Hsia Y, Murray M, et al. (2011) Assessment of pediatric asthma drug use in three European countries; a TEDDY study. Eur J Pediatr 170: 81–92.
10. KVB The Bavarian Association of Statutory Health Insurance Physicians (Kassenärztliche Vereinigung Bayerns).
11. Graubner B (2008) ICD-10-GM Internationale statistische Klassifikation der Krankheiten und verwandter Gesundheitsprobleme, 10. Revision, German Modification, Version 2009. Deutscher Ärzte-Verlag: Köln.
12. WHO (1992) Anatomical Therapeutic Chemical (ATC) Classification Index. Geneva: WHO Collaborating Centre for Drug Statistics Methodology.
13. Rote Liste Service GmbH (2013) FachInfo-Service, Fachinformationsverzeichnis Deutschland (einschließlich EU-Zulassungen).
14. Deutsches Institut für Medizinische Dokumentation und Information (2013) AMIS - öffentlicher Teil.
15. Rote Liste Service GmbH (2013) Rote Liste - Arzneimittelinformationen für Deutschland (einschließlich EU-Zulassungen und bestimmter Medizinprodukte).
16. Bayerisches Landesamt für Statistik und Datenverarbeitung (2013) Bevölkerung Bayern.
17. Elkout H, Helms PJ, Simpson CR, McLay JS (2012) Changes in primary care prescribing patterns for paediatric asthma: a prescribing database analysis. Arch Dis Child 97: 521–525.
18. Choonara I (2013) Rational prescribing is important in all settings. Arch Dis Child 98: 720.
19. De Brasi D, Pannuti F, Antonelli F, de Seta F, Siani P, et al. (2010) Therapeutic approach to bronchiolitis: why pediatricians continue to overprescribe drugs? Ital J Pediatr 36: 67.
20. American Academy of Pediatrics Subcommittee on Diagnosis and Management of Bronchiolitis (2006) Diagnosis and management of bronchiolitis. Pediatrics 118: 1774–1793.

21. Fernandes RM, Bialy LM, Vandermeer B, Tjosvold L, Plint AC, et al. (2013) Glucocorticoids for acute viral bronchiolitis in infants and young children. Cochrane Database Syst Rev 6: CD004878.
22. Gadomski AM, Brower M (2010) Bronchodilators for bronchiolitis. Cochrane Database Syst Rev: CD001266.
23. Hartling L, Fernandes RM, Bialy L, Milne A, Johnson D, et al. (2011) Steroids and bronchodilators for acute bronchiolitis in the first two years of life: systematic review and meta-analysis. BMJ 342: d1714.
24. Ochoa Sangrador C, Gonzalez de Dios J, Research Group of the aBREVIADo Project (2012) Management of acute bronchiolitis in emergency wards in Spain: variability and appropriateness analysis (aBREVIADo Project). Eur J Pediatr 171: 1109–1119.
25. Barben J, Kuehni CE, Trachsel D, Hammer J, Swiss Paediatric Respiratory Research G (2008) Management of acute bronchiolitis: can evidence based guidelines alter clinical practice? Thorax 63: 1103–1109.
26. Parikh K, Hall M, Teach SJ (2014) Bronchiolitis management before and after the AAP guidelines. Pediatrics 133: e1–7.
27. McCowan C, Hoskins G, Neville RG (2007) Clinical symptoms and 'off-label' prescribing in children with asthma. Br J Gen Pract 57: 220–222.
28. Teoh L, Cates CJ, Hurwitz M, Acworth JP, van Asperen P, et al. (2012) Anticholinergic therapy for acute asthma in children. Cochrane Database Syst Rev 4: CD003797.
29. Global Initiative for Asthma (GINA) (2012) Global strategy for asthma management and prevention (Updated 2012).

7

Novel Respiratory Syncytial Virus (RSV) Genotype ON1 Predominates in Germany during Winter Season 2012–13

Julia Tabatabai[1,2], Christiane Prifert[3], Johannes Pfeil[4,5], Jürgen Grulich-Henn[4], Paul Schnitzler[1]*

1 Department of Infectious Diseases, Virology, University of Heidelberg, Heidelberg, Germany, **2** London School of Hygiene and Tropical Medicine, London, United Kingdom, **3** Institute of Virology and Immunobiology, University of Würzburg, Würzburg, Germany, **4** Department of Pediatrics, University of Heidelberg, Heidelberg, Germany, **5** German Centre for Infectious Diseases (DZIF), Heidelberg, Germany

Abstract

Respiratory syncytial virus (RSV) is the leading cause of hospitalization especially in young children with respiratory tract infections (RTI). Patterns of circulating RSV genotypes can provide a better understanding of the molecular epidemiology of RSV infection. We retrospectively analyzed the genetic diversity of RSV infection in hospitalized children with acute RTI admitted to University Hospital Heidelberg/Germany between October 2012 and April 2013. Nasopharyngeal aspirates (NPA) were routinely obtained in 240 children younger than 2 years of age who presented with clinical symptoms of upper or lower RTI. We analyzed NPAs via PCR and sequence analysis of the second variable region of the RSV G gene coding for the attachment glycoprotein. We obtained medical records reviewing routine clinical data. RSV was detected in 134/240 children. In RSV-positive patients the most common diagnosis was bronchitis/bronchiolitis (75.4%). The mean duration of hospitalization was longer in RSV-positive compared to RSV-negative patients (3.5 vs. 5.1 days; $p<0.01$). RSV-A was detected in 82.1%, RSV-B in 17.9% of all samples. Phylogenetic analysis of 112 isolates revealed that the majority of RSV-A strains (65%) belonged to the novel ON1 genotype containing a 72-nucleotide duplication. However, genotype ON1 was not associated with a more severe course of illness when taking basic clinical/laboratory parameters into account. Molecular characterization of RSV confirms the co-circulation of multiple genotypes of subtype RSV-A and RSV-B. The duplication in the G gene of genotype ON1 might have an effect on the rapid spread of this emerging RSV strain.

Editor: Steven M. Varga, University of Iowa, United States of America

Funding: The authors have no support or funding to report.

Competing Interests: The authors have declared that no competing interests exist.

* Email: Paul_Schnitzler@med.uni-heidelberg.de

Introduction

Respiratory syncytial virus (RSV) is the major pathogen of lower respiratory tract infections (RTI) in infants and young children. By the age of 2 years, virtually all children have been infected at least once with RSV [1]. Re-infections are common throughout life; in older children and adults infections are associated with milder disease indicating that RSV induces only partial immunity [2]. Strain variation is thought to contribute to its ability to cause frequent re-infections [3] enabling RSV to remain present at high levels in the population [4]. Viral strains are separated into two major groups based on its genetic and antigenic variability. Several lineages within the subtypes RSV-A and RSV-B co-circulate simultaneously in the population [5] and their relative proportions may differ between epidemics, although RSV-A viruses tend to predominate [6]. The main differences between RSV-A and RSV-B are found in the attachment (G) glycoprotein [7]. The G protein is a type II surface glycoprotein of about 300 amino acids in length, consisting of a cytoplasmic domain, a transmembrane domain and an ectodomain. The G protein is heavily glycosylated with N-linked and O-linked sugars. However, the amino acid sequence positions of potential glycosylation sites are poorly conserved [8].

This protein is able to accommodate drastic changes with the emergence of new variants. Diversity occurs mainly in the two hypervariable regions of the ectodomain which are separated by a highly conserved 13-amino acid (aa) length domain [9]. Sequencing of the second hypervariable region at the C-terminal end of the G gene has been widely used to further subdivide RSV-A and RSV-B into genotypes and facilitated differentiation between RSV isolates. To date, 11 RSV-A genotypes, GA1-GA7, SAA1, NA1-NA2, and ON1 [10–12], and 23 RSV-B genotypes, GB1-GB4, SAB1-SAB3, SAB4, URU1, URU2, BAI - BAXII, and THB [10,13–21] have been described based on nucleotide sequence analysis.

RSV strains show an accumulation of translated amino acid changes over the years, suggesting antigenic drift-based immunity-mediated selection [22]. In 1999, a new RSV-B genotype BA emerged in Buenos Aires, Argentina, containing a 60-nucleotide (nt) duplication in the second hypervariable region of the G gene [23]. In the following ten years, the BA genotype spread worldwide and largely replaced previous described RSV-B genotypes [24]. During the 2010–11 winter season, a novel

RSV-A genotype ON1 with a 72-nt duplication has been reported in Canada [14]. In line with the gradual spread of the BA genotype making it the dominant circulating RSV-B genotype today, the nucleotide duplication of the ON1 genotype might likewise result in a similar selection advantage [25]. There is an increasing number of reports from across the world describing this novel genotype and the following seasons will show its impact on the evolution of RSV-A [6].

In Germany, there is only limited information regarding the molecular epidemiology of RSV, the emergence of novel viral strains and their impact on the course of RSV infection. In the present study, we evaluated hospitalized children below the age of 2 years presenting with acute RTI in the Pediatric Department in Heidelberg, Germany during the winter season 2012–13. We investigated the genetic diversity and patterns of the co-circulating genotypes of Heidelberg RSV-A and RSV-B strains in comparison with other RSV strains circulating worldwide. Furthermore we explored a possible association between individual RSV genotypes and the course of RSV infection by retrospectively analyzing basic clinical and laboratory data.

Materials and Methods

Patients and clinical samples

We retrospectively analyzed children under the age of 2 years admitted to the Pediatric Department at the Heidelberg University Hospital between October 2012 and April 2013 with clinical symptoms of upper or lower respiratory tract infection (RTI) as part of their admission diagnosis or as concomitant symptom. Prior to the transfer to the inpatient unit, nasopharyngeal aspirates (NPA) are obtained and these children are routinely screened for RSV infection using a rapid antigen test in order to inform for isolation strategies. All obtained NPAs (242 samples from 240 children) were collected and stored frozen for further molecular analysis by RSV PCR and phylogenetic analysis. Medical records were reviewed from all children to obtain routine clinical and laboratory data. Patient records were anonymized and de-identified prior to analysis. The Ethical Committee of the University of Heidelberg has approved this study (S-166/2014).

PCR and sequencing

For PCR analysis, RNA was extracted from NPAs using the QIAamp viral RNA mini kit (Qiagen, Hilden, Germany) according to the manufacturer's protocol. Amplification and detection of viral RNA was performed with the RealStar RSV real-time PCR kit (altona Diagnostics, Hamburg, Germany) on a LightCycler 480 instrument II (Roche, Mannheim, Germany). This assay differentiated RSV into subtypes A and B. For sequencing and identification of RSV genotypes, extracted RNA was initially reverse transcribed and cDNA was synthesized using random hexamer primers. Subsequently, PCR targeting the second hypervariable region of the G gene was performed using primer pairs as previously described by Peret et al. [11]. PCR products were sequenced with the same primer pairs previously used for amplification. Overlapping sequences were assembled and edited using the SEQMAN II software of the Lasergene package (DNAstar, Madsion, WI). Nucleotide sequences of the second hypervariable region of the G gene retrieved in this study were deposited in GenBank under accession numbers [KJ710364-KJ710420].

Phylogenetic and deduced amino acid sequence analysis

Multiple sequence alignments and phylogenetic analysis of the second hypervariable region of the G gene were conducted using the Clustal W 1.6 method of MEGA software version 6 [26]. Phylogenetic trees were generated using the maximum-likelihood method and bootstrap values with 1,000 replicates were calculated to evaluate confidence estimates. Reference strains representing known genotypes were retrieved from GenBank (http://www.ncbi.lm.nih.gov) and included in the tree. Pairwise nucleotide distances were calculated to compare the differences within and between genotypes of subgroup RSV-A and RSV-B using MEGA software version 6. Positive selected sites were estimated by use of the Datamonkey Web server (http://www.datamonkey.org) identifying the rates of non-synonymous and synonymous substitutions [27].

Deduced amino acid sequences were translated with the standard genetic code using MEGA software version 6. Alignments of the second hypervariable region of the G protein of Heidelberg RSV-A and RSV-B strains were compared to references strains from GenBank to identify amino acid substitutions. Putative N-glycosylation sites were predicted if the encoded amino acid sequence was Asn-Xaa-Thr/Ser, where Xaa was not a proline and accepted if the glycosylation potential was ≥ 0.5 in NetNGlyc 1.0 server [28]. O-glycosylation was determined using the NetOGlyc 3.1 server and sites were predicted using a G-score ≥ 0.5 [29].

Statistical analysis of epidemiological factors

To describe the temporal distribution of admitted RSV cases, we aggregated RSV results as obtained by PCR by calendar month and week. Demographic and clinical data in our study population was summarized. Group comparisons were performed using $\chi 2$ or Fisher's exact test for categorical variables and by Student's t-test or analysis of variance (ANOVA) for continuous variables, as appropriate. P-values <0.05 were considered statistically significant. Stata/IC13.0 (StataCorp. LP, College Station, TX, USA) was used for all statistical analysis.

Results

Detection of RSV

Between October 2012 and April 2013, a total of 242 samples from hospitalized infants and children were analyzed for RSV infection by PCR resulting in 134 (55.4%) RSV-positive samples. Among these RSV-positive samples, 110 (82.1%) were subgrouped as RSV-A and 24 (17.9%) as RSV-B, respectively. No co-infection for RSV-A and RSV-B was detected. Two children presented twice and were tested RSV-positive at their first admission and RSV-negative at the consecutive admission few weeks later. The distribution of RSV-A and RSV-B per calendar week and month is shown in Fig. 1.

Sequence alignments and phylogenetic analysis

Sequences of the second hypervariable region of the G gene from 97 (72.4%) RSV-A and 15 (11.2%) RSV-B samples were successfully obtained and aligned with representative GenBank sequences of previously published genotypes. Due to a low viral load some RSV-positive samples (n = 22; 16.4%) could not be sequenced. The phylogenetic trees of RSV-A and RSV-B sequences are shown in Figure 2. Heidelberg RSV_A and RSV-B strains clustered into three genotypes for RSV-A and two genotypes for RSV-B, respectively.

The majority of RSV-A strains (n = 73, 75.3%) clustered with strains that were previously assigned to the novel ON1 genotype with a 72-nt duplication, followed by strains clustering with genotype NA1 (n = 23, 31.5%) and one strain clustering with GA5 (Fig. 2A). Sequence homology between Heidelberg sequences and

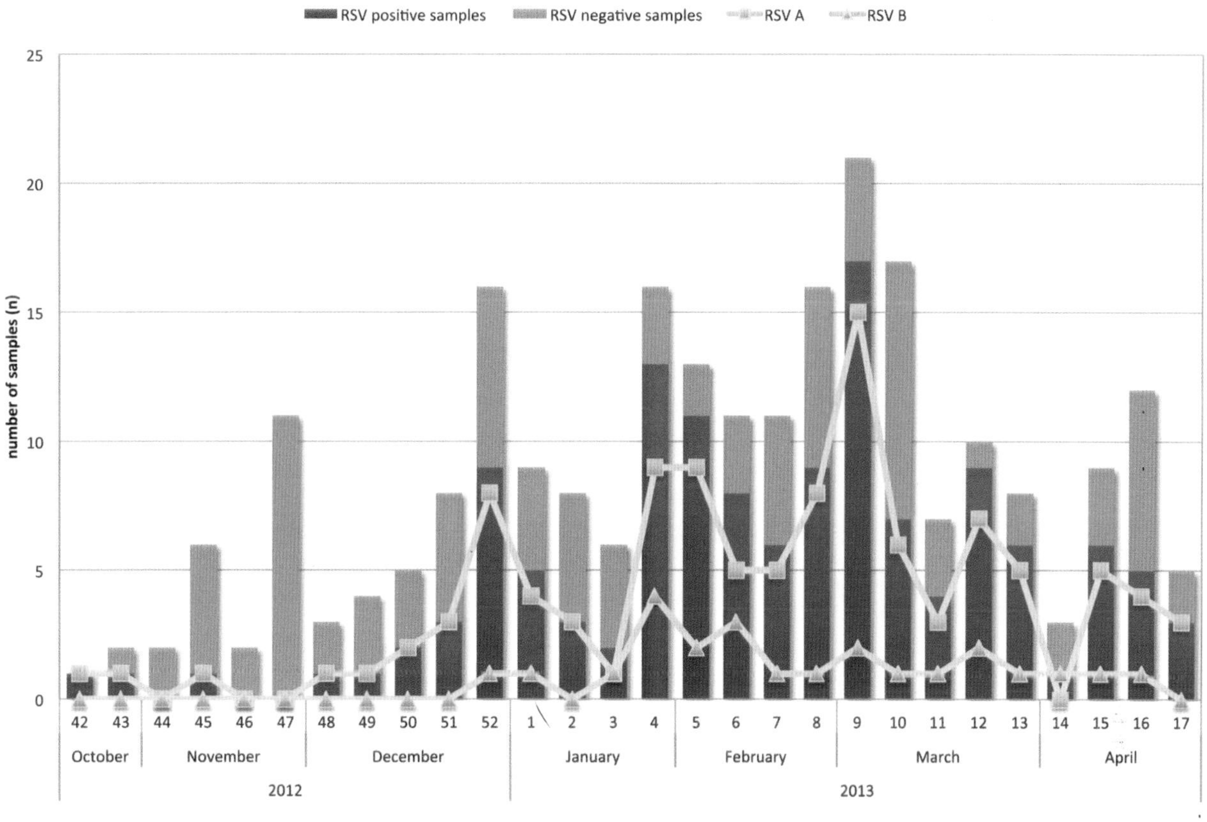

Figure 1. Weekly/monthly distribution of subgroup RSV A/RSV B in children ≤2 years with acute RTI in Heidelberg/Germany, winter season 2012/13.

the ON1 reference strain [JN257693] was ≥96.9% at the nucleotide level and ≥94.1% at the amino acid level. The intragenotypic p-distance was 1.9% for ON1 and 6.2% for NA1 for Heidelberg sequences. The intergenotypic p-distance for ON1 and NA1 was not comparable because of the 72-nt duplication.

All RSV-B strains (n = 15) clustered with strains that were previously assigned to the BA genotype with a 60-nt duplication. In addition, BA strains could be further differentiated into the previously designated genotypes BAIX (n = 10, 66.7%) and BAX (n = 5, 33.3%) (Fig. 2B). Sequence homology between Heidelberg sequences and the BA reference strain (AY333364) was 94.3%–96.6% at the nucleotide level and 87%–95% at the amino acid level. The intergenotypic p-distance for BAIX and BAX was 4.7% for Heidelberg sequences, with an intragenotypic p-distance of 3% for BAIX and 0.8% for BAX.

Deduced amino acid sequence analysis

We aligned and compared Heidelberg RSV-A genotype NA1 and GA5 strains with the A2 reference strain (M11486) (Fig. 3A). The majority of NA1 strains had three predicted N-glycosylation sites at amino acid (aa) positions 237, 251 and 294. However, HD12262 had an additional predicted N-glycosylation site at aa position 242 and HD12188 at aa position 273. A group of 11 isolates lost the N-glycosylation site at aa positions 237 due to a N237D/H substitution. Strain HD12055 lost all N-glycosylation site but the aa position 294. The N-glycosylation site at aa position 250 is characteristic for the GA5 genotype as found in one of the Heidelberg isolates. O-glycosylation patterns varied between Heidelberg isolates with 32±3 sites potentially O-glycosylated (G-score ≥0.5) in NA1 isolates and 23 sites in the one GA5 isolate.

As a consequence of the insertion in the G gene, ON1 genotype strains translate into a polypeptide with a length of 321 amino acids and are thereby lengthened by 24 aa when compared to the A2 reference strain (Fig. 3B). The insertion contains a 23 aa duplicated region. The comparison of Heidelberg ON1 strains with ON1 strains from other countries with reference to the original strain from Canada (JN257693) revealed that Heidelberg isolates can be divided into three sub-clusters: The first sub-cluster (n = 12) comprises isolates closely related to the primary Canadian strain (JN257693) with few mixed substitutions. This sub-cluster also includes one strain with an E308K substitution as previously described in South African strains [JX885730]. The second sub-cluster (n = 28) contained three characteristic substitutions, L274P, L298P and Y304H as previously described in strains from Wuerzburg, Germany [JX912364, JX12364], as well as in strains from Italy and Japan [KC858245, KC587959; AB808774, AB808757]. Furthermore, on group of 13 identical isolates showed a E287K substitution which was unique for Heidelberg strains. The third sub-cluster consists of 28 isolates with a L310P substitution in addition to the three substitutions found in the second sub-cluster and aligned with isolates from Japan, India and Kenya [AB808774, AB808757; KF246641, KF246640; KF587959]. A group of 19 identical strains additionally showed a V303A substitution, which was also seen in strains from Italy, Croatia and India [KC858245, KC587959; KF057865;

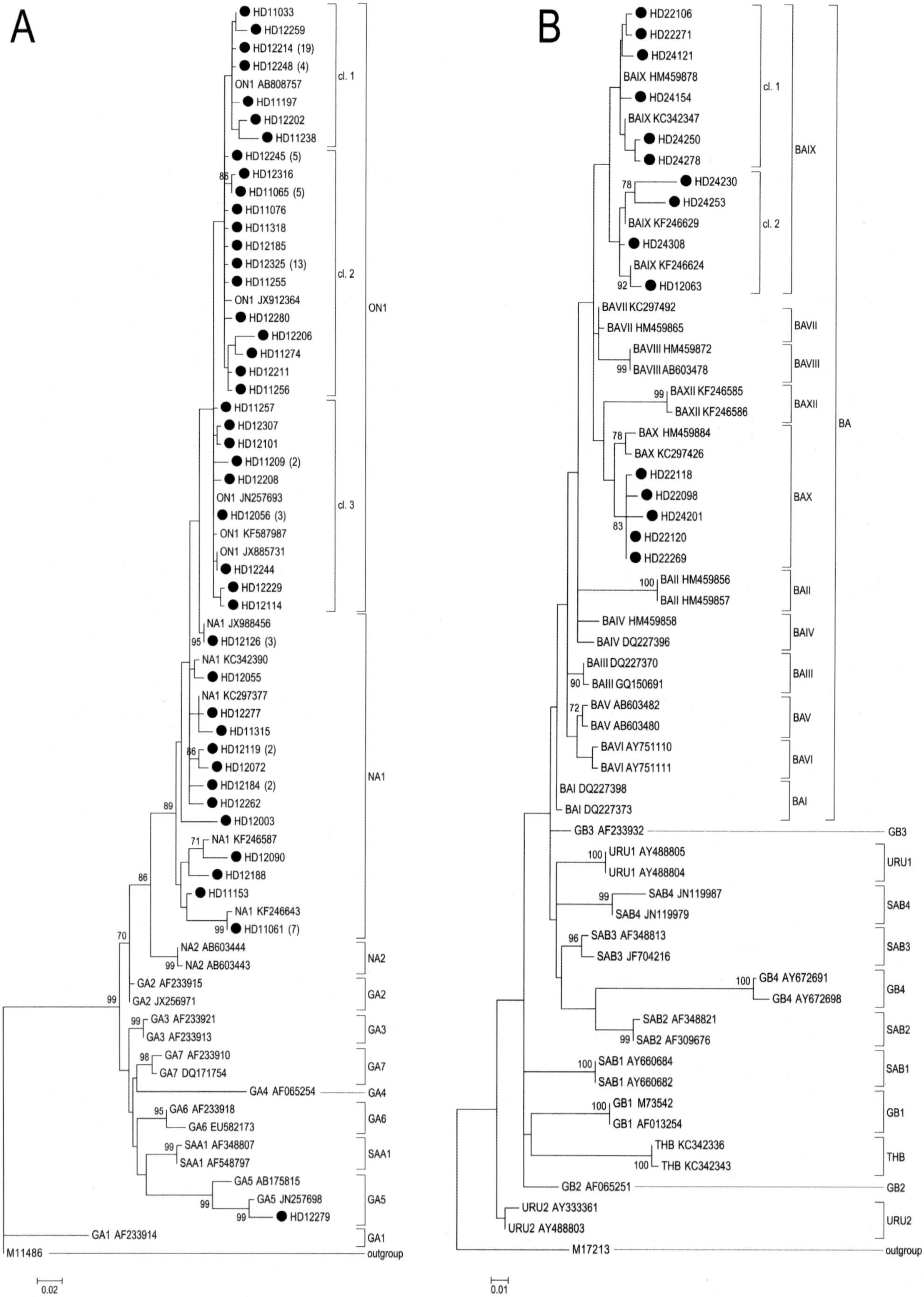
A
HD11033
HD12259
HD12214 (19)
HD12248 (4)
ON1 AB808757
HD11197
HD12202
HD11238
cl. 1
HD12245 (5)
86
HD12316
HD11065 (5)
HD11076
HD11318
HD12185
HD12325 (13)
HD11255
ON1 JX912364
HD12280
HD12206
HD11274
HD12211
HD11256
cl. 2
ON1
HD11257
HD12307
HD12101
HD11209 (2)
HD12208
ON1 JN257693
HD12056 (3)
ON1 KF587987
ON1 JX885731
HD12244
HD12229
HD12114
cl. 3
NA1 JX988456
95
HD12126 (3)
NA1 KC342390
HD12055
NA1 KC297377
HD12277
HD11315
86
HD12119 (2)
HD12072
HD12184 (2)
HD12262
89
HD12003
71
NA1 KF246587
HD12090
HD12188
86
HD11153
NA1 KF246643
99
HD11061 (7)
NA1
70
NA2 AB603444
99
NA2 AB603443
NA2
GA2 AF233915
99
GA2 JX256971
GA2
99
GA3 AF233921
GA3 AF233913
GA3
98
GA7 AF233910
GA7 DQ171754
GA7
GA4 AF065254
GA4
95
GA6 AF233918
GA6 EU582173
GA6
99
SAA1 AF348807
SAA1 AF548797
SAA1
GA5 AB175815
99
GA5 JN257698
99
HD12279
GA5
GA1 AF233914
GA1
M11486
outgroup
0.02
B
HD22106
HD22271
HD24121
BAIX HM459878
HD24154
BAIX KC342347
HD24250
HD24278
cl. 1
78
HD24230
HD24253
BAIX KF246629
HD24308
BAIX KF246624
92
HD12063
cl. 2
BAIX
BAVII KC297492
BAVII HM459865
BAVII
BAVIII HM459872
99
BAVIII AB603478
BAVIII
99
BAXII KF246585
BAXII KF246586
BAXII
78
BAX HM459884
BAX KC297426
HD22118
HD22098
HD24201
83
HD22120
HD22269
BAX
BA
100
BAII HM459856
BAII HM459857
BAII
BAIV HM459858
BAIV DQ227396
BAIV
BAIII DQ227370
90
BAIII GQ150691
BAIII
72
BAV AB603482
BAV AB603480
BAV
BAVI AY751110
BAVI AY751111
BAVI
BAI DQ227398
BAI DQ227373
BAI
GB3 AF233932
GB3
100
URU1 AY488805
URU1 AY488804
URU1
99
SAB4 JN119987
SAB4 JN119979
SAB4
96
SAB3 AF348813
SAB3 JF704216
SAB3
100
GB4 AY672691
GB4 AY672698
GB4
SAB2 AF348821
99
SAB2 AF309676
SAB2
100
SAB1 AY660684
SAB1 AY660682
SAB1
100
GB1 M73542
GB1 AF013254
GB1
THB KC342336
100
THB KC342343
THB
GB2 AF065251
GB2
URU2 AY333361
URU2 AY488803
URU2
M17213
outgroup
0.01

Figure 2. Phylogenetic tree of RSV A/RSV B strains and reference sequences of identified genotypes. Phylogenetic trees for RSV A (A) and RSV B (B) strains were constructed with maximum-likelihood method with 1,000 bootstrap replicates using MEGA 6 software. RSV strains from Heidelberg/Germany are indicated by "●HD" followed by their strain identification number. Number of identical strains is indicated in brackets after the strain identifier. Reference strains representing known genotypes were retrieved from GenBank and included in the tree (labels include accession number). The genotype assignment is shown on the right by brackets. Prototype strains (M11486 for subgroup A and M17213 for subgroup B) were used as an outgroup. Bootstrap values greater than 70% are indicated at the branch nodes. The scale bar represents the number of nucleotide substitutions per site. cl. = cluster.

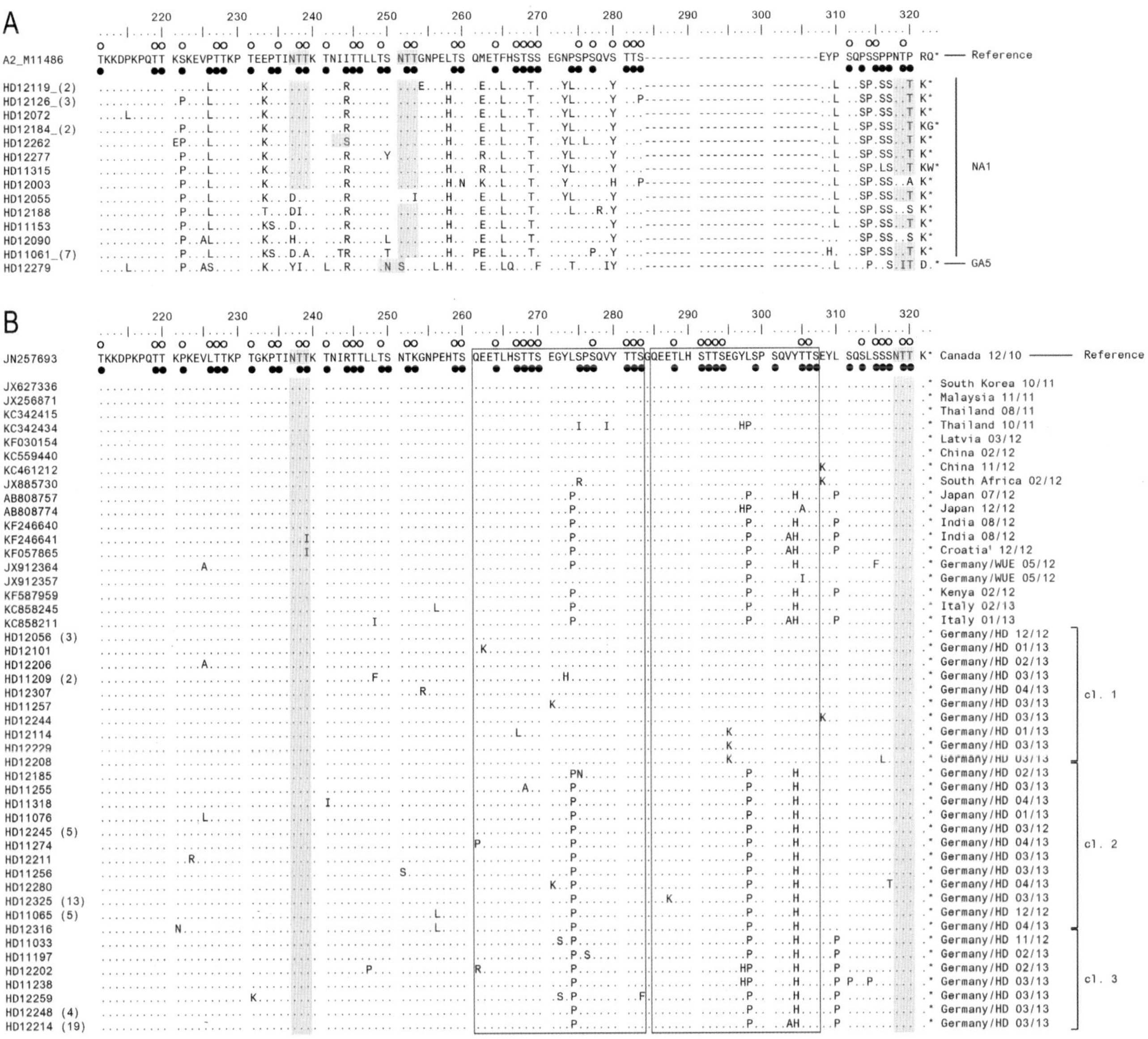

Figure 3. Alignment of deduced amino acid sequences of RSV-A strains. A) Alignment of RSV-A genotype NA1 and GA5 are shown relative to the sequence of prototype strain A2 (GenBank accession number M11486). Alignment of sequences was performed using the Clustal W 1.6 method via MEGA 6 software. The amino acid positions correspond to positions 210 to 298 of the G protein of strain A2. Identical residues are indicated by dots, asterisks indicate the position of stop codons. Number of identical strains is indicated in brackets after the strain identifier in the left column. Gray shading highlights predicted N-glycosylation sites. Unfilled circles indicate predicted O-glycosylation sites of the prototype strain A2; potential O-glycosylation sites of Heidelberg strains are indicated by black dots. The genotype assignment is shown on the right by brackets. B) Alignments are shown relative to the sequence of ON1 strain first described in Canada (GenBank accession number JN257693). Alignment of sequences was performed using the Clustal W 1.6 method via MEGA 6 software. The amino acid positions correspond to positions 210 to 298 of the G protein of the prototype strain A2. Identical residues are indicated by dots, asterisks indicate the position of stop codons. Boxes frame the 23 amino acid duplicated region of the 24 amino acid insertion. Gray shading highlights predicted N-glycosylation sites. Unfilled circles indicate predicted O-glycosylation sites of the Canadian reference ON1 strain; potential O-glycosylation sites of Heidelberg strains are indicated by black dots. On the right hand site, GenBank and Heidelberg strains are labeled with the country and time of occurrence (month/year).

[1] Sequences were published in GenBank only.

HD = Heidelberg; WUE = Wuerzburg, cl. = cluster.

KF246641, KF246640]. However, positive selection analysis of ON1 strains revealed no positive selected site.

All Heidelberg ON1 strains had two predicted N-glycosylation sites at aa positions 237 and 318 and lost the N-glycosylation sites at aa position 251 due to a T251K substitution. ON1 strains showed different patterns of O-glycosylation sites with 31 to 44 predicted sites and showed some new sites when compared to the Ontario reference strain. The 23-aa duplicated region contained a maximum of 10 glycosylation sites as observed in 17 ON1 isolates from Heidelberg.

Heidelberg RSV-B genotype BA strains were compared to BA reference strain from Buenos Aires [AF33364] (Fig. 4). Stop codons were either at aa position 320 for HD24308, HD24250 and HD24278 or at aa position 313 for the remaining BA strains. All BA strains had a K218P, L223P and S247P substitution. The BAIX genotype had a H287Y and a V271A substitution. Furthermore some BAIX strains (sub-cluster 1) had a P291L substitution whereas other BAIX strains (sub-cluster 2) had an I281T substitution. The BAX strains had a P291G substitution.

All Heidelberg RSV B strains had a predicted N-glycosylation site at aa positions 296. However the N-glycosylation site at aa position 310 only fulfilled the typical amino acid patterns but the glycosylation potential calculated by NetOGlyc 3.1 server was below 0.5 in isolates with a stop codon at aa position 313. HD24253 had an additional potential N-glycosylation site at aa position 230. O-glycosylation of BA strains varied between 40 and 47 predicted sites and showed an additional predicted site at aa position 317 in longer strains with a stop codon at aa position 320.

Basic and clinical characteristics of the study cohort

The mean age of the all screened children was 7.9 months and ranged in line with the inclusion criteria between 11 days and 23.8 months. RSV-positive patients were significantly younger compared to RSV-negative patients (t-test; $p < 0.001$). The age group distribution showed that 62.7% RSV-positive children were below 6 months of age. All children had at least a concomitant acute RTI at time of admission; however, in some patients the main clinical diagnosis was non-respiratory (total 12.4%, RSV positive 4.5%). In RSV-positive patients the most common diagnosis was bronchitis/bronchiolitis (75.4%). The mean duration of hospitalization was longer in RSV-positive patients (3.5 vs. 5.1 days; $p < 0.01$).

We performed a group comparison of the main three genotypes (RSV-A: ON1 and NA1; RSV-B: BA) using basic and clinical characteristics of RSV-positive infants and children (Table 1). There were no risk factors for one of the three groups of genotypes identified when looking at the demographic characteristics (age, gender, weight). Furthermore, we could not identify any association between a specific genotype and a more severe course of illness when taking the retrospectively available clinical and laboratory parameters into account.

Discussion

RSV accounts for a significant burden of acute respiratory tract infections particularly in infants and young children in need for hospital care [30]. Patterns of circulating RSV genotypes can provide a better understanding of the molecular epidemiology of RSV infection. In our study, we analyzed the genetic diversity and patterns of co-circulating genotypes of both, subtypes RSV-A and RSV-B, during the winter season 2012–13 in Heidelberg/Germany. RSV was detected in 134 out of 242 samples of which 110 (82.1%) were sub-grouped as RSV-A and 24 (17.9%) as RSV-B, respectively. Phylogenetic analysis revealed that the majority of RSV-A strains (n = 73, 75.3%) clustered with strains of the novel ON1 genotype with a 72-nt duplication first described by Eshaghi et al. in Ontario, Canada in 2010 [14]. In Germany, circulation of this genotype was reported for the first time in Wuerzburg in winter 2011–12 [31]. In line with another study in Europe, this study reports ON1 as the predominant genotype during the RSV epidemic season 2012–13, suggesting a rapid spread of this emerging RSV strain [32,33].

Most RSV cases were detected between December 2012 and April 2013, which is in line with the previously described seasonality of RSV infection in Germany [30]. However, the core season with more than half of all RSV-positive cases was from end-January to mid-March, which can be considered a late pattern of a RSV epidemic season in Germany [22]. Within our study population RSV was detectable in 55.4% of hospitalized children below the age of 2 years emphasizing the need for RSV screening on admission to assure proper management and to prevent nosocomial infections [34].

In our cohort, age group analysis revealed that infants below 6 months of age had the highest infection rates, as expected. Primary RSV infection commonly occurs within the first year of life [13]

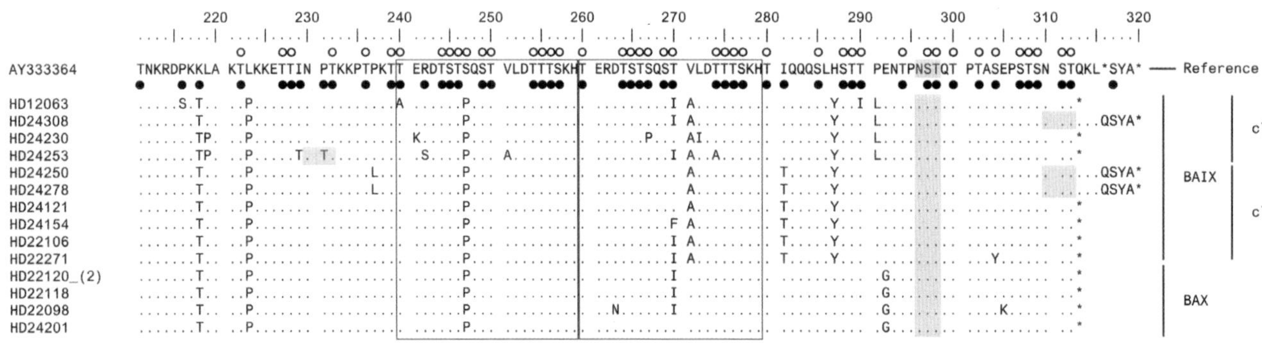

Figure 4. Alignment of deduced amino acid sequences of the second variable region of the G protein of RSV-B strains isolated in Heidelberg/Germany during 2012–2013 winter season. Alignments are shown relative to the sequence of a prototype BA strain (GenBank accession number AY333364). Alignment of sequences was performed using the Clustal W 1.6 method via MEGA 6 software. The amino acid positions correspond to positions 210 to 315 of the G protein of the BA strain. Identical residues are indicated by dots, asterisks indicate the position of stop codons. Number of identical strains is indicated in brackets after the strain identifier in the left column. Boxes frame the 20 amino acid duplication. Gray shading highlights predicted N-glycosylation sites. Open circles indicate predicted O-glycosylation sites of the prototype BA strain; potential O-glycosylation sites of Heidelberg strains are indicated by black dots. Genotypes are shown on the right by brackets.

Table 1. Basic and clinical characteristics of RSV positive children by genotype.

		RSV A*		RSV B	
	RSV positive	ON1	NA1	BA	p-value
	n = 134	n = 73	n = 23	n = 15	
Demographic characteristics					
Age in months, mean ±SD	6.5±6.2	6.4±6.2	5.7±5.6	4.8±5.1	0.63
Age group, n (%)					
0–6 months	84 (62.7)	48 (65.8)	15 (65.2)	10 (66.7)	0.18
>6–12 months	20 (14.9)	7 (9.6)	6 (26.1)	3 (20.0)	
>12–18 months	20 (14.9)	13(17.8)	0 (0.0)	2 (13.3)	
>18–24 months	10 (7.5)	15 (6.9)	2 (8.7)	0 (0.0)	
Gender, n (%)					
Male	83 (61.9)	44 (60.3)	18 (78.3)	9 (60.0)	0.28
Female	51 (38.1)	29 (39.7)	5 (21.7)	6 (40.0)	
Weight in kg, mean ±SD	6.2±2.3	5.9±2.1	7.0±2.7	5.8±2.3	0.11
Leading clinical diagnosis, n (%)					
Non-respiratory	6 (4.5)	4 (5.5)	0 (0.0)	1 (6.7)	0.49
Respiratory	128 (95.5)	69 (94.5)	23 (100.0)	14 (93.3)	
Upper RTI	4 (3.0)	1 (1.4)	1 (4.4)	0 (0.0)	0.61
Bronchitis/Bronchiolitis	101 (75.4)	54 (74.0)	20 (87.0)	12 (80.0)	
Pneumonia	23 (17.2)	14 (19.2)	2 (8.7)	2 (6.7)	
Course of disease					
Symptoms prior to hospitalization in days, mean ±SD	4.2±3.6	3.9±3.1	3.9±2.9	3.8±5.0	0.98
Hospital stay in days, mean ±SD#	5.3±3.9	5.3±3.8	5.5±2.8	4.5±2.1	0.68
Need for intensive care, n (%)	6 (4.5)	4 (5.5)	0 (0.0)	1 (6.7)	0.49
Laboratory parameters on admission					
Hemoglobin in g/dl, mean ±SD	11.7±1.7	11.4±1.5	11.9±1.9	11.7±2.0	0.45
Leucocytes/nl, mean ±SD	11.5±4.7	11.0±4.5	10.1±3.6	10.4±3.8	0.64
Thrombocytes/nl, mean ±SD	434.2±120.5	435.8±130.9	391.5±84.6	467.9±117.4	0.17
C-reactive protein in mg/L, mean ±SD	22.5±37.0	20.1±26.7	22.4±24.5	17.5±17.7	0.88
pCO2 in mmHg, mean ±SD	41.5±8.8	41.6±9.4	42.1±8.4	45.6±8.9	0.44

*RSV A genotype GA5 was not included in this table as this genotype was only present in one patient. In total, 112 of 134 RSV positive patients could be sequenced and a genotype could be determined.

#Hospital stay was only calculated for patients who stayed at least 24 hours in hospital.

SD = standard deviation; RTI = respiratory tract infection, RSV = Respiratory Syncytial Virus.

and the risk of RSV infection decreases with increasing age [22]. The majority of RSV-positive children presented with bronchitis/bronchiolitis followed by pneumonia and the duration of hospitalization was significantly longer compared to RSV-negative patients. However, the median duration of hospital stay of 5 days in RSV-positive patients in this study was shorter compared to previous findings of 7 days [30].

Molecular analysis of RSV-positive samples demonstrated that RSV-A was the predominant subtype which is in line with previous findings of multiple-season studies from Europe and other geographical areas [21,22]. Phylogenetic analysis revealed that the majority of RSV-A strains (n = 73, 75.3%) clustered with strains of the novel ON1 genotype with a 72-nt duplication. Phylogenetic analysis of Tsukagoshi et al. estimated that genotype ON1 evolved from genotype NA1 [35]. Recent estimates place the time of the ON1 emergence around 2008/09 [36,37].

Over the past three epidemic seasons (2010–2013) the prevalence of ON1 strains among all circulating strains varied between the different reports, but there seems to be a trend towards ON1 as the predominating RSV-A strain. In its first description in Ontario/Canada, the genotype ON1 accounted for 10% of RSV-positive samples in the season 2010-11 [14]. In the same season in Thailand, the majority of RSV isolates belonged to NA1, only few isolates belonged to ON1 [20]. One season later in 2011–12, RSV-A genotype ON1 was reported in different studies from Asia, Africa and Europe suggesting a worldwide emergence of the novel RSV-A strain. However, ON1 was only sporadically detected during that time and some countries like Pakistan did not report ON1 among circulating genotypes in 2011–12 [34]. A study from Heidelberg/Germany evaluating the genetic diversity of RSV in an outbreak in a haematology unit in 2012 also did not describe any ON1 strains [38]. In a study from Bejing, China, only one sample from February 2012 out of about 250 sequenced RSV-positive samples between 2007 and 2012 was characterized as ON1 genotype [39]. One report from Wuerzburg/Germany, assigned 10% of the identified strains to genotype ON1 in 2011–

12 [31]. In the past months an increasing number of reports about circulating genotypes in the season 2012–13 were published. In line with the findings in this study, reports from Cyprus, Italy, Kenya and South Korea described ON1 as the predominating genotype in the epidemic season 2012–13 [32,33,36,37]. Our study therefore describes a further cohort in Europe with ON1 as the predominating genotype in 2012–13 suggesting a rapid emergence of this novel strain. Further surveillance of circulating genotypes will be needed to observe the future global distribution of the ON1 strain and its trend to diversify.

The comparison of Heidelberg ON1 strains with ON1 strains from other countries revealed that Heidelberg isolates could be divided into three sub-clusters with characteristic substitutions as previously described in different countries and continents. Similar to the subdivision of RSV-B genotype BA into several sub-genotypes (BA-I – BAXII), this could be a first trend to a diversification of the ON1 genotype. However, none of the sub-clusters had bootstrap values ≥70%. Furthermore, positive selection analysis did not reveal any positively selective sites among ON1 isolates. This is also reflected by two groups of identical isolates (n = 13 and n = 18) of the ON1 genotype, suggesting the absence of selective pressure among the newly emerging strains.

Although the majority of strains was subtyped as RSV-A, 13.4% of all Heidelberg trains were subtyped as RSV-B. All RSV-B strains clustered with strains of the BA genotype with a 60-nt duplication, first described by Trento et al. in Buenos Aires, Argentina in 1999 [23], further differentiating into the genotypes BAIX (n = 10, 66.7%) and BAX (n = 5, 33.3%). Genotype BAIX separated into two sub-clusters: one including the BAIX reference sequence from Japan designated by Dapat et al. [18] who first described this genotype in 2007, and the second including the BAIX reference sequence from India described by Choudhary et al. in 2010 [40]. However, none of the two sub-clusters had bootstrap values ≥70%.

Similar to genotype BA, the nucleotide duplication of the ON1 genotype seems to result in a selection advantage compared to other RSV-A genotypes. Interestingly, despite the emergence of the ON1 virus there is conflicting data concerning the virulence in terms of disease severity [31–33]. In our cohort, retrospective analysis of basic clinical and laboratory parameters such as the duration of hospital stay, the need for intensive care as well as pCO_2 levels on admission did not reveal any association between a specific genotype and disease severity. Further surveillance of circulating RSV genotypes and corresponding clinical data is needed to understand the evolution, transmission and pathogenicity of genotype ON1 RSV infections.

Our study is subject to several limitations: We report the genetic diversity of RSV during one season in winter 2012–13 and a comparison of proportions of circulating genotypes is therefore restricted to other reports from Germany as well as worldwide. Our analysis included hospitalized children with community acquired RSV infection and therefore cannot draw conclusions for the overall population of community acquired RSV infections. However, the cohort of hospitalized children is of particular clinical relevance. Due to the retrospective study design, the evaluation of the association between pathogenicity of RSV infection and genotypes was limited to the available data. Furthermore, we did not include an analysis of further co-infections, which might also have an effect on disease severity in the evaluated study cohort. Further surveillance of the molecular epidemiology for several seasons in combination with prospectively complied clinical data is needed to directly compare the emergence of new variants and their transmissibility and virulence.

In summary, molecular characterization of RSV in Heidelberg, Germany during winter season 2012–13 confirmed the co-circulation of multiple genotypes of subtype RSV-A and RSV-B and the predominance of the novel genotype ON1. In line with the emergence of the BA genotype, it can be hypothesized that genotype ON1 could spread in a similar way and several branches might subdivide into further sub-genotypes. However, we could not find any association between disease severity and this newly emerging RSV-A genotype ON1. Continuing and long-term molecular epidemiological surveys for early detection of circulating and newly emerging genotypes in combination with clinical data are necessary to gain a better understanding of underlying genetic and antigenic mechanisms of RSV infection.

Acknowledgments

We would like to thank all nurses in the Department of Pediatrics, Heidelberg, Germany for collecting respiratory samples and all technicians in the virology diagnostic laboratory Heidelberg, Germany and Benedikt Weissbrich from the virology diagnostic laboratory at the University of Wuerzburg, Germany for excellent technical assistance. Furthermore, we cordially thank our colleague Steffen Geis from the virology diagnostic laboratory Heidelberg for the support in developing the methodology, critical reading of the manuscript as well as for his statistical advice.

Author Contributions

Conceived and designed the experiments: JT CP JGH PS. Performed the experiments: JT CP. Analyzed the data: JT CP JP. Wrote the paper: JT PS.

References

1. Glezen WP, Taber LH, Frank AL, Kasel JA (1986) Risk of primary infection and reinfection with respiratory syncytial virus. Am J Dis Child 140: 543–546.
2. Henderson FW, Collier AM, Clyde WA, Denny FW (1979) Respiratory-syncytial-virus infections, reinfections and immunity. A prospective, longitudinal study in young children. N Engl J Med 300: 530–534. doi: 10.1056/NEJM197903083001004
3. García O, Martín M, Dopazo J, Arbiza J, Frabasile S, et al. (1994) Evolutionary pattern of human respiratory syncytial virus (subgroup A): cocirculating lineages and correlation of genetic and antigenic changes in the G glycoprotein. J Virol 68: 5448–5459.
4. Hall CB, Walsh EE, Long CE, Schnabel KC (1991) Immunity to and frequency of reinfection with respiratory syncytial virus. J Infect Dis163: 693–698.
5. Storch GA, Anderson LJ, Park CS, Tsou C, Dohner DE (1991) Antigenic and genomic diversity within group A respiratory syncytial virus. 163: 858–861.
6. Pretorius MA, van Niekerk S, Tempia S, Moyes J, Cohen C, et al. (2013) Replacement and Positive Evolution of Subtype A and B Respiratory Syncytial Virus G-Protein Genotypes From 1997–2012 in South Africa. J Infect Dis 208: S227–S237. doi: 10.1093/infdis/jit477
7. Anderson LJ, Hierholzer JC, Tsou C, Hendry RM, Fernie BF, et al. (1985) Antigenic characterization of respiratory syncytial virus strains with monoclonal antibodies. J Infect Dis 151: 626–633.
8. Wertz GW, Krieger M, Ball LA (1989) Structure and cell surface maturation of the attachment glycoprotein of human respiratory syncytial virus in a cell line deficient in O glycosylation. J Virol 63: 4767–4776.
9. Johnson PR, Spriggs MK, Olmsted RA, Collins PL (1987) The G glycoprotein of human respiratory syncytial viruses of subgroups A and B: extensive sequence divergence between antigenically related proteins. Proc Natl Acad Sci USA 84: 5625–5629.
10. Peret TC, Hall CB, Schnabel KC, Golub JA, Anderson LJ (1998) Circulation patterns of genetically distinct group A and B strains of human respiratory syncytial virus in a community. J Gen Virol 79 (Pt 9): 2221–2229.
11. Peret TCT, Hall CB, Hammond GW, Piedra PA, Storch GA, et al. (2000) Circulation patterns of group A and B human respiratory syncytial virus genotypes in 5 communities in North America. J Infect Dis 181: 1891–1896. doi: 10.1086/315508
12. Venter M, Madhi SA, Tiemessen CT, Schoub BD (2001) Genetic diversity and molecular epidemiology of respiratory syncytial virus over four consecutive

seasons in South Africa: identification of new subgroup A and B genotypes. J Gen Virol 82: 2117–2124.

13. Shobugawa Y, Saito R, Sano Y, Zaraket H, Suzuki Y, et al. (2009) Emerging Genotypes of Human Respiratory Syncytial Virus Subgroup A among Patients in Japan. J Clin Microbiol 47: 2475–2482. doi: 10.1128/JCM.00115-09
14. Eshaghi A, Duvvuri VR, Lai R, Nadarajah JT, Li A, et al. (2012) Genetic variability of human respiratory syncytial virus A strains circulating in Ontario: a novel genotype with a 72 nucleotide G gene duplication. PLoS ONE 7: e32807. doi: 10.1371/journal.pone.0032807
15. Arnott A, Vong S, Mardy S, Chu S, Naughtin M, et al. (2011) A study of the genetic variability of human respiratory syncytial virus (HRSV) in Cambodia reveals the existence of a new HRSV group B genotype. J Clin Microbiol 49: 3504–3513. doi: 10.1128/JCM.01131-11
16. Blanc A, Delfraro A, Frabasile S, Arbiza J (2005) Genotypes of respiratory syncytial virus group B identified in Uruguay. Arch Virol 150: 603–609. doi: 10.1007/s00705-004-0412-x
17. Trento A, Viegas M, Galiano M, Videla C, Carballal G, et al. (2006) Natural history of human respiratory syncytial virus inferred from phylogenetic analysis of the attachment (G) glycoprotein with a 60-nucleotide duplication. J Virol 80: 975–984. doi: 10.1128/JVI.80.2.975-984.2006
18. Dapat IC, Shobugawa Y, Sano Y, Saito R, Sasaki A, et al. (2010) New Genotypes within Respiratory Syncytial Virus Group B Genotype BA in Niigata, Japan. J Clin Microbiol 48: 3423–3427. doi: 10.1128/JCM.00646-10
19. Baek YH, Choi EH, Song M-S, Pascua PNQ, Kwon H-I, et al. (2012) Prevalence and genetic characterization of respiratory syncytial virus (RSV) in hospitalized children in Korea. Arch Virol 157: 1039–1050. doi: 10.1007/s00705-012-1267-1
20. Khor C-S, Sam I-C, Hooi P-S, Chan Y-F (2013) Displacement of predominant respiratory syncytial virus genotypes in Malaysia between 1989 and 2011. Infect Genet Evol 14: 357–360. doi: 10.1016/j.meegid.2012.12.017
21. Auksornkitti V, Kamprasert N, Thongkomplew S, Suwannakarn K, Theamboonlers A, et al. (2014) Molecular characterization of human respiratory syncytial virus, 2010–2011: identification of genotype ON1 and a new subgroup B genotype in Thailand. Arch Virol 159: 499–507. doi: 10.1007/s00705-013-1773-9
22. Reiche J, Schweiger B (2009) Genetic variability of group A human respiratory syncytial virus strains circulating in Germany from 1998 to 2007. J Clin Microbiol 47: 1800–1810. doi: 10.1128/JCM.02286-08
23. Melero JA, Trento A, Videla C, Galiano M, Carballal G, et al. (2003) Major changes in the G protein of human respiratory syncytial virus isolates introduced by a duplication of 60 nucleotides. J Gen Virol 84: 3115–3120. doi: 10.1099/vir.0.19357-0
24. Trento A, Casas I, Calderón A, Garcia-Garcia ML, Calvo C, et al. (2010) Ten years of global evolution of the human respiratory syncytial virus BA genotype with a 60-nucleotide duplication in the G protein gene. J Virol 84: 7500–7512. doi: 10.1128/JVI.00345-10
25. Valley-Omar Z, Muloiwa R, Hu N-C, Eley B, Hsiao N-Y (2013) Novel respiratory syncytial virus subtype ON1 among children, Cape Town, South Africa, 2012. Emerging Infect Dis 19: 668–670. doi: 10.3201/eid1904.121465
26. Tamura K, Stecher G, Peterson D, Filipski A, Kumar S (2013) MEGA6: Molecular Evolutionary Genetics Analysis version 6.0. Mol Biol Evol 30: 2725–2729. doi: 10.1093/molbev/mst197
27. Delport W, Poon AFY, Frost SDW, Kosakovsky Pond SL (2010) Datamonkey 2010: a suite of phylogenetic analysis tools for evolutionary biology. Bioinformatics 26: 2455–2457. doi: 10.1093/bioinformatics/btq429
28. Gupta R, Jung E, Brunak S (2004) Prediction of N-glycosylation sites in human proteins. NetNGlycServer. Available: http://www.cbs.dtu.dk/services/NetNGlyc/. Accessed: 2014 Apr 6.
29. Julenius K, Mølgaard A, Gupta R, Brunak S (2005) Prediction, conservation analysis, and structural characterization of mammalian mucin-type O-glycosylation sites. Glycobiology 15: 153–164. doi: 10.1093/glycob/cwh151
30. Berner R, Schwoerer F, Schumacher RF, Meder M, Forster J (2001) Community and nosocomially acquired respiratory syncytial virus infection in a German paediatric hospital from 1988 to 1999. Eur J Pediatr 160: 541–547.
31. Prifert C, Streng A, Krempl CD, Liese J, Weissbrich B (2013) Novel respiratory syncytial virus a genotype, Germany, 2011–2012. Emerging Infect Dis 19: 1029–1030. doi: 10.3201/eid1906.121582
32. Panayiotou C, Richter J, Koliou M, Kalogirou N, Georgiou E, et al. (2014) Epidemiology of respiratory syncytial virus in children in Cyprus during three consecutive winter seasons (2010–2013): age distribution, seasonality and association between prevalent genotypes and disease severity. Epidemiol Infect: 1–6. doi: 10.1017/S0950268814000028
33. Pierangeli A, Trotta D, Scagnolari C, Ferreri ML, Nicolai A, et al. (2014) Rapid spread of the novel respiratory syncytial virus A ON1 genotype, central Italy, 2011 to 2013. Euro Surveill 19.
34. Aamir UB, Alam MM, Sadia H, Zaidi SSZ, Kazi BM (2013) Molecular Characterization of Circulating Respiratory Syncytial Virus (RSV) Genotypes in Gilgit Baltistan Province of Pakistan during 2011–2012 Winter Season. PLoS ONE 8: e74018. doi: 10.1371/journal.pone.0074018
35. Tsukagoshi H, Yokoi H, Kobayashi M, Kushibuchi I, Okamoto-Nakagawa R, et al. (2013) Genetic analysis of attachment glycoprotein (G) gene in new genotype ON1 of human respiratory syncytial virus detected in Japan. Microbiol Immunol 57: 655–659. doi: 10.1111/1348-0421.12075
36. Agoti CN, Otieno JR, Gitahi CW, Cane PA, Nokes DJ (2014) Rapid spread and diversification of respiratory syncytial virus genotype ON1, Kenya. Emerging Infect Dis 20: 950–959. doi: 10.3201/eid2006.131438
37. Kim Y-J, Kim D-W, Lee W-J, Yun M-R, Lee HY, et al. (2014) Rapid replacement of human respiratory syncytial virus A with the ON1 genotype having 72 nucleotide duplication in G gene. Infect Genet Evol 26C: 103–112. doi: 10.1016/j.meegid.2014.05.007
38. Geis S, Prifert C, Weissbrich B, Lehners N, Egerer G, et al. (2013). Molecular characterization of a respiratory syncytial virus (RSV) outbreak in a haematology unit, Heidelberg, Germany. J Clin Microbiol 51: 155–162.
39. Cui G, Qian Y, Zhu R, Deng J, Zhao L, et al. (2013) Emerging human respiratory syncytial virus genotype ON1 found in infants with pneumonia in Beijing, China. Emerg Microbes Infect 2: e22. doi: 10.1038/emi.2013.19
40. Choudhary ML, Anand SP, Wadhwa BS, Chadha MS (2013) Genetic variability of human respiratory syncytial virus in Pune, Western India. Infect Genet Evol 20C: 369–377. doi: 10.1016/j.meegid.2013.09.025

8

Rhinitis, Asthma and Respiratory Infections among Adults in Relation to the Home Environment in Multi-Family Buildings

Juan Wang*, **Karin Engvall, Greta Smedje, Dan Norbäck**

Department of Medical Sciences, Uppsala University and University Hospital, Uppsala, Sweden

Abstract

Risk factors for rhinitis, asthma and respiratory infections in the home environment were studied by a questionnaire survey. Totally 5775 occupants (≥18 years old) from a stratified random sample of multi-family buildings in Sweden participated (46%). 51.0% had rhinitis in the last 3 months (current rhinitis); 11.5% doctor diagnosed asthma; 46.4% respiratory infections in the last 3 months and 11.9% antibiotic medication for respiratory infections in the last 12 months. Associations between home environment and health were analyzed by multiple logistic regression, controlling for gender, age and smoking and mutual adjustment. Buildings constructed during 1960–1975 were risk factors for day time breathlessness (OR = 1.53, 95%CI 1.03–2.29). And those constructed during 1976–1985 had more current rhinitis (OR = 1.43, 95%CI 1.12–1.84) and respiratory infections (OR = 1.46, 95%CI 1.21–1.78). Cities with higher population density had more current rhinitis ($p = 0.008$) and respiratory infections ($p < 0.001$). Rented apartments had more current rhinitis (OR = 1.23, 95%CI 1.07–1.40), wheeze (OR = 1.20, 95%CI 1.02–1.41), day time breathlessness (OR = 1.31, 95%CI 1.04–1.66) and respiratory infections (OR = 1.13, 95%CI 1.01–1.26). Living in colder parts of the country was a risk factor for wheeze ($p = 0.03$) and night time breathlessness ($p = 0.002$). Building dampness was a risk factor for wheeze (OR = 1.42, 95%CI 1.08–1.86) and day time breathlessness (OR = 1.57, 95%CI 1.09–2.27). Building dampness was a risk factor for health among those below 66 years old. Odor at home was a risk factor for doctor diagnosed asthma (OR = 1.49, 95%CI 1.08–2.06) and current asthma (OR = 1.52, 95%CI 1.03–2.24). Environmental tobacco smoke (ETS) was a risk factor for current asthma (OR = 1.53, 95%CI 1.09–2.16). Window pane condensation was a risk factor for antibiotic medication for respiratory infections (OR = 1.41, 95%CI 1.10–1.82). In conclusion, rhinitis, asthma and respiratory infections were related to a number of factors in the home environment. Certain building years (1961–1985), building dampness, window pane condensation and odor in the dwelling may be risk factors.

Editor: Oliver Schildgen, Kliniken der Stadt Köln gGmbH, Germany

Funding: The Swedish Research Council Formas supported the study through contract no. 244-2011-222. The funders had no role in study design, data collection and analysis, decision to publish, or preparation of the manuscript.

Competing Interests: The authors have declared that no competing interests exist.

* Email: juan.wang@medsci.uu.se

Introduction

Concern about possible health effects of indoor air pollution has been increasing especially with respects to allergies and asthma. The dwelling is an important indoor environment, since it is where we spend most time, usually 15–16 h per day [1].

Rhinitis can be divided into allergic rhinitis (AR) and non-allergic rhinitis (NAR). AR occurs when an allergen is the trigger for the nasal symptoms. NAR is when obstruction and rhinorrhea occurs in relation to non-allergic, noninfectious triggers, such as changes in the weather, cigarette smoke, etc [2]. Approximately 10%–25% of the world population is affected by AR [3]. The worldwide prevalence of allergic rhinitis among adults has been on the rise since at least 1990 [4–8]. In Sweden, the prevalence of AR increased from 22% to 31% from 1990 to 2008 in young adults [7]. However, less information is available on the prevalence or incidence of NAR. Generally, females [9,10], young adults [10–12], and those with allergic heredity [13,14] are at higher risk of having AR. Allergen sources in the home environment are common, such as from pets [15], cockroaches [12,14], house dust mites, microbiologic agents [16,17], etc. Signs of dampness and indoor molds is another common exposure that has been widely studied in relation to both AR and NAR in home [17–19]. Other factors such as traffic-related air pollution, different lifestyle and socioeconomic conditions are quoted as adjuvant factors for AR [20].

Asthma is the most common chronic respiratory disease in the world. Approximately 300 million people in the world currently have asthma [21]. Epidemiological studies have suggested that the prevalence of asthma in adults is approximately 7–10% in different parts of the western world [22]. The current trend (since 1990's) in the prevalence of asthma among adults is unclear, some studies suggesting that asthma prevalence has stabilized or even decreased [5,7,22], while, others suggesting it is still increasing [4]. However, asthma prevalence among children in many parts of the world is still increasing [23]. Asthma frequently co-exist with rhinitis [3,24–26]. Adult asthma is more common among females [27–29], younger adults [27], and those with allergic heredity [27,29].

Smoking [30,31] and environmental tobacco smoke (ETS) [29,32–34] were found to be associated with asthma or asthma related symptoms. A common finding is the association between observed building dampness and molds and adults' asthma [35]. Exposures related to building dampness can be house dust mites, molds, bacteria, and even chemicals (from the degradation process of building materials). Studies has shown that adults' asthma or asthmatic symptoms were associated with higher levels of cockroach allergen [36], mouse allergen [36], house dust mites [37], fungal [38], airborne bacteria [37], formaldehyde [39,40] and total volatile organic compounds (VOC) [39,40] in dwellings, newly painted indoor surfaces [41], and combustion of wood, coal or biomass fuels [34].

Respiratory infections include infections of the lower and upper respiratory tract, and otitis media [42]. Preventive strategies include attempting to avoid contact with or spreading of infectious agents and covering sneezes and vaccination for influenza and pneumococcal pneumonia [42]. The presence of building dampness and molds are associated with increase in respiratory infections in adults [19,35,42,43]. Air movements in buildings and ventilation are essential for the transmission/spread of infectious diseases. There is some evidence of spread of infections by airborne transmission, such as measles, tuberculosis, chickenpox, influenza, smallpox and severe acute respiratory syndrome (SARS) [44]. There is however insufficient data to specify the minimum ventilation requirements to avoid the spread of infectious diseases via the airborne route [44,45].

The aging population is an important issue in many countries [46]. A better understanding of the health consequences of exposure to different risk factors among elderly, notably to environmental factors, is needed. There are only few studies investigating the influence of environment factors among respiratory health in the elderly [47,48]. Exposure to elevated levels of outdoor air pollution such as particle matter (PM), ozone (O_3), nitrogen dioxide (NO_2) and sulphur dioxide (SO_2) were associated with increased hospital admissions for asthma and chronic obstructive pulmonary disease (COPD) [47]. For indoor environment, the most consistent association was found between increased risk of COPD and exposure to ETS [48].

The first aim of this study was to investigate the prevalence of rhinitis, asthma and respiratory infections among occupants living in multi-family buildings in Sweden. The second of aim was to study occupants' health symptoms in relation to their home environment. The third aim was to study if there is any difference of these associations in relation to occupants' age (comparing those less than or equal to 65 years old with those more than 65 years old).

Material and Methods

Ethics Statement

The study and the consent procedure were approved by the Regional Ethical Committee in Uppsala, Sweden. All participants gave informed consent. An information letter sent together with the questionnaire stated that if the subjects answered and returned the questionnaire it meant they had given informed consent.

Selection of Buildings

The selection of multi-family buildings was performed by Statistics Sweden (SCB) [49]. The buildings were selected by a multi-stage sampling procedure with a first step to select 30 Swedish municipalities out of totally 290 municipalities across Sweden through a stratified random selection according to geographic and demographic characteristics (temperature zone and region), and degree of urbanization. The probability for a municipality to be selected was proportional to the size of the population of the municipality in December 31, 2006. The next step was selection of multi-family buildings from these 30 municipalities. Data on all multi-family buildings and their construction year were obtained from the central building register in Sweden. Stratified random sampling was used to sample buildings based on the construction year in 5 classes (before 1960, 1960–1975, 1976–1985, 1986–1995 and 1996–2005) aiming to get the same number of buildings in each age class. Since most buildings in Sweden are old, there was an over-sampling of new buildings in this study. Totally 690 multi-family buildings were sampled from the 30 municipalities.

Questionnaire and study population

The study population consisted of all adults (≥18 years old) living in the multi-family buildings included in the study. There were totally 8841 apartments and 12488 adults. The questionnaires were developed at Department of Medical Science, Uppsala University, based on previous studies [7,27,50–53]. The number of adults living in each apartment was identified by SCB from the Swedish civil registration register. Each adult (≥18 years) registered in the selected apartments received a personal questionnaire including medicine questions and personal factors. Moreover, one indoor environment questionnaire was sent to each apartment. The postal questionnaire was administered by SCB during the spring 2008. Two reminders were sent to those who did not reply the first time. Totally, 5775 adults participated in the study and returned the medical questionnaire (46%) and 4369 indoor environment questionnaires (49%) were returned.

Environmental questions

The home environment questionnaire included the following questions:

(1) Number of persons living at home;
(2) Ownership of the apartment (own/rented);
(3) Type of ventilation system (mechanical ventilation system/ only natural ventilation);
(4) Current pet-keeping status in the apartment: dog (no/yes); cat (no/yes);
(5) Whether anybody living in the apartment ride a horse or has in another way contact with horses (no/yes);
(6) Current environmental tobacco smoke at home (ETS) (no, if the answer is "never"/yes, if the answer is "daily", "weekly" or "monthly");
(7) Condensation on window panes in winter (no, if the answer is "never"/yes, if the answer is "less than 5 cm", "5–25 cm" or "more than 25 cm");
(8) New indoor painting in the last 12 months (no/yes);
(9) New floor materials in the last 12 months (no/yes);
(10) Any water leakage in the last 12 months (no/yes);
(11) Any floor dampness in the last 12 months (no/yes);
(12) Any visible molds in the last 12 months (no/yes);
(13) Any moldy odor in the last 12 months (no/yes);
(14) Any other odor in the last 12 months (no/yes);
(15) Any damp spot, visible mold or water leakage in the last 5 years (no/yes);
(16) Any technical building investigation of the apartment by a consulting company because of dampness, water damage or mold (no/yes);

One new variable "dampness in the last 12 months" was created based on four questions (which are question (10) – (13)) among all the 16 questions above, named as question (17). The options for this variable are: no, if the answers for the four questions are all "no"; yes, if the answer of any of the four question is "yes".

A dampness index was created based on question (15) and (17), which coded as: 0, both answers are "no"; 1, only one of the answers is "no"; 2, both answers are "yes".

A window-opening index was created based on two questions about window opening habit as follows: a) How often do you usually air the apartment by opening the windows during heating season (from September to April)? There are four options: daily, weekly, monthly and never, which were coded as 1, 2, 3 and 4; b) if you do, how long time? There are four options: the whole day/night, few hours, have cross-draught for a few minutes and never, which were coded as 1, 2, 3 and 4. The window-opening index was coded as: 0, if b) = 4; 1, if a) = 3 and b) = 3; 2, if a) = 2 and b) = 3, or a) = 3 and b = 2, or a) = 1 b) = 3; 3, if a) = 2 and b) = 2; or if a) = 3 and b) = 1, or a) = 2 and b) = 1; 4, if a) = 1 and b) = 2; 5, if a) = 1 and b) = 1. A higher window-opening index indicate more window opening.

Data about construction year of buildings were collected from the National Building Register, Real Property Register and were categorized into 5 groups (-1960/1961–1975/1976–1985/1986–1995/1996–2005). Data about population and area of each municipality were acquired from wikipedia website (http://sv.wikipedia.org/wiki/Lista_%C3%B6ver_Sveriges_kommuner). Population density (number of persons per km^2) were calculated based on population and area of each municipality. Data about temperature zone were collected from a Swedish government report [54], which has 4 catagories: 1, inner part of north Sweden (Norrland); 2, costal part of Norrland and some inner part of Svealand; 3, Svealand (main parts); 4, Göteland (main parts). A higher number indicate a warmer climate.

Personal questions

Medical questions in the personal questionnaire included the following:

(1) Gender (female/male);

(2) Age;

(3) Current rhinitis (Irritating, stuffy or runny nose in the last 3 months). There were three options: often (every week), sometimes, never;

(4) Any wheezing in the chest in the last 12 months (no/yes);

(5) Any daytime attack of time breathlessness at rest in the last 12 months (no/yes);

(6) Any daytime attack of time breathlessness after exercise in the last 12 months (no/yes);

(7) Woken by attack of time breathlessness at any time in the last 12 months (no/yes);

(8) Diagnosed with asthma by a doctor (no/yes);

(9) Asthma attack during the last 12 months (no/yes);

(10) Current asthma medication (no/yes);

(11) Number of respiratory infections (such as cold, throat infection or flu) in the last 3 months (no/yes)? The options were: never (no); 1 time and 2 or more times (yes);

(12) Antibiotic medication because of respiratory infections during the last 12 months (no/yes);

(13) Pollen allergy (no/yes);

(14) Furry pet allergy (no/yes).

The variable daytime breathlessness was created from question (5) and (6) coded as "no" if the answers to both questions is "no", and "yes" if any one of the answers is "yes".

Current asthma was created from question (9) and (10) coded as "no" if the answers to both questions is "no", and "yes" if any one of the answers is "yes".

The variable pollen or furry pet allergy was created from question (13) and (14) coded as "no" if the answers to both questions is "no", and "yes" if any one of the answers is "yes".

The rhinitis variable was further classified into 4 categories: no rhinitis, infection rhinitis, allergic rhinitis and non-allergic rhinitis. Infection rhinitis was defined as having both current rhinitis and any respiratory infections in the last 3 months. Allergic rhinitis was defined as having current rhinitis and pollen of furry pet allergy, but no respiratory infections. Non-allergic rhinitis was defined as having current rhinitis, but no pollen or furry pet allergy and no respiratory infections.

Statistical analysis

All statistical analyses were conducted with STATA 11.0 (STATA Corp, Texas, USA). The prevalence of symptoms and exposures were calculated for total subjects and age stratified groups. Ordinal regression models were used to study associations between current rhinitis, respiratory infections and home environment factors with adjustment for gender, age and current smoking. In the ordinal logistic regression OR is expressed for one step on the scale of the dependent variable. Mutual adjustment were then applied including all significant or nearly significant factors ($p<0.1$) with additional adjustment for gender, age and current smoking. As a next step, associations between different types of rhinitis symptoms and home environment factors were calculated by multi-nominal regression models with adjustment for gender, age and current smoking.

Multiple logistic regression was used to study associations between wheeze, day time breathlessness, night time breathlessness, doctor-diagnosed asthma, current asthma, respiratory infections and antibiotic medication for respiratory infections and home environment factors with adjustment for gender, age and smoking. Mutual adjustment were then applied including all significant or nearly significant factors ($p<0.1$) with additional adjustment for gender, age and current smoking.

In addition, sensitivity analyses were performed, by stratifying for age (≤65 years v.s >65 years old (elderly)).

Age interaction was studied in the mutual adjusted models (≤65 years old v.s elderly). Interaction was tested statistically if there were a marked numerical difference in OR when comparing the occupational active age group with elderly.

Associations were expressed as odds ratios (OR) with a 95% confidence interval (CI) for ordinal regression and logistic regression models. For multi-nominal regression models, associations were expressed as relative risk ratio (RRR) with a 95% confidence interval (CI). In all statistical analysis, two-tailed tests and a 5% level of significance were applied.

Results

Totally, 5775 personal (46%) and 4369 indoor environment questionnaires (49%) were returned. 73 subjects did not fill the question of their gender, and 49 subjects did not fill the question of their of age. Analysis of non-responders was performed by SCB Sweden. SCB Sweden analyzed differences between participants and non-participants based on background factors available from other population registers linked to the census [54]. For privacy reasons we did not have access to all these variables. The participation rate was higher among older persons, especially those older than 60 years. Married persons had a higher participation rate, as compared to those not being married. Moreover, the participation rate was related to degree of urbanization, with a slightly lower participation rate in larger cities and suburban municipalities. The participation rate was slightly lower in older buildings. There was no major difference in participation rate between different municipalities. The differences in participation rate between those being born in Sweden as compared to those foreign-born persons and between those having or not having Swedish citizenship were very small. All of the differences in participation rate were small, except for age and civil status.

The prevalence of smoking, allergy, rhinitis, asthma and respiratory infection symptoms in relation to gender and different age groups are shown in Table 1. In total 56.5% were female, 63.5% were 18 to 65 years old, and 36.5% were more than 65 years old; 12.0% were current smokers; 51.0% had current rhinitis; 17.7% wheeze; 11.7% day time breathlessness; 6.0% night time breathlessness; 11.5% doctor diagnosed asthma; 7.7% current asthma; 46.4% respiratory infections and 11.9% antibiotic medication for respiratory infections. The prevalence of current smoking, pollen allergy, furry pet allergy, current rhinitis, asthma attack, respiratory infections were lower among elderly. Wheeze, day time breathlessness, night time breathlessness were higher among elderly.

Descriptive data on home environment factors are shown in Table 2. Totally, 40.9% were living alone; 50.7% were living in rented apartments; 19.0% had window pane condensation; 14.7% had any dampness in the last 12 months and 19.3% in the last 5 years. Females were more living in rented apartments and more often in certain building years. Compared with subjects ≤65 years old, there were more elderly were living alone. The elderly had less cats, and less contact with horses, less exposure to ETS, less renovation (painting, new floors) and less dampness, visible molds and odors.

The associations between current rhinitis and home environment factors are shown in Table 3 (mutual adjustment). Current rhinitis was more common in those living in buildings constructed during 1976–1985, as compared to older buildings constructed before 1961 (reference category). Moreover, living in densely populated areas, living alone and living in rented apartments were associated with current rhinitis.

When dividing type of rhinitis into three groups (infection-allergic- and non-allergic rhinitis), infection rhinitis was more common among those living in buildings constructed during 1976–1985, as compared with older buildings constructed before 1961 and other buildings constructed after 1985. Moreover, it was more common in densely populated areas, among those living alone, those in rented apartments and in homes with window condensation in winter time. Living alone and window pane condensation were risk factors for allergic rhinitis. Non-allergic rhinitis was more reported among those living in rented apartments (Tables 4).

The associations between wheeze, day time breathlessness, night time breathlessness and home environment factors are shown in Table 5 (mutual adjustment). Wheeze was more common among those living in colder climate zones, in rented apartments and in homes with dampness problems (dampness index). Day time attacks of breathlessness was associated with living in buildings constructed during 1961–1975, in rented apartments, in homes with dampness problems, and in apartments with more window-opening (high window-opening index). The association between day time breathlessness and dampness close to significance for dampness index = 1 ($p = 0.05$). Night time breathlessness was more reported in colder climate zones and in apartments with more window-opening time. The associations between doctor-diagnosed asthma, current asthma and home environment factors are shown in Table 6 (mutual adjustment). Doctor-diagnosed asthma was associated with living in homes with odor, other than moldy odor. Current asthma was more common in homes with ETS and in homes with odor, other than moldy odor.

The associations between respiratory infections, used antibiotic medication for respiratory infections and home environment factors are shown in Table 7 (mutual adjustment). Respiratory infections were associated with living in buildings constructed during 1976–1985, as compared with older buildings constructed before 1960, and in densely populated areas and in rented apartments. Antibiotic medication for respiratory infections was more common in homes with window pane condensation.

Among elderly, current rhinitis was less common among those in homes with dampness problems. Wheeze was more common in rented apartments. Day time attacks of breathlessness was associated with living in homes without mechanical ventilation and more common in homes with high window-opening index. Night time attacks of breathlessness was more reported among those living in colder climate zones. Doctor-diagnosed asthma was more common among those living in rented apartments. Respiratory infections was associated with living in buildings constructed during 1976–1985 and 1996–2005, as compared to older buildings constructed before 1961, and it was more commonly reported in less populated areas. Generally, for these associations OR were numerically higher among elderly as compared to subjects ≤65 years old.

Finally, statistical interaction was tested, comparing elderly with subjects ≤65 years old. There was an age interaction for the association between dampness index and the following health variables: current rhinitis (for interaction, $p = 0.001$), wheeze (for interaction, $p = 0.001$), day time attacks of breathlessness (for interaction, $p = 0.002$), night time attacks of breathlessness (for interaction, $p = 0.004$), doctor-diagnosed asthma (for interaction, $p = 0.024$), current asthma (for interaction, $p = 0.021$) and antibiotic medication for respiratory infections (for interaction, $p = 0.015$). There was a trend for age interaction between apartment ownership and doctor-diagnosed asthma (for interaction, $p = 0.056$). Moreover, there was an age interaction for the association between ownership and antibiotic medication for respiratory infections (for interaction, $p = 0.015$).

Discussions

Associations were demonstrated between home environmental factors in multi-family buildings and adults' rhinitis, asthma and respiratory symptoms. Densely populated areas (urbanization), colder climate zones, rented apartments, building dampness, certain construction years (1961–1975, 1976–1985), odor perception and ETS at home were risk factors for rhinitis, asthma symptoms and respiratory infections.

This study was made during the spring season, which is part of the pollen season in Sweden. Selection bias due to a low response rate can influence epidemiological studies. In this study, we included all subjects (≥18 years old) living in multi-family buildings, with no prior information on their health status. The sample size of this study was reasonably large, and is one of few covering a sample from a whole country. The response rate was not very high (46%). The participation rate was higher among elderly persons, married persons, and slightly lower in larger cities, suburban municipalities and in older buildings. However, we have found no major difference in participation rate between different

Table 1. Data on gender, smoking, allergy, rhinitis, asthma and respiratory infections.

Category	Subcategory	Male n = 2483[b] (%)	Female n = 3219[b] (%)	*p* value[d]	≤65 years old n = 3637[c] (%)	>65 years old n = 2089[c] (%)	*p* value[d]	Total n = 5775 (%)
Female		-	-		54.2	60.4	<0.001	56.5
Current smoking		11.8	12.1	0.728	14.8	7.2	<0.001	12.0
Pollen allergy		23.9	23.7	0.891	28.3	15.7	<0.001	23.8
Furry pet allergy		12.2	11.6	0.505	15.5	5.4	<0.001	11.9
Pollen or furry pet allergy		27.4	27.1	0.847	32.7	17.6	<0.001	27.3
Rhinitis in the last 3 months	Never	49.4	48.7	<0.001	47.4	52.1	0.007	49.0
	Sometimes	41.3	37.2		40.3	36.7		39.1
	Weekly	9.3	14.1		12.3	11.2		11.9
Type of rhinitis	Never	49.6	49.0	0.308	47.6	52.4	<0.001	49.2
	Infection rhinitis	29.9	32.0		34.9	23.5		31.1
	Allergic rhinitis	8.2	7.3		8.3	6.5		7.7
	Non-allergic rhinitis	12.3	11.7		9.2	17.6		12.0
Wheeze in the last 12 months		17.3	17.8	0.642	16.4	19.9	0.001	17.7
Day time breathlessness in the last 12 months		10.8	12.3	0.078	10.3	14.0	<0.001	11.7
Night time breathlessness in the last 12 months		5.7	6.3	0.367	5.9	6.1	0.727	6.0
Doctor diagnosed asthma		9.9	12.6	0.002	12.0	10.3	0.056	11.5
Current asthma[a]		7.0	8.2	0.082	7.5	7.8	0.728	7.7
	Asthma attack	3.1	3.8	0.171	3.9	2.7	0.016	3.5
	Asthma medication	6.3	7.9	0.028	6.9	7.6	0.339	7.2
Respiratory infections in the last 3 months	No infection	53.1	53.9	0.191	48.0	63.1	<0.001	53.6
	One time	36.2	34.3		38.4	29.6		35.1
	Two or more times	10.6	11.8		13.6	7.3		11.3
Used antibiotic medication for respiratory infections in the last 12 months		9.7	13.5	<0.001	11.2	12.9	0.058	11.9

[a]Subjects who have had asthma attacks or have taken asthma medicine during the last 12 months.
[b]Subjects with missing data on gender (n = 73) were excluded.
[c]Subjects with missing data on age (n = 49) were excluded.
[d]*p* value by Chi-square test.

Table 2. Data on home building characteristics and indoor environment factors.

Home environment factors	Subcategory	Male n = 2483[e] (%)	Female n = 3219[e] (%)	*p* value[g]	≤65 years old n = 3637[f] (%)	>65 years old n = 2089[f] (%)	*p* value[g]	Total n = 5775 (%)
Temperature zone[a]	1	2.6	2.7	0.967	2.5	2.8	0.016	2.6
	2	11.0	11.1		10.1	12.6		11.0
	3	52.6	51.9		53.2	50.4		52.1
	4	33.9	34.4		34.2	34.1		34.3
Construction year	-1960	12.9	12.1	0.017	13.6	10.5	<0.001	12.5
	1961–1975	33.7	32.4		34.0	31.0		33.0
	1976–1985	16.8	18.6		17.0	19.1		17.9
	1986–1995	14.6	17.0		15.1	17.5		16.0
	1996–2005	21.9	19.8		20.2	21.9		20.7
Living alone		41.0	40.9	0.991	36.6	48.4	<0.001	40.9
Rented apartments		49.1	52.0	0.031	52.7	47.0	<0.001	50.7
Natural ventilation only		45.7	45.3	0.788	46.5	43.6	0.063	45.4
Have dog		7.5	7.7	0.726	8.1	6.9	0.112	7.7
Have cat		8.0	9.1	0.166	9.7	6.7	<0.001	8.7
Horse contact		3.2	3.6	0.376	4.4	1.8	<0.001	3.5
ETS		11.9	12.0	0.928	13.1	10.2	0.003	12.1
New indoor painting in the last 12 months		18.0	16.3	0.088	19.1	13.6	<0.001	17.1
New floor materials in the last 12 months		9.6	9.5	0.866	10.8	7.4	<0.001	9.5
Window pane condensation		19.4	18.7	0.535	21.3	15.2	<0.001	19.0
Water leakage in the last 12 months		7.1	6.4	0.306	7.4	5.4	0.004	6.7
Floor dampness in the last 12 months		6.3	7.0	0.287	7.6	5.1	<0.001	6.8
Visible molds in the last 12 months		4.0	3.5	0.355	4.5	2.4	<0.001	3.8
Moldy odor in the last 12 months		2.6	2.7	0.799	3.2	1.5	<0.001	2.7
Other odor in the last 12 months		8.2	8.7	0.611	9.2	7.2	0.026	8.5
Any dampness in the last 12 months[b]		15.0	14.4	0.536	16.4	11.4	<0.001	14.7
Any dampness in the last 5 years		20.1	18.5	0.156	21.3	15.3	<0.001	19.3
Consultant investigation for home dampness		15.4	13.9	0.177	15.8	12.4	0.003	14.5
Dampness index[c]	0	74.1	75.4	0.514	72.3	79.5	<0.001	74.7
	1	16.1	15.7		17.1	13.7		15.9
	2	9.7	9.0		10.6	6.9		9.3
Window-opening index[d]	0	2.0	1.8	0.912	2.2	1.4	<0.001	1.9
	1	2.9	2.6		3.1	2.0		2.7
	2	23.4	23.1		24.2	21.8		23.2
	3	11.2	10.8		11.9	9.3		11.0
	4	36.8	37.0		34.6	41.0		37.1

Table 2. Cont.

Home environment factors	Subcategory	Male n = 2483[e] (%)	Female n = 3219[e] (%)	*p* value[g]	≤65 years old n = 3637[f] (%)	>65 years old n = 2089[f] (%)	*p* value[g]	Total n = 5775 (%)
	5	23.5	24.6		23.9	24.5		24.2

[a]Higher number stands for warmer climate.
[b]Subjects have reported one of the following dampness problems: water leakage, floor dampness, visible molds or moldy odor in the last 12 months.
[c]Dampness index, number of "yes" answers to "any dampness in the last 12 months" and "any dampness in the last 5 year": 0, answers were both "no"; 1, only one answer was "yes"; 2, answers were "yes" to both questions.
[d]Higher number stands for more window opening.
[e]Subjects with missing data on gender (n = 73) were excluded.
[f]Subjects with missing data on age (n = 49) were excluded.
[g]*p* value by Chi-square test.

municipalities, between those being born in Sweden as compared to those foreign-born persons, and between those having or not having Swedish citizenships. Furthermore, most of the differences in participation rate were small. The elderly in our study accounted for 36% in our study. It has been shown that elderly population (more than 65 years old) in Sweden are accounting for 23% of the adult population [55]. Elderly in our study were more prone to answer questionnaire, and retired people lives more in apartments other than in single-family buildings in Sweden. Recall bias can be a potential problem in questionnaire surveys. Subjects may overestimate or underestimate their personal symptoms or reports on indoor environment risk factors. However, some factors, such as building constructed year, population density were not collected by questionnaire. Moreover, we found some associations between specific home environmental risk factors and health status, not a similar association for all risk factors. Thus, we don't believe that our conclusions are seriously biased by selection or response errors.

Our study found that subjects living in colder climate zones reported more wheeze and night time breathlessness. This is in agreement with a previous study reported more asthma among Swedish conscripts in the colder parts of northern Sweden [56]. One possible explanation could be less ventilation to save energy.

Living in an area with a higher population density (persons/km^2) was associated with current rhinitis, infection rhinitis and respiratory infections. One study in Swedish preschool children found that asthma prevalence increased by municipality population density measured the same way as in our study [57]. Population density is used as a proxy variable for degree of urbanization. Exposure to traffic air pollution is one factor associated with population density. Outdoor traffic related exposure was related to an increased risk of allergic rhinitis among adults in Italy [58] and in Sweden [59]. The risk for having infections would increase with the increase of population density because of increased probability of spending time in crowded environments.

Despite the low prevalence of ETS in the Swedish homes, we confirmed that ETS at home is still a risk factor for current asthma. ETS in homes is one of the most consistently factors associated with asthma and asthma-related symptoms among adults in homes [34].

Subjects renting their apartment had more current rhinitis, infection rhinitis, wheeze, day time breathlessness and respiratory infections. Renting apartment can be a proxy variable for lower socio-economic status (SES). One Swedish study on multi-family buildings in Stockholm found that dwellers renting their apartments reported more nasal symptoms than those owning their homes, and found a high correlation between different socio-economic factors (apartment ownership, income, education, and occupation) [60]. One study on SES (defined by parental education) and children's respiratory and allergic symptoms conducted in 13 diverse countries found that lower SES was related to decreased prevalence of allergy to aero-allergens [61]. The association between SES and asthma prevalence and incidence in adults is not well understood and is a matter of debate [62]. However, lower SES seems to be associated with more severe asthma or poorly controlled asthma [62]. Asthma prevalence was higher in lower SES groups among adults [63] and among children [61]. In Sweden, a large number of multi-family apartments of all construction periods are rental, owned by the community, with similar living standards and rental costs as private apartments [64]. However families with lower SES are overrepresented in buildings built from 1961–1975, mostly rented and today buildings prioritized for renovation. The influence of

Table 3. Associations between current rhinitis and building characteristics and indoor environment factors analyzed by ordinal regression models.

Factors	Subcategory	All subjects n = 5775 OR(95% CI)[c]	All subjects n = 5775 Mutual adj. OR(95% CI)[d]	≤65 years old, n = 3637[g], Mutual adj. OR(95% CI)[e]	>65 years old n = 2089[g], Mutual adj. OR(95% CI)[f]
Construction year	-1960	1.00	1.00	1.00	1.00
	1961–1975	1.23(1.03,1.46)*	1.12(0.90,1.41)	1.17(0.90,1.52)	1.12(0.73,1.72)
	1976–1985	1.34(1.10,1.63)**	1.43(1.12,1.84)**	1.45(1.07,1.96)*	1.54(0.97,2.46)
	1986–1995	1.18(0.96,1.44)	1.27(0.99,1.63)	1.30(0.96,1.74)	1.32(0.83,2.11)
	1996–2005	1.01(0.83,1.22)	1.15(0.91,1.46)	1.24(0.93,1.64)	1.12(0.71,1.76)
Population density/10000[a]		1.48(1.12,1.97)**	1.61(1.13,2.29)**	1.74(1.14,2.64)*	1.81(0.90,3.64)
Living alone		1.14(1.02,1.27)*	1.25(1.09,1.43)**	1.54(1.30,1.82)***	0.88(0.69,1.11)
Rented apartments		1.33(1.20,1.49)***	1.23(1.07,1.40)**	1.25(1.06,1.48)**	1.21(0.95,1.54)
Window pane condensation		1.23(1.07,1.42)**	1.16(0.98,1.38)	1.15(0.94,1.41)	1.22(0.88,1.68)
Odor, other than moldy odor in the last 12 months		1.21(0.98,1.50)	1.25(0.98,1.60)	1.30(0.97,1.73)	1.03(0.63,1.67)
Dampness index[b]	0	1.00	1.00	1.00	1.00
	1	1.10(0.94,1.28)	1.07(0.88,1.29)	1.32(1.05,1.67)*	0.67(0.46,0.98)*
	2	1.26(1.04,1.53)*	1.19(0.88,1.60)	1.46(1.03,2.06)*	0.64(0.34,1.21)

[a]The ORs were expressed per 10000 increase of the population density (number of persons per km^2).
[b]Dampness index, number of "yes" answers to "any dampness in the last 12 months" and "any dampness in the last 5 year": 0, answers were both "no"; 1, only one answer was "yes"; 2, answers were "yes" to both questions.
[c]Adjusted for gender, age and smoking.
[d]Mutual adjustment models including gender, age and smoking for all subjects (inclusion criteria is $p<0.1$ in total sample).
[e]Mutual adjustment models including gender, age and smoking for younger and middle aged subjects (≤65 years old) (inclusion criteria is $p<0.1$ in total sample).
[f]Mutual adjustment models including gender, age and smoking for elderly (>65 years old) (inclusion criteria is $p<0.1$ in total sample).
[g]Subjects with missing data on age (n = 49) were excluded.
*** $p<0.001$,
** $p<0.01$,
* $p<0.05$.

Table 4. Associations between different types of rhinitis symptoms and building characteristics and indoor environment factors analyzed by multi-nominal logistic regression models.

Factors	Infection rhinitis n = 1568 RRR(95% CI)[a]	Allergic rhinitis n = 388 RRR(95% CI)[a]	Non-allergic rhinitis n = 605 RRR(95% CI)[a]
Construction year 1961–1975[b]	1.09(0.94,1.27)	1.16(0.91,1.48)	1.21(0.99,1.48)
Construction year 1976–1985[c]	1.32(1.11,1.57)**	0.93(0.68,1.28)	1.10(0.86,1.42)
Population density[d]	1.24(1.09,1.42)**	1.08(0.86,1.34)	1.00(0.84,1.20)
Living alone	1.16(1.02,1.33)*	1.37(1.10,1.69)**	1.03(0.85,1.23)
Rented apartments	1.28(1.12,1.46)***	1.16(0.93,1.45)	1.35(1.13,1.63)**
Window pane condensation	1.24(1.04,1.47)*	1.32(1.00,1.75)*	1.13(0.89,1.45)
Dampness index = 2[e]	1.21(0.96,1.53)	1.41(0.98,2.03)	0.98(0.69,1.40)

[a]Adjusted for gender, age and smoking.
[b]Buildings constructed during 1961–1975 compared with buildings constructed before 1960 and during 1986–2005 (excluding buildings constructed during 1976–1985).
[c]Buildings constructed during 1976–1985 compared with buildings constructed before 1960 and during 1986–2005 (excluding buildings constructed during 1961–1975).
[d]Population density (number of persons per km^2) was used as a categorical variable in this analysis: population density >1000 persons/km^2 was compared with population density ≤1000 persons/km^2.
[e]Dampness index, number of "yes" answers to "any dampness in the last 12 months" and "any dampness in the last 5 year": 0, answers were both "no"; 1, only one answer was "yes"; 2, answers were "yes" to both questions. Dampness index = 2 was compared with dampness index = 0 in this analysis.
*** $p<0.001$,
** $p<0.01$,
* $p<0.05$.

Table 5. Associations between wheeze, day time breathlessness, night time breathlessness, building characteristics and indoor environment factors (by logistic regresson models).

Symptoms	Factors	Subcategory	All subjects n = 5775 OR(95% CI)[d]	All subjects n = 5775, mutual adj. OR(95% CI)[e]	≤65 years old n = 3637[h], mutual adj. OR(95% CI)[f]	>65 years old n = 2089[h], mutual adj. OR(95% CI)[g]
Wheeze in the last 12 months	Temperature zone[a]		0.91(0.83,1.01)	0.89(0.80,0.99)*	0.87(0.75,1.00)*	0.90(0.76,1.06)
	Rented apartments		1.35(1.16,1.56)***	1.20(1.02,1.41)*	1.10(0.89,1.35)	1.37(1.06,1.77)*
	Window pane condensation		1.20(0.99,1.43)	1.15(0.95,1.41)	1.13(0.89,1.44)	1.17(0.83,1.65)
	Dampness index[b]	0	1.00	1.00	1.00	1.00
		1	1.16(0.95,1.42)	1.06(0.85,1.33)	1.27(0.96,1.67)	0.77(0.52,1.15)
		2	1.53(1.20,1.94)**	1.42(1.08,1.86)*	1.90(1.38,2.62)***	0.69(0.38,1.22)
Day time breathlessness in the last 12 months	Construction year	-1960	1.00	1.00	1.00	1.00
		1961–1975	1.37(1.03,1.83)*	1.53(1.03,2.29)*	1.47(0.93,2.33)	2.13(0.91,4.99)
		1976–1985	1.25(0.91,1.72)	1.28(0.82,2.01)	1.11(0.65,1.91)	2.20(0.89,5.45)
		1986–1995	1.20(0.87,1.66)	1.39(0.89,2.18)	1.38(0.81,2.36)	1.94(0.78,4.81)
		1996–2005	0.76(0.54,1.05)	1.12(0.71,1.76)	0.95(0.55,1.63)	1.92(0.78,4.71)
	Rented apartments		1.60(1.34,1.90)***	1.31(1.04,1.66)*	1.25(0.93,1.69)	1.45(0.99,2.12)
	Natural ventilation only		1.35(1.12,1.63)**	1.13(0.90,1.42)	1.04(0.77,1.39)	1.47(1.01,2.14)*
	ETS		1.32(1.03,1.70)*	1.15(0.83,1.57)	1.03(0.70,1.54)	1.41(0.82,2.41)
	New indoor painting in the last 12 months		0.79(0.62,1.00)	0.71(0.50,1.01)	0.70(0.45,1.07)	0.76(0.39,1.47)
	New floor materials in the last 12 months		0.75(0.54,1.03)	0.62(0.38,1.00)	0.61(0.35,1.08)	0.62(0.24,1.55)
	Dampness index[b]	0	1.00	1.00	1.00	1.00
		1	1.35(1.07,1.70)*	1.35(1.00,1.81)*	1.44(1.00,2.07)	1.26(0.76,2.10)
		2	1.76(1.34,2.30)***	1.57(1.09,2.27)*	2.18(1.44,3.31)***	0.48(0.19,1.25)
	Window-opening index[c]		1.08(1.01,1.16)*	1.10(1.01,1.20)*	1.06(0.95,1.19)	1.20(1.02,1.40)*
Night time breathlessness in the last 12 months	Temperature zone[a]		0.85(0.74,0.99)*	0.74(0.61,0.90)**	0.76(0.59,0.97)*	0.69(0.50,0.97)*
	Construction year	-1960	1.00	1.00	1.00	1.00
		1961–1975	1.65(1.11,2.44)*	1.19(0.70,2.01)	1.39(0.76,2.57)	0.93(0.32,2.67)
		1976–1985	1.44(0.93,2.22)	1.23(0.69,2.18)	1.18(0.59,2.35)	1.54(0.51,4.64)
		1986–1995	1.42(0.91,2.22)	1.04(0.57,1.89)	0.95(0.45,1.99)	1.39(0.47,4.15)
		1996–2005	0.64(0.39,1.05)	0.55(0.29,1.05)	0.53(0.24,1.17)	0.63(0.19,2.06)
	Rented apartments		1.66(1.31,2.09)***	1.34(0.98,1.84)	1.27(0.85,1.89)	1.51(0.87,2.62)
	Natural ventilation only		1.25(0.97,1.62)	0.99(0.72,1.35)	1.02(0.69,1.50)	0.99(0.56,1.73)
	New indoor painting in the last 12 months		0.68(0.49,0.96)*	0.64(0.40,1.01)	0.53(0.31,0.92)*	0.95(0.42,2.19)
	Window pane condensation		1.35(1.02,1.80)*	1.10(0.76,1.59)	1.01(0.65,1.58)	1.28(0.64,2.55)
	Dampness index[b]	0	1.00	1.00	1.00	1.00
		1	1.41(1.04,1.90)*	1.10(0.72,1.68)	1.27(0.77,2.09)	0.87(0.39,1.92)
		2	1.46(1.01,2.13)*	1.60(0.96,2.64)	2.63(1.46,4.36)**	-
	Window-opening index[c]		1.12(1.02,1.24)*	1.18(1.04,1.34)*	1.13(0.97,1.32)	1.26(0.99,1.61)

[a]The ORs were expressed per 1 unit increase for temperature zone.
[b]Dampness index, number of "yes" answers to "any dampness in the last 12 months" and "any dampness in the last 5 year": 0, answers were both "no"; 1, only one answer was "yes"; 2, answers were "yes" to both questions.
[c]The ORs were expressed per 1 unit increase for window-opening index.
[d]Adjusted for gender, age and smoking.
[e]Mutual adjustment models including gender, age and smoking for all subjects (inclusion criteria is $p<0.1$ in total sample).
[f]Mutual adjustment models including gender, age and smoking for subjects ≤65 years old (inclusion criteria is $p<0.1$ in total sample).
[g]Mutual adjustment models including gender, age and smoking for subjects >65 years old (inclusion criteria is $p<0.1$ in total sample).
[h]Subjects with missing data on age (n = 49) were excluded.
*** $p<0.001$,
** $p<0.01$,
* $p<0.05$.

ownership on health in our study may also depend upon differences in building maintenance, e.g. a lack of control over the home environment because of renting rather than owning.

Our study found that reported building dampness (dampness index) was associated with wheeze and day time breathlessness. This finding is consistent with another Swedish study among adults living in multi-family buildings [65]. Building dampness problems in homes is associated with increased asthma prevalence, which has been shown in former studies [35,43,66,67]. A cohort study found that new onset of adult asthma was related to dampness/molds in dwellings in Europe, and concluded that the population-attributable risk was 3–14% for observed dampness/molds [68]. One meta-analysis showed that wheeze among adults were associated with damp homes, and concluded that building dampness and molds were associated with approximately 30–50% increases in a variety of respiratory and asthma-related health outcomes [43]. Building dampness is related to a complex mix of exposures, including house dust mite allergens [69], microbial agents [70,71], bacteria [71–73], chemical emissions from degradation of building materials [74] as well as microbial volatile organic compounds (MVOC) [71].

Window pane condensation was associated with infection rhinitis, allergic rhinitis and antibiotic medication for respiratory infections. Window pane condensation is usually a marker of poor ventilation and a predictor of high relative air humidity (RH) indoors. A Japanese study found that window pane condensation in homes of female university students was related to wheeze symptoms [75]. Exhaled nitric oxide (NO) levels were associated with home window pane condensation among non-sensitized (skin prick tests for IgE sensitization) school children aged [76]. NO is a method introduced for non-invasive monitoring of airway inflammation.

We found that certain construction periods were associated with more respiratory illness. Buildings constructed from 1961–1975 were associated with more day time breathlessness. Buildings constructed from 1976–1985 were associated with more current

Table 6. Associations between doctor-diagnosed asthma, current asthma, building characteristics and indoor environment factors analyzed by logistic regression models.

Symptoms	Factors	Subcategory	All subjects n = 5775 OR(95% CI)[d]	All subjects n = 5775, mutual adj. OR(95% CI)[e]	≤65 years old n = 3637[h], mutual adj. OR(95% CI)[f]	>65 years old n = 2089[h], mutual adj. OR(95% CI)[g]
Doctor-diagnosed asthma	Temperature zone[b]		0.90(0.80,1.01)	0.95(0.83,1.08)	0.86(0.74,1.01)	1.16(0.90,1.50)
	Rented apartments		1.24(1.04,1.47)*	1.13(0.93,1.38)	0.97(0.76,1.23)	1.69(1.15,2.46)**
	Odor, other than moldy odor in the last 12 months		1.52(1.12,2.06)**	1.49(1.08,2.06)*	1.66(1.15,2.39)**	1.04(0.50,2.16)
	Dampness index[c]	0	1.00	1.00	1.00	1.00
		1	1.10(0.87,1.39)	1.14(0.87,1.49)	1.32(0.98,1.80)	0.67(0.36,1.25)
		2	1.34(1.01,1.78)*	1.20(0.79,1.81)	1.48(0.95,2.33)	0.50(0.15,1.66)
Current asthma[a]	Temperature zone[b]		0.89(0.78,1.02)	0.90(0.75,1.06)	0.78(0.64,0.95)*	1.25(0.90,1.74)
	Construction year	-1960	1.00	1.00	1.00	1.00
		1961–1975	1.17(0.84,1.62)	1.08(0.72,1.63)	0.99(0.62,1.58)	1.32(0.53,3.27)
		1976–1985	1.10(0.76,1.58)	1.02(0.64,1.62)	0.96(0.56,1.64)	1.26(0.47,3.35)
		1986–1995	1.09(0.75,1.59)	0.88(0.55,1.42)	0.73(0.42,1.28)	1.29(0.49,3.40)
		1996–2005	0.70(0.48,1.03)	0.70(0.43,1.13)	0.75(0.44,1.30)	0.60(2.12,1.72)
	Rented apartment		1.32(1.07,1.62)**	1.05(0.81,1.36)	0.95(0.69,1.29)	1.45(0.90,2.32)
	ETS		1.43(1.06,1.92)*	1.53(1.09,2.16)*	1.43(0.94,2.17)	1.79(0.97,3.34)
	New indoor painting in the last 12 months		0.73(0.54,0.98)*	0.69(0.47,0.99)*	0.69(0.45,1.04)	0.61(0.27,1.37)
	Odor, other than moldy odor in the last 12 months		1.64(1.15,2.33)**	1.52(1.03,2.24)*	1.71(1.10,2.65)*	1.05(0.43,2.52)
	Dampness index[c]	0	1.00	1.00	1.00	1.00
		1	1.14(0.86,1.52)	1.29(0.93,1.79)	1.57(1.07,2.29)*	0.76(0.37,1.58)
		2	1.50(1.08,2.08)*	1.14(0.68,1.92)	1.62(0.93,2.82)	0.22(0.03,1.63)

[a]subjects who have had asthma attacks or have taken asthma medicine during the last 12 months.
[b]The ORs were expressed per 1 unit increase for temperature zone.
[c]Dampness index, number of "yes" answers to "any dampness in the last 12 months" and "any dampness in the last 5 year": 0, answers were both "no"; 1, only one answer was "yes"; 2, answers were "yes" to both questions.
[d]Adjusted for gender, age and smoking.
[e]Mutual adjustment models including gender, age and smoking for all subjects (inclusion criteria is $p<0.1$ in total sample).
[f]Mutual adjustment models including gender, age and smoking for subjects ≤65 years old (inclusion criteria is $p<0.1$ in total sample).
[g]Mutual adjustment models including gender, age and smoking for subjects >65 years old (inclusion criteria is $p<0.1$ in total sample).
[h]Subjects with missing data on age (n = 49) were excluded.
*** $p<0.001$,
** $p<0.01$,
* $p<0.05$.

Table 7. Associations between respiratory infections (by ordinal regression models), antibiotic medication for respiratory infections (by logistic regression models), building characteristics and indoor environment factors.

Symptoms	Factors	Subcategory	All subjects n = 5775 OR(95% CI)[d]	All subjects n = 5775, mutual adj. OR(95% CI)[e]	≤65 years old n = 3637[h], mutual adj. OR(95% CI)[f]	>65 years old n = 2089[h], mutual adj. OR(95% CI)[g]
Respiratory infections in the last 3 months	Construction year	-1960	1.00	1.00	1.00	1.00
		1961–1975	1.06(0.89,1.26)	1.07(0.90,1.28)	1.07(0.87,1.31)	1.11(0.79,1.56)
		1976–1985	1.41(1.17,1.71)***	1.46(1.21,1.78)***	1.33(1.06,1.68)*	1.87(1.30,2.69)**
		1986–1995	1.07(0.88,1.30)	1.08(0.88,1.31)	1.03(0.81,1.31)	1.25(0.86,1.80)
		1996–2005	1.09(0.91,1.31)	1.12(0.93,1.35)	0.97(0.78,1.21)	1.56(1.09,2.22)*
	Population density[a]		1.57(1.19,2.09)**	1.72(1.30,2.29)***	1.68(1.20,2.34)**	2.21(1.27,3.87)**
	Rented apartments		1.11(1.00,1.23)	1.13(1.01,1.26)*	1.13(0.99,1.29)	1.14(0.94,1.37)
Antibiotic medication for respiratory infections in the last 12 months	Population density[a]		1.67(1.08,2.58)*	1.63(0.94,2.85)	1.96(0.99,3.90)	1.53(0.58,4.09)
	Rented apartments		1.22(1.03,1.44)*	1.13(0.91,1.40)	1.46(1.10,1.92)**	0.84(0.59,1.20)
	Window pane condensation		1.33(1.08,1.64)**	1.41(1.10,1.82)**	1.49(1.09,2.03)*	1.23(0.78,1.94)
	Odor, other than moldy odor in the last 12 months		1.42(1.05,1.92)*	1.23(0.85,1.80)	1.20(0.75,1.91)	1.22(0.64,2.35)
	Dampness index[b]	0	1.00	1.00	1.00	1.00
		1	1.25(1.00,1.57)	1.08(0.80,1.47)	1.29(0.90,1.86)	0.77(0.42,1.39)
		2	1.43(1.08,1.89)*	1.40(0.92,2.12)	1.84(1.14,2.97)*	0.63(0.24,1.64)
	Window-opening index[c]		1.06(0.99,1.14)	1.09(1.00,1.18)	1.05(0.95,1.17)	1.13(0.97,1.31)

[a]The ORs were expressed per 10000 increase of the population density (number of persons per km^2).
[b]Dampness index, number of "yes" answers to "any dampness in the last 12 months" and "any dampness in the last 5 year": 0, answers were both "no"; 1, only one answer was "yes"; 2, answers were "yes" to both questions.
[c]The ORs were expressed per 1 unit increase for window-opening index.
[d]Adjusted for gender, age and smoking.
[e]Mutual adjustment models including gender, age and smoking for all subjects (inclusion criteria is $p<0.1$ in total sample).
[f]Mutual adjustment models including gender, age and smoking for subjects ≤65 years old (inclusion criteria is $p<0.1$ in total sample).
[g]Mutual adjustment models including gender, age and smoking for subjects >65 years old (inclusion criteria is $p<0.1$ in total sample).
[h]Subjects with missing data on age (n = 49) were excluded.
*** $p<0.001$,
** $p<0.01$,
* $p<0.05$.

rhinitis, infection rhinitis and respiratory infections in the last 3 months. Our age classification of multi-family buildings were based on major changes in buildings technology in Sweden. Buildings from 1961–1975 were constructed during a building boom in suburbs of large cities rented by poorer people. They were mostly poor quality high-rise buildings with basements and only exhaust ventilation. These buildings have been reported to have the highest prevalence of dampness problems [77]. The next generation of multi-family buildings (constructed during 1976–1985) was influenced by energy saving demands, with many changes in construction techniques and new building materials [64]. The drastic increase of the oil price in 1974 initiated energy saving measures to reduce energy consumption in buildings during this period. Moreover, in 1977 self-level mortar containing the protein casein were introduced and used in Swedish buildings from 1977–1983. Due to severe indoor environmental problems this mortar was not used after 1983. Studies have shown that the problem was due to dampness causing chemical emissions such as ammonia and sulfhydryl compounds [78]. Later research identified another odorous compound, 2-acetophenone, emitted from the casein containing mortar. The compound is produced by degradation of the amino acid tryptophan [79]. It has a raw stuffy smell, and has been identified as a compound causing malodour in wine [80] and green tea [81]. The emission of ammonia from the mortar is known to cause blackening of parquet floors and degradation of acrylate polymers in water based glue and the plasticizer di-di-ethyl-hexyl-phthlate (DEHP) in polyvinylchloride (PVC) floor materials, causing emission of 2-etyl-1-hexanol to indoor air [82]. Epidemiological studies have shown that subjects staying in buildings with this type of mortar, and with emission of ammonia and 2-etyl-1-hexanol have a higher prevalence of mucosal inflammation and sick building syndrome [82] and asthma [74]. Thus, multifamily buildings constructed 1976-1984 had particular indoor exposures and were the first generation of buildings in Sweden with low ventilation due to increased energy saving demand and testing of new building materials on a large scale. This may have resulted in an impaired indoor environment leading to the elevated levels of health problems observed in this study.

More window-opening time (higher window-opening index) was associated increased risk of day time breathlessness and night time breathlessness. A review article concluded that higher ventilation rate was associated with less report of asthma or asthma-related symptoms [45]. The negative association between window-opening time and respiratory symptoms in our study is unclear. Polluted outdoor air entering the indoor environment when opening windows could be one explanation. However, this study included all multi-family buildings of the whole country, not only a small polluted area of Sweden. Another possible reason would be that those with asthma problems tried to improve ventilation situation by opening window more often (limitation of the cross sectional design).

We found associations between other odor perception (moldy odor was included in the dampness index) and doctor-diagnosed asthma and current asthma. Experimental studies have shown that odor thresholds are similar in asthmatic and non-asthmatic subjects [83]. Negative or positive attitudes to the odors may (cognitive bias) influence the occurrence of irritative symptoms on experimental exposure to odorous compounds [84]. As our results were based on mutual adjustment models, it is less likely that differences in personal factors or attitudes would have biased our results. Odor perception in our study may be an indicator of poor ventilation. Increased ventilation was found to be associated with less report of odor among university students in computer classrooms [85]. Reported odor was related to higher levels of total fungal DNA in Swedish daycare centers in Sweden [86]. Pungent odor, musty odor and stuffy odor in multi-family buildings in Sweden were associated with asthma symptoms among adults [65]. Self-report of odor perceptions in dwellings were also found to be associated with SBS among adults in China [87]. Thus, odor perception can be associated with different types of exposure and can be of importance for asthma.

New indoor painting in the last 12 months was negatively associated with current asthma, and there was a same trend for its association with night time breathlessness in our study. One former study found that self-reported domestic exposure to newly painted surfaces in the last 12 months in Swedish homes was positively associated with adults' nocturnal breathlessness [41]. The reason for the opposite finding in our study is not clear. Maybe some other activities that related to indoor painting improved the indoor environment but was not measured in our study. Paint used in indoor environment has becoming more and more environmental friendly with less and less chemical emissions, especially in developed countries like Sweden. One study compared new paint and conventional paint and found a significant increase in wheeze and breathlessness during use of conventional paint, but not with the new paint [88]. Painting is usually a part of a major renovation in buildings, which could benefit health by creating a better indoor environment with strategies of removing dust, house dust mites, molds etc.

The elderly in our study reported less pollen allergy, furry pet allergy, current rhinitis and respiratory infections in the last 3 months. The prevalence of environmental factors were also different. Two review articles have summarized articles on environment factors and respiratory health among the elderly [47,48]. The first review summarized 59 articles about the adverse respiratory effects of outdoor air pollution among individuals >65 years [47]. The second review included 33 relevant publications about exposure to major indoor air pollutants and respiratory diseases [48]. Few studies are available on adverse effects of building dampness and molds in relation to respiratory symptoms among subjects above 60 years [48]. Building dampness (dampness index) were associated with current rhinitis, wheeze, day time breathlessness, current asthma and used antibiotic medication for respiratory infections in the last 12 months among subjects less than or equal to 65 years old in our study (born during1943–2008), but no significant association were found among subjects more than 65 years old (born before 1943). The possible explanation for our finding could be that the effects of dampness problems and renting apartments were different between elderly and others in Sweden. The elderly in our study was born before 1943, and others were born during 1943 to 1990. The major increase in atopic diseases in Sweden started among those being born in the early 1960's and later [56,89]. The era with a lot of new chemical products started in the 1940s'. The elderly in our study was grown in a different environment (more exposed to a farming environment) compared with those younger (less than or equal to 65 years old), and which may make the elderly becoming less sensitive to building dampness and molds later in life. Sweden was a rural society in the old time and those born early were more often living on farms when they were young. Farming life experience in childhood was associated with a reduced risk of atopic sensitization [90] and less adult-onset of asthma [91].

Conclusions

Factors in multi-family dwellings, especially rented apartments, certain building years (especially 1961–1985), building dampness and molds, window pane condensation and odor perceptions at home can be risk factors for rhinitis, asthma and respiratory infections. Preventive measures could include avoiding building dampness and molds, repairing those buildings built during the 1961–1985 and increase ventilation flow in indoor environment.

Acknowledgments

Thanks to Boverket-The Swedish National Board of Housing, Building and Planning. Moreover, the authors would like thank all participants.

Author Contributions

Conceived and designed the experiments: KE. Performed the experiments: KE. Analyzed the data: JW. Contributed reagents/materials/analysis tools: KE GS DN. Contributed to the writing of the manuscript: JW KE GS DN.

References

1. Brasche S, Bischof W (2005) Daily time spent indoors in German homes—baseline data for the assessment of indoor exposure of German occupants. Int J Hyg Environ Health 208: 247–253.
2. Tran NP, Vickery J, Blaiss MS (2011) Management of rhinitis: allergic and non-allergic. Allergy Asthma Immunol Res 3: 148–156.
3. Bousquet J, Van Cauwenberge P, Khaltaev N (2001) Allergic rhinitis and its impact on asthma. J Allergy Clin Immunol 108: S147–334.
4. de Marco R, Cappa V, Accordini S, Rava M, Antonicelli L, et al. (2012) Trends in the prevalence of asthma and allergic rhinitis in Italy between 1991 and 2010. Eur Respir J 39: 883–892.
5. Verlato G, Corsico A, Villani S, Cerveri I, Migliore E, et al. (2003) Is the prevalence of adult asthma and allergic rhinitis still increasing? Results of an Italian study. J Allergy Clin Immunol 111: 1232–1238.
6. Braunstahl GJ (2009) United airways concept: what does it teach us about systemic inflammation in airways disease? Proc Am Thorac Soc 6: 652–654.
7. Bjerg A, Ekerljung L, Middelveld R, Dahlen SE, Forsberg B, et al. (2011) Increased prevalence of symptoms of rhinitis but not of asthma between 1990 and 2008 in Swedish adults: comparisons of the ECRHS and GA(2)LEN surveys. PLoS One 6: e16082.

8. Chinn S, Jarvis D, Burney P, Luczynska C, Ackermann-Liebrich U, et al. (2004) Increase in diagnosed asthma but not in symptoms in the European Community Respiratory Health Survey. Thorax 59: 646–651.
9. Eriksson J, Ekerljung L, Ronmark E, Dahlen B, Ahlstedt S, et al. (2012) Update of prevalence of self-reported allergic rhinitis and chronic nasal symptoms among adults in Sweden. Clin Respir J 6: 159–168.
10. Nihlen U, Greiff L, Montnemery P, Lofdahl CG, Johannisson A, et al. (2006) Incidence and remission of self-reported allergic rhinitis symptoms in adults. Allergy 61: 1299–1304.
11. Warm K, Backman H, Lindberg A, Lundback B, Ronmark E (2012) Low incidence and high remission of allergic sensitization among adults. J Allergy Clin Immunol 129: 136–142.
12. Ng TP, Tan WC (1994) Epidemiology of allergic rhinitis and its associated risk factors in Singapore. Int J Epidemiol 23: 553–558.
13. Radon K, Gerhardinger U, Schulze A, Zock JP, Norback D, et al. (2008) Occupation and adult onset of rhinitis in the general population. Occup Environ Med 65: 38–43.
14. Nyembue TD, Jorissen M, Hellings PW, Muyunga C, Kayembe JM (2012) Prevalence and determinants of allergic diseases in a Congolese population. Int Forum Allergy Rhinol 2: 285–293.
15. Bener A, Mobayed H, Sattar HA, Al-Mohammed AA, Ibrahimi AS, et al. (2004) Pet ownership: its effect on allergy and respiratory symptoms. Eur Ann Allergy Clin Immunol 36: 306–310.
16. Araki A, Kanazawa A, Kawai T, Eitaki Y, Morimoto K, et al. (2012) The relationship between exposure to microbial volatile organic compound and allergy prevalence in single-family homes. Sci Total Environ 423: 18–26.
17. Jaakkola MS, Quansah R, Hugg TT, Heikkinen SA, Jaakkola JJ (2013) Association of indoor dampness and molds with rhinitis risk: A systematic review and meta-analysis. J Allergy Clin Immunol 132: 1099–1110.e1018.
18. Kurt E, Metintas S, Basyigit I, Bulut I, Coskun E, et al. (2009) Prevalence and Risk Factors of Allergies in Turkey (PARFAIT): results of a multicentre cross-sectional study in adults. Eur Respir J 33: 724–733.
19. Kilpelainen M, Terho EO, Helenius H, Koskenvuo M (2001) Home dampness, current allergic diseases, and respiratory infections among young adults. Thorax 56: 462–467.
20. Wang DY (2005) Risk factors of allergic rhinitis: genetic or environmental? Ther Clin Risk Manag 1: 115–123.
21. Bahadori K, Doyle-Waters MM, Marra C, Lynd L, Alasaly K, et al. (2009) Economic burden of asthma: a systematic review. BMC Pulm Med 9: 24.
22. Lotvall J, Ekerljung L, Ronmark EP, Wennergren G, Linden A, et al. (2009) West Sweden Asthma Study: prevalence trends over the last 18 years argues no recent increase in asthma. Respir Res 10: 94.
23. Anandan C, Nurmatov U, van Schayck OC, Sheikh A (2010) Is the prevalence of asthma declining? Systematic review of epidemiological studies. Allergy 65: 152–167.
24. Yorgancioglu A, Ozdemir C, Kalayci O, Kalyoncu AF, Bachert C, et al. (2012) ARIA (Allergic Rhinitis and its Impact on Asthma) achievements in 10 years and future needs. Tuberk Toraks 60: 92–97.
25. Cruz AA, Popov T, Pawankar R, Annesi-Maesano I, Fokkens W, et al. (2007) Common characteristics of upper and lower airways in rhinitis and asthma: ARIA update, in collaboration with GA(2)LEN. Allergy 62 Suppl 84: 1–41.
26. Bousquet J, Annesi-Maesano I, Carat F, Leger D, Rugina M, et al. (2005) Characteristics of intermittent and persistent allergic rhinitis: DREAMS study group. Clin Exp Allergy 35: 728–732.
27. Janson C, Anto J, Burney P, Chinn S, de Marco R, et al. (2001) The European Community Respiratory Health Survey: what are the main results so far? European Community Respiratory Health Survey II. Eur Respir J 18: 598–611.
28. Leynaert B, Sunyer J, Garcia-Esteban R, Svanes C, Jarvis D, et al. (2012) Gender differences in prevalence, diagnosis and incidence of allergic and non-allergic asthma: a population-based cohort. Thorax 67: 625–631.
29. Lee YL, Hsiue TR, Lee CH, Su HJ, Guo YL (2006) Home exposures, parental atopy, and occurrence of asthma symptoms in adulthood in southern Taiwan. Chest 129: 300–308.
30. Backman H, Hedman L, Jansson SA, Lindberg A, Lundback B, et al. (2014) Prevalence trends in respiratory symptoms and asthma in relation to smoking - two cross-sectional studies ten years apart among adults in northern Sweden. World Allergy Organ J 7: 1.
31. Bjerg A, Ekerljung L, Eriksson J, Olafsdottir IS, Middelveld R, et al. (2013) Higher risk of wheeze in female than male smokers. Results from the Swedish GA 2 LEN study. PLoS One 8: e54137.
32. Meszaros D, Burgess J, Walters EH, Johns D, Markos J, et al. (2014) Domestic airborne pollutants and asthma and respiratory symptoms in middle age. Respirology.
33. Nadif R, Matran R, Maccario J, Bechet M, Le Moual N, et al. (2010) Passive and active smoking and exhaled nitric oxide levels according to asthma and atopy in adults. Ann Allergy Asthma Immunol 104: 385–393.
34. Jie Y, Ismail NH, Jie X, Isa ZM (2011) Do indoor environments influence asthma and asthma-related symptoms among adults in homes? a review of the literature. J Formos Med Assoc 110: 555–563.
35. WHO (2009). WHO Guidelines for Indoor Air Quality: Dampness and Mould. Geneva: World Health Organization.
36. Chew GL, Carlton EJ, Kass D, Hernandez M, Clarke B, et al. (2006) Determinants of cockroach and mouse exposure and associations with asthma in families and elderly individuals living in New York City public housing. Ann Allergy Asthma Immunol 97: 502–513.
37. Bjornsson E, Norback D, Janson C, Widstrom J, Palmgren U, et al. (1995) Asthmatic symptoms and indoor levels of micro-organisms and house dust mites. Clin Exp Allergy 25: 423–431.
38. Hulin M, Moularat S, Kirchner S, Robine E, Mandin C, et al. (2013) Positive associations between respiratory outcomes and fungal index in rural inhabitants of a representative sample of French dwellings. Int J Hyg Environ Health 216: 155–162.
39. Norback D, Bjornsson E, Janson C, Widstrom J, Boman G (1995) Asthmatic symptoms and volatile organic compounds, formaldehyde, and carbon dioxide in dwellings. Occup Environ Med 52: 388–395.
40. Hulin M, Simoni M, Viegi G, Annesi-Maesano I (2012) Respiratory health and indoor air pollutants based on quantitative exposure assessments. Eur Respir J 40: 1033–1045.
41. Wieslander G, Norback D, Bjornsson E, Janson C, Boman G (1997) Asthma and the indoor environment: the significance of emission of formaldehyde and volatile organic compounds from newly painted indoor surfaces. Int Arch Occup Environ Health 69: 115–124.
42. Fisk WJ, Eliseeva EA, Mendell MJ (2010) Association of residential dampness and mold with respiratory tract infections and bronchitis: a meta-analysis. Environ Health 9: 72.
43. Fisk WJ, Lei-Gomez Q, Mendell MJ (2007) Meta-analyses of the associations of respiratory health effects with dampness and mold in homes. Indoor Air 17: 284–296.
44. Li Y, Leung GM, Tang JW, Yang X, Chao CY, et al. (2007) Role of ventilation in airborne transmission of infectious agents in the built environment - a multidisciplinary systematic review. Indoor Air 17: 2–18.
45. Sundell J, Levin H, Nazaroff WW, Cain WS, Fisk WJ, et al. (2011) Ventilation rates and health: multidisciplinary review of the scientific literature. Indoor Air 21: 191–204.
46. Christensen K, Doblhammer G, Rau R, Vaupel JWAgeing populations: the challenges ahead. (2009) The Lancet 374: 1196–1208.
47. Bentayeb M, Simoni M, Baiz N, Norback D, Baldacci S, et al. (2012) Adverse respiratory effects of outdoor air pollution in the elderly. Int J Tuberc Lung Dis 16: 1149–1161.
48. Bentayeb M, Simoni M, Norback D, Baldacci S, Maio S, et al. (2013) Indoor air pollution and respiratory health in the elderly. J Environ Sci Health A Tox Hazard Subst Environ Eng 48: 1783–1789.
49. The Swedish National Board of Housing Building and Planning (2009) Statistiska urval och metoder i Bovekets projekt BETSI. Sweden: The Swedish National Board of Housing, Building and Planning.
50. Norback D, Bjornsson E, Janson C, Palmgren U, Boman G (1999) Current asthma and biochemical signs of inflammation in relation to building dampness in dwellings. Int J Tuberc Lung Dis 3: 368–376.
51. Burney PG, Luczynska C, Chinn S, Jarvis D (1994) The European Community Respiratory Health Survey. Eur Respir J 7: 954–960.
52. Andersson K (1998) Epidemiological approach to indoor air problems. Indoor Air 8: 32–39.
53. Engvall K, Norrby C, Norback D (2003) Ocular, nasal, dermal and respiratory symptoms in relation to heating, ventilation, energy conservation, and reconstruction of older multi-family houses. Indoor Air 13: 206–211.
54. The Swedish National Board of Housing Building and Planning (2009) Enkätundersökning om boendes upplevda inomhusmiljö och ohälsa - resultat från projektet BETSI. Sweden: The Swedish National Board of Housing, Building and Planning.
55. Statistics Sweden (2009) The furture population of Sweden 2009–2060. Demographic reports.
56. Aberg N (1989) Asthma and allergic rhinitis in Swedish conscripts. Clin Exp Allergy 19: 59–63.
57. Broms K, Norback D, Eriksson M, Sundelin C, Svardsudd K (2009) Effect of degree of urbanisation on age and sex-specific asthma prevalence in Swedish preschool children. BMC Public Health 9: 303.
58. de Marco R, Poli A, Ferrari M, Accordini S, Giammanco G, et al. (2002) The impact of climate and traffic-related NO2 on the prevalence of asthma and allergic rhinitis in Italy. Clin Exp Allergy 32: 1405–1412.
59. Lindgren A, Stroh E, Nihlen U, Montnemery P, Axmon A, et al. (2009) Traffic exposure associated with allergic asthma and allergic rhinitis in adults. A cross-sectional study in southern Sweden. Int J Health Geogr 8: 25.
60. Engvall K, Hult M, Corner R, Lampa E, Norback D, et al. (2010) A new multiple regression model to identify multi-family houses with a high prevalence of sick building symptoms "SBS", within the healthy sustainable house study in Stockholm (3H). Int Arch Occup Environ Health 83: 85–94.
61. Gehring U, Pattenden S, Slachtova H, Antova T, Braun-Fahrlander C, et al. (2006) Parental education and children's respiratory and allergic symptoms in the Pollution and the Young (PATY) study. Eur Respir J 27: 95–107.
62. Le Moual N, Jacquemin B, Varraso R, Dumas O, Kauffmann F, et al. (2013) Environment and asthma in adults. Presse Med 42: e317–333.
63. Basagana X, Sunyer J, Kogevinas M, Zock JP, Duran-Tauleria E, et al. (2004) Socioeconomic status and asthma prevalence in young adults: the European Community Respiratory Health Survey. Am J Epidemiol 160: 178–188.
64. Engvall K, Norrby C, Bandel J, Hult M, Norback D (2000) Development of a multiple regression model to identify multi-family residential buildings with a high prevalence of sick building syndrome (SBS). Indoor Air 10: 101–110.

65. Engvall K, Norrby C, Norback D (2001) Asthma symptoms in relation to building dampness and odour in older multifamily houses in Stockholm. Int J Tuberc Lung Dis 5: 468–477.
66. Bornehag CG, Sundell J, Bonini S, Custovic A, Malmberg P, et al. (2004) Dampness in buildings as a risk factor for health effects, EUROEXPO: a multidisciplinary review of the literature (1998–2000) on dampness and mite exposure in buildings and health effects. Indoor Air 14: 243–257.
67. Wang J, Li B, Yu W, Yang Q, Wang H, et al. (2014) Rhinitis Symptoms and Asthma among Parents of Preschool Children in Relation to the Home Environment in Chongqing, China. PLoS One 9: e94731.
68. Norback D, Zock JP, Plana E, Heinrich J, Svanes C, et al. (2013) Mould and dampness in dwelling places, and onset of asthma: the population-based cohort ECRHS. Occup Environ Med 70: 325–331.
69. Zock JP, Jarvis D, Luczynska C, Sunyer J, Burney P (2002) Housing characteristics, reported mold exposure, and asthma in the European Community Respiratory Health Survey. J Allergy Clin Immunol 110: 285–292.
70. Bush RK, Portnoy JM, Saxon A, Terr AI, Wood RA (2006) The medical effects of mold exposure. J Allergy Clin Immunol 117: 326–333.
71. Sahlberg B, Gunnbjornsdottir M, Soon A, Jogi R, Gislason T, et al. (2013) Airborne molds and bacteria, microbial volatile organic compounds (MVOC), plasticizers and formaldehyde in dwellings in three North European cities in relation to sick building syndrome (SBS). Sci Total Environ 444: 433–440.
72. Nevalainen A, Seuri M (2005) Of microbes and men. Indoor Air 15 Suppl 9: 58–64.
73. Zhang X, Zhao Z, Nordquist T, Larsson L, Sebastian A, et al. (2011) A longitudinal study of sick building syndrome among pupils in relation to microbial components in dust in schools in China. Sci Total Environ 409: 5253–5259.
74. Norback D, Wieslander G, Nordstrom K, Walinder R (2000) Asthma symptoms in relation to measured building dampness in upper concrete floor construction, and 2-ethyl-1-hexanol in indoor air. Int J Tuberc Lung Dis 4: 1016–1025.
75. Takaoka M, Norback D (2011) The Home Environment of Japanese Female University Students - Association with Respiratory Health and Allergy. Indoor and Built Environment 20: 369–376.
76. Janson C, Kalm-Stephens P, Foucard T, Norback D, Alving K, et al. (2005) Exhaled nitric oxide levels in school children in relation to IgE sensitisation and window pane condensation. Respir Med 99: 1015–1021.
77. Engvall K, Norrby C, Norback D (2001) Sick building syndrome in relation to building dampness in multi-family residential buildings in Stockholm. Int Arch Occup Environ Health 74: 270–278.
78. Lundholm M, Lavrell G, Mathiasson L (1990) Self-leveling mortar as a possible cause of symptoms associated with "sick building syndrome". Arch Environ Health 45: 135–140.
79. Hoenicke K, Simat TJ, Steinhart H, Christoph N, Kohler HJ, et al. (1999) Determination of tryptophan and tryptophan metabolites in grape must and wine. Adv Exp Med Biol 467: 671–677.
80. Schmarr HG, Ganss S, Sang W, Potouridis T (2007) Analysis of 2-aminoacetophenone in wine using a stable isotope dilution assay and multidimensional gas chromatography-mass spectrometry. J Chromatogr A 1150: 78–84.
81. Kumazawa K, Masuda H (1999) Identification of potent odorants in Japanese green tea (Sen-cha). J Agric Food Chem 47: 5169–5172.
82. Wieslander G, Norback D, Nordstrom K, Walinder R, Venge P (1999) Nasal and ocular symptoms, tear film stability and biomarkers in nasal lavage, in relation to building-dampness and building design in hospitals. Int Arch Occup Environ Health 72: 451–461.
83. Caccappolo E, Kipen H, Kelly-McNeil K, Knasko S, Hamer RM, et al. (2000) Odor perception: multiple chemical sensitivities, chronic fatigue, and asthma. J Occup Environ Med 42: 629–638.
84. Andersson L, Claeson AS, Ledin L, Wisting F, Nordin S (2013) The influence of health-risk perception and distress on reactions to low-level chemical exposure. Front Psychol 4: 816.
85. Norback D, Nordstrom K (2008) An experimental study on effects of increased ventilation flow on students' perception of indoor environment in computer classrooms. Indoor Air 18: 293–300.
86. Cai GH, Broms K, Malarstig B, Zhao ZH, Kim JL, et al. (2009) Quantitative PCR analysis of fungal DNA in Swedish day care centers and comparison with building characteristics and allergen levels. Indoor Air 19: 392–400.
87. Wang J, Li B, Yang Q, Yu W, Wang H, et al. (2013) Odors and sensations of humidity and dryness in relation to sick building syndrome and home environment in Chongqing, China. PLoS One 8: e72385.
88. Beach JR, Raven J, Ingram C, Bailey M, Johns D, et al. (1997) The effects on asthmatics of exposure to a conventional water-based and a volatile organic compound-free paint. Eur Respir J 10: 563–566.
89. Aberg N, Hesselmar B, Aberg B, Eriksson B (1995) Increase of asthma, allergic rhinitis and eczema in Swedish schoolchildren between 1979 and 1991. Clin Exp Allergy 25: 815–819.
90. Leynaert B, Neukirch C, Jarvis D, Chinn S, Burney P, et al. (2001) Does living on a farm during childhood protect against asthma, allergic rhinitis, and atopy in adulthood? Am J Respir Crit Care Med 164: 1829–1834.
91. Varraso R, Oryszczyn MP, Mathieu N, Le Moual N, Boutron-Ruault MC, et al. (2012) Farming in childhood, diet in adulthood and asthma history. Eur Respir J 39: 67–75.

9

Aetiology of Acute Febrile Episodes in Children Attending Korogwe District Hospital

Coline Mahende[1,2]*, Billy Ngasala[2], John Lusingu[1], Allvan Butichi[1], Paminus Lushino[1], Martha Lemnge[1], Zul Premji[2]

1 Korogwe Research Laboratory, National Institute for Medical Research, Tanga, Tanzania, **2** Department of Medical Entomology and Parasitology, School of Public Health, Muhimbili University of Health and Allied Sciences, Dar es Salaam, Tanzania

Abstract

Introduction: Although the burden of malaria in many parts of Tanzania has declined, the proportion of children with fever has not changed. This situation underscores the need to explore the possible causes of febrile episodes in patients presenting with symptoms at the Korogwe District Hospital (KDH).

Methods: A hospital based cross-sectional study was conducted at KDH, north-eastern Tanzania. Patients aged 2 to 59 months presenting at the outpatient department with an acute medical condition and fever (measured axillary temperature ≥37.5°C) were enrolled. Blood samples were examined for malaria parasites, human immunodeficiency virus (HIV) and bacterial infections. A urine culture was performed in selected cases to test for bacterial infection and a chest radiograph was requested if pneumonia was suspected. Diagnosis was based on both clinical and laboratory investigations.

Results: A total of 867 patients with a median age of 15.1 months (Interquartile range 8.6–29.9) were enrolled from January 2013 to October 2013. Respiratory tract infections were the leading clinical diagnosis with 406/867 (46.8%) of patients diagnosed with upper respiratory tract infection and 130/867 (15.0%) with pneumonia. Gastroenteritis was diagnosed in 184/867 (21.2%) of patients. Malaria infection was confirmed in 72/867 (8.3%) of patients. Bacterial infection in blood and urine accounted for 26/808 (3.2%) infections in the former, and 66/373 (17.7%) infections in the latter. HIV infection was confirmed in 10/824 (1.2%) of patients. Respiratory tract infections and gastroenteritis were frequent in patients under 36 months of age (87.3% and 91.3% respectively). Co-infections were seen in 221/867 (25.5%) of patients. The cause of fever was not identified in 65/867 (7.5%) of these patients.

Conclusions: The different proportions of infections found among febrile children reflect the causes of fever in the study area. These findings indicate the need to optimise patient management by developing malaria and non-malaria febrile illnesses management protocols.

Editor: Ana Paula Arez, Instituto de Higiene e Medicina Tropical, Portugal

Funding: The study was sponsored by Swedish International Development Cooperation Agency (SIDA) through Muhimbili University of Health and Allied Sciences. The funders had no role in study design, data collection and analysis, decision to publish, or preparation of the manuscript.

Competing Interests: The authors have declared that no competing interests exist.

* Email: cbdmahende@yahoo.co.uk

Introduction

More than half of the children presenting at health facilities in Africa are estimated not to have a malaria infection [1,2]. The lack of knowledge on the prevalence of the causative agents of other febrile illnesses, the limited access to affordable diagnostic tests as well as the fear of overlooking a life threatening malaria infection, result in most febrile cases being treated and managed as malaria [3,4].

Fever commonly accompanies a wide range of childhood illnesses and if the patient is not properly managed, this can have potentially serious outcomes including death [5]. In malaria endemic countries, febrile episodes are commonly associated with malaria infection [6,7]. As current epidemiological data indicates a decline in malaria infections in many parts of sub Saharan Africa, including Tanzania, other causative agents of febrile illnesses should be investigated [8,9].

Acute febrile episodes are caused by various pathogenic organisms (such as viruses and bacteria), and infections with these agents result in patients presenting with clinical symptoms which resemble those of a malaria infection [10]. An accurate clinical diagnosis without laboratory confirmation can be difficult to make and misleading [11,12]. Despite efforts by the World Health Organisation (WHO) to improve the diagnosis of malaria through its updated integrated management of childhood illness (IMCI) guidelines, confirmatory diagnosis of malaria is still not adequately carried out. In routine practice, clinicians have continued prescribing antimalarial drugs to malaria negative patients [13,14]. As IMCI approach is apparently not specific on the diagnosis of non-malarial febrile illnesses [15]. This results in the inappropriate use of antimalarial drugs, possible development of antimicrobial drug resistance and also elevates treatment costs due to unnecessary prescriptions. Incorrect prescriptions may leave patients untreated, thereby unnecessarily increasing morbidity and mortality in these resource poor settings [16].

There is limited data on the epidemiological causes of febrile illnesses (other than malaria) among outpatient children, as well as a lack of reliable surveillance data in Tanzania. A recent study conducted in Tanzania found that malarial infections were no longer a major cause of fever among outpatient children [17]. Disease-specific studies among febrile patients have been conducted in few settings across Sub Saharan Africa. These studies focused mainly on malaria, bacteraemia and human immunodeficiency virus (HIV) infection among inpatients [18–20].

Information on the prevalence of local infections, that is based on diagnosis using both clinical presentation and laboratory confirmatory tests is critical for correct management of both malarial and non-malarial febrile illnesses. The main objective of this study was to describe the common causes of fever in children presenting at an outpatient department at the Korogwe District Hospital, north-eastern Tanzania.

Methods

Study area

The study was conducted at Korogwe District Hospital (KDH) in Korogwe District, Tanga Region, north-eastern part of Tanzania. The Korogwe District has a population of approximately 73,275 children under the age of five years according to the Tanzanian population and housing census of 2012 [21]. The District has a population growth rate of 2.7% per annum [21]. The environment is characterised by daily temperatures varying from 18°C to 20°C during the rainy season and 26°C to 30°C during the dry season. The annual rainfall ranges from 700–1000 mm with long rainy seasons extending from March to May. The majority of the inhabitants reside in rural settings, practicing subsistence farming and informal trade. The hospital receives 6000 (2010 estimates) children under the age of five years as outpatients annually. The most common clinical diagnoses among children under the age of five years have been malaria, pneumonia, gastroenteritis, septicaemia, anaemia and diarrhoea (Korogwe District Medical Officer, personal communication).

The prevalence of *Plasmodium falciparum* malaria parasitaemia from the community in lowland villages has decreased from 78% in 2003 to 13% in 2008, whereas in the highland villages, the decrease was from 25% to 3% during the same time period [22]. The prevalence of HIV infection among women attending the antenatal clinic at KDH was 2.5% for 2010 [23]. Pneumococcal and rotavirus vaccines were introduced into Tanzania in January 2013 as part of the Expanded Program on Immunization. Vaccine coverage for other vaccines in the Expanded Program on Immunization (EPI) has been above 80%. These vaccines include; Bacille Calmette–Guérin, pentavalent vaccine (diphtheria–tetanus–pertussis, hepatitis B and haemophilus influenza type B), poliovirus and measles vaccines.

Study population

Sick children aged between 2 and 59 months presenting at KDH outpatient department were assessed for study eligibility from January 2013 to October 2013. Enrolment took place Mondays to Fridays every week. The inclusion criteria were: children aged 2 to 59 months of age presenting at KDH with an acute medical condition and a history of fever in the last 48 hours or measured axillary temperature of ≥37.5°C. The visit should be their first consultation for the present problem. Patients younger than 2 months of age were excluded in the study. Patients were excluded if they had planned admissions (e.g. elective surgery), trauma/injury, if they required an emergency intervention or if they had taken antimalarial drugs and/or antibiotics within the last seven days.

Ethics statement

The study obtained ethical clearance with reference number NIMR/HQ/R.8a/Vol.1X/1373 from the Tanzanian Medical Research Coordinating Committee. A written informed consent form was issued and signed by the parent/legal guardian of every child enrolled in the study.

Study procedure

A detailed medical history and a thorough clinical examination were performed on each patient and this information was recorded on a standardised Case Report Form (CRF). This information included: demographic information, clinical history and physical examination data (including weight, axillary temperature and respiratory rate). A chest radiograph was requested if pneumonia was suspected. A clinical diagnosis was made based on the presenting signs and symptoms according to the IMCI guidelines [24]. This ensured that patients could be appropriately managed according to national standard practice while laboratory tests were being processed. Patients who had positive culture results were contacted and the necessary required treatment provided. The Final diagnosis was based on both the clinical presentation and the laboratory findings for malaria microscopy, bacteriology, radiology and HIV testing.

Laboratory investigations

A maximum of 5 mL venous blood for laboratory investigations was drawn from every patient once inclusion criteria had been met. Each blood draw was conducted aseptically in order to avoid contamination. The venipuncture site was disinfected with 70% isopropyl alcohol and allowed to dry prior to blood drawing.

Diagnosis of Plasmodium species and *Borrelia* parasitic infection

Thick and thin blood smears were prepared (in duplicate) from the blood collected in the ethylene diamine tetra acetic acid (EDTA) tubes. The thin film was fixed with methanol and blood slides were stained with a 5% Giemsa solution for identification and quantitation of asexual *Plasmodium falciparum* and other *Plasmodium* species. The blood slides were read by two expert microscopists and in case of discrepancy, a third reading was performed. Asexual parasites were counted against 200 (500 if parasite count was <10) white blood cells. A blood slide was considered negative for *Plasmodium* species if no parasites were seen in at least 100 oil-immersion high power fields on the thick film. During examination of the slides for *Plasmodium* species, *Borrelia* species were also screened. *Borrelia* species are seen as spirochaetes under microscopy.

Differential complete blood count

Blood collected in anticoagulated EDTA tubes was analysed for differential complete blood count using automated MS4s haematology analyser (Melet Schloesing Diamond Diagnostics, USA).

Aerobic blood culturing

Blood collected in commercially available BD BACTEC PEDS PLUS culture bottles were incubated in an automated blood culture system BACTEC 9050 (Becton Dickinson, Sparks, Maryland, USA). A single blood culture bottle was used per patient. The minimal volume inoculated was 2 mL (3 mL was an ideal volume) and blood culture bottles were incubated for a maximum of five days (unless they flag positive). The BACTEC 9050 detects positive cultures based on CO_2 production. Blood culture bottles which flagged positive were cultured on standard media with the use of routine microbiological techniques. Analytical Profile Index (API) biochemical test kit (BioMérieux, France) and/or serological tests were used to confirm suspected pathogens.

Definition of positive and negative culture

A blood culture was considered positive when: a definite pathogen was isolated (e.g. *Streptococcus pneumoniae*, *Streptococcus agalactiae*, *Streptococcus pyogenes*, *Haemophilus influenzae*, *Salmonella* species), a bacteria that could be either a pathogen or a contaminant was isolated within 48 hours of blood culture incubation (e.g. *Escherichia coli*, *Klebsiella pneumoniae*, *Staphylococcus aureus*, *Enterococcus faecalis* group D). Blood cultures were considered to be negative if there were no bacteria isolated after five days incubation.

Definition of contamination

A blood culture was considered to be contaminated if one or more of the following organisms were identified; coagulase-negative *Staphylococcus* species, *Corynebacterium* species, *alpha- or gamma-hemolytic streptococci*, *Micrococcus* species, *Bacillus* species and *Propionibacterium* species. However, a definitive diagnosis of a contaminant was decided by a clinician based on the clinical presentation of the patient due to the fact that these organisms could be the cause of an opportunistic infection.

Urine culturing

Urine was collected from patients presenting with fever, dysuria and/or no obvious cause of fever on clinical examination. A midstream urine was collected in a sterile container. The perineum was swabbed with chlorhexidine and the sample was collected using a sterile urine collector for the younger patients who were not able to follow instructions. Urinalysis by dipstick (URiScan, YD Diagnostics, Korea) was used for presumptive diagnosis of urinary tract infections for early initiation of therapy while urine cultures were being processed. The urine was cultured by inoculation onto cysteine lactose electrolyte deficient agar, MacConkey agar and sheep blood agar. An API biochemical test kit (BioMérieux, France) was used to confirm suspected pathogens. A definitive diagnosis of urinary tract infection was based on the isolation of a bacteria pathogen from the positive culture containing $>10^5$ colony-forming units (CFU)/ml [25].

Antimicrobial susceptibility testing

The Kirby-Bauer disc diffusion method was used for in-vitro antimicrobial susceptibility testing for all pathogenic bacterial isolates from blood and urine cultures. The testing was performed on the following antimicrobial agents; amoxicillin, chloramphenicol, ceftriaxone, ciprofloxacin, co-trimoxazole, gentamicin and penicillin. Reading and interpretation of zone sizes was performed using criteria stipulated by the Clinical and Laboratory Standards Institute (CLSI).

Human immunodeficiency virus (HIV) testing

HIV antibody testing was performed after patients were informed and counselled as per the National Health Guidelines. Blood drawn from patients was tested for the presence of HIV-1 and HIV-2 antibodies according to the National HIV rapid testing algorithm using the Determine HIV-1/2 Assay Kit (Abbott Laboratories, Abbott Park, IL, USA) [26]. If this was positive, confirmation was carried out using the Uni-Gold HIV (Trinity Biotech, Bray, Co Wicklow, Ireland). For children under the age of 18 months, HIV testing was performed using HIV-1 RNA PCR.

Case definitions

Fever was defined as history of abnormally high body temperature as reported by the parent/guardian and/or measured axillary temperature ≥37.5°C on presentation. Malaria infection was defined as fever with the presence of asexual *Plasmodium falciparum* parasites in a blood smear confirmed by microscopy. Bacteremia was defined as fever with isolation of pathogenic bacteria from blood culture. Anaemia was defined as haemoglobin concentration below 9.3 g/dL. Clinical diagnoses of respiratory infections and gastroenteritis were defined according to the IMCI guidelines [24].

Data management and statistical analysis

Data management involved double entry and validation using Microsoft Access 2007. Data analysis was done by STATA version 11.2 (Stata Corp LP, College Station, Texas, USA). Variables were summarized as frequencies and proportions and medians and inter-quartile ranges, as appropriate. Data was compared using the chi-square (X^2) test when comparing proportions. Odds ratios (OR) and 95% confidence intervals (95% CI) were calculated as appropriate. The value of $p<0.05$ was considered statistically significant.

Results

Demographic characteristics of the study population

A total of 1380 patients attending the outpatient department at KDH from January 2013 to October 2013 were screened. Of these, 867/1380 (62.8%) were febrile children who were eligible for enrolment (Figure 1). The median age was 15.1 months (Interquartile range (IQR): 8.6–29.9) and girls comprised of 459/867 (52.9%) patients as shown on Table 1. Median axillary body temperature was 38.1°C (IQR 37.5–38.7). The common presenting clinical symptoms other than fever were cough 411/867 (47.4%) and diarrhoea 174/867 (20.1%).

Malaria infection

Malaria infection due to *Plasmodium falciparum* was confirmed in 72/867 (8.3%, 95%CI, 6.5–10.1) of the patients identified by thick and thin blood smears. Anaemia was found in 226/841 (26.9%) patients, of whom 36/226 (15.9%) had malaria which increased the risk of anaemia (OR: 3.6 [95%CI: 2.1–6.1] p<0.01). No other *Plasmodia* species or *Borrelia* species were found. Overlap of clinical symptoms was observed among patients with malaria infection; 14/72 (19.4%) and 4/72 (5.6%) patients had clinical symptoms of respiratory tract infections and gastroenteritis respectively.

Bacteremia

Blood cultures were collected and analysed from 808 patients, of which 26/808 (3.2%, 95%CI, 1.9–4.4) were positive for pathogenic bacterial growth. *Salmonella typhi* was the predominant

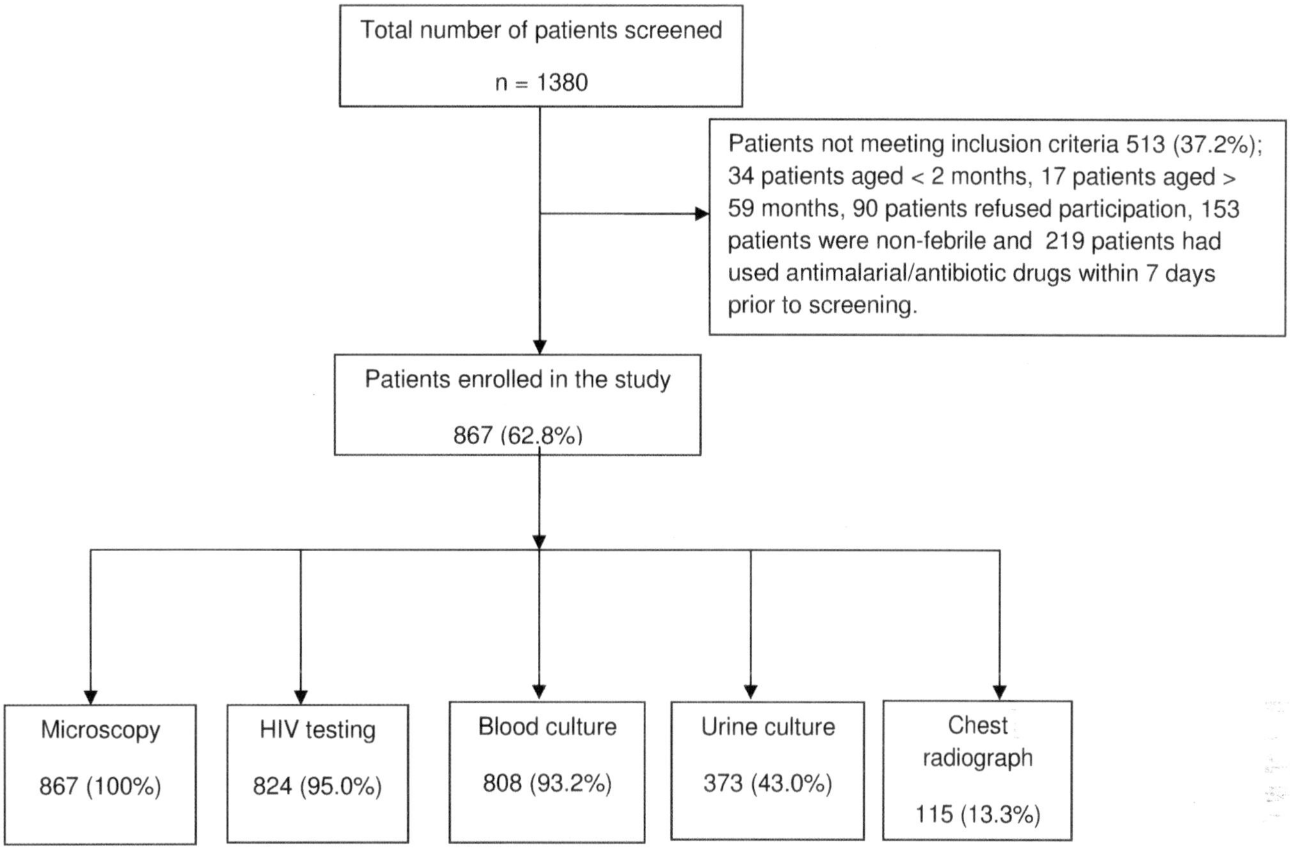

Figure 1. Study flow diagram of patient enrollment at KDH and the investigations performed.

bacteria isolated in 17/26 (65.4%) of cases followed by *Streptococcus pneumoniae* 4/26 (15.4%) as shown in Table 1.

Urinary tract infection

A Urinary tract infection was confirmed in 66/373 (17.7%, 95%CI, 14.0–22.0) of patients and there was no significant association with gender (36 boys, 30 girls, $X^2 = 0.074$, $P = 0.786$). The most commonly isolated bacteria were *Escherichia coli* 37/66 (56.1%) followed by *Klebsiella pneumoniae* 7/66 (10.6%), *Staphylococcus aureus* 6/66 (9.1%) and *Proteus mirabilis* 5/66 (7.6%).

HIV infection

HIV testing was performed in 824/867 (95.0%) patients and among them, 10/824 (1.2%, 95%CI, 0.6–2.2) were confirmed positive for infection with HIV. None of the HIV infected patients had either a malarial or a bacterial infection.

Clinical diagnoses

Respiratory tract infections. Upper respiratory tract infections were the most common clinical diagnoses presenting in 406/867 (46.8%, 95%CI, 43.5–50.2) of patients. Pneumonia was clinically diagnosed in 130/867 (15.0%, 95%CI, 12.7–17.5) of patients. Pneumonia confirmed by chest radiograph was accounted in 54/130 (41.5%) of these cases and five patients had diagnosis of severe pneumonia. *Salmonella typhi* (n = 2) and *Escherichia coli* (n = 1) were isolated from single blood cultures of patients with upper respiratory tract infections. *Streptococcus pneumoniae* (n = 1) and *Staphylococcus aureus* (n = 1) were isolated from single blood cultures of patients with pneumonia diagnosis. One patient was suspected to have pulmonary tuberculosis from clinical symptoms and chest radiograph results.

Gastroenteritis. Gastroenteritis was diagnosed in 184/867 (21.2%, 95%CI, 18.5–24.1) of patients. Dysentery was diagnosed in 6 patients. *Salmonella typhi* (n = 6) and non-typhi salmonella (n = 1) were isolated from the blood cultures of patients with gastroenteritis.

Other infections. Other infections are summarised on Table 1. The cause of fever could not be identified in 65/867 (7.5%, 95%CI, 5.8–9.5) of the patients.

Distribution of diagnoses according to age. The majority of the patients under the age of 36 months presented with respiratory tract infections 468/536 (87.3%). The second most common diagnosis was gastroenteritis 168/184 (91.3%) and thirdly, urinary tract infections 57/66 (86.4%). Malaria infection 8/72 (11.1%) was less common in patients under the age of 12 months (Figure 2).

Diagnosis of hospitalised patients

Following enrolment, 141/867 (16.3%) patients were hospitalised, of whom 2/141 (1.4%) died from severe pneumonia and upper respiratory tract infection. Malaria infection was a leading cause of admission with 53/141 (37.6%) of patients, followed by pneumonia 35/141 (24.8%), gastroenteritis 27/141 (19.1%) and other infections as indicated in Figure 3.

Co- infections

Co-infections were common and were observed in 221/867 (25.5%, 95%CI, 22.6–28.5) of the patients. Urinary tract

Table 1. Demographic characteristics, clinical diagnosis and laboratory findings of patients enrolled at KDH.

Patient characteristics	n, n/N	Proportions (%)
Gender		
Girls	408	47.1
Age		
2–11 months	356	41.1
12–35 months	370	42.7
36–59 months	141	16.3
Fever		
Duration of fever in days, median (IQR)	2 (1–2)	-
Axillary temperature ≥37.5°C	627	72.3
Common symptoms		
Cough	411	47.4
Diarrhoea	174	20.1
Difficulty breathing	97	11.2
Clinical diagnosis		
Respiratory infections		
Upper respiratory tract infection	406/867	46.8
Pneumonia	130/867	15
Pulmonary Tuberculosis	1/867	0.1
Asthma	19/867	2.2
Gastroenteritis	184/867	21.2
Dysentery	6/867	0.7
Otitis media	5/867	0.6
Fungal infections	6/867	0.7
Skin infections/soft tissue infections	33/867	3.8
Other infections	44/867	5.1
Laboratory findings		
Plasmodium falciparum	72/867	8.3
Geometric mean parasitemia (range)	37635 (159–1656400)	-
Human immunodeficiency virus	10/824	1.2
Anaemia	226/841	26.9
Blood culture positive	26/808	3.2
Non-typhi salmonella	2/26	7.7
Salmonella typhi	17/26	65.4
Streptococcus pneumoniae	4/26	15.4
Other†	3/26	11.5
Urine culture	66/373	17.7
Escherichia coli	37/66	56.1
Klebsiella pneumoniae	7/66	10.6
Proteus mirabilis	5/66	7.6
Other‡	17/66	25.7
Pyrexia of Unknown Origin	65/867	7.5

†*Escherichia coli* (1), *Enterobacter cloacae* (1), *Staphylococcus* aureus (1).
‡*Acinetobacter baumanii* (1), *Citrobacter koseri* (1), *Pseudomonas aeruginosa* (2), *Staphylococcus aureus* (6) *Staphylococcus saprophyticus* (3), *Streptococcus faecalis* (1), *Streptococcus mitis* (1), *Streptococcus viridans* (2).

infections were present in 33/436 (7.6%) patients with respiratory tract infections and in 19/184 (10.3%) patients with gastroenteritis (Figure 4). Five patients had multiple diagnoses of urinary tract infection, respiratory tract infection and gastroenteritis. Among patients with malaria, 8/72 (11.1%) patients had urinary tract infections. Sixty patients had both respiratory tract infections as well as gastroenteritis.

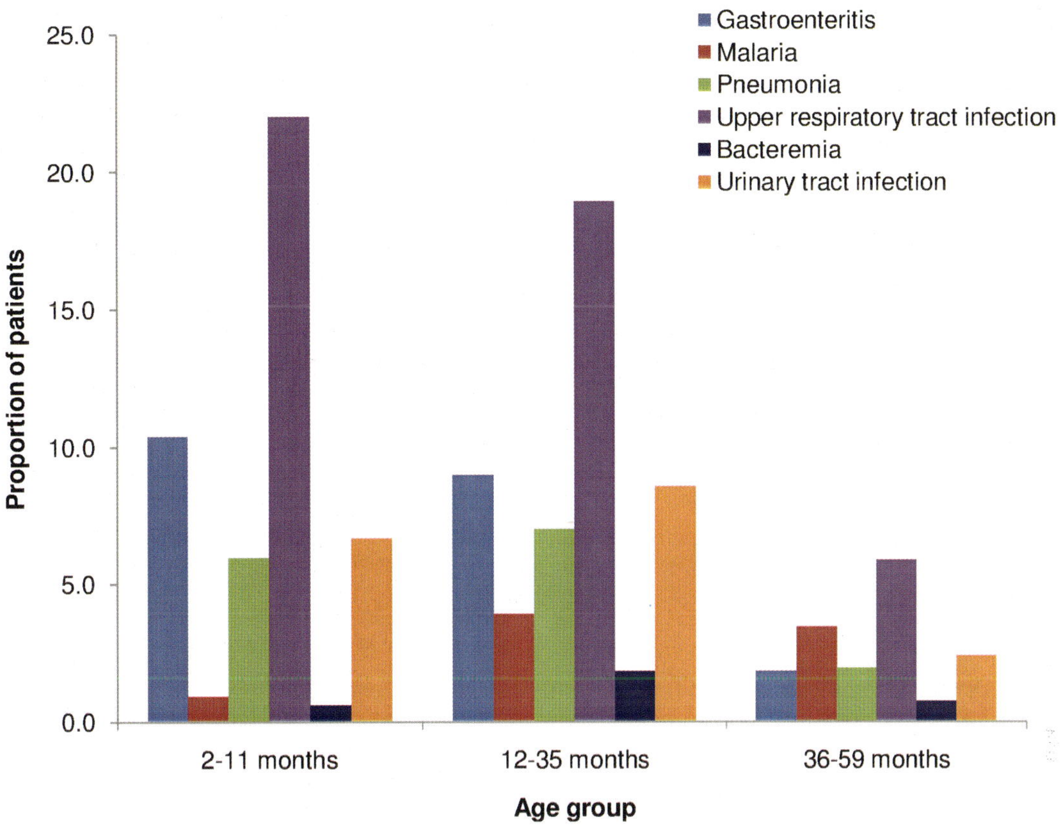

Figure 2. Distribution of common diagnosis according to age group.

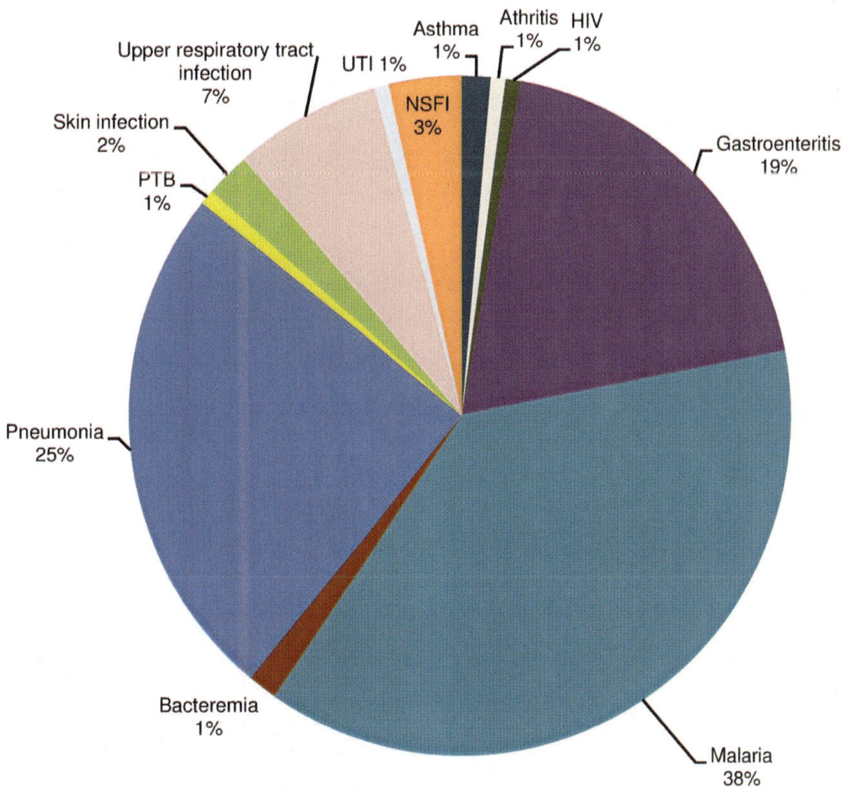

Figure 3. Distribution of illnesses among hospitalised patients at KDH (n = 141).

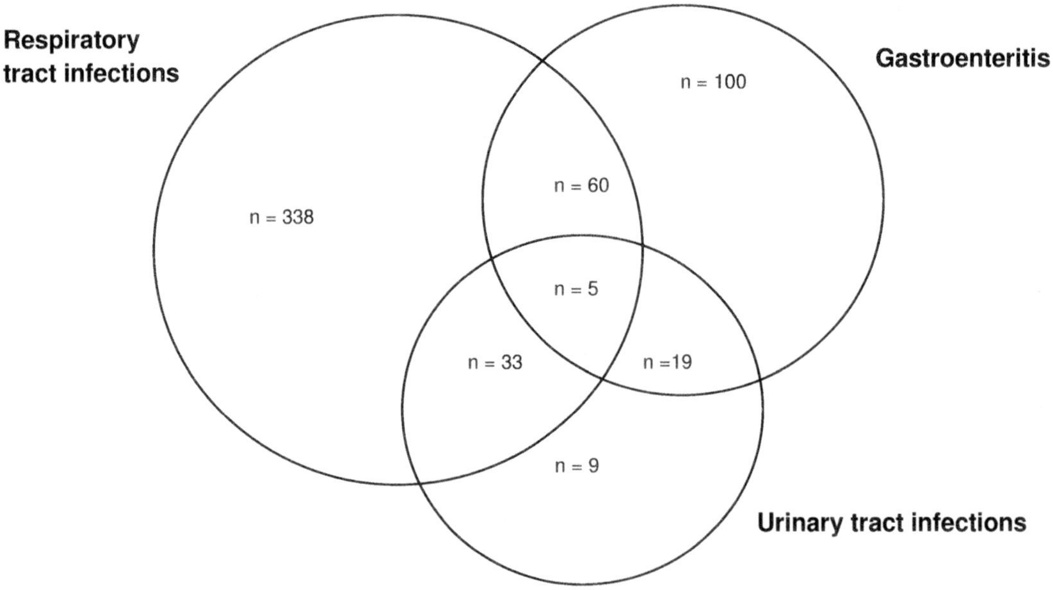

Figure 4. Co-infections of common diagnosis.

Antimicrobial susceptibility pattern

Gram negative bacterial isolates demonstrated good susceptibility to ciprofloxacin (80%–100%), moderate susceptibility to gentamicin (50%–72%) and poor susceptibility to amoxicillin, chloramphenicol and co-trimoxazole (3%–14%). *Escherichia coli* and *Klebsiella pneumoniae* demonstrated poor susceptibility to ceftriaxone (35.1% and 14.3% respectively). *Klebsiella pneumoniae* was the only Gram negative bacteria with good susceptibility to chloramphenicol (71.4%). The Gram positive bacterial isolates were observed to have good susceptibility to ceftriaxone and chloramphenicol (75%–100%) and poor susceptibility to co-trimoxazole and penicillin (0%–50%).

Discussion

This study has been able to contribute information on the prevalence of the possible causes of common febrile episodes among children less than five years of age, attending an outpatient department at KDH in north-eastern Tanzania. Over three quarters of children presenting with fever were under the age of 36 months and the majority had respiratory tract infections and gastroenteritis as the leading clinical diagnosis. Younger children under the age of 36 months tend to be more vulnerable to infections due to their immature immunity, different modes of exposure to pathogenic organisms and possibly due to a low rate of immunisation [27,28].

Plasmodium falciparum malaria, invasive community-acquired bacteria and HIV infections were uncommon among febrile children in the study with a prevalence of 8.3%, 3.2% and 1.2%, respectively. These findings are consistent with other studies on the declining malaria and community-acquired bacterial infections in the region [29,30]. The low malaria prevalence rate might partly be due to current interventions which include use of insecticide treated nets, the wide availability of effective antimalarial drugs, residual spraying and change of malaria vector behaviour [31,32]. This underscores the importance of the rational use of antibiotic and antimalarial drugs in evidence based medicine among less severely ill patients in order to counteract the problem of drug resistance.

This study found an increasing prevalence of *Salmonella typhi* among young children compared with that of non-typhi salmonella. These findings are in keeping with those of Biggs and colleagues, who found similar changing pattern of bacterial infections where *Salmonella typhi* compared with non-typhi salmonella was more common in lower malaria prevalent areas [20]. The observed prevalence of *Salmonella typhi* indicates the presence of typhoid fever among these young rural patients. The following critical measures can be implemented in preventing typhoid fever in this resource poor area through improving the quality of life. This can be done by ensuring good sanitation, safe water supply and public health education on personal as well as food hygiene.

Amoxicillin, chloramphenicol and co-trimoxazole are the most widely available antimicrobial agents in the community. These were shown to demonstrate poor susceptibility to the leading Gram negative bacterial isolates from both blood and urine cultures. Ciprofloxacin was effective but not recommended for use in children under the age of five years [33,34]. The findings support previously published work and emphasize the increasing problem of antimicrobial drug resistance [35,36]. Specific identification of bacteria causing infections is important for understanding and monitoring of antimicrobial drug resistance patterns. This will ensure patients especially children are provided with appropriate and effective treatment.

The prevalence of urinary tract infections in this study was higher among children under 36 months of age and these patients were often co-infected. The lack of access to clean water and good sanitation in this rural community might be the reason for the higher prevalence of infections observed. As in most studies conducted on urinary tract infections, *Escherichia coli* were found to be the predominant isolate. This study did not find any significant difference in gender among children with urinary tract infection. The burden of urinary tract infections in young children living in developing countries remains undefined, despite being the most common bacterial infections in childhood. The diagnosis of urinary tract infection is important in young children since if left untreated can cause nephrourologic abnormalities and impaired renal function in future [37]. With an increase in the prevalence of urinary tract infections among young children, findings from this study recommend routine urine testing of febrile children from rural communities where living conditions are poor [17,36].

Half of the febrile children in the study were clinically diagnosed with respiratory tract infections and nearly a quarter had gastroenteritis making these the leading clinical diagnoses. The observations were more frequent in children under the age of 36 months. The majority of respiratory tract infections and diarrhoea in children are known to be of viral origin [38–40,40–42]. A recent study conducted in Tanzanian children has indicated nearly half of acute respiratory infections were caused by respiratory viruses [17]. Unfortunately, antibiotics are routinely and continuously used to treat these viral infections, contributing to the increase burden of antimicrobial drug resistance. The current study provides preliminary data for future evidence-based research on respiratory and enteric viruses in the community.

Co-infections were observed in a quarter of the patients, mostly among those with urinary tract infections, respiratory tract infections and gastroenteritis. Existence of multiple infections is a challenging issue when developing fever management guidelines, especially in poor rural areas which are usually at higher risks of numerous kinds of infections [43]. This study has underlined the prevalence of co-infections that exist among patients enrolled in the study area.

The causative agents of febrile infections documented in this study can be considered as representative of the causes of fever in this specific area. Despite recommendations by WHO on the parasitological evidence for malaria treatment, management of fever cases in Tanzania is still challenging [44,45]. Furthermore, IMCI guidelines remain unspecific for the management of non-malaria febrile illnesses. Evidence based findings on bacterial infections from the current study can contribute to the revision of clinical algorithms for management of febrile illnesses. There is a need for guidelines that would assist in the management of non-malarial febrile illnesses given the declining malaria trend. Febrile illnesses, especially in children, require proper management so as to avoid unnecessary morbidity and mortalities, antimicrobial abuse and unnecessary expense. Investment in diagnostic facilities, such as adequate microbiology laboratories, qualified and trained laboratory personnel is needed. Furthermore, availability of rapid diagnostic tests for malaria, bacterial and viral infections, is required for rapid and accurate diagnoses of paediatric infections. A possible recommendation is that fever surveillance be conducted along side the existing malaria surveillance systems in future clinical research on vaccines and drugs.

The study had a number of limitations. Firstly, the study was conducted for the period of ten months and therefore could not assess seasonality of febrile episodes. Secondly, the study relied on verbal information provided by parents and guardians on the prior use of antimalarial drugs and antibiotics. This means that some of the children enrolled may well have been on antimicrobial therapy and this will have contributed to the low yield of positive cultures. In addition, the collection of only a single blood culture is known to reduce the possibility of isolating the organisms present in the bloodstream. The volume of blood inoculated into culture bottles was sometimes low due to difficulty in getting venous access especially from young patients and this might have contributed to the low bacterial yield. The study could not provide evidence-based data on respiratory and enteric viruses which are thought to cause majority of respiratory tract infections and diarrhoea in young children. Causative agents of zoonosis among outpatient children from this particular study community were not investigated. Understanding their prevalence would be of advantage despite not being investigated routinely at health facilities in the country.

Acknowledgments

We would like to thank all children and their parents/guardians who participated in the study. We thank Korogwe District Hospital management, NIMR employees; Samwel Gesase, Samuel Sembuche, Monica Billa and Boniface Eustack for their clinical assistance; Neema Malle, Theresia Joseph and Thabita Joseph for blood drawing and sample collection; Geofrey Lyimo, Jerome Msamba, Jackson Kimaro and Grayson Mwakalindile for chest radiographs; Zeno Manjulungu, Peter Gondwe, Gerson Goodluck Maro, Martin George, Joyce Mbwana and Lincoln Malle for laboratory sample analysis; Mohammed Mapondela, Neema Barua and Mary Lukindo for database and data entry; Filbert Francis and Brunno Mmbando for statistical assistance. We thank RTS,S project, PATH-MVI and Afrique-One Project for their support during the study. We thank NIMR Director General for permission to publish this work.

Author Contributions

Conceived and designed the experiments: CM BN JL AB PL ML ZL. Performed the experiments: CM AB PL. Analyzed the data: CM BN JL. Contributed reagents/materials/analysis tools: CM BN JL. Contributed to the writing of the manuscript: CM. Reviewed the manuscript and provided critical inputs: CM BN JL AB PL ML ZL. Read and approved the final manuscript: CM BN JL AB PL ML ZL.

References

1. Gething PW, Kirui VC, Alegana VA, Okiro EA, Noor AM, et al. (2010) Estimating the number of paediatric fevers associated with malaria infection presenting to Africa's public health sector in 2007. PLoS Med 7: e1000301. doi:10.1371/journal.pmed.1000301
2. Osei-Kwakye K, Asante KP, Mahama E, Apanga S, Owusu R, et al. (2013) The benefits or otherwise of managing malaria cases with or without laboratory diagnosis: the experience in a district hospital in Ghana. PLoS One 8: e58107.;PONE-D-12-26544 [pii]. doi:10.1371/journal.pone.0058107
3. Archibald LK, Reller LB (2001) Clinical microbiology in developing countries. Emerg Infect Dis 7: 302–305. doi:10.3201/eid0702.700302
4. Gwer S, Newton CR, Berkley JA (2007) Over-diagnosis and co-morbidity of severe malaria in African children: a guide for clinicians. Am J Trop Med Hyg 77: 6–13. 77/6_Suppl/6 [pii].
5. Petit PL, van Ginneken JK (1995) Analysis of hospital records in four African countries, 1975–1990, with emphasis on infectious diseases. J Trop Med Hyg 98: 217–227.
6. Ye Y, Madise N, Ndugwa R, Ochola S, Snow RW (2009) Fever treatment in the absence of malaria transmission in an urban informal settlement in Nairobi, Kenya. Malar J 8: 160. 1475-2875-8-160 [pii]; doi:10.1186/1475-2875-8-160
7. Hertz JT, Munishi OM, Sharp JP, Reddy EA, Crump JA (2013) Comparing actual and perceived causes of fever among community members in a low malaria transmission setting in northern Tanzania. Trop Med Int Health 18: 1406–1415. doi:10.1111/tmi.12191
8. D'Acremont V, Lengeler C, Genton B (2010) Reduction in the proportion of fevers associated with Plasmodium falciparum parasitaemia in Africa: a systematic review. Malar J 9: 240. 1475-2875-9-240 [pii]; doi:10.1186/1475-2875-9-240
9. Rutta AS, Francis F, Mmbando BP, Ishengoma DS, Sembuche SH, et al. (2012) Using community-owned resource persons to provide early diagnosis and treatment and estimate malaria burden at community level in north-eastern Tanzania. Malar J 11: 152. 1475-2875-11-152 [pii]; doi:10.1186/1475-2875-11-152
10. Were T, Davenport GC, Hittner JB, Ouma C, Vulule JM, et al. (2011) Bacteremia in Kenyan children presenting with malaria. J Clin Microbiol 49: 671–676. JCM.01864-10 [pii]; doi:10.1128/JCM.01864-10
11. Petti CA, Polage CR, Quinn TC, Ronald AR, Sande MA (2006) Laboratory medicine in Africa: a barrier to effective health care. Clin Infect Dis 42: 377–382. CID37615 [pii]; doi:10.1086/499363
12. Urdea M, Penny LA, Olmsted SS, Giovanni MY, Kaspar P, et al. (2006) Requirements for high impact diagnostics in the developing world. Nature 444 Suppl 1: 73–79. nature05448 [pii]; doi:10.1038/nature05448

13. Strom GE, Haanshuus CG, Fataki M, Langeland N, Blomberg B (2013) Challenges in diagnosing paediatric malaria in Dar es Salaam, Tanzania. Malar J 12: 228. 1475-2875-12-228 [pii]; doi:10.1186/1475-2875-12-228
14. Moon AM, Biggs HM, Rubach MP, Crump JA, Maro VP, et al. (2014) Evaluation of In-Hospital Management for Febrile Illness in Northern Tanzania before and after 2010 World Health Organization Guidelines for the Treatment of Malaria. PLoS One 9: e89814. doi:10.1371/journal.pone.0089814; PONE-D-13-35569 [pii].
15. World Health Organisation (WHO) (2010) Guidelines for the treatment of malaria, 2nd edition.
16. Reyburn H, Mbatia R, Drakeley C, Carneiro I, Mwakasungula E, et al. (2004) Overdiagnosis of malaria in patients with severe febrile illness in Tanzania: a prospective study. BMJ 329: 1212. bmj.38251.658229.55 [pii]; doi:10.1136/bmj.38251.658229.55
17. D'Acremont V, Kilowoko M, Kyungu E, Philipina S, Sangu W, et al. (2014) Beyond malaria–causes of fever in outpatient Tanzanian children. N Engl J Med 370: 809–817. doi:10.1056/NEJMoa1214482
18. Nadjm B, Amos B, Mtove G, Ostermann J, Chonya S, et al. (2010) WHO guidelines for antimicrobial treatment in children admitted to hospital in an area of intense Plasmodium falciparum transmission: prospective study. BMJ 340: c1350.
19. Crump JA, Ramadhani HO, Morrissey AB, Msuya LJ, Yang LY, et al. (2011) Invasive bacterial and fungal infections among hospitalized HIV-infected and HIV-uninfected children and infants in northern Tanzania. Trop Med Int Health 16: 830–837. doi:10.1111/j.1365-3156.2011.02774.x
20. Biggs HM, Lester R, Nadjm B, Mtove G, Todd JE, et al. (2014) Invasive salmonella infections in areas of high and low malaria transmission intensity in Tanzania. Clin Infect Dis 58: 638–647. cit798 [pii]; doi:10.1093/cid/cit798
21. National Bureau of Statistics Ministry of Finance Tanzania (2013) 2012 Population and housing census.
22. Mmbando BP, Vestergaard LS, Kitua AY, Lemnge MM, Theander TG, et al. (2010) A progressive declining in the burden of malaria in north-eastern Tanzania. Malar J 9: 216. 1475-2875-9-216 [pii]; doi:10.1186/1475-2875-9-216
23. Schmiegelow C, Minja D, Oesterholt M, Pehrson C, Suhrs HE, et al. (2013) Malaria and fetal growth alterations in the 3(rd) trimester of pregnancy: a longitudinal ultrasound study. PLoS One 8: e53794. doi:10.1371/journal.-pone.0053794; PONE-D-12-29446 [pii].
24. World Health Organisation (WHO) (2005) Intergrated Managemnet of Childhood Illness.
25. Kwon JH, Fausone MK, Du H, Robicsek A, Peterson LR (2012) Impact of laboratory-reported urine culture colony counts on the diagnosis and treatment of urinary tract infection for hospitalized patients. Am J Clin Pathol 137: 778–784. 137/5/778 [pii]; doi:10.1309/AJCP4KVGQZEG1YDM
26. National Aids Control Programme Ministry of Health and Social Welfare Tanzania (2012) Guideline for HIV testing.
27. Liu L, Johnson HL, Cousens S, Perin J, Scott S, et al. (2012) Global, regional, and national causes of child mortality: an updated systematic analysis for 2010 with time trends since 2000. Lancet 379: 2151–2161. S0140-6736(12)60560-1 [pii]; doi:10.1016/S0140-6736(12)60560-1
28. Hamilton JL, John SP (2013) Evaluation of fever in infants and young children. Am Fam Physician 87: 254–260. d10789 [pii].
29. Mmbando BP, Vestergaard LS, Kitua AY, Lemnge MM, Theander TG, et al. (2010) A progressive declining in the burden of malaria in north-eastern Tanzania. Malar J 9: 216. 1475-2875-9-216 [pii]; doi:10.1186/1475-2875-9-216
30. Mtove G, Amos B, Nadjm B, Hendriksen IC, Dondorp AM, et al. (2011) Decreasing incidence of severe malaria and community-acquired bacteraemia among hospitalized children in Muheza, north-eastern Tanzania, 2006–2010. Malar J 10: 320. 1475-2875-10-320 [pii]; doi:10.1186/1475-2875-10-320
31. Murray CJ, Rosenfeld LC, Lim SS, Andrews KG, Foreman KJ, et al. (2012) Global malaria mortality between 1980 and 2010: a systematic analysis. Lancet 379: 413–431. S0140-6736(12)60034-8 [pii]; doi:10.1016/S0140-6736(12)60034-8
32. Aregawi MW, Ali AS, Al-mafazy AW, Molteni F, Katikiti S, et al. (2011) Reductions in malaria and anaemia case and death burden at hospitals following scale-up of malaria control in Zanzibar, 1999–2008. Malar J 10: 46. 1475-2875-10-46 [pii]; doi:10.1186/1475-2875-10-46
33. The United Republic of Tanzania MoHaSW (2007) Standard Treatment Guidelines (STG) and The National Essential Medicines List (NEMLIT) for Mainland Tanzania (Page 6).
34. Choi SH, Kim EY, Kim YJ (2013) Systemic use of fluoroquinolone in children. Korean J Pediatr 56: 196–201. doi:10.3345/kjp.2013.56.5.196
35. Thriemer K, Ley B, Ame S, von SL, Pak GD, et al. (2012) The burden of invasive bacterial infections in Pemba, Zanzibar. PLoS One 7: e30350. doi:10.1371/journal.pone.0030350; PONE-D-11-19140 [pii].
36. Msaki BP, Mshana SE, Hokororo A, Mazigo HD, Morona D (2012) Prevalence and predictors of urinary tract infection and severe malaria among febrile children attending Makongoro health centre in Mwanza city, North-Western Tanzania. Arch Public Health 70: 4. 0778-7367-70-4 [pii]; doi:10.1186/0778-7367-70-4
37. Montini G, Tullus K, Hewitt I (2011) Febrile urinary tract infections in children. N Engl J Med 365: 239–250. doi:10.1056/NEJMra1007755
38. Feikin DR, Njenga MK, Bigogo G, Aura B, Aol G, et al. (2013) Viral and bacterial causes of severe acute respiratory illness among children aged less than 5 years in a high malaria prevalence area of western Kenya, 2007–2010. Pediatr Infect Dis J 32: e14–e19. doi:10.1097/INF.0b013e31826fd39b
39. Niang MN, Diop OM, Sarr FD, Goudiaby D, Malou-Sompy H, et al. (2010) Viral etiology of respiratory infections in children under 5 years old living in tropical rural areas of Senegal: The EVIRA project. J Med Virol 82: 866–872. doi:10.1002/jmv.21665
40. Bonkoungou IJ, Haukka K, Osterblad M, Hakanen AJ, Traore AS, et al. (2013) Bacterial and viral etiology of childhood diarrhea in Ouagadougou, Burkina Faso. BMC Pediatr 13: 36. 1471-2431-13-36 [pii]; doi:10.1186/1471-2431-13-36
41. Sire JM, Garin B, Chartier L, Fall NK, Tall A, et al. (2013) Community-acquired infectious diarrhoea in children under 5 years of age in Dakar, Senegal. Paediatr Int Child Health 33: 139–144. doi:10.1179/2046905512Y.0000000046
42. Moyo SJ, Gro N, Matee MI, Kitundu J, Myrmel H, et al. (2011) Age specific aetiological agents of diarrhoea in hospitalized children aged less than five years in Dar es Salaam, Tanzania. BMC Pediatr 11: 19. 1471-2431-11-19 [pii]; doi:10.1186/1471-2431-11-19
43. Alemu A, Shiferaw Y, Addis Z, Mathewos B, Birhan W (2013) Effect of malaria on HIV/AIDS transmission and progression. Parasit Vectors 6: 18. 1756-3305-6-18 [pii]; doi:10.1186/1756-3305-6-18
44. Mubi M, Kakoko D, Ngasala B, Premji Z, Peterson S, et al. (2013) Malaria diagnosis and treatment practices following introduction of rapid diagnostic tests in Kibaha District, Coast Region, Tanzania. Malar J 12: 293. 1475-2875-12-293 [pii]; doi:10.1186/1475-2875-12-293
45. Baltzell K, Elfving K, Shakely D, Ali AS, Msellem M, et al. (2013) Febrile illness management in children under five years of age: a qualitative pilot study on primary health care workers' practices in Zanzibar. Malar J 12: 37. 1475-2875-12-37 [pii]; doi:10.1186/1475-2875-12-37

10

Children with Chronic Suppurative Lung Disease Have a Reduced Capacity to Synthesize Interferon-Gamma *In Vitro* in Response to Non-Typeable *Haemophilus influenzae*

Susan J. Pizzutto[1]*, Stephanie T. Yerkovich[1,2,3], John W. Upham[3,4], Belinda J. Hales[5], Wayne R. Thomas[5], Anne B. Chang[1,6,7]

1 Menzies School of Health Research, Charles Darwin University, Brinkin, Northern Territory, Australia, **2** Queensland Lung Transplant Service, The Prince Charles Hospital, Chermside, Queensland, Australia, **3** School of Medicine, The University of Queensland, St Lucia, Queensland, Australia, **4** Department of Respiratory Medicine, Princess Alexandra Hospital, Wooloongabba, Queensland, Australia, **5** Telethon Kids Institute, The University of Western Australia, Crawley, Western Australia, Australia, **6** The Department of Respiratory Medicine, Royal Children's Hospital, Herston, Queensland, Australia, **7** Queensland Children's Medical Research Institute, Royal Children's Hospital, Herston, Queensland, Australia

Abstract

Chronic suppurative lung disease (CSLD) is characterized by the presence of a chronic wet or productive cough and recurrent lower respiratory infections. The aim of this study was to identify features of innate, cell-mediated and humoral immunity that may increase susceptibility to respiratory infections in children with CSLD. Because non-typeable *Haemophilus influenzae* (NTHi) is commonly isolated from the airways in CSLD, we examined immune responses to this organism in 80 age-stratified children with CSLD and compared their responses with 51 healthy control children. Cytokines involved in the generation and control of inflammation (IFN-γ, IL-13, IL-5, IL-10 at 72 hours and TNFα, IL-6, IL-10 at 24 hours) were measured in peripheral blood mononuclear cells challenged *in vitro* with live NTHi. We also measured circulating IgG subclass antibodies (IgG_1 and IgG_4) to two *H. influenzae* outer membrane proteins, P4 and P6. The most notable finding was that PBMC from children with CSLD produced significantly less IFN-γ in response to NTHi than healthy control children whereas mitogen-induced IFN-γ production was similar in both groups. Overall there were minor differences in innate and humoral immune responses between CSLD and control children. This study demonstrates that children with chronic suppurative lung disease have an altered systemic cell-mediated immune response to NTHi *in vitro*. This deficient IFN-γ response may contribute to increased susceptibility to NTHi infections and the pathogenesis of CSLD in children.

Editor: John S. Tregoning, Imperial College London, United Kingdom

Funding: SP is funded by an Australian National Health and Medical Research Council postgraduate scholarship (1038415); AC (grant 545216) and JU (grant 511019) funded by Australian National Health and Medical Research Council practitioner fellowships (https://www.nhmrc.gov.au). The study was funded by Channel 7 Children's Research Foundation (grant 13688; http://www.crf.org.au) and supported by Australian National Health and Medical Research Council Center for Research Excellence for Lung Health of Aboriginal and Torres Strait Islander (grant 1040830). The funders had no role in study design, data collection and analysis, decision to publish, or preparation of the manuscript.

Competing Interests: The authors have declared that no competing interests exist.

* Email: susan.pizzutto@menzies.edu.au

Introduction

Bronchiectasis and chronic suppurative lung disease (henceforth collectively termed CSLD) describe a syndrome of persistent or recurrent respiratory symptoms predominantly characterized by chronic productive or wet cough. CSLD is increasingly recognized as an important chronic respiratory disorder affecting children [1–4] and adults [5] globally and may represent a precursor to bronchiectasis [1].

Non-typeable *Haemophilus influenzae* (NTHi) are Gram-negative bacteria commonly associated with chronic upper and lower respiratory disease. It is the dominant species isolated from the lower airways of children and adults with chronic respiratory symptoms [6–8]. However, NTHi is also a commensal organism in healthy adults [9] and children [10] and as healthy adults and children both develop antibodies against NTHi [11,12], the relationship between host and bacterium and the transition from commensal organism to pathogen is likely influenced by a complex interaction of host and bacterial factors.

One such host factor identified as important in adults is the cell-mediated immune response. Altered NTHi-specific cytokine responses, including Th2-skewed cytokine profiles have been reported in adults (>50 years of age) with established bronchiectasis or COPD and impaired lung function [11,13]. However, it is unclear whether these alterations were involved in disease induction, or rather arose as a consequence of systemic inflammation in adults with chronic, severe disease [14,15]. A study in children with milder disease of short duration may help elucidate some of these unresolved issues.

In the absence of published data to explain the susceptibility of some children to recurrent lower respiratory infections, we characterized systemic immune responses to NTHi in children with CSLD and healthy children. Our key outcome measures included NTHi-specific cytokine profiles (24 hour and 72 hour) *in vitro* and serum antibodies specific for the *H. influenzae* outer membrane proteins (OMP) P4 and P6. In this study we describe these profiles and identify key differences which may contribute to an increased susceptibility to lower respiratory infections in children.

Materials and Methods

Study population and sample collection

Eighty children (aged≤10 years) undergoing chest computed tomography (CT) scan and flexible bronchoscopy for suspected CSLD (CSLD group) and 51 age-matched children without acute infection or clinical history of respiratory or chronic illness (healthy control, HC group) were prospectively recruited (2008–2011) from the Royal Darwin Hospital (RDH), Darwin, Northern Territory (NT), Australia.

All children in the study group were clinically stable (absence of respiratory exacerbation) at the time of sample collection. Blood and bronchoalveolar lavage (BAL) for clinical and research investigations were collected at the time of intravenous access (i.e. at the start of general anesthesia), prior to chest CT scan/ bronchoscopy. Clinical and socio-demographic data were collected using standardized data collection forms. Routine clinical investigations [1] were performed using the regional reference laboratory (RDH) and subsequently two children were excluded from analysis following a diagnosis of primary immunodeficiency (final n = 80). Radiographic diagnosis of bronchiectasis was made by the pediatric respiratory physician (AC). *Haemophilus influenzae*, *Streptococcus pneumoniae* and *Moraxella catarrhalis* culture and identification were performed by our laboratory (diagnostic threshold $>10^4$ CFU/ml [6]). *Pseudomonas aeruginosa* and *Klebsiella pneumoniae* culture and identification were performed by the diagnostic laboratory at the Royal Darwin Hospital.

Healthy controls (absence of a history of chronic respiratory, other non-respiratory illness and no acute illness within 4 weeks) were enrolled primarily through RDH elective surgery list. They did not have the same clinical work up as the CSLD group (including chest CT, bronchoscopy) as these investigations were not clinically indicated for their procedure. Blood was collected under the same conditions as described for the group with CSLD, prior to any procedure. BAL was not collected from the control children.

The Human Research Ethics Committee (Northern Territory Department of Health and Menzies School of Health Research) approved this study (#07/63). The children were enrolled following written informed consent from the parent/carer.

NTHi preparation

A single NTHi strain originally isolated from the sputum of an adult with pneumonia (confirmed by the Phadebact Haemophilus Test (Bactus AB, Huddinge, Sweden) and by PCR [16]) was used for this study. The immunogenicity of this strain and optimization of culture conditions were first determined in peripheral blood mononuclear cell (PBMC) cultures from healthy adults. A pilot study of 19 additional NTHi strains indicated that the strain used in this study was representative of NTHi-specific cytokine responses in a healthy adult.

NTHi was grown on chocolate agar plates overnight at 37°C, 5% CO_2. Brain heart infusion broth supplemented with hemin (30 mg/L), nicotinamide adenine dinucleotide (30 mg/L) and glycerol (4%) was inoculated with isolated colonies and incubated with shaking at 37°C overnight. This starter culture was used to inoculate a large volume broth culture and grown to an optical density at 600 of 0.47 units. Single use aliquots were stored in 20% heat-inactivated fetal bovine serum (FBS) at −80°C. The same batch of NTHi was used in all experiments. Viability was quantified by plating serial dilutions on chocolate agar and batch viability was routinely monitored.

Peripheral Blood Mononuclear Cell (PBMC) isolation

Venous blood was collected into preservative-free heparin and processed within 2 hours. PBMC were isolated by centrifugation over Ficoll-Paque Plus (GE Healthcare Bio-Sciences AB, Sweden) and cryopreserved in liquid nitrogen in 10%DMSO/heat-inactivated FBS. These techniques have been successfully used in studies of immune function in large human cohorts [17,18]. Matched plasma for antibody analysis was stored at −80°C.

PBMC challenge assays

In order to measure adaptive, cell mediated immune function, PBMC were resuspended in AIM-V serum-free medium (Gibco Life Technologies, Australia) supplemented with 2-mercaptoethanol (0.04 mM final concentration), and cultured in duplicate at 2.5×10^5 cells per well in 96 well plates with either live NTHi (4×10^6 CFU/ml final concentration), PHA (2 μg/ml; Sigma, Missouri, USA) or medium alone for 72 hours at 37°C, 5% CO_2. IFNγ, IL-13, IL-5 and IL-10 were measured in supernatant collected at 72 hours. Where sufficient cells were available, innate immune responses (IL-6, TNFα and early IL-10) were also assessed. PBMC were cultured in RPMI 1640 with 10% non-heat inactivated FCS and NTHi (4×10^6 and 4×10^5 CFU/ml final concentration), or medium alone for 24 hours at 37°C, 5% CO_2. Supernatants were collected and stored at 4°C for up to 7 days prior to cytokine quantification.

Quantification of cytokines

Cytokines were measured from the 72 and 24 hour culture supernatants using dissociation-enhanced lanthanide fluorescent immunoassays (DELFIA) as described previously [19]. Quantitative standard curves were generated from serial dilutions of recombinant human cytokine proteins and included on each plate. The limit of detection for all cytokines was 10 pg/ml; samples with concentrations below the limit of detection were assigned the value of 1 pg/ml. The data is presented as delta concentrations (amount of cytokine from NTHi challenge minus nil challenge). Children were identified as responders if cytokine production was at least two-fold greater than the nil treatment or two-fold above the assay limit of detection (whichever was greater).

Immunoglobulin levels

IgG_1 and IgG_4 specific for the recombinant outer-membrane proteins (OMP) P4 and P6 from *H. influenzae* were quantified from plasma by Dissociation Enhanced Lanthanide Fluorescent Immunoassay (DELFIA; PerkinElmer) as previously described [20,21]. Negative control plasma for each OMP/antibody combination were included on each plate. Plasma IgE was measured using ELISA. Children were identified as responders if their antibody level was at least two-fold greater than the mean concentration of the negative control plasma.

Data analysis

For the primary analysis, the children were stratified by age (< 18, 18–36, 37–60 and >60 months) and the data analyzed according to respiratory diagnosis (healthy control or CSLD). As a secondary analysis, the age groups were combined and potential confounding factors of the data identified and assessed in the analysis. For the secondary analysis, only cytokines which maintained a statistical difference following correction for potential confounding factors are described.

Statistical analysis was performed using STATA 13 (StataCorp, USA) and a p-value <0.05 was considered statistically significant. Group differences (by age, diagnosis of CSLD and cultural background) were assessed by the Mann-Whitney U test and categorical data were assessed by Fisher's exact test. Cytokine and antibody data were non-parametric and are presented as median with interquartile range. Potential factors that might confound analysis of the immunologic data were identified (cultural background, clinical characteristics) and regression analysis used to investigate their effects.

Results

Study population

The demographic characteristics of the children are shown in table 1. All of the children in the current study came from a similar geographic region, northern Australia. High generational cultural diversity is a characteristic of the population in this region and studies to determine the influence of race on the immune response are not feasible. Despite this, we found that a high proportion of children in the CSLD group were identified by their parent as having Indigenous Australian ancestry, thus we have grouped children as either having known Indigenous Australian ancestry (described as Indigenous descent) or with no, or unknown, Indigenous Australian ancestry (non-Indigenous descent).

Children with CSLD have altered 72 hour NTHi-cytokine profiles

We detected IFN-γ, IL-13 and IL-10 in the NTHi-challenged PBMC culture supernatants from almost all children (figure 1a). Whilst the number of IL-5 responders was comparatively low, the CSLD group had almost 2-fold more responders than the HC group.

For the three older age groups, PBMC from children with CSLD produced significantly less IFN-γ compared with HC children but no significant difference between groups were present in the <18 month age group (figure 1a). When all age groups were combined, IFN-γ production was also significantly lower in the CSLD group compared to HC (median (IQR) 876 (145–2536) versus 7861 (1939–17840) pg/ml, age-adjusted $p<0.001$; table S1).

In the HC group there was a dramatic upward trajectory in IFNγ production between the <18 month age group and the 18–36 month age groups (median 845 versus 8115 pg/ml; $p=0.06$) and this level of production remained high in the older children. In contrast, IFNγ production in children with CSLD <18 months of age was similar to that seen in children with CSLD in the 18–36 month age group (median 928 versus 678 pg/ml; $p=0.36$) and also similar to that seen in the older age groups (figure 1b).

Furthermore, children with CSLD aged <18 months produced higher amounts of the Th2 associated cytokine IL-13 than the age-matched HC children (median 63 versus 19 ng/ml; $p=0.03$). In contrast, IL-13 production was similar in CSLD and HC children in each of the three older age groups. The production of IL-5 and

Table 1. Demographic characteristics of the population by age group.

		<18 months		18–36 months		37–60 months		>60 months	
		HC	CSLD	HC	CSLD	HC	CSLD	HC	CSLD
n		6	18	9	38	14	12	22	12
Age in months	median	8	14	26	26	51	47	81	82
	(IQR)	(5–13)	(10–15)	(24–35)	(21–29)	(46–56)	(40–54)	(66–107)	(71–106)
	p value#	0.09		0.19		0.21		0.59	
Male	n (%)	5 (83)	9 (50)	8 (89)	22 (58)	6 (43)	5 (42)	12 (55)	6 (50)
Indigenous descent	n (%)	0	13 (72)	5 (56)	36 (95)	6 (43)	12 (100)	4 (18)	12 (100)

#analysis of age between HC and CSLD at each age group.

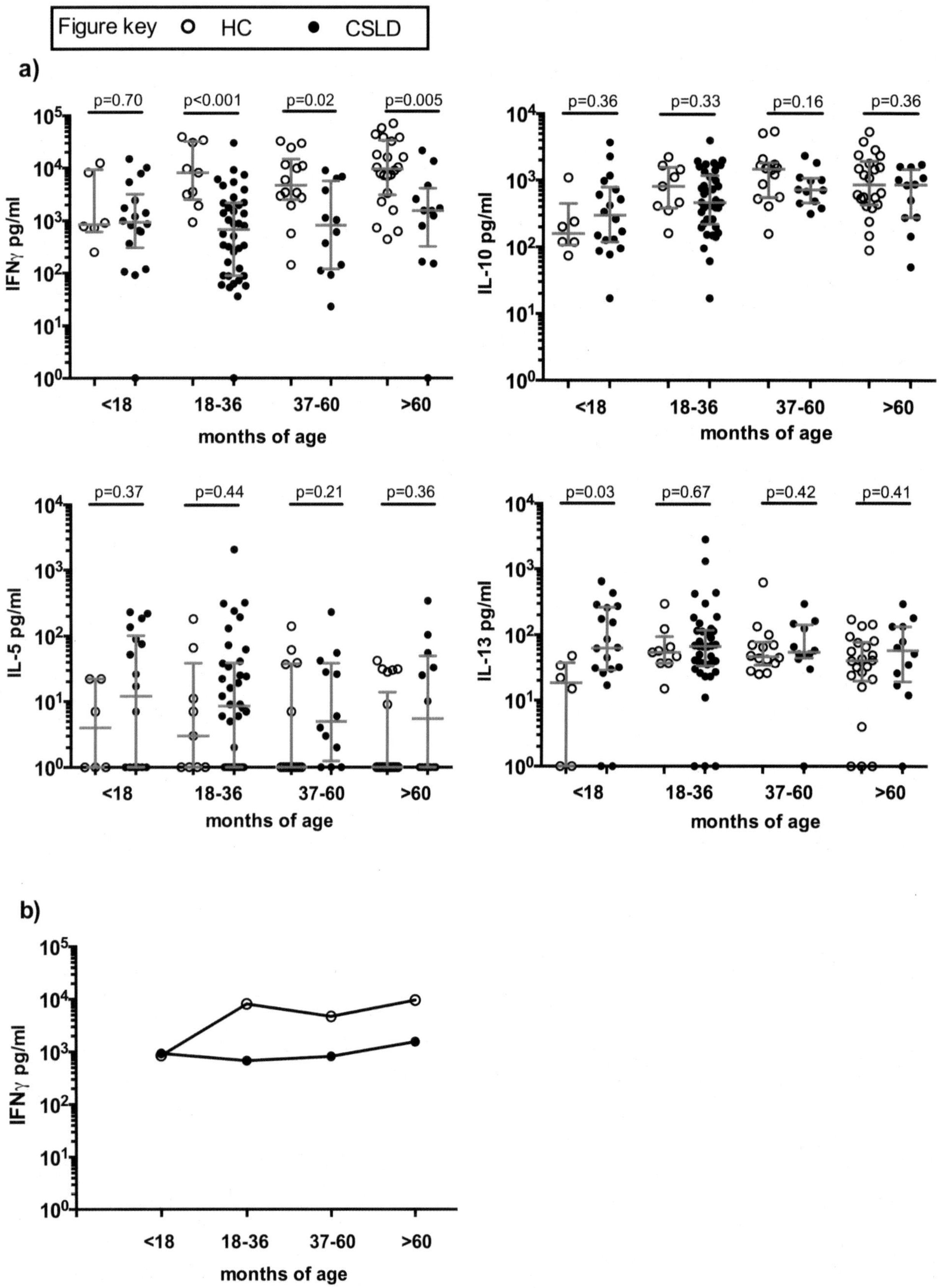

Figure 1. Adaptive (72 hour) cytokine production to NTHi. a) In vitro cytokine production by HC (open circles) and CSLD (filled circles) PBMC following 72 hour challenge with NTHi. Delta concentration (NTHi challenge minus nil challenge) with median and IQR. b) Trajectory of adaptive (72 hour) IFN-γ production to NTHi with age. In vitro cytokine production by HC (open circles) and CSLD (filled circles) PBMC following 72 hour challenge with NTHi. Median (delta) concentration, pg/ml.

IL-10 did not differ between the CSLD and HC groups across any age group.

We used the non-specific mitogen PHA to test the global capacity for cytokine production and found minimal differences between CSLD and HC children (figure 2). These data indicate that the reduced capacity to synthesise IFN-γ observed in CSLD children aged >18 months is specific to NTHi and cannot be attributed to a generalised impairment in the capacity of T-cell and natural killer cells to produce these cytokines.

As CSLD was found to be prevalent in children of Indigenous descent, we investigated if this contributed to the differences in IFN-γ observed between children with CSLD and HC children. We found that Indigenous children with CSLD produced significantly less IFN-γ than age-matched Indigenous HC children (median 703 versus 3497 pg/ml; $p<0.001$) and non-Indigenous HC children (median 703 versus 10017 pg/ml $p<0.001$) (table 2). Finally, using regression analysis, Indigenous descent was not an independent predictor of IFN-γ production (table S1).

Innate (24 hour) cytokine responses to NTHi

Because innate immunity may modulate adaptive immunity, we examined the strength and nature of the innate immune response to NTHi by measuring IL-6, TNFα and IL-10 production in 24 hour NTHi-stimulated PBMC (figure 3). Measurable quantities of the cytokines were produced by almost all children. Children with CSLD aged18–36 months produced less IL-6 and TNFα than HC children, but these differences were not observed in the three other age groups. IL-10 production at 24 hours was similar across all groups. When all age groups were combined, the CSLD group produced less IL-6 than the HC group (median (IQR) 5527 (3131–8733) versus11425 (4835–18458) pg/ml, age-adjusted $p = 0.007$; table S1).

As found with the 72 hour cytokine data, none of the 24 hour cytokine data varied in relation to Indigenous descent (table 2).

Serum antibodies specific for H. influenzae outer membrane proteins P4 and P6

Most children had measurable serum IgG_1 to both P4 and P6. The number producing detectable levels of IgG_4 was low. Only minor differences were observed between the children with CSLD and the HC children (figure 4).

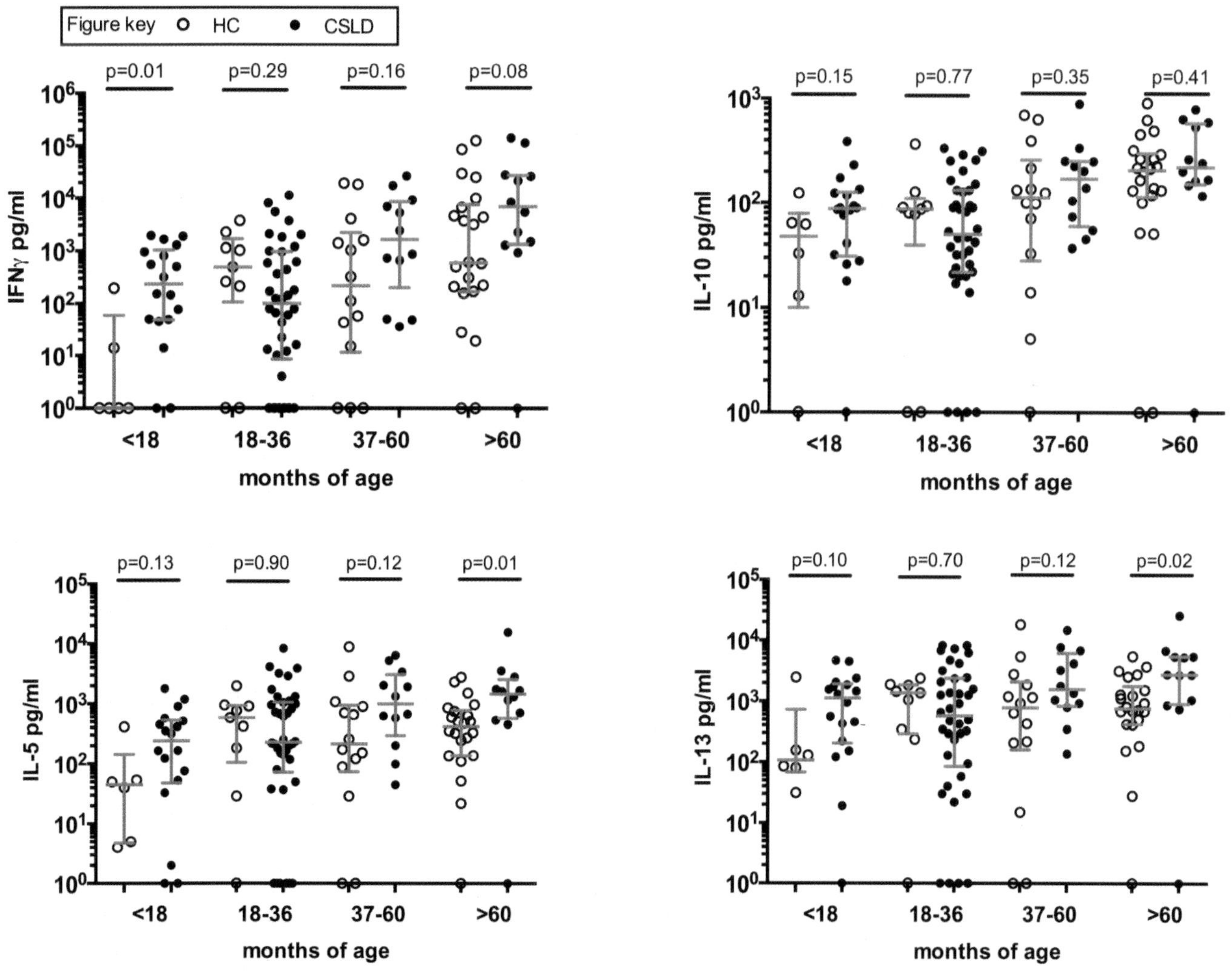

Figure 2. Adaptive (72 hour) cytokine production to PHA. In vitro cytokine production by HC (open symbols) and CSLD (filled symbols) PBMC following 72 hour challenge with the non-specific mitogen PHA. Delta concentration (NTHi challenge minus nil challenge) with median and IQR.

Table 2. Cytokine production (pg/ml; median (IQR)) from NTHi-challenged PBMC from children ≥18 months; HC Indigenous descent n = 15, HC non-Indigenous descent n = 30, CSLD Indigenous descent n = 60, CSLD non-Indigenous descent n = 2.

		Indigenous descent	non-Indigenous descent	p#
IFN-γ (72 hr)	HC	3497 (1939–33950)	10017 (3331–24437)	0.36
	CSLD	703 (102–2190)	557, 3858**	n/a*
	p##	**<0.001**	n/a*	
IL-13 (72 hr)	HC	44 (37–123)	46 (25–66)	0.36
	CSLD	65 (33–129)	50, 69**	n/a*
	p##	0.76	n/a*	
IL-5 (72 hr)	HC	0 (0–37)	0 (0–3)	0.07
	CSLD	7 (0–40)	0, 9**	n/a*
	p##	0.54	n/a*	
IL-10 (72 hr)	HC	562 (352–1454)	1336 (555–2230)	**0.03**
	CSLD	682 (279–1109)	391, 467**	n/a*
	p##	0.83	n/a*	
TNF (24 hr)	HC	656 (541–1094)	1556 (727–2086)	0.10
	CSLD	588 (226–1267)	181, 533**	n/a*
	p##	0.53	n/a*	
IL-6 (24 hr)	HC	7154 (4221–18458)	12819 (8966–17698)	0.18
	CSLD	6563 (3701–10969)	2304, 2736**	n/a*
	p##	0.38	n/a*	

#Analysis between Indigenous and non-Indigenous descent.
##analysis between HC and CSLD.
*p value not calculated due to small numbers.
**absolute values for the 2 participants.

Effect of patient and clinical characteristics on cytokine response

Although all children were clinically stable at the time of sample collection, 45% were receiving maintenance antibiotics for CLSD or chronic suppurative otitis media, a common co-morbidity in this population. BAL culture showed lower airway infection (growth of ≥10^4 colony-forming units (CFU)/mL of any pathogen using standard culture methods) in 21 (25.6%) children. NTHi was the most common pathogen identified (24% of children), followed by *Streptococcus pneumoniae* (5%) and *Moraxella catarrhalis* (5%), *Pseudomonas aeruginosa* (2.5%) and *Klebsiella pneumoniae* (1%). Serum total IgE was similar between healthy controls (HC) (median 449 ng/ml; IQR 73–1142 ng/ml) and the CSLD group (641 ng/ml; 149–1623 ng/ml) (p = 0.07). All but one child were up to date with their childhood vaccination schedule. Using regression analysis, Mann-Whitney U test or Spearman's rank order correlation, we investigated whether these characteristics of the children with CSLD at the time of sample collection could explain variations in NTHi-induced cytokine production. The observed NTHi-stimulated cytokine responses were not associated with antibiotic use (including azithromycin), current isolation of NTHi or other respiratory pathogens in the BAL, evidence of parasitic infection (strongyloides), serum IgE and inflammatory cell counts in BAL and blood (table S2).

Discussion

Despite advances in the prevention and management of pediatric respiratory infections, CSLD remains a problem in children and adults globally. This prospective, cross-sectional study is the first to compare NTHi-driven innate, cell-mediated and humoral immune responses across a large group of children with CSLD (n = 80) and healthy control children (n = 51). The most notable finding was that, in children aged ≥18 months, PBMC from those with CSLD produced significantly less IFN-γ than PBMC from their healthy peers. In contrast, in children aged <18 months, those with CSLD produced more IL-13 than the healthy control children. We found comparatively minor differences in humoral and innate immune responses. These data are consistent with our hypothesis that impaired cell mediated immune responses may contribute to the pathogenesis of CSLD in children.

Immune development begins in utero [22,23]. Various environmental, respiratory and immune pressures drive the maturation of the Th1 response from the Th2-dominated response of neonates [24–26]. By 18 months of age there is a substantial rise in IFN-γ function [27] and a delay in the development of the IFN-γ response may predict Th2-associated disorders in childhood [28]. IFN-γ, primarily secreted by T lymphocytes and natural killer cells, is integral to the orchestration of antiviral and antibacterial activity and is a dominant Th1 cytokine. Furthermore impaired IFN-γ responses have been implicated in the pathogenesis of rhinovirus-induced asthma exacerbations in adults [29]. Whilst our study was not designed to investigate the mechanistic process of immune maturation, our findings have highlighted a disparity between children with CSLD and HC children in age-related IFN-γ and IL-13 production. We found a log-fold increase in IFN-γ production between HC aged <18 months compared to those > 18 months. The capacity to produce IFN-γ remained high in the older age groups. These data are consistent with normal maturation of the Th1 response through early childhood. This age-related increase in IFN-γ response observed in the HC

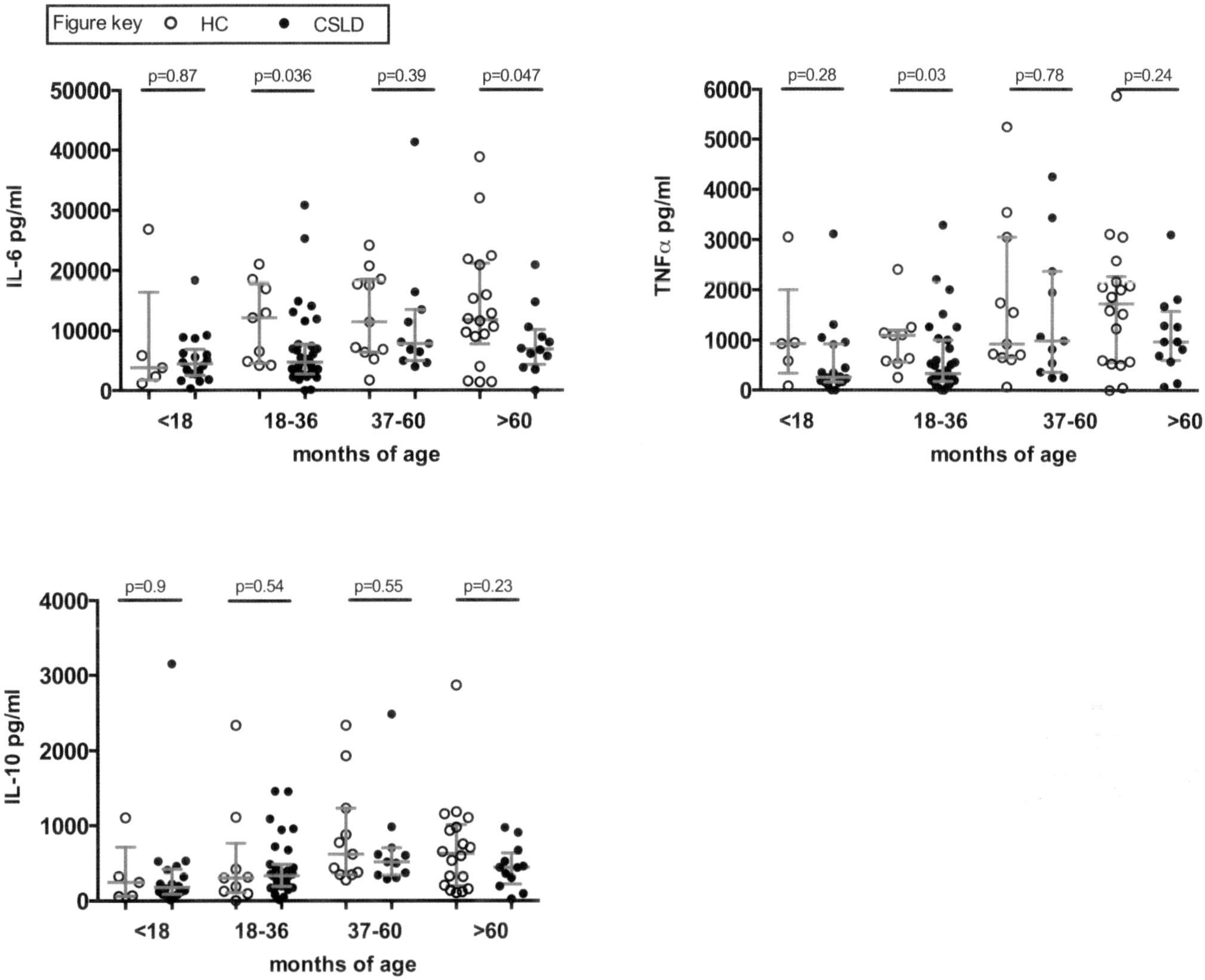

Figure 3. Innate (24 hour) cytokine production. In vitro cytokine production by HC (open circles) and CSLD (filled circles) PBMC following 24 hour challenge with NTHi. Delta concentration (NTHi challenge minus nil challenge) with median and IQR.

children was not reflected in the children with CSLD. Children < 18 months of age with CSLD had a similar capacity for NTHi-specific IFN-γ production as their HC peers, however unlike the HC group, the CSLD group maintained a significantly lower capacity for IFN-γ production over subsequent increasing age groups. Conversely, IL-13 production was significantly higher in younger children with CSLD, with no significant difference between the two groups in older children. Whilst future longitudinal studies are required, these data support the notion that normal maturation of the cell mediated immune response is impaired in children who develop CSLD.

We also examined cytokines representative of innate immune responses in PBMC challenged for 24 hours with NTHi reasoning that altered innate immunity might provide a mechanism for altered adaptive immunity. No studies have previously addressed this issue in children with CSLD. IL-6 is an important cytokine in facilitating the transition from the innate to the adaptive response and is also important for the resolution of acute inflammation (reviewed in Jones [30]). The low IL-6 response to NTHi which we observed in children with CSLD as a group and in the 18–36 month age group is consistent with our data demonstrating an impaired cell-mediated immune response. That TNFα production was also low in 18–36 month CSLD children may point to an immaturity or impaired function of innate immune cells such as monocytes or dendritic cells. Immaturity of such antigen presenting cells would also account for low IFN-γ responses to antigenic stimulation via impaired IL-12 or IL-27 pathways [31]. The possible contribution of IL-6 and other Th1-polarising cytokines, including IL-12 and IL-27, to the pathogenesis of NTHi infections and chronic inflammation requires exploration in future longitudinal studies.

P4 and P6 are highly conserved, immunogenic outer membrane proteins ubiquitously expressed on *H. influenzae*. Given the association of OMP antibodies with protection from NTHi infection in animal models [32] and the association of low P4 and P6 IgG_1 titres with asthma and atopy, in children [20], we investigated if children with CSLD were deficient in NTHi-specific antibodies, especially since clinical investigations found no deficiency in total IgG or any IgG subgroup overall. Consistent with published data [20,21], most children in our study produced IgG_1 to P4 and P6 whilst the number of children (CSLD and HC) producing IgG_4 to either antigen was low. In contrast to published

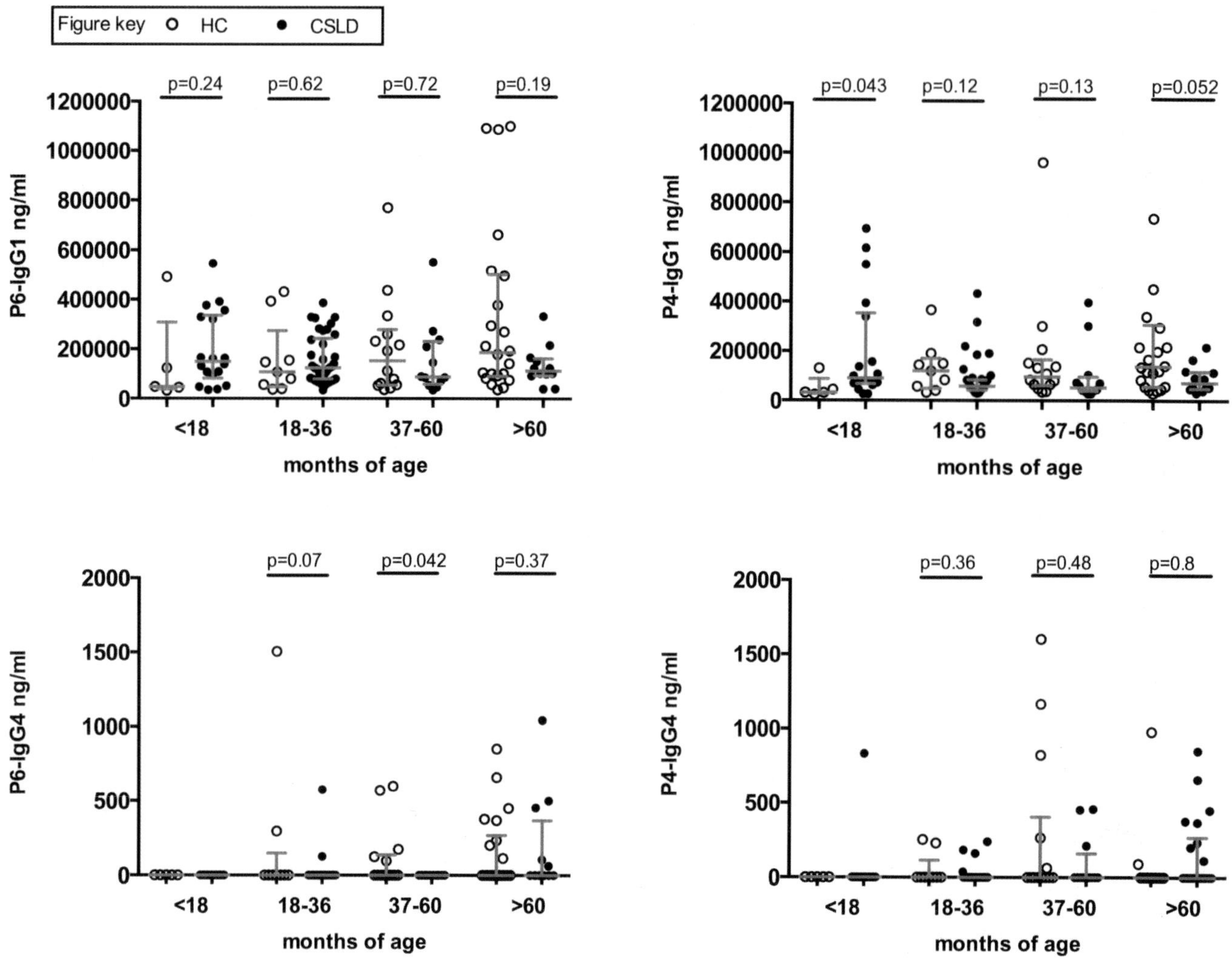

Figure 4. Serum IgG1 and IgG4 to outer membrane proteins P4 and P6. HC (open circles) and CSLD (filled circles). Concentration with median and inter-quartile range.

data of children with Th2-associated disorders asthma and atopy [20] we found no significant difference in P4 and P6 IgG1 levels between children with CLSD and HC children. These results plus the comparable levels of early (24 hour) and later (72 hour) IL-10 responses support the hypothesis that non-protective immunity to NTHi in children with CSLD is more closely linked to aberrant cell-mediated immune function rather than the humoral arm of the immune response.

Our finding that children with CLSD have an impaired IFN-γ response to NTHi has some interesting parallels with that described in adults with the chronic respiratory conditions associated with infection (COPD and bronchiectasis). In these studies involving smaller cohorts, King and colleagues demonstrated that persistent or recurrent lower respiratory infection with NTHi in adults with COPD (n = 39) or bronchiectasis (n = 16) was associated with high IL-13 production in the airways and low systemic IFN-γ production [13,11]. These studies provide important data on the pathogenesis of NTHi infection in adults, however extrapolation of this data to the pediatric setting may not be appropriate. The strengths of our study, which also distinguish it from the adult studies, lie in our large sample size of young children with early onset chronic disease. 75% of our total cohort (n = 80) were aged <3.5 years and had comparatively mild disease of recent onset. The effect of age, chronic inflammation, airway remodeling and pollutants on immune responses is well documented [33–36]. Thus studying CSLD in children with early stage disease may be more instructive to understanding the early pathogenesis of bronchiectasis. The differences in immune function described in the current study are more likely to be involved in disease initiation rather than an effect of chronic disease and long standing tissue damage.

It is now evident that the airways are colonized with microbial flora and that respiratory illness is frequently characterized by changes in the normal microbiota [9]. Furthermore emerging evidence suggests that normal immune profiles vary between populations; children from regions of high pathogen burden have functionally distinct immune profiles compared with children from regions of low burden [23,24]. Whilst all of the children in our study came from a similar geographic location, a large proportion of our CSLD group identified with an Indigenous Australian ancestry. Many factors beyond the scope of this study may contribute to this disparity including both biological and socio-economic determinants of health. We undertook several approaches to ensure that the differences in cytokine profiles were a result of the CSLD and not merely explained by the demographics of the population.

There are numerous host and environmental factors which may influence the immune response thus, whilst our current study has novel findings, we acknowledge some limitations. We chose to use NTHi because it is the most common bacterium in children with CSLD but it was beyond the scope of our study to examine if other pathogens also induce low IFN-γ responses. Secondly it is a cross-sectional study thus we cannot explain the cause or the effect of the observed impaired IFN-γ response in children with CSLD. Also, the association between systemic and local airway responses is unknown as limited cell numbers obtained from BAL precluded measurement of IFN-γ production by airway T-cells in our study. Nonetheless, our findings suggest that altered systemic immune responses are characteristic of CSLD, and we would argue that both local and systemic immunity are likely to be important in defending the lungs from respiratory pathogens.

In conclusion, this is the first study to compare NTHi-driven innate, cell-mediated and humoral immune responses between a large group of children with CSLD and HC children. Our key finding is that the ability to induce protective cell mediated immune responses against NTHi is compromised in children with CSLD. We found clear evidence of impaired IFN-γ responses by PBMC, *in vitro*, in children with CSLD and limited evidence of impaired innate and humoral responses. Furthermore, whilst our data on young infant responses is preliminary it suggests that this impairment begins at an early age. This study has important implications for research into management strategies for children at risk of CSLD. Effective management strategies require an understanding of host responses to respiratory pathogens and the contribution of these responses to the pathogenesis of chronic infection. Future intervention studies that can improve cell mediated immune responses along with longitudinal studies examining the relative contributions of delayed immune development, and high microbial load to the pathophysiology of CSLD in children, are required.

Supporting Information

Table S1 a) Linear regression model of IFN-γ production at 72 hours. b) Linear regression model of IL-13 production at 72 hours. c) Linear regression model of IL-10 production at 72 hours. d) Linear regression model of IL-6 production at 24 hours.

Table S2 Analysis of patient characteristics on NTHi-specific cytokine production. # p value from analysis by Mann-Whitney U test, ## p value from analysis by ANOVA, ### p value from analysis by Spearman's rank order correlation.

Acknowledgments

We thank the participating children and their families. We thank Clare McKay and Lesley Versteegh for their assistance with participant recruitment and sample collection. We thank the staff of Royal Darwin Hospital, in particular Dr Paul Bauert (Maternal and Child Health), Dr Brian Spain (Anesthetics) and the Radiology staff, for their critical support of our research.

Author Contributions

Conceived and designed the experiments: SJP STY JWU BJH WRT ABC. Performed the experiments: SJP STY. Analyzed the data: SJP STY. Contributed reagents/materials/analysis tools: SJP STY JWU BJH WRT ABC. Contributed to the writing of the manuscript: SJP STY JWU BJH WRT ABC.

References

1. Chang A, Bell S, Byrnes C, Grimwood K, Holmes P, et al. (2010) Chronic suppurative lung disease and bronchiectasis in children and adults in Australia and New Zealand. Med J Aust 193: 356–365.
2. Karadag B, Karakoc F, Ersu R, Kut A, Bakac S, et al. (2005) Non-cystic-fibrosis bronchiectasis in children: A persisting problem in developing countries. Respiration 72: 233–238.
3. Singleton R, Morris A, Redding G, Poll J, Holck P, et al. (2000) Bronchiectasis in Alaska Native children: Causes and clinical courses. Pediatr Pulmonol 29: 182–187.
4. Twiss J, Metcalfe R, Edwards E, Byrnes C (2005) New Zealand national incidence of bronchiectasis "too high" for a developed country. Arch Dis Child 90: 737–740.
5. Kelly MG, Murphy S, Elborn JS (2003) Bronchiectasis in secondary care: a comprehensive profile of a neglected disease. Eur J Intern Med 14: 488–492.
6. Hare K, Grimwood K, Leach A, Smith-Vaughan H, Torzillo P, et al. (2010) Respiratory bacterial pathogens in the nasopharynx and lower airways of Australian Indigenous children with bronchiectasis. J Pediatr 157: 1001–1005.
7. Kapur N, Grimwood K, Masters IB, Morris PS, Chang AB (2012) Lower airway microbiology and cellularity in children with newly diagnosed non-CF bronchiectasis. Pediatr Pulmonol 47: 300–307.
8. King PT, Holdsworth SR, Freezer NJ, Villanueva E, Holmes PW (2007) Microbiologic follow-up study in adult bronchiectasis. Respir Med101: 1633–1638.
9. Hilty M, Burke C, Pedro H, Cardenas P, Bush A, et al. (2010) Disordered Microbial Communities in Asthmatic Airways. PLoS ONE 5: e8578.
10. Dunne EM, Smith-Vaughan HC, Robins-Browne RM, Mulholland EK, Satzke C (2013) Nasopharyngeal microbial interactions in the era of pneumococcal conjugate vaccination. Vaccine 31: 2333–2342.
11. King PT, Hutchinson PE, Johnson PD, Holmes PW, Freezer NJ, et al. (2003) Adaptive Immunity to Nontypeable Haemophilus influenzae. Am J Respir Crit Care Med 167: 587–592.
12. Wiertsema SP, Corscadden KJ, Mowe EN, Zhang G, Vijayasekaran S, et al. (2012) IgG Responses to Pneumococcal and Haemophilus Influenzae Protein Antigens Are Not Impaired in Children with a History of Recurrent Acute Otitis Media. PLoS ONE 7: e49061.
13. King PT, Lim S, Pick A, Ngui J, Prodanovic Z, et al. (2013) Lung T-cell responses to nontypeable Haemophilus influenzae in patients with chronic obstructive pulmonary disease. J Allergy Clin Immunol 131: 1314–1321.e1314.
14. Chalmers JD, Smith MP, McHugh BJ, Doherty C, Govan JR, et al. (2012) Short- and Long-Term Antibiotic Treatment Reduces Airway and Systemic Inflammation in Non–Cystic Fibrosis Bronchiectasis. Am J Respir Crit Care Med186: 657–665.
15. Zheng L, Tipoe G, Lam W, Leung R, Ho J, et al. (2000) Up-regulation of circulating adhesion molecules in bronchiectasis. Eur Resp J 16: 691–696.
16. Pickering J, Binks MJ, Beissbarth J, Hare KM, Kirkham L-AS, et al. (2013) A PCR high-resolution melt for the rapid differentiation of nontypable Haemophilus influenzae and Haemophilus haemolyticus. J Clin Micro.
17. Heaton T, Rowe J, Turner S, Aalberse RC, de Klerk N, et al. (2005) An immunoepidemiological approach to asthma: identification of in-vitro T cell response patterns associated with different wheezing phenotypes in children. Lancet 365: 142–149.
18. Prescott SL, Macaubas C, Smallacombe T, Holt BJ, Sly PD, et al. (1999) Development of allergen-specific T-cell memory in atopic and normal children. Lancet 353: 196–200.
19. Rowe J, Heaton T, Kusel M, Suriyaarachchi D, Serralha M, et al. (2004) High IFN-γ production by CD8+ T cells and early sensitization among infants at high risk of atopy. The J Allergy Clin Immunol 113: 710–716.
20. Hales BJ, Chai LY, Elliot CE, Pearce LJ, Zhang G, et al. (2012) Antibacterial antibody responses associated with the development of asthma in house dust mite-sensitised and non-sensitised children. Thorax 67: 321–327.
21. Hales BJ, Pearce LJ, Kusel MMH, Holt PG, Sly PD, et al. (2008) Differences in the antibody response to a mucosal bacterial antigen between allergic and non-allergic subjects. Thorax 63: 221–227.
22. Ege MJ, Bieli C, Frei R, van Strien RT, Riedler J, et al. (2006) Prenatal farm exposure is related to the expression of receptors of the innate immunity and to atopic sensitization in school-age children. J Allergy Clin Immunol 117: 817–823.
23. Lisciandro JG, Prescott SL, Nadal-Sims MG, Devitt CJ, Richmond PC, et al. (2012) Neonatal antigen-presenting cells are functionally more quiescent in children born under traditional compared with modern environmental conditions. J Allergy Clin Immunol 130: 1167–1174.
24. Lisciandro JG, Prescott SL, Nadal-Sims MG, Devitt CJ, Pomat W, et al. (2012) Comparison of neonatal T regulatory cell function in Papua New Guinean and Australian newborns. Pediatr Allergy Immunol 23: 173–180.
25. Pfefferle PI, Büchele G, Blümer N, Roponen M, Ege MJ, et al. (2010) Cord blood cytokines are modulated by maternal farming activities and consumption

of farm dairy products during pregnancy: The PASTURE Study. J Allergy Clin Immunol 125: 108–115.
26. Schaub B, Liu J, Höppler S, Schleich I, Huehn J, et al. (2009) Maternal farm exposure modulates neonatal immune mechanisms through regulatory T cells. J Allergy Clin Immunol 123: 774–782.
27. Yerkovich ST, Wikstrom ME, Suriyaarachchi D, Prescott SL, Upham JW, et al. (2007) Postnatal Development of Monocyte Cytokine Responses to Bacterial Lipopolysaccharide. Pediatr Res 62: 547–552
28. Tulic MK, Andrews D, Crook ML, Charles A, Tourigny MR, et al. (2012) Changes in thymic regulatory T-cell maturation from birth to puberty: Differences in atopic children. The J Allergy Clin Immunol 129: 199–206.
29. Message SD, Laza-Stanca V, Mallia P, Parker HL, Zhu J, et al. (2008) Rhinovirus-induced lower respiratory illness is increased in asthma and related to virus load and Th1/2 cytokine and IL-10 production. Proc Nat Acad Sci 105: 13562–13567.
30. Jones SA (2005) Directing Transition from Innate to Acquired Immunity: Defining a Role for IL-6. J Immunol 175: 3463–3468.
31. Upham JW, Lee PT, Holt BJ, Heaton T, Prescott SL, et al. (2002) Development of Interleukin-12-Producing Capacity throughout Childhood. Infect Immun 70: 6583–6588.
32. Hotomi M, Ikeda Y, Suzumoto M, Yamauchi K, Green BA, et al. (2005) A recombinant P4 protein of Haemophilus influenzae induces specific immune responses biologically active against nasopharyngeal colonization in mice after intranasal immunization. Vaccine 23: 1294–1300.
33. Arnold C, Wolf J, Brunner S, Herndler-Brandstetter D, Grubeck-Loebenstein B (2011) Gain and Loss of T Cell Subsets in Old Age—Age-Related Reshaping of the T Cell Repertoire. J Clin Immunol 31: 137–146.
34. Holt PG, Upham JW, Sly PD (2005) Contemporaneous maturation of immunologic and respiratory functions during early childhood: Implications for development of asthma prevention strategies. J Allergy Clin Immunol 116: 16–24.
35. Barnes PJ, Celli BR (2009) Systemic manifestations and comorbidities of COPD. Eur Resp J 33: 1165–1185.
36. Zhu X, Gadgil AS, Givelber R, George MP, Stoner MW, et al. (2009) Peripheral T Cell Functions Correlate with the Severity of Chronic Obstructive Pulmonary Disease. J Immunol 182: 3270–3277.

11

S. mansoni Bolsters Anti-Viral Immunity in the Murine Respiratory Tract

Sebastian Scheer[1,2,3¤], Christine Krempl[4], Carsten Kallfass[5], Stefanie Frey[6], Thilo Jakob[6], Gabriel Mouahid[7], Hélène Moné[8], Annette Schmitt-Gräff[9], Peter Staeheli[5], Marinus C. Lamers[1]*

1 Max Planck Institute of Immunobiology and Epigenetics, Freiburg, Germany, **2** International Max Planck Research School of Molecular and Cellular Biology, Freiburg, Germany, **3** University of Freiburg, Freiburg, Germany, **4** Institute of Virology and Immunology, University of Wuerzburg, Wuerzburg, Germany, **5** Institute for Virology, Department of Medical Microbiology and Hygiene, University Medical Center Freiburg, Freiburg, Germany, **6** Allergy Research Group, Department of Dermatology, University Medical Center Freiburg, Freiburg, Germany, **7** Univ. Perpignan Via Domitia, Ecologie et Evolution des Interactions, UMR 5244, F-66860, Perpignan, France, **8** CNRS, Ecologie et Evolution des Interactions, UMR 5244, F-66860, Perpignan, France, **9** Institute of Pathology, University of Freiburg, Freiburg, Germany

Abstract

The human intestinal parasite *Schistosoma mansoni* causes a chronic disease, schistosomiasis or bilharzia. According to the current literature, the parasite induces vigorous immune responses that are controlled by Th2 helper cells at the expense of Th1 helper cells. The latter cell type is, however, indispensable for anti-viral immune responses. Remarkably, there is no reliable literature among 230 million patients worldwide describing defective anti-viral immune responses in the upper respiratory tract, for instance against influenza A virus or against respiratory syncitial virus (RSV). We therefore re-examined the immune response to a human isolate of *S. mansoni* and challenged mice in the chronic phase of schistosomiasis with influenza A virus, or with pneumonia virus of mice (PVM), a mouse virus to model RSV infections. We found that mice with chronic schistosomiasis had significant, systemic immune responses induced by Th1, Th2, and Th17 helper cells. High serum levels of TNF-α, IFN-γ, IL-5, IL-13, IL-2, IL-17, and GM-CSF were found after mating and oviposition. The lungs of diseased mice showed low-grade inflammation, with goblet cell hyperplasia and excessive mucus secretion, which was alleviated by treatment with an anti-TNF-α agent (Etanercept). Mice with chronic schistosomiasis were to a relative, but significant extent protected from a secondary viral respiratory challenge. The protection correlated with the onset of oviposition and TNF-α-mediated goblet cell hyperplasia and mucus secretion, suggesting that these mechanisms are involved in enhanced immune protection to respiratory viruses during chronic murine schistosomiasis. Indeed, also in a model of allergic airway inflammation mice were protected from a viral respiratory challenge with PVM.

Editor: Jie Sun, Indiana University, United States of America

Funding: SS was supported by the Fonds National de la Recherche, Luxembourg (http://www.fnr.lu) (PHD-08-045-RE). The funders had no role in study design, data collection and analysis, decision to publish, or preparation of the manuscript.

Competing Interests: The authors have declared that no competing interests exist.

* Email: rinuslamers@t-online.de

¤ Current address: The Biomedical Research Centre, University of British Columbia, Vancouver, Canada

Introduction

Immunity to intracellular pathogens like viruses and mycobacteria is ensured by type I immune responses. These responses are dependent on and characterised by IFN-γ [1]. In contrast, infestation with helminths, including that by the parasitic trematode worms of the genus *Schistosoma*, typically elicits host type-II immune responses that are characterised by a massive production of the cytokines IL-4, IL-5 and IL-13 [2,3]. These cytokines are thought to inhibit the induction of type I immune responses [1,3,4]. Helminthic infections are moreover often brought in context with a generalised immune regulation or suppression. Improved hygienic conditions, in which helminth infections have become rare, are now often implied in diseases that are caused by unbalanced immune system activity, like autoimmune diseases and allergy. This is subsumised in the hygiene hypothesis [5]. In this passed-on framework of mutually exclusive immune response types and generalised immunosuppression in worm infestation, anti-viral and anti-mycobacterial responses should be severely hampered in areas with a high spread of *Schistosoma* parasites. However, an unambiguous disease pattern was not found [6,7].

Schistosomiasis or bilharzia is a chronic and, when untreated, finally lethal parasitic disease; approximately 230 million people worldwide require treatment yearly [8]. Murine schistosomiasis caused by *S. mansoni* resembles human schistosomiasis in many, but not all respects [9]. The pathogenesis involves a passage of the helminth through several organ systems and elicits several types of immune defence mechanisms. An initial Th1-biased host immune response is induced by the invasion of the infectious cercariae. The immature worms (schistosomula) travel through the lungs and liver to their final destination in the portal veins, where they mate. Around 6 weeks after entry, egg deposition by the worm pairs starts. The Th1-biased immune response converts into a Th2-

biased response, and is accompanied by a regulatory (suppressive) response with the production of the prototypical cytokine IL-10 [10]. Eggs must travel through the walls of vessel and gut to reach the gut lumen and to leave the host to continue their life cycle. The passage through the gut wall affects its integrity, requiring repair mechanisms and an increased anti-bacterial response, and is accompanied by extensive inflammation. Repair mechanisms are induced by IL-4 and IL-13 [11], whereas defence to extracellular bacteria is dependent on Th17 responses with the signature cytokine IL-17 [12]. Not all eggs make it to the gut lumen. Many are flushed into the liver or are stuck in the gut wall, where they are then encapsulated by a fibrotic granulomatous response.

Coinfection studies in animal models which could have shed light on the anomalous comorbidity situation were also not conclusive and often difficult to interpret: hepatotropic viruses like HCV and LCMV target an organ, which is stressed by the granulomatous reaction and which is extremely sensitive to cytopathologic effects of TNF-α and IL-12 [13–15].

The lack of expected comorbidities and the ambiguous animal coinfection studies are puzzling in the light of the predominant immunological dogmas. More study is required, with emphasis on systemic effects. The observations also raise the question, whether, from an evolutionary point of view, the parasitic relationship does not only have an unfavourable, but also a certain beneficial effect on the host [16]. Further, recent evidence points to the (gut) microbiome as a modulator of immune responses, also in distant locations like the airways, to respiratory viruses [17,18].

In the present study we infected mice, without antibiotic treatment, with a human isolate of *S. mansoni* from Oman. We tested the immune response in the chronic phase of the disease, to viruses with tropism for tissues that are not directly targeted in schistosomiasis. Hereto we have chosen the respiratory tract viruses pneumonia virus of mice (PVM) [19] and influenza A [20]. We show that a primary, chronic infection with the Omani isolate induces strong, coexistent, and systemic cytokine secretion of the Th1, Th2, and Th17 type. In particular, high serum levels of TNF-α were found that induced a low-grade inflammatory response and a marked hyperplasia of mucus-producing cells in the lung. Under these conditions, mice were relatively well protected from a secondary infectious challenge with the pneumotropic viruses influenza A and PVM. This suggests that chronic schistosomiasis can provide a beneficial effect on the host by reducing the susceptibility to respiratory viral infections.

Materials and Methods

Ethics Statement

Animal experimentation was approved by the local animal welfare authority (Regierungspräsidium Freiburg, Abt. 3, Referat 35; reference: AZ.: 35/9185.81/G-08/104), based on local law and animal ethics regulations (Tierschutzgesetz: http://www.gesetze-im-internet.de/bundesrecht/tierschg/gesamt.pdf). The health status of the mice was scored with some modifications according to Morton and Griffiths [21]. Criteria used for termination were: appearance (grooming, starey coat, posture, dehydration, crusty eyes or nose); body weight (slight (<5%), moderate (5–10%), moderate with decreased appetite (10–20%), severe (>20%); clinical symptoms (breathing rate, heart rate, body temperature, diarhoea, anaemia); handling (alertness, agressiveness, irritability); and behaviour (self-mutilation). Animal condition was monitored on a daily basis, if necessary, at shorter intervals. Mice were sacrificed by asphyxia in carbondioxide.

Mice

Mice were bred and kept in the SPF animal facility of the Max-Planck-Institute of Immunobiology and Epigenetics or of the Virology Department of the University of Freiburg, without antibiotic treatment. B6.A2G-*Mx1* mice carrying functional Mx1 alleles were previously described [20].

Infections

S. mansoni. An Omani human isolate [22] was maintained using *Biomphalaria* species as intermediate hosts. Mice were anaesthetized with Ketamine/Xylazine (0.1 mg resp. 0.5 mg/mouse) and exposed to 80–90 cercariae via the shaved belly method [23]. Infection efficiency was ~75% (number of cercariae left after 1 h of exposure/number of input cercariae). Mice were infected at 10–11 weeks of age.

Influenza. Mice were anaesthetized with Ketamine/Xylazine and infected intranasally (i.n.) with either influenza A strain hvPR8 or strain PR8. For influenza A strain hvPR8 (a highly virulent variant of A/PR/8/34 [20]) Mx1-competent mice received 60 or 200 pfu in 50 µl MEM. Mx1-competent control mice received 5×10^5 U hybrid human IFN-αB/D one day before virus challenge. For influenza A strain PR8 C57BL/6J mice (Mx1-deficient) received 2000 pfu i.n. in 50 µl MEM. Challenge was at 10–12 weeks after primary infection with *S. mansoni*. Control mice were left untreated until the infection with influenza virus.

PVM. Mice were anaesthetized with isoflurane (Baxter) and infected i.n. with either 200 or 2000 pfu of PVM clone 15 (ATCC) in 80 µl MEM medium. Virus titers were determined as described previously [24]. Viral challenge was at 12 weeks after primary infection with *S. mansoni*, unless stated otherwise. Control mice were infected at 12–15 weeks of age.

After infection, mice were observed daily and weighed at indicated time points at the same time of day.

Treatment with Etanercept

Mice received Etanercept (a kind gift of Pfizer Germany) at 4 mg/kg body weight intraperitoneally at the indicated time points.

Immunisation with OVA

Mice were immunised i.p. with 20 µg chicken egg ovalbumin (OVA; grade V; Sigma-Aldrich) in 200 µl Alum (4 mg/ml in PBS; Imject Alum Adjuvant; ThermoScientific), at day 0, 7 and 14. Two weeks later, the mice were treated 3 times at daily intervals with aerosolised OVA (1% w/v OVA in PBS) for 20 min [25]. 24 h after the last treatment, the mice were either sacrificed and analysed, or infected with 200 pfu/mouse of PVM.

Broncho-alveolar lavage (BAL)

Lungs were lavaged with 4×800 µl PBS. The BAL fluid (BALF) of the first lavage was used for quantification of cytokines. The cells of the lavages from one mouse were pooled, counted, and used for analysis or *ex vivo* stimulation.

Organs

After BAL, the right half of the lung was dissected, chopped in pieces (<1 mm^3) and digested for 1 h with 25 µg/ml Liberase DL and 10 µg/ml DNase I (both Roche) in HBSS medium. The cell suspension was treated with Gey's solution to deplete erythrocytes, washed, filtered through a 100 µm mesh, and used for flow cytometry. The left half of the lung was snap-frozen and stored at −80°C until analysis.

For the assessment of virus entry, lungs were instilled with 800 µl 4% formalin and kept in 4% formalin for 2 h at room temperature. Afterwards, the lungs were washed with PBS, tumbled for 24 h in 30% sucrose at 4°C, washed with PBS, embedded in OCT, and kept at 4°C for another 24 h before storage at −80°C.

Muc5ac and Muc5b expression

Lungs were snap frozen in liquid nitrogen and stored at −80°C. For RNA extraction, the tissue was extracted with TriReagent (Sigma), and the RNA was immediately reverse transcribed with SuperScript III (Invitrogen) using random hexamers as primers. Quantitative PCR analysis was performed with a Lightcycler (Roche), 18S RNA was used as internal standard. Primers used were described earlier [26].

Cytokine analysis

Serum and BALF were stored at −80°C and analysed for IL-2, IL-4, IL-5, IL-6, IL-10, IL-12p70 (IL-12), IL-13, IL-17, GM-CSF, MIP-1α (CCL3), TNF-α, and IFN-γ applying the Pro Cytokine Assay with the Bio-Plex 200 System (both Bio-Rad). IFN-α was determined with the Premium ELISA kit (eBioscience). To gauge expression of IFN-β, Mx-1-competent mice harbouring a reporter for IFN-β [27] were infected with *S. mansoni*. 12 weeks after infection mice were sacrificed, and luciferase activity in lung tissue was determined as described [27].

Endotoxin determination

Endotoxin levels in the serum of mice was determined by LAL assay (QCL-1000, LONZA).

Flow cytometry

Single-cell suspensions of organs were treated with Gey's solution where appropriate, and washed with PBS/3% FCS. The cells were preincubated with 20 µg anti-CD16/32 antibody (clone 2.4G2), washed and stained with a combination of fluorochrome-labelled monoclonal antibodies (all steps at 4°C). Antibodies were from BD Biosciences {name [alternative name] clone)} {TCRβ (H57-597); CD4 (RM4-5 or GK1.5), CD5 ([Ly-1] 53–7.3), CD8 (53–6.7), CD11b (M1/70); CD11c (HL3), CD11c (IM7), CD19 (1D3), Siglec F (E50-2440), NK1.1 (PK136), Ly6G (1A8)}, eBioscience {I-Ab [MHC class II] AF6-120.1), H-2K^b [MHC class I] AF6-88.5.5.3), CD3e (eBio500A2 or 145-2C11), CD25 (PC61.5), CD27 (LG.7F9), CD45 (30-F11), CD90.2 (53–2.1), F4/80 (BM8), Ly6C (HK1.4)}, and MD Bioproducts {T1-ST2 (DJ8)}. Samples were processed on a LSR II flow cytometer equipped for 10-parameter acquisition, and analysed with TreeStar FlowJo software (version 9.5).

Characterization of ILCs and lung interstitial leukocytes

Lungs were digested as above and ILCs were prepared and characterised as described [28] using the lineage markers CD11c, CD3, B220, TCRβ, CD5, CD27, NK1.1 and CD11b. Lineage^{neg} cells were considered ILCs when they were positive for the markers CD45, CD90, CD25 and T1-ST2. Data shown are from 10, 8, 8, and 14 animals for control mice and from 10, 5, 6, and 4 animals for *S. mansoni*-infected mice at 0, 4, 7, and 10 days post infection with PVM, respectively.

Histology

Sections of paraffin-embedded lungs were stained with H&E or PAS and analysed for columnar cell hyperplasia, goblet cell hyperplasia, atypica, degenerative changes, epithelial necrosis (for the assessment of involvement of the bronchial mucosa), fibrosis, and inflammation (for the assessment of interstitial disease). Sections were scored blindly by one experienced observer. Scoring was as follows: 0: normal; 1: minor; 2: intermediate; 3: markedly increased pathology. Sections of OCT-embedded lungs were fixed with 75% acetone/25% methanol, rehydrated with PBS, blocked with anti-CD16/32 antibody (clone 2.4G2) and stained with rabbit anti-PVM-antibody specific for the PVM-G protein [24]. They were then washed, blocked with 5% goat serum and counter-stained with goat Alexa555-conjugated anti-rabbit IgG (Invitrogen). The sections were embedded with ProLong Gold Antifade containing DAPI (Invitrogen) and analysed on a Zeiss Imager Z1 at 10× magnification (Zeiss, Plan-Apochromat, 0.17) with a Zeiss AxioCam MRc. Data was acquired and processed with Zeiss Axiovision software (release 4.8.2).

Statistics

Significant differences between two groups were estimated using the unpaired t test with Welch correction for data with Gaussian distribution (passed assumption method of Kolmogorov and Smirnov), and the Mann-Whitney test for data with non-Gaussian distribution. Significant differences between three groups were estimated using two-way ANOVA with Bonferroni post-test. Statistical relevance was indicated in the plots when significant ($p \leq 0.05$).

Results

Systemic cytokine response in C57BL/6 mice infected with *Schistosoma mansoni*

In our studies we used a recent human isolate of *S. mansoni*, which originated from Oman [22,29]. We first established the optimal number of cercariae that caused chronic schistosomiasis in C57Bl/6 mice (Fig. S1). 70–75 cercariae per mouse, infected at 9–10 weeks of age, was considered optimal. Herewith a moderate, chronic course of the disease was established that resembled Henderson's moderate splenomegaly syndrome (MSS) of mouse schistosomiasis [30], and that allowed the study of secondary infections in the chronic phase of the disease. Survival at 16 weeks of age was more than 95% in a large group of animals that were infected at different time points during this study. Serum cytokine profiles were also established. As expected, a slight increase in IFN-γ levels was seen immediately after infection, indicative of Th1-type immune responsiveness. Significant Th2-type responsiveness was seen from week 7 of infection onwards, after the onset of oviposition, with IL-4 and IL-5 rising ahead of IL-13. Also, IL-17 and IL-2 levels rose significantly after week 7. We found very high systemic levels of the proinflammatory cytokines IFN-γ, TNF-α and GM-CSF after week 7, which challenges the idea of mutually exclusive immune responses (Fig. 1). IL-10 showed small peaks of activity at week 1, 4, and 8, which most likely reflected a reaction to inflammatory processes after skin and lung passage of the schistosomula, and egg passage into the gut [31].

These findings were not dependent on the Th1-prone mouse strain C57BL/6J; in Th2-prone BALB/c mice we obtained similar data, with the exception of GM-CSF, which did not increase (Fig. S2).

We also analysed the ability of T cells from spleen and mesenteric and pulmonary (mediastinal) lymph nodes to secrete cytokines after polyclonal stimulation. The T cells produced high levels of the Th1-type cytokines *in vitro*, also later in the infection (Table S1). However, the increase of Th1 cytokines was less profound than those of Th2 cytokines, in agreement with previous reports [3].

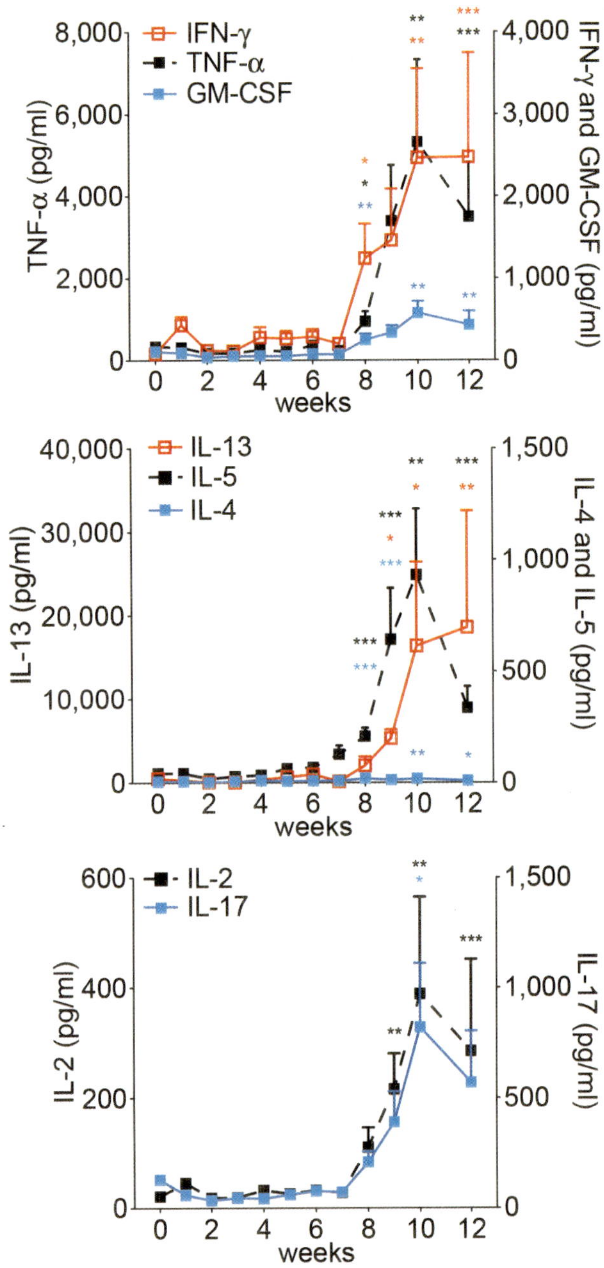

Figure 1. Serum cytokine levels of C57BL/6J mice infected with *S. mansoni*. Cytokine levels were determined at indicated time points after infection. The data points represent means from 4–10 mice. Error bars represent SEM. Significant differences between each time point and control mice (day 0) are marked: *, $p \leq 0.05$; **, $p \leq 0.01$; ***, $p \leq 0.001$.

The high levels of serum IFN-γ, but not those for TNF-α during an infection with *S. mansoni* is dependent on ligands for TLR2 and/or TLR4, because in mice deficient for both TLRs serum IFN-γ was low throughout the infection (Fig. S3). In IL-12Rβ2-deficient mice neither a systemic IFN-γ, nor a TNF-α response was found (Fig. S3). We could not detect increased systemic levels of endotoxin in mice that were infected with *S. mansoni* (Fig. S4).

We conclude that the immune response in C57BL/6 mice to a chronic infection with *S. mansoni* is not polarised systemically. High levels of the signature Th1 cytokine IFN-γ are dependent on TLR2 or 4 ligands, both TNF-α and IFN-γ are dependent on IL12Rβ2.

Influence of chronic schistosomiasis on the lung environment

The epithelial barrier layer of the lung reacts to environmental stimuli with the production of alarmins like IL-33 and GM-CSF [32–34], which attract dendritic cells. These cytokines also stimulate innate lymphoid cells in the lung (ILCs [35,36]) to produce IL-5 and IL-13, which create an intensely Th2-prone environment, and to produce amphiregulin, which is important for the integrity of the barrier layer [37]. We studied the steady state conditions in the lung during the infection with *S. mansoni* (Fig. 2). Analysis of the broncho-alveolar lavage fluid (BALF) showed a transient increase in the Th1 cytokines IFN-γ, TNF-α and IL-12 at week 5 post infection. At this time point schistosomula have passed through the lungs and establish in the portal system. Thereafter, IFN-γ fell below normal levels, while TNF-α and IL-12 remained significantly increased throughout the measurement period. The Th2 cytokines IL-5 and IL-13 increased steadily from week 2 onwards; IL-4 was only increased late in infection. IL-10 was increased around week 5 post infection, while the stress cytokines IL-6 and MIP-1α were significantly increased late in infection (Fig. 2A). Thus, also in the BALF we registered concomitant, not mutually exclusive Th1 and Th2 immune responses during the infection with *S. mansoni*.

We also analysed the cellular composition of the BALF (Fig. 2B). Total cell numbers of eosinophils were increased throughout the infection, with an early peak at week 2 of infection. The number of $CD4^{pos}$ and $CD8^{pos}$ T cells and NK cells were increased late in infection. *In vitro* TNF-αsecretion by $CD4^{pos}$ and $CD8^{pos}$ T cells was doubled late in infection (Fig. 2C). The epithelial cell layer of the airway showed discrete signs of an increased barrier function with mucus-producing goblet cell hyperplasia, columnar cell hyperplasia, and light perivascular and peribronchial infiltrates (Fig. 2D and Fig. S5A). Furthermore, as signs of increased immunological alertness we saw a marked increase in the expression of MHC class I and II on $CD45^{pos}$ $CD11b^{pos}$ $SiglecF^{neg}$ interstitial lung cells (Fig. 3B, left panels). We did not find an expansion of ILCs, rather we observed a relative contraction of this cell population (Fig. S6A).

We conclude that in murine schistosomiasis a low-grade inflammation is found in the lung with strong signs of an increased barrier function.

Muc5a expression is increased in mice with chronic schistosomiasis and is inhibited by depletion of TNF-α

Goblet cell hyperplasia can be induced, among others, by IL-13 [38] and TNF-α [39,40]. A hallmark of goblet cell hyperplasia is the increased production of the gel-forming mucin Muc5ac [41,42]. We determined Muc5ac mRNA levels in lungs of mice infected with *S. mansoni* and in control mice. Muc5ac mRNA levels were 10× times higher in infected mice compared to control mice. As expected [42], only a moderate induction of the levels of Muc5b was found in infected animals. We treated mice with soluble TNF-receptor (Etanercept) [43] to explore the role of TNF-α in the increased mucus production. After treatment of the mice (starting at week 11 of infection), mRNA for Muc5ac returned to baseline levels (Fig. 4). Thus, we conclude that TNF-α is essential for pulmonary goblet cell hyperplasia in chronic schistosomiasis.

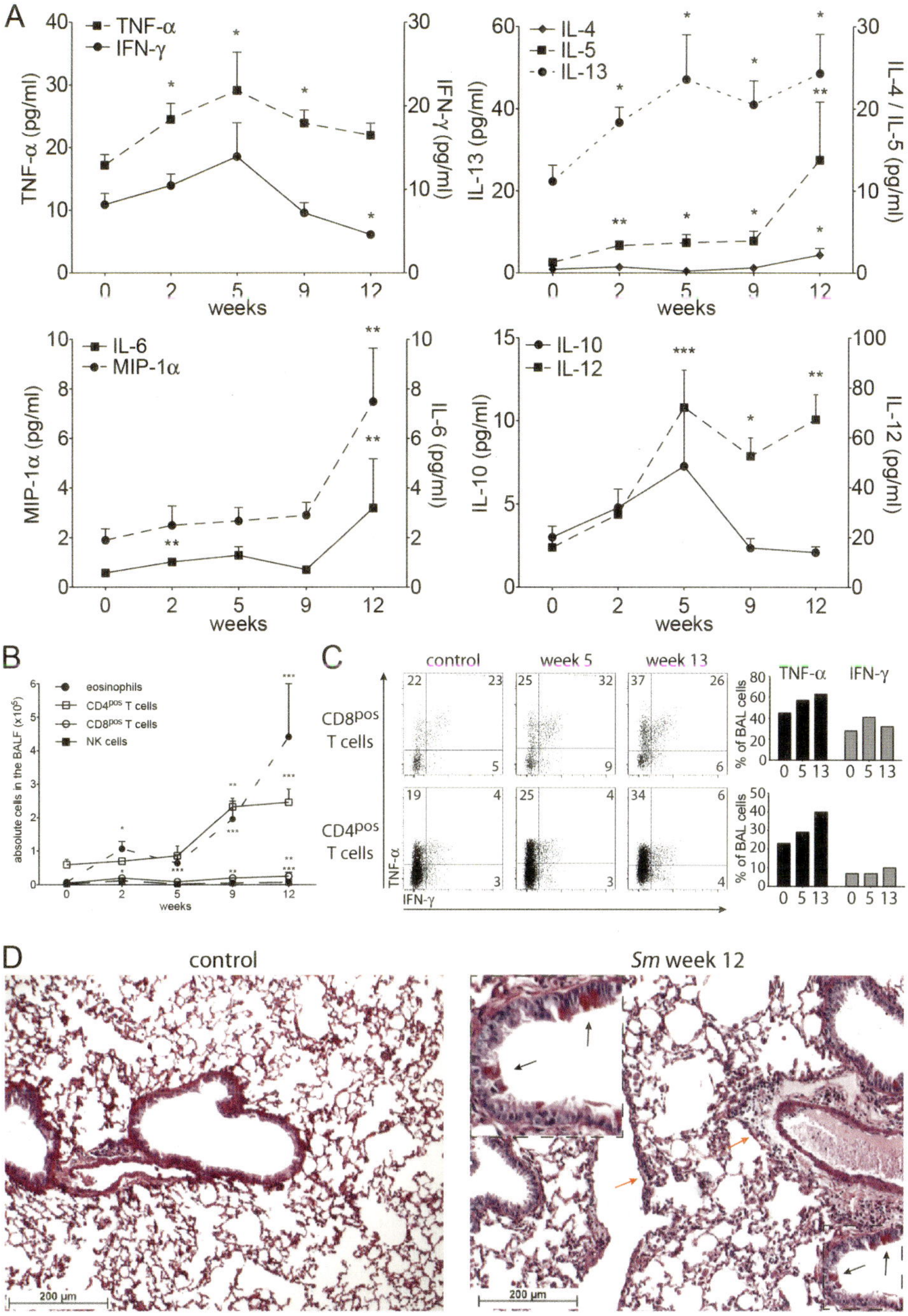

Figure 2. Immuno- and histopathology of lungs of C57BL/6J mice with schistosomiasis. A, BALF cytokine levels at indicated time points after infection with *S. mansoni*. Data was cumulatively acquired from 6–9 mice in 3–4 experiments; **B**, Number of different cell types in the BALF of mice with schistosomiasis, at indicated times after infection. Data points represent means of 13 (week 0 of infection), 4 (week 2), 7 (week 5), 9 (week 9) and 14 mice (week 12) in 2–5 individual experiments. **C**, Potential of $CD4^{pos}$ and $CD8^{pos}$ BALF cells to produce IFN-γ and TNF-α 4 hrs after stimulation with PMA/Ionomycin/Brefeldin A, cells taken at the indicated time points after infection, left panels (FACS plots) show intracellular stainings, right plots (bar graphs) show a quantitative rendition of the FACS data; data shown is representative for 3 individual experiments with 3 mice each. **D**, Section of the lung (H&E staining) of a control animal (left) and a mouse 12 wks after infection with *S. mansoni* (right), insert shows goblet cell hyperplasia (black arrows) and light cellular infiltrates (red arrow). Sections are representative for 3 mice each; Error bars represent SEM. Significant differences between each time point and control mice (day 0) are marked: *, $p \leq 0.05$; **, $p \leq 0.01$; ***, $p \leq 0.001$.

Coinfection of mice with chronic schistosomiasis with influenza A virus

Increased production of Muc5ac has recently been shown to protect from severe infection with influenza virus [44]. We therefore tested the resistance of mice with chronic schistosomiasis to a secondary infection with influenza. We first used influenza A virus strain hvPR8, which is lethal to normal mice, even if they can express the influenza virus resistance gene Mx1 [45]. However, such mice are protected against hvPR8, if they are pretreated with a single dose of type I IFN [20], because expression of Mx1 is

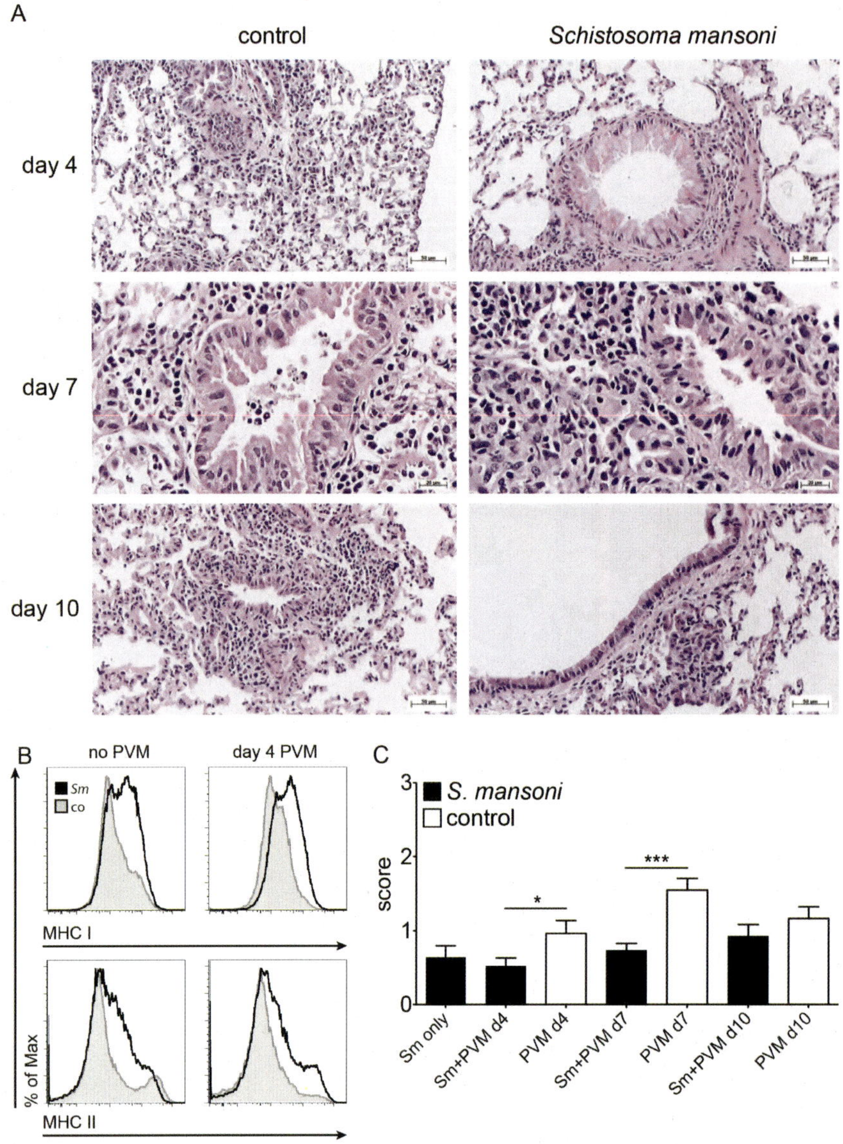

Figure 3. Immuno- and histopathology of lungs of C57BL/6J mice with a coinfection of *S. mansoni* and PVM. A, Section of the lung (H&E staining) of control animals (left) and mice 12 wks after infection with *S. mansoni* (right), at indicated time points after infection with PVM (200 pfu/mouse). **B**, FACS profiles of the expression of MHC class I and II antigens on interstitial CD45^{pos} CD11b^{pos} SiglecF^{neg} lung cells of mice with chronic schistosomiasis (12 weeks) and control animals, before and 4 days after challenge with PVM, shaded grey: control mice, black line: mice with schistosomiasis. The data shown are pooled samples from 3 mice and is representative for 9 mice in 3 individual experiments; **C**, Combined histopathological score of mice treated as described in panel A, at the indicated time points after challenge with PVM. Bars represent the mean results from 2–3 mice per group. Scoring: 0: normal; 1: minor; 2: intermediate; 3: markedly increased pathology; Error bars represent SEM. Significant differences are marked: *, $p \leq 0.05$; **, $p \leq 0.01$; ***, $p \leq 0.001$.

regulated by type I and type III interferons [46]. We found no evidence for the presence of IFN-αin the BALF of mice infected with *S. mansoni* (Fig. 5A). Further, IFN-β-reporter mice [27] that were chronically infected with *S. mansoni* showed no evidence for enhanced production of IFN-β in the lungs. However, IFN-β was significantly enhanced in liver and to a lesser extent in the kidney (Fig. S7). We infected Mx1-competent mice in the chronic phase of schistosomiasis with 60 pfu of influenza A strain hvPR8. Mice infected with *S. mansoni*, without pretreatment with IFN, were significantly protected from a challenge with hvPR8, and they survived longer when compared to non-infected (*S. mansoni*-free) controls (Fig. 6A,B). When the challenge dose of influenza virus was increased to 200 pfu per animal, animals with chronic schistosomiasis were still relatively protected and survived longer than control animals (Fig. 6C,D). From these experiments we conclude that infection with *S. mansoni* offers a relative, but significant protection from influenza virus, which is independent of IFN production.

To gauge the role of Muc5ac, we treated Mx1-deficient mice that were infected *S. mansoni* 10 weeks previously with Etanercept or PBS 3 and 1 day before, and also 1 and 3 days after infection with influenza A virus strain PR8 (2000 pfu/mouse). Control mice which were not infected with *S. mansoni* were treated similarly. As expected, control mice were not protected from infection (Fig. 6E,F). However, mice with chronic schistosomiasis were significantly protected with less weight loss and enhanced survival.

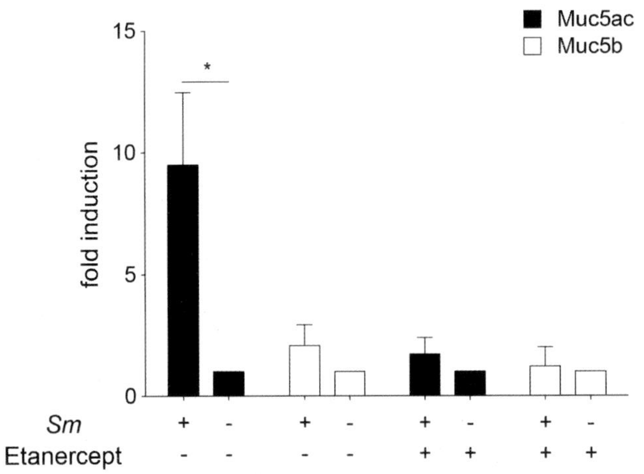

Figure 4. Muc5ac and Muc5b expression in the lungs of mice with chronic schistosomiasis before and after treatment with Etanercept. At 11 week of infection with *S. mansoni*, mice were treated 3 times, every other day, with 4 mg/kg body weight, intraperitoneally. Lungs were taken at day 6 of treatment. Error bars represent SEM. Significant differences between each time point and control mice (day 0) are marked: *, $p \leq 0.05$.

Treatment with Etanercept abrogated protection, which indicates that the reduced virulence of influenza A virus in mice with chronic schistosomiasis is mediated by a TNF-α-induced goblet cell hyperplasia and enhanced Muc5ac synthesis.

Coinfection of mice with chronic schistosomiasis with pneumonia virus of mice (PVM)

We also performed coinfection experiments with *S. mansoni*-infected mice and the respiratory virus PVM to validate our findings with a second pneumoviral infection. 12 weeks after infection with *S. mansoni*, mice were challenged intranasally with a sublethal dose (200 pfu/mouse) of PVM. C57BL/6 mice without *S. mansoni* showed, as expected [47], signs of disease and a significant loss of weight 8–9 days after infection, followed by a recovery. In contrast, mice infected with *S. mansoni* 12 weeks before viral challenge did not show additional signs of disease and did not lose weight (Fig. 7A). Viral challenge shortly after infection with *S. mansoni* did not cause protection (Fig. 7B), in fact, reproducible protection was only found after week 8 of infection (data not shown). Whereas viral challenge with 2000 pfu/mouse was lethal in control mice, mice with chronic (12 weeks) schistosomiasis survived this type of challenge, but they did show signs of disease (Fig. 7C,D). Sublethally infected T cell-deficient mice fail to clear the virus, but they are able to exert some virus control, and the virus load can stay constant over weeks without extensive disease or weight loss [47]. The reported dominant Th2 response and immune regulatory activity in the chronic phase of schistosomiasis prompted the question, whether mice with schistosomiasis controlled or cleared the virus. Fig. 7E shows that mice with schistosomiasis carried a significantly reduced ($p \leq 0.01$) viral burden at day 7 post PVM infection and were able to clear the infection. Immunohistochemical staining of the lungs corroborated this finding (Fig. 7F).

Before viral challenge we found increased levels of TNF-α, IL-5, and IL-13 in the BALF of mice with chronic schistosomiasis compared to healthy controls (Fig. 2A, week 12 and Fig. 5A, day 0). At day 4 after viral challenge we found significantly higher levels of TNF-α, IL-5 and IL-13 in mice with chronic schistosomiasis, whereas at day 7 control animals had significantly higher levels of IFN-γ and IL-6, but lower levels of IL-13. At day 10 after challenge, the titers of TNF-α, IL-5 and IL-13 remained high in *Schistosoma*-infected mice and were significantly increased compared to control animals, all of which showed falling titers for all measured cytokines. As expected [48], IFN-α, a type I interferon, was markedly increased at day 7 after viral challenge in the BALF of control animals, but was not increased in *Schistosoma*-infected mice (Fig. 5A).

$CD4^{pos}$ T cells, $CD8^{pos}$ T cells, NK cells, and eosinophils were present in significantly higher numbers at all times after viral challenge in the BALF of *Schistosoma*-infected mice when compared to control animals, with the exception of day 7 and 10, where we found highly increased numbers of NK cells in control mice (Fig. 5B). At day 4 after viral challenge, expression of MHC class I and II antigens on interstitial $CD45^{pos}$ $CD11b^{pos}$ $SiglecF^{neg}$ lung cells was only marginally increased in control mice, while the expression stayed high in mice with chronic schistosomiasis (Fig. 3B).

The protective effect of bilharzia on subsequent viral challenge was not found in mice that were infected 12 weeks prior with single-sex cercariae (Fig. S8), which indicates that the eggs - rather than the worm itself - induce protection.

Histopathology in mice infected with PVM

We scored the extent of histopathology of the bronchial mucosae and of the lung parenchyma before and after challenge with PVM (Fig. 3A). The combined score is shown in Fig. 3C (scores for the individual parameters are shown in Fig. S5, B–F). Early in the infection with PVM (day 0 (Fig. 2D) and day 4 (Fig. 3A and S5B)), mice with chronic schistosomiasis had marked goblet cell hyperplasia, which disappeared later on. At day 4 and 7 after viral challenge, the combined score was significantly lower in *Schistosoma*-infected mice when compared to controls.

Inflammatory processes with a strong Th2 component can protect from viral attack

Another factor that can lead to increased Muc5ac production is an increased level of IL-13 in the lungs [38], as is found in pulmonary inflammatory processes, in particular in those with a strong Th2 component. Indeed, in a model of allergic airway inflammation [25] we saw type II inflammatory responses similar to those in the lungs of mice with schistosomiasis, but more pronounced. Levels of IL-5 in serum were high (Fig. 8A). In BALF high levels of IL-4, IL-5 and IL-13 were found (Fig. 8B). We found increased numbers of $CD4^{pos}$ and $CD8^{pos}$ T cells, NK cells, and eosinophils in BALF (Fig. 8C). The expression of MHC class I, but not of MHC class II antigens on $CD45^{pos}$ $CD11b^{pos}$ $SiglecF^{neg}$ interstitial lung cells was increased (Fig. 8D). When challenged with 200 pfu/mouse PVM, ovalbumin-immunised and -challenged mice were protected from loss of weight and signs of disease (Fig. 8E). At day 7 after viral challenge these mice had significantly lower viral titres than the control mice (Fig. 8F).

Discussion

In this work we studied the immunological influence of murine schistosomiasis on a subsequent challenge with a respiratory virus. Mice that are chronically infected with an human Omani isolate of *S. mansoni* are relatively, but significantly protected from a viral respiratory challenge with low doses of influenza A virus or pneumonia virus of mice (PVM), and they survived challenges with normally lethal doses. The protection is caused by

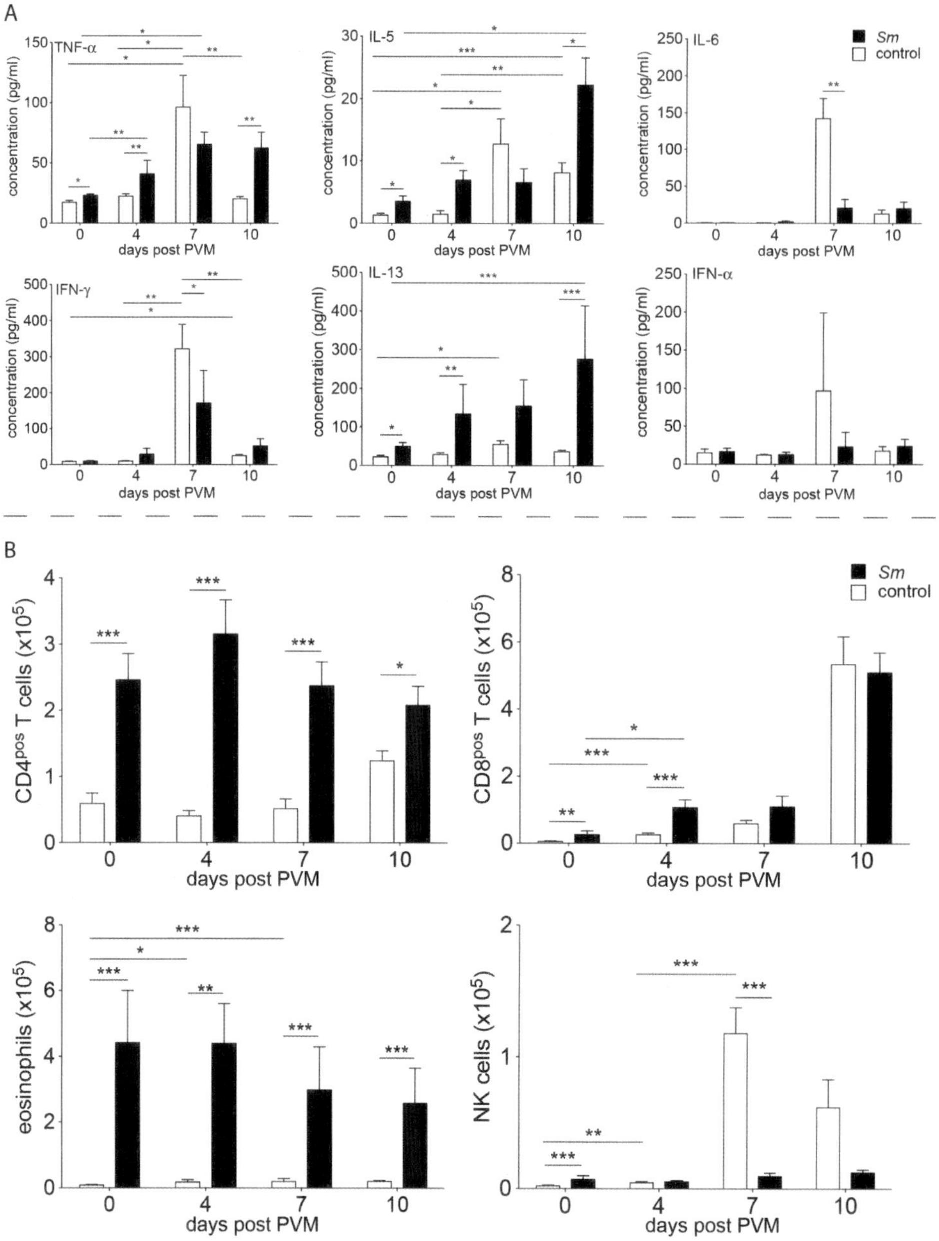

Figure 5. Analysis of BALF and lung tissue of C57BL/6J mice with schistosomiasis and control mice before (day 0) and at indicated time points after infection with PVM (200 pfu/mouse). Filled columns: mice with schistosomiasis, empty columns: control mice. **A**, Cytokine levels. Bars represent data from 7–15 mice in 3–5 individual experiments; **B**, Cell counts for different cell types ($CD4^{pos}$ T cells, $CD8^{pos}$ T cells, eosinophils and NK cells) in the BALF of mice that were infected only with PVM (empty columns), or with *S. mansoni* and challenged 12 wks later with PVM (filled columns) and control mice (empty columns at day 0). Data are from 9–15 mice in 4–5 individual experiments. Error bars represent SEM. Significant differences are marked: *, $p \leq 0.05$; **, $p \leq 0.01$; ***, $p \leq 0.001$.

TNF-α-mediated goblet cell hyperplasia and concomitant Muc5ac production in the lungs of *S. mansoni*-infected mice.

Th1- besides Th2- and Th17-mediated immunity in murine schistosomiasis

S. mansoni is thought to induce primarily Th2 immune responses in the chronic, egg-depositing stage of the disease [2,10]. Indeed, *Schistosoma* eggs themselves are considered important drivers of Th2 responses, through principles secreted by them: IPSE-alpha-1 [49] and omega-1 [50,51]. Th2 responses are thought to inhibit Th1 responses, either by direct inhibition or by a relative deficiency for the appropriate inducing cytokine. A careful analysis of the systemic (serum) cytokine levels in mice chronically infected with the Omani isolate revealed that type 1 (IFN-γ, TNF-α, GM-CSF), type 2 (IL-5, IL-13, to a lesser degree IL-4), and type 17 (IL-17) cytokines coexisted throughout the infection. The cytokines rose to high levels from week 8 of infection onwards. When probed for potency, $CD4^{pos}$ and $CD8^{pos}$ T cells from the spleen and mesenteric lymph nodes produced high levels of IFN-γ and TNF-α, besides IL-4, IL-13 and IL-17. The increase in production of Th2 cytokines was percentually higher than those of Th1 cytokines. IL-4 and IL-13 are

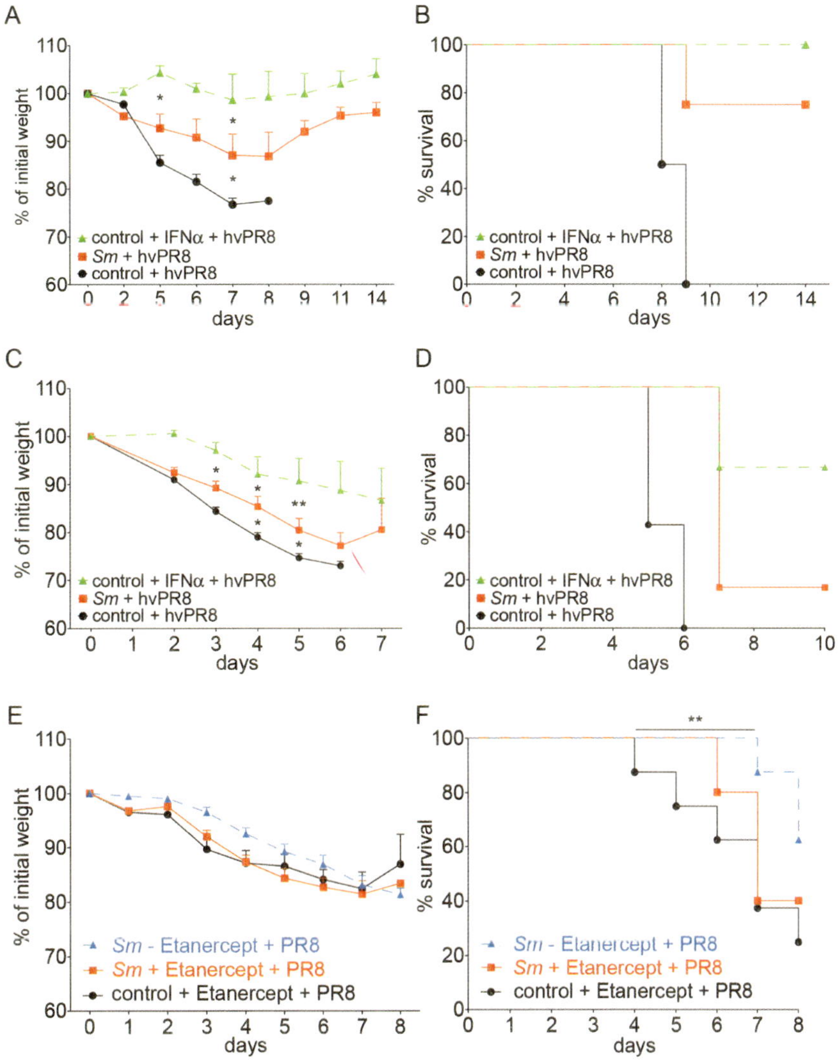

Figure 6. Coinfection experiments with *S. mansoni*-infected C57BL/6J mice and Influenza A virus. A–D: Analysis of C57BL/6 mice carrying functional Mx1 alleles (B6.A2G-*Mx1*) after infection with *S. mansoni* and influenza A virus (strain hvPR8). **E–F**: Analysis of wild-type, MX-1-deficient C57BL/6 mice after infection with *S. mansoni* and influenza A virus (strain PR8). **A**, Relative weight loss of mice with chronic schistosomiasis (10 wks; red) and control animals (black) at indicated times after challenge with 60 pfu/mouse of hvPR8. Some control mice received 50.000 U IFN-α, given one day before challenge with hvPR8 (green). Data points were cumulatively acquired from 3–4 mice in each group in one experiment. Error bars represent SEM; **B**, Survival curves of mice in Fig. 6A. **C**, Relative weight loss of mice with chronic schistosomiasis (10 wks, red) and control animals (black) at indicated time points after challenge with 200 pfu/mouse of hvPR8. Some control mice received 50.000 U IFN-α, given one day before challenge with hvPR8 (green). Data points were cumulatively acquired from 7 mice in each group in one experiment; **D**, Survival curves of mice in Fig. 6C; **E**, Relative weight loss of mice with chronic schistosomiasis (10 wks; red, treated with Etanercept, blue, not treated, black, control animals treated with Etanercept) at indicated time points after challenge with 2000 pfu/mouse. Data points were cumulatively acquired from 7, 5 and 7 mice in each group, respectively, in one experiment; **F**, Survival curves of mice in Fig. 6E; Error bars represent SEM. Significant differences are marked: *, $p \leq 0.05$; **, $p \leq 0.01$; ***, $p \leq 0.001$, nd: below detection limit of 10 pfu.

indispensible in the gut to initiate tissue repair mechanisms [11] and to expel worm eggs [52], and IL-17 is necessary for protection from bacterial attack through the battered gut wall [53,54]. TNF-α, IL-13 and IL-17 can all induce mucin production, both in the intestines and in the airways. Mucins play an important role in worm expulsion, Muc5ac can expell and harm certain nematodes [55]. Remarkably, for intestinal goblet cell hyperplasia in schistosomiasis signalling by IL-4/IL-13 is dispensible [56].

Thelper cell polarisation

The notion that Th1 or Th2 polarisation occurs in a systemic fashion was strongly influenced by early studies on leishmaniasis. These showed an exclusive responsiveness and a different immunity, depending on the strain of mice (C57BL/6 and BALB/c) [57]. We compared C57BL/6 and BALB/c mice in their systemic response to *S. mansoni* and could not find fundamental differences. Can we explain previous, discordant results of other groups? First, some reports are compatible with our results [58], and in a meta-analysis, Yu et al. [59] found significantly increased TNF-α and IL-4 levels in human patients with schistosomiasis. Second, we did not infect with the commonly used Puerto Rican strain of *S. mansoni*. However, the Omani strain caused a disease that resembled the moderate splenomegaly syndrome (MSS) of mice [30], with very few eggs being dispersed

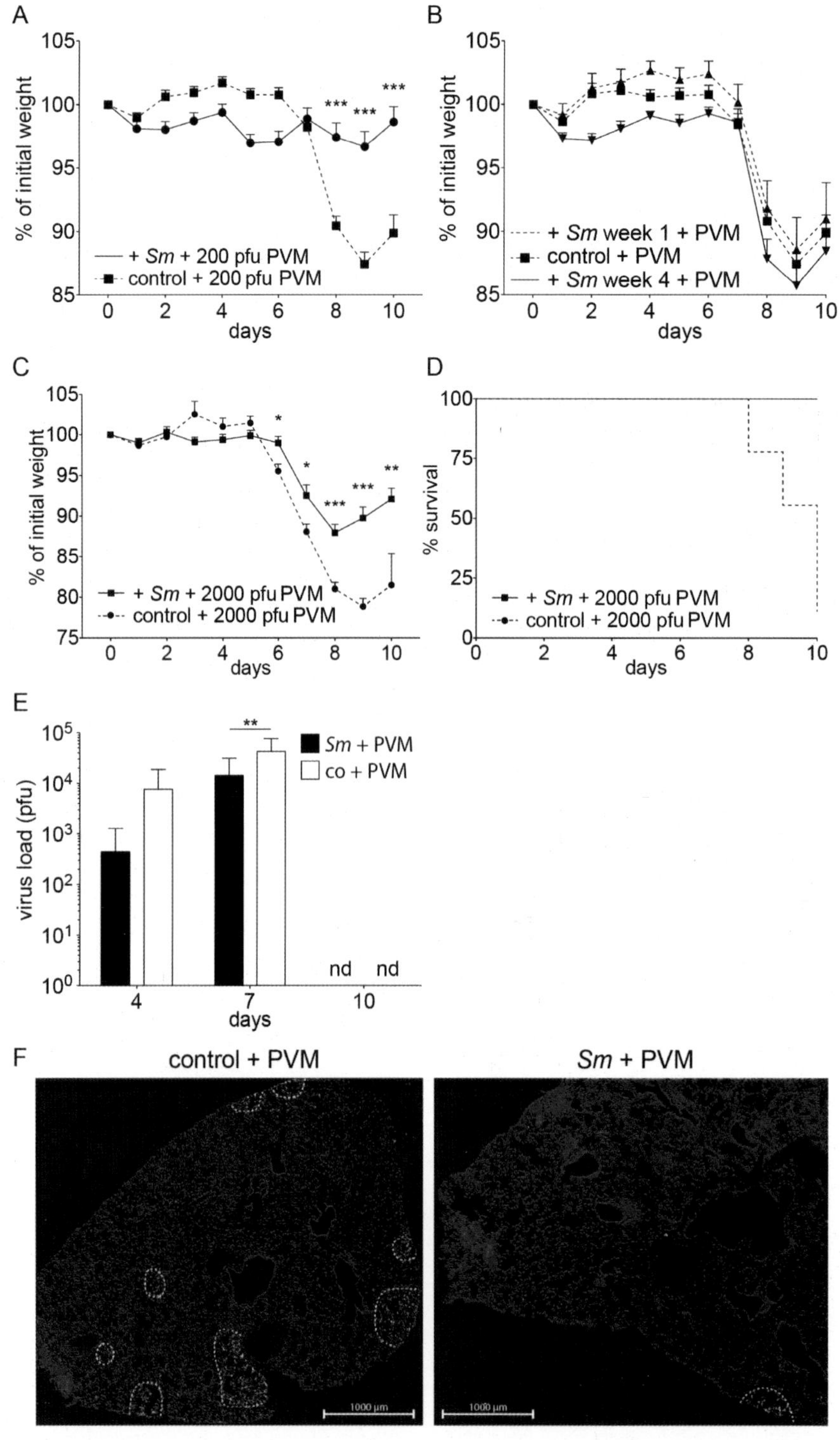

Figure 7. Coinfection experiments with *S. mansoni*-infected C57BL/6J mice and pneumonia virus of mice (PVM). A, Relative weight loss of mice with chronic schistosomiasis (12 wks) and control animals at indicated times after a sublethal dose (200 pfu/mouse) of PVM. Data are from 30–38 mice in 7–8 experiments. **B**, Relative weight loss of mice at the indicated time points after challenge with 200 pfu/mouse of PVM, at 1 and 4 weeks after infection with *S. mansoni*. The data are cumulative from 15 (week 1), 6 (week 4), and 52 (control) mice representative of 3, 1 and 12 experiments, respectively; **C**, Relative weight loss of mice with chronic schistosomiasis (12 weeks) and control animals at indicated time points after a lethal dose (2000 pfu/mouse) of PVM. The data are cumulative from 10 mice in 2 individual experiments; **D**, Survival curves of mice in Fig. 7C; **E**, Viral load, expressed as pfu, in the right lobes of the lungs of mice, treated as described in Fig. 7A, at day 4, 7 and 10 after challenge with PVM. Bars represent data from 9–15 mice in 2–4 individual experiments; **F**, Lungs of mice as described in Fig. 7A were taken at day 4, fixed with paraformaldehyde and stained with an antibody directed against the G-protein of PVM. The infected areas are enclosed with dashed lines. Images are representative for 6 sections from 3 individual mice per group; Error bars represent SEM. Significant differences between groups at one time point are marked: *, $p \leq 0.05$; **, $p \leq 0.01$; ***, $p \leq 0.001$, nd: below detection limit.

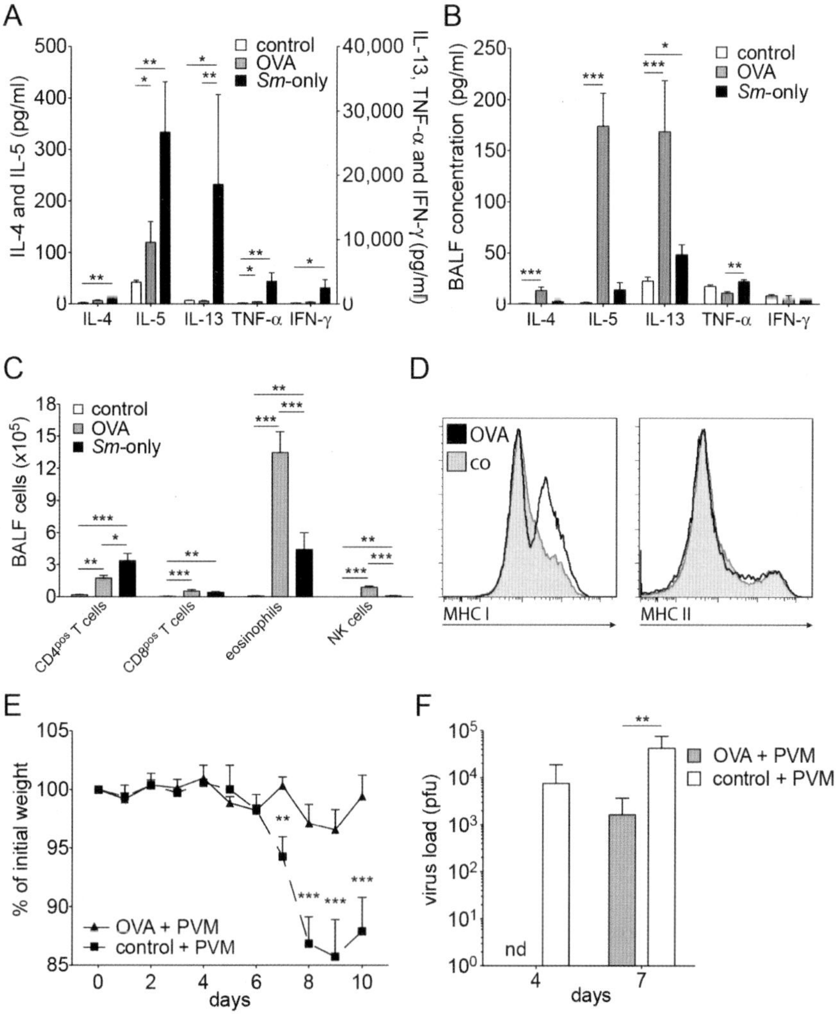

Figure 8. Resistance of C57BL/6 mice with inflammatory airway processes to challenge with PVM. A, **B**, Cytokine levels in the serum (A) and BALF (B) 24 h after the last of 3 consecutive days of aerosolised OVA of OVA-immunised mice (C57BL/6J) compared to mice infected with *S. mansoni* and control mice. The data shown are pooled from 4–8 mice in 3 individual experiments; **C**, Number of cells of various cell types in the BALF of mice 24 h after the last of 3 consecutive days of treatment with aerosolised OVA of OVA-immunised mice (C57BL/6J) compared to mice infected with *S. mansoni* and control mice. The data are from 10–14 mice in 3–5 individual (depending on the time point) experiments; **D**, FACS profiles of the expression of MHC class I and II antigens on interstitial CD45^{pos} CD11b^{pos} SiglecF^{neg} lung cells of C57BL/6J mice 24 h after the last of 3 consecutive days of aerosolised OVA challenge of OVA-immunised mice (thick lines) and control mice (shaded grey). Data shown is representative for 6 mice from 2 experiments; **E**, Relative weight loss of OVA-immunised mice (C57BL/6J) challenged with a sublethal dose (200 pfu/mouse) of PVM 24 h after the last of 3 consecutive days of aerosolised OVA and control mice at the indicated times after challenge. The data are cumulative from 10–16 mice in 3 individual experiments. The controls were obtained separately and are the same as in Fig. 7A. **F**, Viral load, expressed as pfu, in the right lobes of the lungs of mice, treated as described in Fig. 8E, at day 4 and 7 after challenge with PVM. The controls were obtained separately and are the same as in Fig. 7E. The data from OVA-immunised mice are derived from 2 and 3 mice (day 4 and 7, respectively). Error bars represent SEM. nd: not detectable. Significant differences are marked: *, $p \leq 0.05$; **, $p \leq 0.01$; ***, $p \leq 0.001$.

to the lungs. Third, in some studies mice were treated with antibiotics, which are known to significantly affect the microbiome and therewith the immune response [17,18,60]. We did not find evidence for a systemic bacterial spread or LPS in the blood of infected mice [61]. Fourth, in many experiments, mice were not followed beyond week 8, only 2 weeks after the onset of oviposition Fifth, the majority of conclusions relied on experiments in which *ex vivo* production of cytokines by polyclonally stimulated T cells was measured [3,62]. In this approach the potential activity rather than actual activity of regional T cells is gauged [63]. We strongly support the idea, that regional immune cells can exert exclusive regional functions, for instance the production of Th2 cytokines in the gut. These facilitate egg transition through the gut and limit inflammation in the gut [60]. Finally, the concept of mutually exclusive responses slowly becomes cracks: recent studies point towards a more plastic view on the response [64,65], and cell fate seems to be fixed rather early in the differentiation pathway of a T cell. In this concept, specifically responsive cells can be called upon later, when demand is present [66,67]. Early systemic Th1 responses in *S. mansoni* could function as a stabilisator of the enhancer "landscape", allowing continuous access to a Th1-prone cell pool [68]. Indeed, several groups found evidence for dual or hybrid types of helper T cells [69–71]. We therefore argue that our model of murine schistosomiasis resembles early infection in human, in which, like in our model, Th1, Th2 and Th17 cells coexist.

The role of TNF-α in schistosomiasis

High levels of TNF-α and IFN-γ are often implied in the pathogenesis of a severe form of human schistosomiasis, the hepato-splenic form [72], which could resemble Henderson's hypersplenomegaly syndrome (HSS). As outlined, we do not find evidence for HSS in our model. Also in the mild form, hepatic involvement in mice is more pronounced than in benign cases of human schistosomiasis. Also in MSS increased levels of TNF-α are found in liver tissue [73]. In mice both protective and deleterious effects have been described for TNF-α, together with evidence that granuloma-induced TNF production is necessary for the maturation of the adult worms [74,75].

Pulmonary milieu in murine schistosomiasis

In chronic murine schistosomiasis the lungs show low-grade inflammatory processes, with goblet cell hyperplasia and increased production of the gel-forming mucin Muc5ac (see Fig. S9 for a graphical summary of our data). Early in the infection Th1 cytokines were found in BALF, they stayed high with the exception of IFN-γ. Th2 cytokines also rose early, with the exception of IL-4. Pathology in our model was less pronounced than in that described by Crosby et al. [58], which could well be explained by the lower number of parasite eggs found in the lungs of our mice. The sustained high levels of IL-13 and IL-5 without a joined increase of IL-4 suggests that they were not derived from Th2-type helper cells, but rather from ILC2-type cells [76,77]. However, we saw a relative decrease in number of ILCs during the course of schistosomiasis, likely arguing against an activated state of the ILCs [37]. Instead, our results indicate that sustained high levels of systemic TNF-α were primarily responsible for the goblet cell hyperplasia.

Coinfection studies with *S. mansoni* and influenza virus or PVM

In this *Schistosoma*-moulded milieu respiratory viruses do not spread as easily as in a healthy environment. PMV did not expand as rapidly and was cleared with a lower expenditure of $CD8^{pos}$ cytotoxic T cells, and therefore with less airway inflammation and involvement. As a consequence, a lower combined histopathology score was found. The virulent influenza virus strain hvPR8 is lethal to normal (Mx-competent) mice, unless they are pretreated with type-I or type III interferons, which induce the indispensible Mx protein. Mice with chronic schistosomiasis were to a certain extent resistant to strain hvPR8, indicating that the infection with *S. mansoni* had either induced the production of type I or type III interferons or that other protective mechanisms, like the production of Muc5ac [44], were active. We were unable to detect significant amounts of IFN-α by ELISA in mice with schistosomiasis, and reporter mice for IFN-β did not show any significant involvement of IFN-β. Therefore, we conclude that type I interferons did not play a significant role in the observed protection, although we cannot completely exclude the involvement of type III interferons [78]. High levels of isolated production of Muc5ac in the lung, as found in Muc5ac-transgenic mice, protects from infection with influenza A virus [44]. In these studies Muc5ac production was increased by a factor of 20, in our studies, mice with chronic schistosomiasis had a ten-fold induction of Muc5ac. Treatment of the mice with Etanercept revealed that upstream TNF-α was responsible for this induction. Indeed, Mx1-deficient mice with chronic schistosomiasis were relatively, but not absolutely protected from an infection with influenza A virus, and the protection was lost after treatment with Etanercept.

TNF-α does not seem to affect viral replication in primary infections [47,79,80]. However, TNF has a significant effect on immunopathology: it negatively regulates the extent of pathology [79], or increases pathology [80], depending on virus strain and study design. Therefore we favour the notion that was put forward by Ehre et al. [44]: mucus alone is sufficient to sequester virus and reduce viral entry into the lung cells. Less cytotoxic T cells were needed for viral control, which resulted in reduced tissue damage.

The role of TNF-α in Muc5ac expression and goblet cell hyperplasia

TNF-α has a direct influence on Muc5ac transcription via the NF-κB pathway, and it induces expression of the EGFR [40]. NF-κB further modulates IL-13Rα1-signalling [81]. Both the IL-13Rα1 and the EGFR are essential in the development of goblet cell hyperplasia. It is debated, whether these factors work in parallel or whether engagement of the EGFR is making the goblet cell receptive for consecutive IL-13 signalling [82]. We saw that short-time treatment of mice with Etanercept, i.e. neutralising TNF-α in the continuing presence of IL-13, inhibited Muc5ac expression and interfered with protection to viral challenge. This suggests a role for TNF-α that is independent of IL-13. Indeed, it was clearly shown that the mere transgenic expression of Muc5ac, without the involvement of (IL-13-driven) inflammatory responses, is protective in influenza infections [44].

Factors influencing protection

The increased resistance to viral attack and the increased immunological "alertness" in the lungs of mice with schistosomiasis is not dependent on worm passage through the lungs, because infections with single-sex cercariae did not protect from viral attack. Protection is reliably found after week eight of infection, thus after the onset of oviposition. This coincides with the first deposition of eggs in the liver and the subsequent granulomatous reaction, but more importantly, also the passage of the eggs through the intestinal wall. This causes considerable damage, leads to inflammation, the secretion of high amounts of IL-17, and a noticeable change in the stool constitution with first some, later more - and also bloody - mucoid stool. Conditions in the gut of mice with schistosomiasis are therefore very different from normal. Already under normal conditions, bacterial products can enter the body, enhance systemic innate immunity [36], and exert considerable influence also in distant compartments like the lung. Effective immunity to influenza virus is dependent on the existing microbiome [17,18], with bacterial products of gram-positive bacteria and certain TLR-ligands (TLR2,-3,-4 or -9) as active principle, even when rectally applied [17]. Abt *et al.* showed that interferon-induced genes were responsible for this kind of protection [18]. We could show, that systemic IFN-γ responses were absent in TLR2,4-double-deficient mice with schistosomiasis. In IL-12Rβ2-deficient mice both IFN-γ and TNF-αwere absent, pointing to an IL-12/IFN-γ axis in protection in mice with schistosomiasis.

Allergic inflammation and viral infections

We then asked whether pulmonary inflammatory processes in general could lead to protection. We found that in a mouse model of asthma mice were protected from viral attack by PVM, to a similar degree as found in mice with schistosomiasis. Indeed, conditions in the lung were to a large degree comparable, with a strong Th2 component in the inflammation. These results were not unexpected, Th2 cytokines, in particular IL-13, are potent inducers of goblet cell hyperplasia and Muc5ac production and thus protective in viral attacks. Remarkably, in the recent pandemic influenza (H1N1) infection, asthma was independently associated with a lower risk of dying during hospitalisation [83]. We interpret these results as a reflection of an increased immune alertness, with goblet cell hyperplasia and Muc5ac production. This response will initially protect the host from pneumotropic viruses, but in chronic conditions it may be detrimental for the host because of ensuing, debilitating chronic inflammatory processes like COPD [84].

Other helminths will exert other effects

We do not think that our findings can be transferred to all helminth infections. In infections in which the parasite deploys systemic immunosuppression, as does for instance *Heligmosomoides polygyrus* [85,86], or induces only a weak Th1 response, the outcome can be different. Indeed, two recent articles supported this notion. In a murine model, infection with *H. polygyrus* and *S. mansoni* eggs (a complete infectious cycle was not tested) could reactivate the mouse γ-herpes virus MHV68 *in vivo*, via an IL-4- and Stat6-dependent pathway[87]. In a second study, *Trichinella spiralis* and *H polygyrus* both could inhibit specific T-cell responses to murine norovirus, or to influenza virus (only tested with *T. spiralis*). Immune modulation was shown to be dependent on a Stat6-dependent alternative activation of macrophages and their secreted product Ym1 [88]. In both cases, Th2-type immune responses are induced, without previous Th1-type immunity. Unfortunately, no data were provided for the lung environment.

In schistosomiasis, we did not find evidence for a generalised immune suppression. The similarity of *S. mansoni*-induced and allergen-induced pulmonary inflammation rather predicts a more severe course, when allergy and schistosomiasis coexist. The immune regulatory activity of T regulatory cells and IL-10 is therefore most likely secondary to inflammation and antigen-specific [54]. Remarkably, in schistosomiasis, a disease with at least 200 million people a year needing treatment, little tenable information is available regarding comorbidities. Of course, many variables can influence the outcome of coinfections, as discussed extensively by Abruzzi and Fried [6].

In conclusion, our results shed a new light both on the biology of schistosomiasis and the immune response to the parasite. Contrary to previous reports, we do not find the immune responses to be polarised systemically, but they reflect local need for defence. From an evolutionary point of view, the parasite would initially benefit from an increased barrier function towards common pathogens like respiratory tract viruses.

Supporting Information

Figure S1 Determination of the optimal cercarial dose of *S. mansoni* that leads to a chronic disease. A, five C57BL/6J mice were exposed to different number of cercariae and analysed 12 weeks after infection for worm burden (Δ), worm pairs (◆), infection rate (○) and weight of liver (■) and spleen (□). **B**, total number of eggs/liver 12 weeks after infection, relative to the cercarial dose. Data points represent mean data from 3–7 mice in one experiment. Error bars represent SEM. Grey zones indicate the optimal cercarial dose we have used in further experiments to obtain a chronic course of the disease.
(TIF)

Figure S2 Serum cytokine levels in BALB/cJ mice at indicated time points after infection with *S. mansoni*. A, signature Th1 cytokines IFN-γ and TNF-α and **B, D**, signature Th2 cytokines IL-5, IL-13 and IL-4 were measured, as well as **C, D**, IL-6, IL-17 and IL-2. The data points represent means from 2–7 mice. Error bars represent SEM. Significant differences between each time point and control mice (day 0) are marked: *, $p \le 0.05$; **, $p \le 0.01$; ***, $p \le 0.001$.

Figure S3 Serum IFN-γ(A) and TNF-α(B) levels in C57BL/6J (black line), TLR2$^{-/-}$/4$^{-/-}$ (green line) and IL-12Rβ2$^{-/-}$ (blue dotted line) mice at indicated time points after infection with *S. mansoni*. Error bars represent SEM. Significant differences between each time point and control mice (day 0) are marked: *, $p \le 0.05$; **, $p \le 0.01$; ***, $p \le 0.001$.

Figure S4 Serum endotoxin levels in C57BL/6 mice at indicated time points after infection with *S. mansoni*. Serum endotoxin levels were determined by LAL assay. The data points represent means from 11, 4 and 12 mice at week 0, 5, and 12, respectively. Error bars represent SEM. ANOVA analysis (Kruskall-Wallis): p = 0.0488.

Figure S5 Histo-pathological scores of the lungs of C57BL/6J mice with chronic schistosomiasis. A, basal values at 12 weeks after infection with *S. mansoni*; **B–F**, scores of mice with schistosomiasis (12 wks; black) and control animals (white) at indicated times after a sublethal dose (200 pfu/mouse) of PVM. Columns represent mean results from 2–3 mice per group. Error bars represent SEM. Scoring: 0: normal; 1: minor; 2: intermediate; 3: markedly increased. Absence of bars represents normal (0) scoring.

Figure S6 Analysis of ILCs in the lungs of control mice and at indicated time points after infection with *S. mansoni*. ILCs were prepared from the right lobes of the lungs. **A**, gating strategy. Lin: Lineage markers. The plots are representative for n = 10 (control), 4 (week 2), 2 (week 5), 4 (week 9) and 10 (week 12) mice. **B**, total number of cells that are Lin-negative and positive for the markers CD25, CD90 and T1-ST2. Significant differences between groups are marked: *, $p \le 0.05$; **, $p \le 0.01$; ***, $p \le 0.001$.

Figure S7 Type I interferon levels in mice infected with *S. mansoni* at week 12 of infection. A, IFN-α levels in BALF; **B**, IFN-β levels in indicated organs (RLU: relative luciferase units) Error bars represent SEM. Significant differences between each time point and control mice (day 0) are marked: *, $p \le 0.05$; ***, $p \le 0.001$.

Figure S8 Coinfection experiments with *S. mansoni*-infected mice and pneumonia virus of mice (PVM). Mice were i.n. challenged at day 0 with 200 pfu of virus. Relative weight loss of C57BL/6J mice infected with 100 cercariae of a single sex (cercariae obtained from snails infected with only 1 miracidium) (12 wks) and control animals at indicated times. Data are pooled from 13 mice in 2 experiments. Error bars represent SEM. Significant differences between data points from normal and single sex infection with *S. mansoni* are marked: *, $p \le 0.05$; **, $p \le 0.01$.

Figure S9 Graphical summary. Representation of pulmonary conditions. Upper left: normal condition. Upper right: chronic schistosomiasis. Lower left: infection with a respiratory virus. Lower right: secondary infection with a respiratory virus in chronic schistosomiasis.

Table S1 ***Ex vivo*** **stimulation of cells.** Pulmonary lymph nodes (pLN), spleens and mesenteric lymph nodes (mLN) were taken from mice on the C57BL/6J background and single cell suspensions were prepared. At week 0 not enough cells could be prepared from the pLN to perform *in vitro* stimulation. Cells were then incubated for 4 h in complete medium containing phorbol 12-myristate 13-acetate (PMA, 20 ng/ml), Ionomycin (500 ng/ml) and Brefeldin A (1 µg/ml). Cells were stained extracellularly and, after fixation, stained intracellularly with fluorochrome-labelled anti-TNF-α (MP6-XT22), anti-IFN-γ (XMG1.2), anti-IL-4 (11B11) and anti IL-13 (eBio13A), using the IntraSure fixation and permeabilisation kit (all from BD Biosciences, except for anti IL-13, which was from eBioscience). The percentage of cells positive for the indicated cytokine is given.
(TIF)

Acknowledgments

We thank Drs. Markus Simon, Stefan Martin and Peter Nielsen for critically reading the manuscript and for fruitful discussions; Sandra Groß (MPI-IE), Kristin Hauck and Theresa Kreuzahler (University of Wuerzburg) for excellent technical assistance.

Author Contributions

Conceived and designed the experiments: SS HM PS MCL. Performed the experiments: SS C. Krempl C. Kallfass SF GM HM AS-G PS MCL. Analyzed the data: SS C. Krempl TJ GM HM AS-G PS MCL. Contributed reagents/materials/analysis tools: C. Krempl GM HM AS-G PS. Wrote the paper: SS TJ PS MCL.

References

1. Zhu J, Paul WE (2008) CD4 T cells: fates, functions, and faults. Blood 112: 1557–1569. doi: 10.1182/blood-2008-05-078154.
2. Dunne DW, Cooke A (2005) A worm's eye view of the immune system: consequences for evolution of human autoimmune disease. Nat Rev Immunol 5: 420–426. doi: 10.1038/nri1601.
3. Pearce EJ, Caspar P, Grzych J-M, Lewis FA, Sher A (1991) Downregulation of Th1 cytokine production accompanies induction of Th2 responses by a parasitic helminth, Schistosoma mansoni. J Exp Med 173: 159–166. doi: 10.1084/jem.173.1.159.
4. Mosmann TR, Coffman RL (1989) TH1 and TH2 cells: different patterns of lymphokine secretion lead to different functional properties. Annu Rev Immunol 7: 145–173. doi: 10.1146/annurev.iy.07.040189.001045.
5. Strachan DP (1989) Hay fever, hygiene, and household size. BMJ 299: 1259.
6. Abruzzi A, Fried B (2011) Coinfection of Schistosoma (Trematoda) with Bacteria, Protozoa and Helminths. Adv Parasitol 77: 1–85. doi: 10.1016/B978-0-12-391429-3.00005-8.
7. Salgame P, Yap GS, Gause WC (2013) Effect of helminth-induced immunity on infections with microbial pathogens. Nat Immunol 14: 1118–1126. doi: 10.1038/ni.2736.
8. WHO | Schistosomiasis Fact sheet # 115 (2012) WHO | Schistosomiasis Fact sheet # 115. WHO.
9. Fallon PG (2000) Immunopathology of schistosomiasis: a cautionary tale of mice and men. Immunology Today 21: 29–35.
10. Fallon PG, Mangan NE (2007) Suppression of TH2-type allergic reactions by helminth infection. Nat Rev Immunol 7: 220–230. doi: 10.1038/nri2039.
11. Brunet LR, Finkelman FD, Cheever AW, Kopf MA, Pearce EJ (1997) IL-4 protects against TNF-alpha-mediated cachexia and death during acute schistosomiasis. J Immunol 159: 777–785.
12. Herbert DR, Orekov T, Roloson A, Ilies M, Perkins C, et al. (2010) Arginase I suppresses IL-12/IL-23p40-driven intestinal inflammation during acute schistosomiasis. J Immunol 184: 6438–6446. doi: 10.4049/jimmunol.0902009.
13. Actor JK, Shirai M, Kullberg MC, Buller RM, Sher A, et al. (1993) Helminth infection results in decreased virus-specific CD8+ cytotoxic T-cell and Th1 cytokine responses as well as delayed virus clearance. Proc Natl Acad Sci USA 90: 948–952.
14. Araujo MI, Bliss SK, Suzuki Y, Alcaraz A, Denkers EY, et al. (2001) Interleukin-12 promotes pathologic liver changes and death in mice coinfected with Schistosoma mansoni and Toxoplasma gondii. Infect Immun 69: 1454–1462. doi: 10.1128/IAI.69.3.1454-1462.2001.
15. Edwards MJ, Buchatska O, Ashton M, Montoya M, Bickle QD, et al. (2005) Reciprocal immunomodulation in a schistosome and hepatotropic virus coinfection model. J Immunol 175: 6275–6285.
16. Van Valen L (1973) A new Evolutionary law. Evolutionary Theory 1: 1–30.
17. Ichinohe T, Pang IK, Kumamoto Y, Peaper DR, Ho JH, et al. (2011) Microbiota regulates immune defense against respiratory tract influenza A virus infection. Proc Natl Acad Sci USA 108: 5354–5359. doi: 10.1073/pnas.1019378108.
18. Abt MC, Osborne LC, Monticelli LA, Doering TA, Alenghat T, et al. (2012) Commensal bacteria calibrate the activation threshold of innate antiviral immunity. Immunity 37: 158–170. doi: 10.1016/j.immuni.2012.04.011.
19. Krempl CD, Collins PL (2004) Reevaluation of the virulence of prototypic strain 15 of pneumonia virus of mice. J Virol 78: 13362–13365. doi: 10.1128/JVI.78.23.13362-13365.2004.
20. Grimm D, Staeheli P, Hufbauer M, Koerner I, Martínez-Sobrido L, et al. (2007) Replication fitness determines high virulence of influenza A virus in mice carrying functional Mx1 resistance gene. Proc Natl Acad Sci USA 104: 6806–6811. doi: 10.1073/pnas.0701849104.
21. Morton D, Griffiths P (1985) Guidelines on the recognition of pain, distress and discomfort in experimental animals and an hypothesis for assessment. Veterinary Record 116: 431–436. doi: 10.1136/vr.116.16.431.
22. Mouahid G, Idris MA, Verneau O, Théron A, Shaban MMA, et al. (2012) A new chronotype of Schistosoma mansoni: adaptive significance. Trop Med Int Health 17: 727–732. doi: 10.1111/j.1365-3156.2012.02988.x.
23. Standen OD (1953) The penetration of the cercariae of Schistosoma mansoni into the skin and lymphatics of the mouse. Trans R Soc Trop Med Hyg 47: 292–298.
24. Krempl CD, Wnekowicz A, Lamirande EW, Nayebagha G, Collins PL, et al. (2007) Identification of a novel virulence factor in recombinant pneumonia virus of mice. J Virol 81: 9490–9501. doi: 10.1128/JVI.00364-07.
25. Kool M, Soullié T, van Nimwegen M, Willart MAM, Muskens F, et al. (2008) Alum adjuvant boosts adaptive immunity by inducing uric acid and activating inflammatory dendritic cells. J Exp Med 205: 869–882. doi: 10.1084/jem.20071087.
26. Wu CA, Peluso JJ, Shanley JD, Puddington L, Thrall RS (2008) Murine Cytomegalovirus Influences Foxj1 Expression, Ciliogenesis, and Mucus Plugging in Mice with Allergic Airway Disease. Am J Pathol 172: 714–724. doi: 10.2353/ajpath.2008.070462.
27. Lienenklaus S, Cornitescu M, Zietara N, Łyszkiewicz M, Gekara N, et al. (2009) Novel reporter mouse reveals constitutive and inflammatory expression of IFN-beta in vivo. J Immunol 183: 3229–3236. doi: 10.4049/jimmunol.0804277.
28. Chang Y-J, Kim HY, Albacker LA, Baumgarth N, McKenzie ANJ, et al. (2011) Innate lymphoid cells mediate influenza-induced airway hyper-reactivity independently of adaptive immunity. Nat Immunol 12: 631–638. doi: 10.1038/ni.2045.
29. Morgan JAT, Dejong RJ, Adeoye GO, Ansa EDO, Barbosa CS, et al. (2005) Origin and diversification of the human parasite Schistosoma mansoni. Mol Ecol 14: 3889–3902. doi: 10.1111/j.1365-294X.2005.02709.x.
30. Henderson GS, Nix NA, Montesano MA, Gold D, Freeman GL, et al. (1993) Two distinct pathological syndromes in male CBA/J inbred mice with chronic Schistosoma mansoni infections. Am J Pathol 142: 703–714.
31. Scheer S, Gross S, Mouahid G, Moné H, Lamers MC (2014) A novel tool to identify the relative contribution of lymphoid cell types that contribute to IL-10 production during the infection with Schistosoma mansoni: The TIGER index. J Immunol Meth 406: 66–73. doi: 10.1016/j.jim.2014.03.008.
32. Willart MAM, Deswarte K, Pouliot P, Braun H, Beyaert R, et al. (2012) Interleukin-1α controls allergic sensitization to inhaled house dust mite via the epithelial release of GM-CSF and IL-33. J Exp Med 209: 1505–1517. doi: 10.1084/jem.20112691.
33. Lambrecht BN, Hammad H (2009) Biology of lung dendritic cells at the origin of asthma. Immunity 31: 412–424. doi: 10.1016/j.immuni.2009.08.008.
34. Pichery M, Mirey E, Mercier P, Lefrançais E, Dujardin A, et al. (2012) Endogenous IL-33 is highly expressed in mouse epithelial barrier tissues, lymphoid organs, brain, embryos, and inflamed tissues: in situ analysis using a novel Il-33-LacZ gene trap reporter strain. J Immunol 188: 3488–3495. doi: 10.4049/jimmunol.1101977.
35. Neill DR, Wong SH, Bellosi A, Flynn RJ, Daly M, et al. (2010) Nuocytes represent a new innate effector leukocyte that mediates type-2 immunity. Nature 464: 1367–1370. doi: 10.1038/nature08900.
36. Mjösberg JM, Trifari S, Crellin NK, Peters CP, van Drunen CM, et al. (2011) Human IL-25- and IL-33-responsive type 2 innate lymphoid cells are defined by expression of CRTH2 and CD161. Nat Immunol 12: 1055–1062. doi: 10.1038/ni.2104.
37. Monticelli LA, Sonnenberg GF, Abt MC, Alenghat T, Ziegler CGK, et al. (2011) Innate lymphoid cells promote lung-tissue homeostasis after infection with influenza virus. Nat Immunol 12: 1045–1054. doi: 10.1038/ni.2131.
38. Zhen G, Park S-W, Nguyenvu LT, Rodriguez MW, Barbeau R, et al. (2007) IL-13 and epidermal growth factor receptor have critical but distinct roles in epithelial cell mucin production. Am J Resp Cell Mol Biol 36: 244–253. doi: 10.1165/rcmb.2006-0180OC.
39. Lora JM, Zhang DM, Liao SM, Burwell T, King AM, et al. (2005) Tumor necrosis factor-alpha triggers mucus production in airway epithelium through an

IkappaB kinase beta-dependent mechanism. J Biol Chem 280: 36510–36517. doi: 10.1074/jbc.M507977200.
40. Thai P, Loukoianov A, Wachi S, Wu R (2008) Regulation of airway mucin gene expression. Annu Rev Physiol 70: 405–429. doi: 10.1146/annurev.physiol.70.113006.100441.
41. Young HWJ, Williams OW, Chandra D, Bellinghausen LK, Pérez G, et al. (2007) Central role of Muc5ac expression in mucous metaplasia and its regulation by conserved 5′ elements. Am J Resp Cell Mol Biol 37: 273–290. doi: 10.1165/rcmb.2005-0460OC.
42. Evans CM, Kim K, Tuvim MJ, Dickey BF (2009) Mucus hypersecretion in asthma: causes and effects. Curr Opin Pulm Med 15: 4–11. doi: 10.1097/MCP.0b013e32831da8d3.
43. Peppel K, Crawford D, Beutler B (1991) A tumor necrosis factor (TNF) receptor-IgG heavy chain chimeric protein as a bivalent antagonist of TNF activity. J Exp Med 174: 1483–1489.
44. Ehre C, Worthington EN, Liesman RM, Grubb BR, Barbier D, et al. (2012) Overexpressing mouse model demonstrates the protective role of Muc5ac in the lungs. Proc Natl Acad Sci USA 109: 16528–16533. doi: 10.1073/pnas.1206552109.
45. Horisberger MA, Staeheli P, Haller O (1983) Interferon induces a unique protein in mouse cells bearing a gene for resistance to influenza virus. Proc Natl Acad Sci USA 80: 1910–1914.
46. Holzinger D, Jorns C, Stertz S, Boisson-Dupuis S, Thimme R, et al. (2007) Induction of MxA gene expression by influenza A virus requires type I or type III interferon signaling. J Virol 81: 7776–7785. doi: 10.1128/JVI.00546-06.
47. Frey S, Krempl CD, Schmitt-Gräff A, Ehl S (2008) Role of T cells in virus control and disease after infection with pneumonia virus of mice. J Virol 82: 11619–11627. doi: 10.1128/JVI.00375-08.
48. Buchholz UJ, Ward JM, Lamirande EW, Heinze B, Krempl CD, et al. (2009) Deletion of nonstructural proteins NS1 and NS2 from pneumonia virus of mice attenuates viral replication and reduces pulmonary cytokine expression and disease. J Virol 83: 1969–1980. doi: 10.1128/JVI.02041-08.
49. Schramm G, Mohrs K, Wodrich M, Doenhoff MJ, Pearce EJ, et al. (2007) Cutting edge: IPSE/alpha-1, a glycoprotein from Schistosoma mansoni eggs, induces IgE-dependent, antigen-independent IL-4 production by murine basophils in vivo. J Immunol 178: 6023–6027.
50. Steinfelder S, Andersen JF, Cannons JL, Feng CG, Joshi M, et al. (2009) The major component in schistosome eggs responsible for conditioning dendritic cells for Th2 polarization is a T2 ribonuclease (omega-1). J Exp Med 206: 1681–1690. doi: 10.1084/jem.20082462.
51. Everts B, Perona-Wright G, Smits HH, Hokke CH, van der Ham AJ, et al. (2009) Omega-1, a glycoprotein secreted by Schistosoma mansoni eggs, drives Th2 responses. J Exp Med 206: 1673–1680. doi: 10.1084/jem.20082460.
52. Marillier RG, Brombacher TM, Dewals B, Leeto M, Barkhuizen M, et al. (2010) IL-4Rα-responsive smooth muscle cells increase intestinal hypercontractility and contribute to resistance during acute Schistosomiasis. Am J Physiol Gastrointest Liver Physiol 298: G943–G951.
53. Korn T, Bettelli E, Oukka M, Kuchroo VK (2009) IL-17 and Th17 Cells. Annu Rev Immunol 27: 485–517. doi: 10.1146/annurev.immunol.021908.132710.
54. Perona-Wright G, Lundie RJ, Jenkins SJ, Webb LM, Grencis RK, et al. (2012) Concurrent bacterial stimulation alters the function of helminth-activated dendritic cells, resulting in IL-17 induction. J Immunol 188: 2350–2358. doi: 10.4049/jimmunol.1101642.
55. Hasnain SZ, Evans CM, Roy M, Gallagher AL, Kindrachuk KN, et al. (2011) Muc5ac: a critical component mediating the rejection of enteric nematodes. J Exp Med 208: 893–900. doi: 10.1084/jem.20102057.
56. Marillier RG, Michels C, Smith EM, Fick LC, Leeto M, et al. (2008) IL-4/IL-13 independent goblet cell hyperplasia in experimental helminth infections. BMC Immunol 9: 11. doi: 10.1186/1471-2172-9-11.
57. Heinzel FP, Sadick MD, Holaday BJ, Coffman RL, Locksley RM (1989) Reciprocal expression of interferon gamma or interleukin 4 during the resolution or progression of murine leishmaniasis. Evidence for expansion of distinct helper T cell subsets. J Exp Med 169: 59–72. doi: 10.1084/jem.169.1.59.
58. Crosby A, Jones FM, Southwood M, Stewart S, Schermuly R, et al. (2010) Pulmonary vascular remodeling correlates with lung eggs and cytokines in murine schistosomiasis. Am J Respir Crit Care Med 181: 279–288. doi: 10.1164/rccm.200903-0355OC.
59. Yu L, Sun X, Yang F, Yang J, Shen J, et al. (2012) Inflammatory cytokines IFN-γ, IL-4, IL-13 and TNF-α alterations in schistosomiasis: a meta-analysis. Parasitol Res 110: 1547–1552. doi: 10.1007/s00436-011-2661-4.
60. Hooper LV, Littman DR, Macpherson AJ (2012) Interactions between the microbiota and the immune system. Science 336: 1268–1273. doi: 10.1126/science.1223490.
61. Khosravi A, Yáñez A, Price JG, Chow A, Merad M, et al. (2014) Gut microbiota promote hematopoiesis to control bacterial infection. Cell Host Microbe 15: 374–381. doi: 10.1016/j.chom.2014.02.006.
62. McKee A, Pearce E (2004) CD25(+)CD4(+) cells contribute to Th2 polarization during helminth infection by suppressing Th1 response development. J Immunol 173: 1224–1231.
63. Liu F, Whitton JL (2005) Cutting edge: re-evaluating the in vivo cytokine responses of CD8+ T cells during primary and secondary viral infections. J Immunol 174: 5936–5940.
64. Wei G, Wei L, Zhu J, Zang C, Hu-Li J, et al. (2009) Global mapping of H3K4me3 and H3K27me3 reveals specificity and plasticity in lineage fate determination of differentiating CD4+ T cells. Immunity 30: 155–167. doi: 10.1016/j.immuni.2008.12.009.
65. O'Shea JJ, Paul WE (2010) Mechanisms underlying lineage commitment and plasticity of helper CD4+ T cells. Science 327: 1098–1102. doi: 10.1126/science.1178334.
66. Vahedi G, Takahashi H, Nakayamada S, Sun H-W, Sartorelli V, et al. (2012) STATs Shape the Active Enhancer Landscape of T Cell Populations. Cell 151: 981–993. doi: 10.1016/j.cell.2012.09.044.
67. Kanno Y, Vahedi G, Hirahara K, Singleton K, O'Shea JJ (2012) Transcriptional and epigenetic control of T helper cell specification: molecular mechanisms underlying commitment and plasticity. Annu Rev Immunol 30: 707–731. doi: 10.1146/annurev-immunol-020711-075058.
68. Xu J, Smale ST (2012) Designing an enhancer landscape. Cell 151: 929–931. doi: 10.1016/j.cell.2012.11.007.
69. Gallo E, Katzman S, Villarino AV (2012) IL-13-producing Th1 and Th17 cells characterize adaptive responses to both self and foreign antigens. Eur J Immunol 42: 2322–2328. doi: 10.1002/eji.201142227.
70. Cosmi L, Liotta F, Maggi E, Romagnani S, Annunziato F (2011) Th17 cells: new players in asthma pathogenesis. Allergy 66: 989–998. doi: 10.1111/j.1398-9995.2011.02576.x.
71. Peine M, Rausch S, Helmstetter C, Fröhlich A, Hegazy AN, et al. (2013) Stable T-bet(+)GATA-3(+) Th1/Th2 hybrid cells arise in vivo, can develop directly from naive precursors, and limit immunopathologic inflammation. PLoS Biol 11: e1001633. doi: 10.1371/journal.pbio.1001633.
72. Mwatha JK, Kimani G, Kamau T, Mbugua GG, Ouma JH, et al. (1998) High levels of TNF, soluble TNF receptors, soluble ICAM-1, and IFN-gamma, but low levels of IL-5, are associated with hepatosplenic disease in human schistosomiasis mansoni. J Immunol 160: 1992–1999.
73. Adewusi OI, Nix NA, Lu X, Colley DG, Secor WE (1996) Schistosoma mansoni: relationship of tumor necrosis factor-alpha to morbidity and collagen deposition in chronic experimental infection. Exp Parasitol 84: 115–123. doi: 10.1006/expr.1996.0097.
74. Davies SJ, Grogan JL, Blank RB, Lim KC, Locksley RM, et al. (2001) Modulation of blood fluke development in the liver by hepatic CD4+ lymphocytes. Science 294: 1358–1361. doi: 10.1126/science.1064462.
75. Davies SJ, Lim KC, Blank RB, Kim J-H, Lucas KD, et al. (2004) Involvement of TNF in limiting liver pathology and promoting parasite survival during schistosome infection. Int J Parasitol 34: 27–36. doi: 10.1016/j.ijpara.2003.10.010.
76. Spits H, Cupedo T (2012) Innate lymphoid cells: emerging insights in development, lineage relationships, and function. Annu Rev Immunol 30: 647–675. doi: 10.1146/annurev-immunol-020711-075053.
77. Price AE, Liang H-E, Sullivan BM, Reinhardt RL, Eisley CJ, et al. (2010) Systemically dispersed innate IL-13-expressing cells in type 2 immunity. Proc Natl Acad Sci USA 107: 11489–11494. doi: 10.1073/pnas.1003988107.
78. Mordstein M, Michiels T, Staeheli P (2010) What have we learned from the IL28 receptor knockout mouse? J Interferon Cytokine Res 30: 579–584. doi: 10.1089/jir.2010.0061.
79. Damjanovic D, Divangahi M, Kugathasan K, Small C-L, Zganiacz A, et al. (2011) Negative regulation of lung inflammation and immunopathology by TNF-α during acute influenza infection. Am J Pathol 179: 2963–2976. doi: 10.1016/j.ajpath.2011.09.003.
80. Szretter KJ, Gangappa S, Lu X, Smith C, Shieh W-J, et al. (2007) Role of host cytokine responses in the pathogenesis of avian H5N1 influenza viruses in mice. J Virol 81: 2736–2744. doi: 10.1128/JVI.02336-06.
81. Chapoval SP, Al-Garawi A, Lora JM, Strickland I, Ma B, et al. (2007) Inhibition of NF-kappaB activation reduces the tissue effects of transgenic IL-13. J Immunol 179: 7030–7041.
82. Curran DR, Cohn L (2010) Advances in mucous cell metaplasia: a plug for mucus as a therapeutic focus in chronic airway disease. Am J Resp Cell Mol Biol 42: 268–275. doi: 10.1165/rcmb.2009-0151TR.
83. de Miguel-Diez J, Carrasco-Garrido P, Hernández-Barrera V, Rodríguez-Rodríguez P, Puente-Maestu L, et al. (2012) Hospitalizations from pandemic influenza (pH1N1) infections among patients with asthma or COPD in Spain. J Infect 65: 95–98. doi: 10.1016/j.jinf.2012.03.003.
84. Decramer M, Janssens W, Miravitlles M (2012) Chronic obstructive pulmonary disease. Lancet 379: 1341–1351. doi: 10.1016/S0140-6736(11)60968-9.
85. Allen JE, Maizels RM (2011) Diversity and dialogue in immunity to helminths. Nat Rev Immunol 11: 375–388. doi: 10.1038/nri2992.
86. Grainger JR, Smith KA, Hewitson JP, McSorley HJ, Harcus Y, et al. (2010) Helminth secretions induce de novo T cell Foxp3 expression and regulatory function through the TGF-β pathway. J Exp Med 207: 2331–2341. doi: 10.1084/jem.20101074.
87. Reese TA, Wakeman BS, Choi HS, Hufford MM, Huang SC, et al. (2014) Helminth infection reactivates latent -herpesvirus via cytokine competition at a viral promoter. Science 345: 573–577. doi: 10.1126/science.1254517.
88. Osborne LC, Monticelli LA, Nice TJ, Sutherland TE, Siracusa MC, et al. (2014) Virus-helminth coinfection reveals a microbiota-independent mechanism of immunomodulation. Science 345: 578–582. doi: 10.1126/science.1256942.

Persistent and Compartmentalised Disruption of Dendritic Cell Subpopulations in the Lung following Influenza A Virus Infection

Deborah H. Strickland[1¶], Vanessa Fear[1], Seth Shenton[1,2], Mathew E. Wikstrom[1], Graeme Zosky[1,3], Alexander N. Larcombe[1], Patrick G. Holt[1,4], Cassandra Berry[2], Christophe von Garnier[1,5¶], Philip A. Stumbles[1,2*¶]

1 Telethon Institute for Child Health Research and Centre for Child Health Research, University of Western Australia, Perth, W.A., Australia, **2** School of Veterinary and Life Sciences, Murdoch University, Perth, W.A., Australia, **3** School of Medicine, University of Tasmania, Hobart, Tasmania, Australia, **4** Queensland Children's Medical Research Institute, University of Queensland, Brisbane, Qld., Australia, **5** Pulmonary Medicine, Bern University Hospital and Department of Clinical Research, Berne University, Berne, Switzerland

Abstract

Immunological homeostasis in the respiratory tract is thought to require balanced interactions between networks of dendritic cell (DC) subsets in lung microenvironments in order to regulate tolerance or immunity to inhaled antigens and pathogens. Influenza A virus (IAV) poses a serious threat of long-term disruption to this balance through its potent pro-inflammatory activities. In this study, we have used a BALB/c mouse model of A/PR8/34 H1N1 Influenza Type A Virus infection to examine the effects of IAV on respiratory tissue DC subsets during the recovery phase following clearance of the virus. In adult mice, we found differences in the kinetics and activation states of DC residing in the airway mucosa (AMDC) compared to those in the parenchymal lung (PLDC) compartments. A significant depletion in the percentage of AMDC was observed at day 4 post-infection that was associated with a change in steady-state $CD11b^+$ and $CD11b^-$ AMDC subset frequencies and significantly elevated CD40 and CD80 expression and that returned to baseline by day 14 post-infection. In contrast, percentages and total numbers of PLDC were significantly elevated at day 14 and remained so until day 21 post-infection. Accompanying this was a change in $CD11b^+$and $CD11b^-$ PLDC subset frequencies and significant increase in CD40 and CD80 expression at these time points. Furthermore, mice infected with IAV at 4 weeks of age showed a significant increase in total numbers of PLDC, and increased CD40 expression on both AMDC and PLDC, when analysed as adults 35 days later. These data suggest that the rate of recovery of DC populations following IAV infection differs in the mucosal and parenchymal compartments of the lung and that DC populations can remain disrupted and activated for a prolonged period following viral clearance, into adulthood if infection occurred early in life.

Editor: Ulrich A. Maus, Hannover School of Medicine, Germany

Funding: This work was supported by the National Health and Medical Research Council of Australia (APP ID 211912, 437200; www.nhmrc.gov.au). The funders had no role in study design, data collection and analysis, decision to publish, or preparation of the manuscript.

* Email: p.stumbles@murdoch.edu.au

¶ These authors contributed equally to this work.

Introduction

Continuous exposure of the respiratory tract to environmental antigens poses a major challenge to the maintenance of local immunological homeostasis at this site. Inhaled foreign proteins and pathogens must be efficiently screened by the immune system for their potential "danger" to the host and either ignored in the case of harmless proteins (ignorance or tolerance), or translated into signals for induction of innate and adaptive immunity in the case of pathogens such as respiratory viruses. There is a close association between respiratory viral infections, bronchiolitis, wheezing and development of allergic asthma, particularly a subset of susceptible infants and children [1]. Human Rhinovirus (HRV), Respiratory Syncytial Virus (RSV) and Influenza A Virus (IAV) have high burdens of hospitalisation in children younger than 5 years, and particularly in those under 2 years of age [2,3]. Airways inflammation resulting from viral infections in infancy have been linked to wheezing in pre-school years, with associations for IAV, RSV and to a lesser extent other respiratory viral infections being documented [4-6]. Although the development of allergic asthma involves a complex series of interactions between genes and environment, there is data associating respiratory viral infections and atopy to the development of asthma, particularly in children with atopic sensitisation by the age of 2 years [3]. While the underlying pathogenesis of virally induced allergic asthma remains unclear, experimental evidence suggests that viral infections disrupt tolerance to aeroallergens across mucosal barriers together with enhanced pro-allergic immune responses [7,8].

Under normal circumstances, immunological homeostasis within the respiratory tract is maintained via the surveillance activities of local dendritic cell (DC) populations. These are distributed within respiratory tissues as integrated networks, playing a crucial role in sampling of inhaled antigens including viruses and allergens and in the initiation of subsequent tolerance and/or adaptive T cell-mediated immune responses in draining lymph nodes (DLN) [9]. Earlier observations from our group in a rat model were the first to demonstrate the rapid expansion of airway mucosal DC (AMDC) during acute viral (parainfluenza) infection, and the apparent persistence of this response beyond viral clearance [10]. This was subsequently confirmed in a mouse RSV model with respect to whole lung DC and similar observations have been reported in humans for nasal mucosal DC populations in children post RSV and HRV infections [11,12]. Given the key role that these frontline DC populations in local immune surveillance for all classes of environmental antigens, their long-term disruption following viral infection has significant implications in regards to maintenance of general immunological homeostasis within the respiratory tract. With this in mind we have sought to confirm and extend these earlier observational studies, aiming to more comprehensively identify which DC subsets are susceptible to the effects of virus, and in which precise tissue microenvironments within the respiratory tree; moreover we have extended the studies to encompass immunologically immature weanling animals, similar to the age range described above for maximal susceptibility to severe virus associated airways inflammation in humans.

Early studies in rodent models demonstrated the capacity of respiratory tract DC to direct the outcome of $CD4^+$ T cell responses to inhaled allergens and a number of subsequent studies have confirmed the essential requirement for DC migration to DLN for induction of $CD4^+$ T cell mediated allergic airways inflammation and asthmatic syndromes [13,14]. Furthermore, our previous work in rodents identified a subdivision of function based on anatomical location, with AMDC being functionally distinct from their counterparts in parenchymal lung tissue, most likely due to micro-environmental differences between these anatomical locations [15,16]. Consistent with airway mucosal surfaces being the first site of exposure to inhaled allergens and viruses, AMDC show high levels of endocytic activity and rapid turn-over and drainage to airway DLN, defining their proposed role as "gatekeepers" for the initiation of adaptive immunity to inhaled allergens and pathogens [15,17-19].

A number of DC subsets have been described in rodents and humans with differing capacities to influence naïve and memory $CD4^+$ and $CD8^+$ T cell responses [20]. In the mouse, major populations of classical (also termed "myeloid" or "conventional") DC (cDC) and plasmacytoid DC (pDC) have been identified, as well as a number of cDC subsets with distinct phenotypic and transcriptional profiles [21]. In the mouse respiratory tract, two dominant cDC subsets based on the reciprocal expression of CD11b and the alpha (E) integrin CD103 have been described, whereby $CD11b^{lo}$ ($CD103^+$) DC express tight junction proteins, reside within the airway epithelium and increase in numbers during allergic airways inflammation, while the $CD11b^{hi}$ ($CD103^-$) subset readily produces a number of chemokines that regulate $CD4^+$ T cell activity [16,22,23]. During IAV infection, both DC subsets have been shown to be infected and be capable of presenting viral antigens to T cells, however the $CD11b^{lo}$ subset appears to be the predominant subset for migration to DLN and for either direct or cross-presentation of viral antigens to $CD8^+$ T cells although, other subsets in tissue and DLN are likely to be involved [24–27]. In addition to cDC, other non-myeloid lineages such as plasmacytoid DC (pDC) in lungs, as well as resident lymphoid-origin DC in DLN, may also play important roles in initiating T cell immunity to IAV [27–29].

In this study we have characterised the impact of IAV infection on the frequency and activation of cDC in anatomical compartments of the respiratory tract of BALB/c mice following IAV infection. IAV infection was shown to have a differential impact on DC numbers and activation status in airway mucosal and parenchymal lung tissues, which represent two anatomically and immunologically distinct compartments of the respiratory tract. Furthermore, IAV infection of juvenile mice induced long-term alterations on the frequency and activation states of parenchymal lung DC subsets that persisted into adulthood.

Results

Clinical features of the BALB/c mouse model of influenza A virus (IAV) infection

An adult BALB/c mouse model of IAV infection was established, using intranasal (i.n.) delivery of an optimised dose of the mouse-adapted A/PR/8/34 (H1N1) type A influenza virus (IAV). Using this protocol, mice developed peak clinical symptoms on d9 to d10 post-infection (p.i.) as evidenced by body weight loss (Fig. 1A) and clinical score (Fig. 1B), with mice recovering to pre-infection clinical score and weight by d14 and d21 p.i. respectively. Lung tissue viral titres were elevated at d3 p.i. and completely resolved by d14 p.i. (Fig. 1C). Lung mechanics were also altered at d4 p.i., with IAV infected mice showing increased airway resistance at functional residual capacity (FRC) ($p<0.001$), which was maintained throughout inflation up to 20 cmH_2O transrespiratory pressure ($p<0.001$) (Fig. 1D, left panel). Similarly, IAV infected mice had increased tissue damping (0 cm H_2O, $p<0.01$) (Fig. 1D, middle panel) and tissue elastance (0 cm H_2O, $p = 0.002$; 20 cm H_2O, $p<0.001$) (Fig. 1D, right panel), although at high pressures there was no difference in tissue damping between influenza infected mice and controls.

Total cell counts in bronchoalveolar lavage fluids (BALF) from IAV infected mice showed a significant increase at d4 p.i. ($p < 0.01$), and peak increase at d7 p.i. ($p<0.01$), when compared to control mice, declining by d14 p.i. but still remaining significantly elevated above control levels at d21 p.i. ($p<0.05$). (Fig. 2A) Differential cell counts of BALF showed significantly elevated macrophage numbers at d4 p.i. ($p<0.01$) that mirrored the kinetics of total cell counts (Fig. 2B). An early neutrophil response was observed, with a peak at d4 p.i. ($p<0.0001$) that declined but remained significantly elevated above control levels at d14 p.i. ($p<0.05$), and at d21 p.i. ($p<0.05$) (Fig. 2C). Total lymphocyte counts were also significantly elevated by d4 p.i. ($p<0.0001$) with a peak at d7 p.i. ($p<0.0001$), declining but remaining significantly elevated above control levels at d14 and d21 p.i. ($p<0.0001$). (Fig. 2D). Calculation of the percentage of each cell type in BALF showed a significant decrease in the percentage of macrophages from d4 to d21 p.i. (Fig. 2E), and significant increases in the percentages of neutrophils (Fig. 2F) and lymphocytes (Fig. 2G) over the same time period.

Cytokine levels in BALF showed significantly elevated IFNα (Fig. 3A) and KC (Fig. 3B) levels at d4 p.i. ($p<0.05$) that declined to control levels by d14 for IFNα, whereas KC remained elevated until d21p.i. ($p<0.05$). G-CSF showed a biphasic response, being significantly elevated at d4 and d7 p.i. ($p<0.0001$), returning to baseline levels at d14 p.i. and significantly increasing again at d21 p.i. ($p<0.0001$) (Fig. 3C). IL-12 p40 (but not IL-12p70, data not

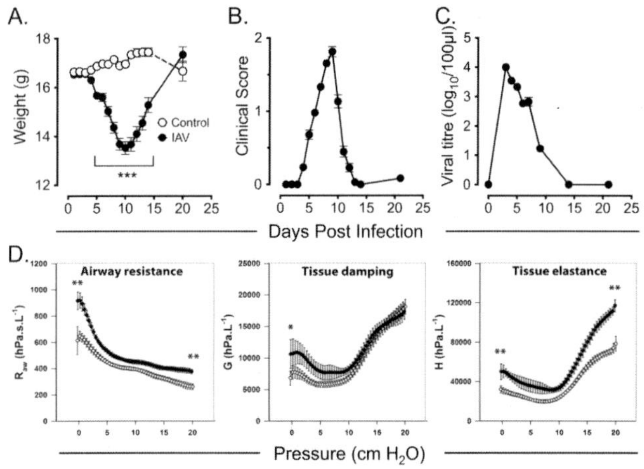

Figure 1. Clinical features of the adult BALB/c mouse model of A/PR8/34 H1N1 influenza A virus (IAV) infection. Eight week-old female BALB/c mice were inoculated i.n. with 1×10^2 $TCID_{50}$ A/PR/8/34 influenza A virus (IAV) in PBS and assessed at the indicated time points over the following 21 days for *(A)* body weight *(B)* clinical score and *(C)* lung tissue viral titres. Data are mean +/− SEM of groups of 20 to 60 mice per time point for weight measurements and clinical score, and 5 mice per time point for lung viral titres. Control mice received equivalent volumes of virus-free DMEM i.n. at day 0. *(D)* Measurement of airway resistance, tissue damping and tissue elastance at transrespiratory pressure during slow inflation manoeuvres up to 20cm H_2O in influenza infected mice (closed circles) and controls (open circles) at day 4 post infection. Influenza infected mice had impairments in Raw, G and H. Asterisks indicate statistical significance of IAV infected as compared to control mice as described in Materials and Methods. Data are means +/− SEM of 4 mice per group. * = $p<0.05$; ** = $p<0.01$; *** = $p<0.001$.

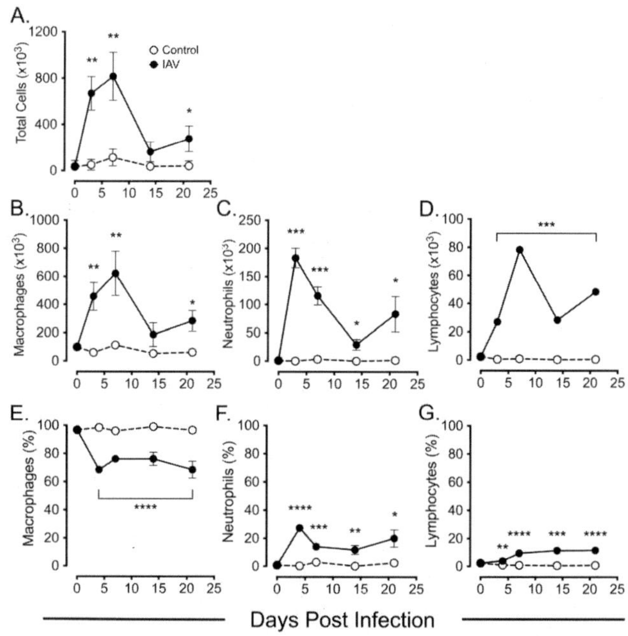

Figure 2. Bronchoalveolar lavage fluid (BALF) differential cell counts following IAV infection. Groups of 8 week old BALB/c mice were infected with IAV i.n. and BALF harvested on day 0 (pre-infection) and at the indicated time post-infection and assessed for total numbers of *(A)* total cells, *(B)* macrophages, *(C)* neutrophils and *(D)* lymphocytes and for percentages of cells by differential Leishman's staining for *(E)* macrophages, *(F)* neutrophils and *(G)* lymphocytes as described in Materials and Methods. Control mice received equivalent volumes of virus-free DMEM i.n. at day 0. Results are mean +/− SEM for 5 mice at each time point. * = $p<0.05$; ** = $p<0.01$; *** = $p<0.001$; **** = $p<0.0001$.

shown) was significantly elevated at d4 and d7 p.i. ($p<0.0001$), declining but remaining significantly elevated at d21 p.i. ($p<0.05$) (Fig. 3D). Both IL-10 (Fig. 3E) and IFNγ (Fig. 3F) were significantly elevated ($p<0.05$) at d7 p.i., returning to control levels by d14 p.i.

Kinetics of airway mucosal and lung parenchymal DC subsets following acute IAV infection

Our previous mouse studies have identified functionally distinct populations of DC in the airway mucosa (AMDC) and parenchymal lung (PLDC), with AMDC displaying more rapid turnover rates (<12 h) compared to PLDC (>7 days) and more rapid activation in response to aeroallergen challenge [15,16]. Given that acute IAV infection is characterised by early infection and replication of the virus in epithelial cells of the airway mucosa, we initially examined the population dynamics of AMDC compared to their more peripheral PLDC counterparts following IAV infection. AMDC and PLDC were identified by flow cytometry using co-staining of tracheal and parenchymal lung tissue respectively for CD11c and MHC class II (I-A/E) as previously described [15], allowing gating of $CD11c^+$ I-A/E^{hi} AMDC and PLDC following IAV infection (Figs. 4A and 4D). This combination of markers also allowed identification of $CD11c^+$ I-A/E^{low} parenchymal lung macrophages (PLMac) [15], which were also tracked over the same time course post-IAV infection (Fig. 4G). In addition, as expression of I-A/E may possibly have modulated after IAV infection, we confirmed that these phenotypes remained stable by substituting the mouse DC marker CD205 for I-A/E (Fig. S1). A time course analysis of tracheal tissue showed a significant depletion of AMDC as a percentage of total cells ($p<0.01$) (Fig. 4A and 4B), but not total cell numbers (Fig. 4C), at day 4 p.i. with the percentages of AMDC returning to baseline levels by d7-14 p.i. In contrast, percentages (Fig. 4D and 4E) and total numbers (Fig. 4F) of PLDC in peripheral lung tissue remained unchanged from controls at d4 p.i., but were then significantly increased above control levels from d14 p.i ($p<0.05$). Over the same time-course, a decrease in percentages (Fig. 4G and 4H) and total numbers (Fig. 4I) of PLMac was observed from d4 p.i., with a significant decrease in the percentage of PLMac at d4 and d14 p.i. ($p<0.01$), returning to near-baseline levels at d21 p.i.

In addition to anatomical location, we and others have shown that the myeloid marker CD11b functionally divides mouse lung DC, with $CD11b^{hi}$ and $CD11b^{lo}$ DC subsets showing different rates of capture and trafficking of inhaled antigens in the steady-state and during allergic inflammatory airways disease [15,16,30]. Furthermore, the $CD11b^{lo}$ DC subset has been shown to be important for clearance of IAV and to have distinct functional properties in terms of T cell recruitment and activation [22,23]. In the current study, analysis of CD11b expression on respiratory tract DC populations following IAV infection showed a compartmentalised change. In the airway mucosa, IAV infection induced a significant decrease in the percentage of $CD11b^{lo}$ AMDC (Fig. 5A), and corresponding increase in the percentage of $CD11b^{hi}$ AMDC (Fig. 5B) at d4 and d7 p.i., returning to control levels for each subset at d14 p.i. Similarly, IAV infection also induced a decrease in the percentage of $CD11b^{lo}$ PLDC (Fig. 5C), and increase in the percentage of $CD11b^{hi}$ PLDC at d7 p.i. (Fig. 5D). However, in contrast to AMDC, changes in CD11b

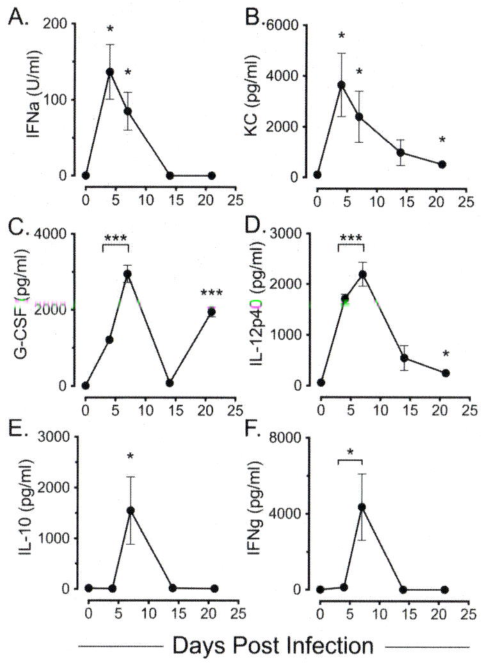

Figure 3. BALF cytokine analysis following IAV infection. Mice were infected with IAV i.n. and BALF fluids harvested at the indicated time points and assessed for *(A)* IFNα by bioassay as described in Materials and Methods, and by multiplex immunoassay assay for *(B)* KC, *(C)* G-CSF *(D)* IL-12 p40, *(E)* IL-10 and *(F)* IFNγ. Results shown are means +/− SEM of duplicate samples for 3 mice at each time point. Statistical significances were calculated for infected mice relative to control (d0) mice. * = $p<0.05$; *** = $p<0.001$.

expression on PLDC persisted, remaining significantly changed from control PLDC until d21 p.i. (Fig. 5C and 5D).

In summary, IAV infection induced a transient derangement of AMDC percentages and CD11b expression that generally resolved by d14 p.i., whereas these alterations persisted in PLDC. Therefore, restoration of homeostasis of DC populations following IAV infection is rapidly regulated at the mucosal surfaces of the conducting airways, but remains disrupted in the lung parenchymal compartment.

Expression of co-stimulatory markers on respiratory tract DC following acute IAV infection

We next examined the expression of the co-stimulatory markers CD40, CD80 and CD86 on AMDC and PLDC following IAV infection as indicators of cellular activation status. We have previously shown that CD40 is an early activation marker of AMDC, being upregulated in the early stages of allergic airways disease [16]. For AMDC, the percentages of cells expressing CD40 (Fig. 6A) and CD80 (Fig. 6B) were significantly increased at d4 p.i. when compared to control AMDC (Fig. S2), generally returning to control levels by d14 p.i. Although baseline expression levels of CD86 were constitutively high on AMDC, expression of this marker was also significantly upregulated at d4 p.i., returning to control levels by d7- d14 p.i. (Fig. 6C). For PLDC, CD40 (Fig. 6D) and CD80 (Fig. 6E) were upregulated at d4 p.i. (Fig. S2) and, in contrast to AMDC, remained elevated until d21 p.i. Again, as for AMDC, CD86 expression was constitutively high on PLDC and was further upregulated from d4 to d14 p.i., returning to normal levels by d21 p.i. (Fig. 6F). Expression of these co-stimulatory markers was equally distributed amongst the $CD11b^{lo}$ and $CD11b^{hi}$ AMDC and PLDC subsets (data not shown).

In summary, AMDC showed a rapid and transient increase in co-stimulatory molecules following IAV infection that returned to baseline levels by d14 p.i., whereas PLDC showed a persistent increase in these molecules on both the $CD11b^{lo}$ and $CD11b^{hi}$ subsets. Therefore, control of DC activation following IAV infection is rapidly regulated in the airway mucosa, but remains dysregulated in the lung parenchymal compartment.

Frequency and activation status of respiratory tract APC populations following early-life IAV infection

We next addressed the question of the long-term impact of IAV on respiratory tract APC populations after early-life virus infection. To investigate this, post-weaning (28 day-old) BALB/c mice were infected with a weight-adjusted dose of IAV as described in the Materials and Methods, and tracheal and lung tissue isolated 35 days later (i.e. as 8 week-old adults) to examine AMDC and PLDC cell frequencies and their activation status. Early-life IAV infection resulted in a clinical syndrome that was very similar to that shown for adult mice (see Fig. 1B), with clinical scores peaking and declining at similar time-points p.i. (data not shown). Analysis of tracheal tissue of mice infected at 28 days of age and analysed as adults showed no significant difference in percentages or total numbers of AMDC compared to control mice (Fig. 7A and 7B), however significant increases were observed in the percentage of cells expressing CD40 ($p<0.01$) and CD86 ($p<0.01$) (Fig. 7C). In contrast, analysis of peripheral lung tissue showed significantly elevated percentages ($p<0.01$, data not shown) and total numbers ($p<0.05$) of PLDC compared to control mice (Fig. 7D and 7E), and significantly up-regulated percentages of cells expressing CD40 and CD80 ($p<0.01$) (Fig. 7F). Analysis of PLMac showed a significant increase in the percentage of cells ($p<0.05$, data not shown), but no significant increases in the percentages or total numbers of cells (Fig. 7G and 7H), and significant increases in the proportions of cells expressing CD40 and CD80 (Fig. 7I). Furthermore, a small but significant decrease in the intensity of MHC Class II expression was observed on PLDC ($p<0.01$), and a significant increase on PLMac ($p<0.001$) (Fig. S3).

In summary, early life IAV infection induced increases in PLDC numbers and increased expression of co-stimulatory molecules on AMDC, PLDC and PLMac that persisted into adulthood. These data indicate that restoration of respiratory APC homeostasis is persistently disrupted if IAV infection occurs in early life.

Discussion

This study examined the acute and long-term effects of A/PR8/34 H1N1 IAV infection on the depletion, reconstitution kinetics and activation state of DC populations in mucosal and parenchymal lung compartments. Uniquely, these were examined both in adult and juvenile mice for airway mucosal and parenchymal lung tissue sites, representing the two major anatomical compartments of the respiratory tract. We have argued previously that these sites differ in their induction and effector immunoregulatory functions in the mouse RT [15,16]. In this study, we have explored the hypothesis that these sites will respond differentially to IAV infection, and that the impact of IAV on immunological homeostasis in the RT will vary as a function of the age of infection.

An adult BALB/c mouse model of IAV infection was established utilising a sub-lethal dose of A/PR8/34, in which clinical signs peaking at days 8 to 9 p.i., with viral titres and lung

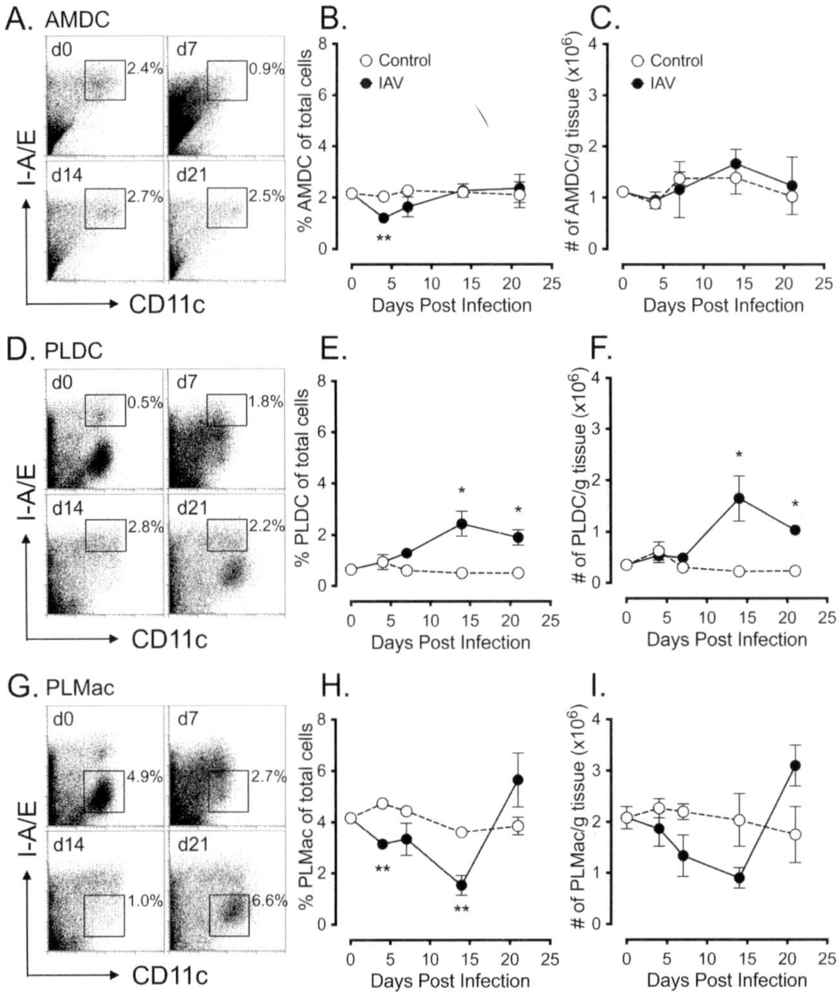

Figure 4. Kinetics of airway mucosal and parenchymal lung DC changes following IAV infection. *(A)* Representative FACS profiles showing gating for AMDC at the indicated time points p.i. *(B and C)* AMDC percentage frequencies *(B)* and total numbers *(C)* following IAV infection for control (open circles) and IAV infected mice (closed circles). *(D)* Representative FACS profiles showing gating for PLDC at the indicated time points p.i. *(E and F)* PLDC percentage frequencies *(E)* and total numbers *(F)* following IAV infection for control (open circles) and IAV infected mice (closed circles). *(G)* Representative FACS profiles showing gating for PLMac at the indicated time points p.i. *(H and I)* PLMac percentage frequencies *(H)* and total numbers *(I)* following IAV infection for control (open circles) and IAV infected mice (closed circles). Data are means +/− SEM for 3 independent infection experiments using pools of tissue from 3 to 4 mice for each experiment. * = $p<0.05$; ** = $p<0.01$.

histopathology reverting to background levels by day 14 p.i. Influenza infection resulted in significant and physiologically important deficits in lung mechanics of the conducting airways, peripheral airways and lung parenchyma that were maintained at high lung volume. Mice showed altered lung physiological responses at the peak of IAV infection, which was associated with the maximum of the neutrophil influx into alveolar space. These data are consistent with previous studies using the A/Mem/1/71(H3N1) strain of influenza virus in BALB/c mice, which showed heightened AHR at day 4 p.i. which had normalised by day 20 p.i. [31]. The acute phase of viral infection was also characterised by peak influxes of lymphocytes and neutrophils into BAL fluid as well as IFNα, the neutrophil chemoattractant KC (CXCL1) and IL-12 p70, which declined by day 14 p.i. The neutrophil response in particular was of interest, as these cells had not return to baseline levels by day 14 when virus had been cleared, and began to increase again by day 14. Interestingly, this second wave of neutrophil influx occurred without a concurrent increase in KC or detectable viral titres in lung tissue, suggesting a secondary recruitment response independent of these factors was taking place. The reason for this is unclear, as we saw no indirect evidence of secondary bacterial infection in the mice, further supported by a lack of Type 1 IFN responses in BAL fluids after day 9 p.i., however this would need to be confirmed by bacteriology. However, the bi-phasic neutrophil response did correlate with a bi-phasic G-CSF response in BALF. This growth factor is a potent regulator of haemopoeisis, and mediates neutrophil activation and survival [32]. It is possible that failure to correctly regulate G-CSF in the resolution phase of disease may lead to persistent neutrophil recruitment and activation and incomplete resolution of the inflammatory response. Recently, Narasaraju *et al.* showed a role for macrophages in limiting neutrophil influxes into lavage fluids following PR8 infection [33]. These late and persistent increases in inflammatory cells in BAL suggest that inflammation may never be fully resolved after IAV infection in BALB/c mice, which is consistent with what has been previously proposed and which may in part explain post-infective

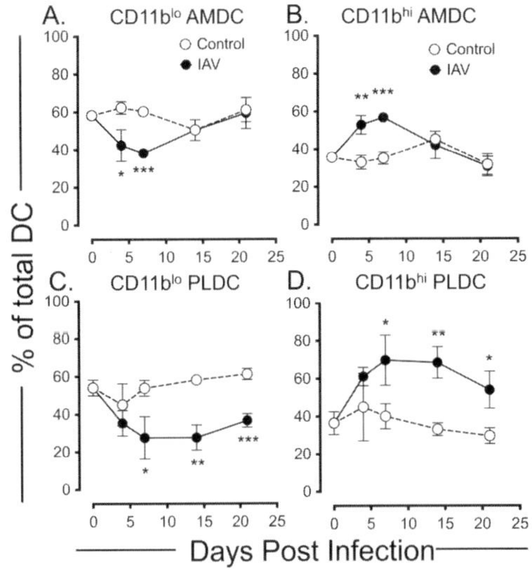

Figure 5. Time course of changes in the expression of CD11b on respiratory DC subsets in anatomical compartments of the respiratory tract following IAV infection. *(A and B)* Percentage frequency of CD11b^{lo} AMDC *(A)* and CD11b^{hi} AMDC *(B)* amongst total AMDC (gated as per Fig. 4A) in IAV infected (closed circles) and control mice (open circles). *(C and D)* Percentage frequency of CD11b^{lo} PLDC *(A)* and CD11b^{hi} PLDC *(B)* amongst total PLDC (gated as per Fig. 4D) in IAV infected (closed circles) and control mice (open circles). Data are means +/− SEM for 3 independent infection experiments using pools of tissue from 3 to 4 mice for each experiment. * = $p<0.05$; ** = $p<0.01$; *** = $p<0.001$.

bronchial hyperreactivity that may persist in humans for weeks or months after influenza infection [34,35].

A key objective of the current study was to examine the kinetics of changes in numbers and activation status of DC, in different anatomical compartments of the mouse respiratory tract after influenza infection. This was based on our previous mouse studies showing that AMDC displayed more rapid turnover rates and were activated early in response to aeroallergen challenge compared to their PLDC counterparts [15,16]. We reasoned that the responses of DC in these two compartments would differ given that AMDC are in intimate contact with airway epithelial cells, which represent the first site of influenza infection and replication, whereas PLDC reside within the alveolar septal walls that represent a distinct microenvironment that may be influenced by inflammatory responses later in the course of infection [36]. Dendritic cells play an important role in the initiation of anti-viral T cell responses, rapidly migrating to draining lymph nodes during early infection and being critical for the activation of both CD4$^+$ and CD8$^+$ viral-specific T cell responses that are essential for viral clearance and resolution of inflammation [27,36,37]. The findings of this study are in accordance with this, as we found that AMDC were being activated to express costimulatory markers early after infection, that correlated with induction of high levels of IAV-specific CD8$^+$ T cell proliferation and IFNγ production in draining lymph nodes at day 4 p.i. (Wikstrom, Stumbles, unpublished observations). Interestingly, associated with this was a significant decrease in the numbers of AMDC at day 4 p.i. but recovery by day 14 p.i., suggesting either cell death, or enhanced migration of AMDC to draining lymph nodes after IAV infection, consistent with the previous findings of others for pulmonary viral infections [37]. Previously we have shown that mouse AMDC and PLDC can be subdivided based on expression of the myeloid

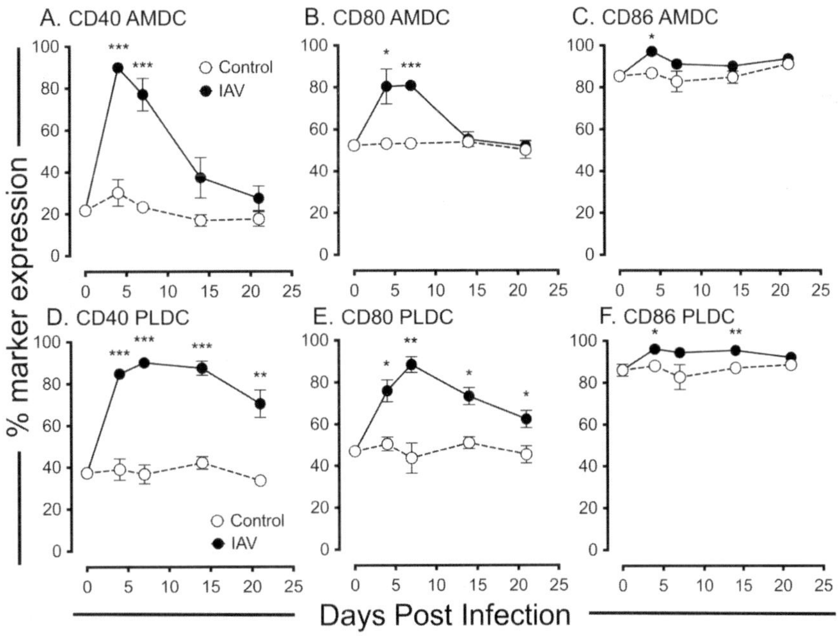

Figure 6. Expression of the co-stimulatory molecules CD40, CD80 and CD86 on respiratory DC subsets in anatomical compartments of the respiratory tract following IAV infection. *(A–C)* Time-course of expression of CD40 *(A)*, CD80 *(B)* and CD86 *(C)* on AMDC expressed as a percentage of cells expressing each marker of the total AMDC population (gated as per Fig. 4A). *(D–F)* Time-course of expression of CD40 *(D)*, CD80 *(E)* and CD86 *(F)* on PLDC expressed as a percentage of cells expressing each marker of the total PLDC population (gated as per Fig. 4D). Data are means +/− SEM for 3 independent infection experiments using pools of tissue from 3 to 4 mice for each experiment. The percentage expression of each marker was calculated based on histogram gates set using matching isotype control antibodies for each marker (Fig. S2) * = $p<0.05$; ** = $p<0.01$; *** = $p<0.001$.

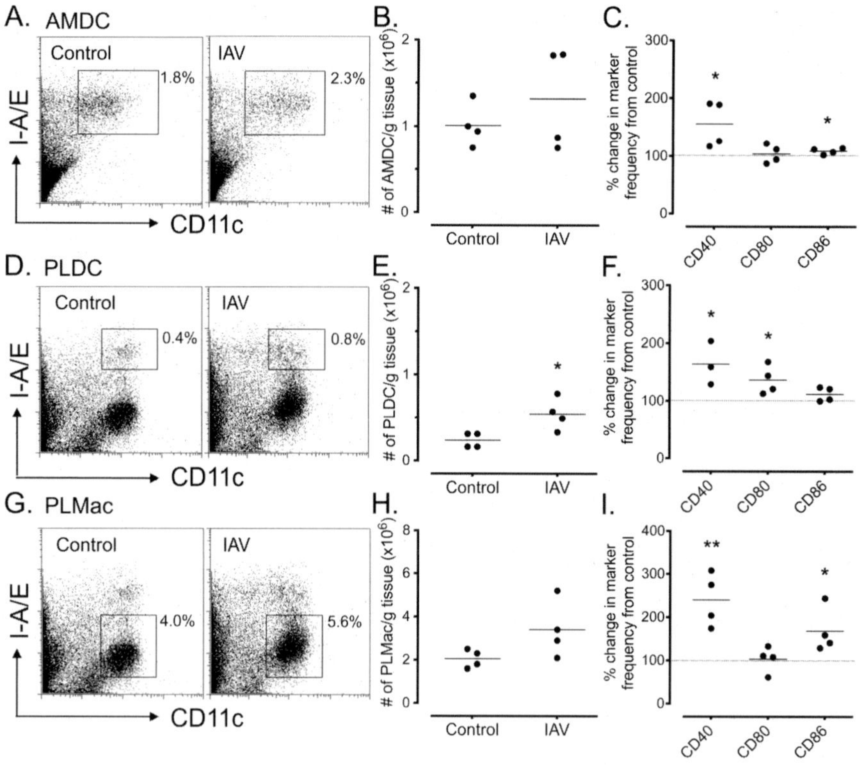

Figure 7. Long-term changes in total cell numbers of, and co-stimulatory molecule expression by, of respiratory APC populations following IAV infection in early life. Juvenile (28 day old) BALB/c mice were infected i.n. with a weight-adjusted dose of IAV as described in Materials and Methods, then respiratory tissues harvested 35 days later as 8 week-old adults. *(A)* Representative FACS profiles showing gating for AMDC in tracheal tissue of control (left) and IAV infected mice (right). *(B and C)* Total AMDC numbers *(B)* and percentage changes in co-stimulatory marker expression *(C)*, expressed a percentage change from control mice. *(D)* Representative FACS profiles showing gating for PLDC in parenchymal lung tissue of control (left) and IAV infected mice (right). *(E and F)* Total PLDC numbers *(E)* and percentage changes in co-stimulatory marker expression *(F)*, expressed a percentage change from control mice. *(G)* Representative FACS profiles showing gating for PLMac in parenchymal lung tissue of control (left) and IAV infected mice (right). *(H and I)* Total PLMac numbers *(H)* and percentage changes in co-stimulatory marker expression *(I)*, expressed a percentage change from control mice. Data are shown for 4 independent infection experiments, using pools of tissue from 4 to 5 mice for each experiment. * = $p<0.05$; ** = $p<0.01$.

marker CD11b into CD11b^{hi} and CD11b^{lo} subsets that show different rates of capture of inhaled antigens *in vivo* [16,30]. Others have shown that the CD11b^{lo} subset, that co-expresses the surface marker CD103, is important in capturing viral antigens and migrating to draining lymph nodes for the activation of CD4^{+} and CD8^{+} T cells. This capacity also resides within the CD11b^{hi} subset, although to a lesser extent [26]. Furthermore, CD11b^{lo} and CD11b^{hi} DC in the mouse RT have been shown to express differing arrays of chemokines and have been proposed to play differing roles in lung homeostasis, with the CD11b^{lo} (CD103^{+}) subset expressing tight junction proteins and may play a major regulatory role in allergen-induced lung inflammation [22,23]. The findings in this study that the relative proportions of CD11b^{hi} PLDC remain persistently elevated amongst the PLDC population after viral clearance. The reason for this disrupted balance in CD11b-expressing subsets was not determined in the current study, but may relate to altered recruitment kinetics or local maturation of CD11b^{hi} and CD11b^{lo} subsets. In this regard, Lin et al., described a population of inflammatory CCR2^{+} monocyte-derived DC recruited during acute IAV infection, that have a similar phenotype to the PLDC observed in our study (CD11c+ MHC Class II^{+} CD11b^{hi}) [38]. Thus, these cells may be contributing to the enhanced proportions of CD11b^{+} PLDC that persist following IAV infection in our study. Disruptions to the balance of CD11b-expressing PLDC subsets, along with persistent elevation of co-stimulatory molecule expression on these cells, may have important implications for immune homeostasis at this site given that maintaining a balance in these subsets of DC is likely to be important for the correct regulation of T cell immunity to inhaled allergens. In this regard, it is of interest to note that IAV infection has been associated with enhanced IgE production and CD4^{+} T cell sensitisation to inhaled allergens, an effect linked to altered function of respiratory dendritic cells [7,39–41]. Furthermore, IAV has been shown to disrupt the induction of T and B cell tolerance to inhaled antigens that normally occurs following exposure to inert proteins in immunologically naïve mice [8]. It is interesting to speculate that these observations may be linked to the findings in the current study of persistently increased proportions of activated CD11b^{hi} PLDC following IAV infection, that may act to promote aberrant local CD4^{+} T cell activation to inhaled allergens in lung tissue.

Finally, we examined the impact of IAV infection in juvenile mice at the age of 28 days old, representing the post-weaning age of human infants. Juvenile mice infected with a weight-adjusted, adult-equivalent dosage of IAV developed a clinical disease of similar severity to adults, with peak clinical signs and resolution of symptoms occurring at the same time points. When these mice were examined at day 35 p.i., an age at which is mice are considered to have reached adult maturity, we observed persistent and significant increases in the numbers and activation status of parenchymal lung DC and Mac populations, but not in their airway mucosal counterparts. This was particularly evident for the PLMac populations, which displayed marked increases in MHC Class II, CD40 and CD86 expression above control mice, and for PLDC that displayed increased numbers and persistent CD40 and CD80 upregulation. Activation of PLMac was also observed in the adult model prior during the course of IAV infection, most likely as a result of TLR7 binding by viral components and NLR (NOD-like receptor) inflammasome activation [42]. Whether persistent PLMac and PLDC activation in juvenile and adult mice is a result of sustained TLR or NLR signalling, or some other sustained inflammatory response is unclear. However, this could have important down-stream consequences for immune homeostasis at in the lung, given that interactions between macrophages and DC are important for dampening DC function and T cell reactivity in parenchymal lung tissue and that long-lived APC expressing elevated levels of MHC Class II could act as depots for allergen persistence and reactivation of allergen-specific T cells [43,44].

In conclusion, in this study we have demonstrated that A/PR8/34 H1N1 IAV infection of BALB/c mice has differential effects on DC populations in differing anatomical locations of the respiratory tract, with persistent derangement in the numbers and activation states of DC in the parenchymal lung compartment as compared to the airway mucosa. Furthermore, these disruptions persisted for several weeks after clearance of the virus in adult mice, and persisted into adulthood in mice that were infected with IAV in early life. These data indicate that IAV has a severe and long-term impact on the balance and activation state of respiratory DC and other APC subsets, potentially disrupting the fine balance of immunological homeostatic mechanisms required for the prevention of respiratory inflammatory diseases to inert antigens.

Materials and Methods

Mice and Viral Inoculations

Ethics statement. All animal experiments were conducted in strict accordance with the recommendations of the National Health and Medical Research Council of Australia, Guidelines to Promote the Wellbeing of Animals used for Scientific Research. All procedures were approved by the Telethon Institute for Child Health Research Animal Experimentation Ethics Committee (permit numbers: 139 and 256) and Murdoch University Animal Ethics Committee (permit number: N2569/13). Intranasal (i.n.) viral inoculations were performed under light inhaled Isofluorane anaesthesia. Mice were sacrificed by i.p. injection of 100μl of Phenobarbitone Sodium performed under inhaled Isofluorane anaesthesia, with all efforts made to minimise animal suffering.

Specific pathogen free female BALB/c mice were obtained from the Animal Resources Centre (Perth, W.A., Australia) and used at either 28 days (juvenile) or 8 weeks (adult) of age. The mouse-adapted influenza H1N1 A/PR/8/34 virus was from the American Type Tissue Culture Collection and prepared in allantoic fluid of 9-day old embryonated hens eggs. Stock virus was sub-passaged through Mardin-Darby canine kidney (MDCK) cells in Dulbecco's modified Eagle's medium (DMEM; Gibco, Sydney, Australia), harvested as tissue culture supernatant and viral titres determined by cytopathic effects on MDCK cells and expressed as the mean $\log_{10}$ tissue culture infective dose that kills 50% of the cells ($TCID_{50}$) over a 5-day incubation period. Adult mice were inoculated intranasally (i.n.) under light inhalation anaesthesia with 0.5×10^2 $TCID_{50}$ PR8 diluted in 50μl DMEM [45]. Juvenile mice were obtained post-weaning and inoculated i.n. using a weight-for-age adjusted volume of 0.5×10^2 $TCID_{50}$ PR8/50μl adjusted to 2.5μl per gram body weight. Mock-infected control mice received matched volumes of virus-free DMEM tissue culture medium by i.n. inoculation.

Animal Monitoring and Clinical Assessments

Mice were weighed daily during the acute period of infection (d0 to d14) and then every second day until day 21. Clinical disease scores were also assessed according ot the following criteria: 0-healthy; 1-barely ruffled fur; 2-ruffled fur, active; 3-ruffled fur, inactive; 4-ruffled fur, inactive, hunched. Mice were euthanized at indicated time points and lung tissue harvested for assessment of viral titres. Lung-tissue viral titres were determined by the $TCID_{50}$ assay described above, using 20% dilutions of clarified lung tissue homogenates. Results are expressed as $\log_{10}$ $TCID_{50}$/100μl of lung tissue homogenate. Broncho-alveolar lavage fluid (BALF) was harvested by slowly infusing and withdrawing 1 ml of PBS containing 20mg/ml bovine serum albumin (CSL, Victoria, Australia) and 35 mg/ml lidocaine (Sigma, St Louis, USA) from the lungs three times, and the cells pelleted and prepared for total cell counts and differential cell counts as previously described [46]. Briefly, the percentage of each cell type as identified by Leishman's stain (macrophage, neutrophil, lymphocyte) was calculated as a proportion of 300 counted cells, and this figure used to derive total numbers of each subset based on the total BALF cell count. The BALF supernatants were stored at -80°C for cytokine analysis. All cytokines were measured in undiluted BALF using a Bio-Plex Pro Mouse Cytokine Grp 1 Panel 23-Plex assay and Bio-Plex MAGPIX plate reader (BIO-RAD, USA) apart from acid stable Type I IFN (IFNα), which was measured by bioassay using encephalomyocarditis virus-induced cytopathic effect (CPE) of L929 monolayers as previously described [47].

Lung Function Testing

Lung mechanics were measured as described previously [48]. Briefly, mice (4 per experimental group) were anaesthetised by i.p. injection of a solution containing 40 $mg.mL^{-1}$ ketamine and 2 $mg.mL^{-1}$ xylazine at a dose of 0.1 mL.10 g^{-1} body weight. Mice were surgically tracheotomised and connected to a mechanical ventilator (tidal volume, 8 mL.kg-1; frequency, 450 breaths.min-1, PEEP, 2 cmH_2O). Following standardisation of lung volume history the ventilator was paused and a pseudorandom oscillatory signal (4-38 Hz) was delivered to the tracheal cannula by a loudspeaker via a wavetube of known impedance. A positive pressure was then applied via the wavetube in order to slowly (15–20s) inflate the lung up to 20 cmH_2O transrespiratory pressure. The oscillatory signal was applied throughout this manoeuvre in order to track changes in lung mechanics from functional residual capacity (FRC) to total lung capacity (TLC). A respiratory system impedance spectrum was then generated for each 0.5 s data epoch of the inflation manoeuvre. Data from each of these spectra was then fit to a 4 parameter mathematical model with constant phase tissue impedance which allowed us to partition lung mechanics into parameters representing airway resistance (Raw, resistance of the conducting airways), tissue damping (G, resistance of the small peripheral airways were airflow occurs by diffusion) and tissue elastance (H, stiffness of the lung parenchyma) [49].

Isolation and Preparation of Respiratory Tract Tissues

Lungs were perfused to isolate tracheal (airway mucosal) and parenchymal lung tissue and prepare single cell suspensions as previously described [50]. In brief, trachea or lungs were collected from pools of five mice and single-cell suspensions prepared by type IV collagenase digestion (1.5 mg/ml; Worthington Biochemical, Lakewood, NJ) with type I DNAse (0.1 mg/ml; Sigma

Aldrich). DLN (upper paratracheal and parathymic) were pooled separately from the same groups of mice, finely chopped with a scalpel, and digested with type IV collagenase and type I DNAse. All digestions and washes were performed in glucose sodium potassium buffer (11 mM D-glucose, 5.5 mM KCl, 137 mM NaCl, 25 mM Na_2HPO_4, 5.5 mM $NaH_2PO_4.2H_2O$) with debris and RBCs removed as previously described [51].

Analysis of Cell Surface Markers by Flow Cytometry

After preparation of single-cell suspensions, FcR were routinely blocked using 2.4G2 (BD Biosciences) for 10 min on ice to prevent non-specific binding of phenotyping antibodies subsequently added. Airway, lung and draining lymph node DC populations were identified in tracheal digests using combinations of fluorochrome labelled mAbs (all from BD Biosciences, NSW, Australia except where indicated) to mouse CD11c (clone N418), I-A/I-E (clone 2G9), CD205 (DEC205; Serotec, Oxford, UK), CD11b (clone M1/70), CD40 (clone 3/23), CD80 (clone 16-10A1) and CD86 (clone GL1). All labelling was performed in glucose sodium potassium buffer containing 0.2% BSA for 30 min on ice. All Abs were used as direct conjugates to FITC, Phycoerythrin (PE), PE-Cy7, allophycocyanin (APC), APC-Cy7, or biotin as required. Where appropriate, biotinylated antibodies were detected with Streptavidin conjugated PE-Cy5 (BD Biosciences). Appropriately matched and conjugated IgG isotype controls (BD Biosciences) were used in all experiments, and cytometer compensation settings were adjusted using single-stained controls for each experiment. Samples were collected using a FACSCalibur or LSRII flow cytometer (BD Biosciences) and analyzed using FlowJo software (TreeStar, Ca, USA).

Determination of Total Cell Counts

Total counts for AMDC, PLDC and PLMac were determined on the basis of tissue weight and total cell yield for each tissue (trachea and peripheral lung), and then calculated on the basis of the total percentage of each DC type as determined by FACS. Values are expresses as number of cells/g tissue according to the formula: (% frequency x total cells/g tissue)/100.

Statistical Analysis

Two-tailed, unpaired Student's t tests assuming equal variance were employed to calculate significances (GraphPad Prism, CA, USA), with *p*-values <0.05 considered statistically significant. Statistical significance is indicated as follows: * = $p<0.05$; ** = $p<0.01$; *** = $p<0.001$; **** = $p<0.0001$.

Supporting Information

Figure S1 CD205 and CD11c staining of respiratory tissues. Tracheal (A) and parenchymal lung tissue (B and C) cells were prepared as per Methods, labelled for CD11c and CD205 and analysed by flow cytometry at the indicated time points after IAV infection. Representative dot plots of 3 experiments for each time point are shown, with AMDC (A), PLDC (B) and PLMac (C) gated as indicated.

Figure S2 Expression levels of co-stimulatory markers on AMDC and PLDC at d4 post-IAV infection. Adult BALB/c mice were infected with IAV and 4 days later (representing a time point of peak expression of each marker) tracheal and lung tissue were prepared for flow cytometry analysis for each marker on AMDC (A) and PLDC (B). Representative histograms (of 3 experiments) are shown for control and IAV infected mice, showing isotype controls (grey shaded) and specific marker (solid black) expression.

Figure S3 Changes in MHC Class II (I-A/E) expression on respiratory APC of adult mice following IAV infection at 4 weeks of age. Mice were infected with IAV at 4 weeks of age and respiratory tissue harvested 35 days later. The mean fluorescence intensity (MFI) of I-A/E expression on AMDC (A), PLDC (B) and PLMac (C) was then determined for IAV infected mice (black line) and control mice (grey shade), and expressed as a percentage change in MFI of IAV infected mice as compared to control mice (D). Histograms are representative of 4 independent experiments using pooled tissue from 5 mice in each, gated on DC populations as shown in Fig. S1. Panel D shows cumulative data of 4 independent experiments using pools of tissue from 5 mice in each experiment.

Acknowledgments

We thank Miranda Smith, Elizabeth Bozanich, Jenny Thomas, Siew Ping Lau and Sylvia Napoli for their excellent technical assistance during this study.

Author Contributions

Conceived and designed the experiments: PAS DHS CvG VF PGH GZ ANL. Performed the experiments: VF SS MEW GZ ANL CB. Analyzed the data: PAS DHS CvG MEW GZ VF SS CB. Contributed reagents/materials/analysis tools: PAS DHS CB GZ ANL. Wrote the paper: PAS DHS CvG VF MEW GZ.

References

1. Gern JE (2008) Viral respiratory infection and the link to asthma. Pediatr Infect Dis J 27: S97–103.
2. Iwane MK, Edwards KM, Szilagyi PG, Walker FJ, Griffin MR, et al. (2004) Population-based surveillance for hospitalizations associated with respiratory syncytial virus, influenza virus, and parainfluenza viruses among young children. Pediatrics 113: 1758–1764.
3. Kusel MM, de Klerk NH, Kebadze T, Vohma V, Holt PG, et al. (2007) Early-life respiratory viral infections, atopic sensitization, and risk of subsequent development of persistent asthma. J Allergy Clin Immunol 119: 1105–1110.
4. Lemanske RF Jr, Jackson DJ, Gangnon RE, Evans MD, Li Z, et al. (2005) Rhinovirus illnesses during infancy predict subsequent childhood wheezing. J Allergy Clin Immunol 116: 571–577.
5. Sigurs N, Gustafsson PM, Bjarnason R, Lundberg F, Schmidt S, et al. (2005) Severe respiratory syncytial virus bronchiolitis in infancy and asthma and allergy at age 13. Am J Respir Crit Care Med 171: 137–141.
6. Stein RT, Sherrill D, Morgan WJ, Holberg CJ, Halonen M, et al. (1999) Respiratory syncytial virus in early life and risk of wheeze and allergy by age 13 years. Lancet 354: 541–545.
7. Al-Garawi AA, Fattouh R, Walker TD, Jamula EB, Botelho F, et al. (2009) Acute, but not resolved, influenza A infection enhances susceptibility to house dust mite-induced allergic disease. J Immunol 182: 3095–3104.
8. Tsitoura DC, Kim S, Dabbagh K, Berry G, Lewis DB, et al. (2000) Respiratory infection with influenza A virus interferes with the induction of tolerance to aeroallergens. J Immunol 165: 3484–3491.
9. Holt P, Strickland D, Wikström M, Jahnsen F (2008) Regulation of immunological homeostasis in the respiratory tract. Nature reviews Immunology 8: 142–194.
10. McWilliam AS, Marsh AM, Holt PG (1997) Inflammatory infiltration of the upper airway epithelium during Sendai virus infection: involvement of epithelial dendritic cells. J Virol 71: 226–236.
11. Beyer M, Bartz H, Horner K, Doths S, Koerner-Rettberg C, et al. (2004) Sustained increases in numbers of pulmonary dendritic cells after respiratory syncytial virus infection. J Allergy Clin Immunol 113: 127–133.
12. Gill MA, Palucka AK, Barton T, Ghaffar F, Jafri H, et al. (2005) Mobilization of plasmacytoid and myeloid dendritic cells to mucosal sites in children with respiratory syncytial virus and other viral respiratory infections. J Infect Dis 191: 1105–1115.

13. Stumbles PA, Thomas JA, Pimm CL, Lee PT, Venaille TJ, et al. (1998) Resting respiratory tract dendritic cells preferentially stimulate T helper cell type 2 (Th2) responses and require obligatory cytokine signals for induction of Th1 immunity. J Exp Med 188: 2019–2031.
14. Lambrecht B, Hammad H (2010) The role of dendritic and epithelial cells as master regulators of allergic airway inflammation. Lancet 376: 835–878.
15. von Garnier C, Filgueira L, Wikström M, Smith M, Thomas JA, et al. (2005) Anatomical location determines the distribution and function of dendritic cells and other APCs in the respiratory tract. J Immunol 175: 1609–1618.
16. von Garnier C, Wikstrom ME, Zosky G, Turner DJ, Sly PD, et al. (2007) Allergic airways disease develops after an increase in allergen capture and processing in the airway mucosa. J Immunol 179: 5748–5759.
17. McWilliam AS, Napoli S, Marsh AM, Pemper FL, Nelson DJ, et al. (1996) Dendritic cells are recruited into the airway epithelium during the inflammatory response to a broad spectrum of stimuli. J Exp Med 184: 2429–2432.
18. Stumbles PA, Strickland DH, Pimm CL, Proksch SF, Marsh AM, et al. (2001) Regulation of dendritic cell recruitment into resting and inflamed airway epithelium: use of alternative chemokine receptors as a function of inducing stimulus. J Immunol 167: 228–234.
19. Wikstrom M, Stumbles P (2007) Mouse respiratory tract dendritic cell subsets and the immunological fate of inhaled antigens. Immunology and cell biology 85: 182–190.
20. Heath W, Carbone F (2009) Dendritic cell subsets in primary and secondary T cell responses at body surfaces. Nature immunology 10: 1237–1281.
21. Miller J, Brown B, Shay T, Gautier E, Jojic V, et al. (2012) Deciphering the transcriptional network of the dendritic cell lineage. Nature immunology 13: 888–899.
22. Beaty SR, Rose CE Jr, Sung SS (2007) Diverse and potent chemokine production by lung CD11b^{high} dendritic cells in homeostasis and in allergic lung inflammation. J Immunol 178: 1882–1895.
23. Sung SS, Fu SM, Rose CE Jr, Gaskin F, Ju ST, et al. (2006) A major lung CD103 (alphaE)-beta7 integrin-positive epithelial dendritic cell population expressing Langerin and tight junction proteins. J Immunol 176: 2161–2172.
24. Moltedo B, Li W, Yount J, Moran T (2011) Unique type I interferon responses determine the functional fate of migratory lung dendritic cells during influenza virus infection. PLoS pathogens 7(11): e1002345.
25. Ho AW, Prabhu N, Betts RJ, Ge MQ, Dai X, et al. (2011) Lung CD103^{+} dendritic cells efficiently transport influenza virus to the lymph node and load viral antigen onto MHC class I for presentation to CD8 T cells. J Immunol 187: 6011–6021.
26. Kim TS, Braciale TJ (2009) Respiratory dendritic cell subsets differ in their capacity to support the induction of virus-specific cytotoxic CD8^{+} T cell responses. PLoS One 4: e4204.
27. GeurtsvanKessel CH, Willart MA, van Rijt LS, Muskens F, Kool M, et al. (2008) Clearance of influenza virus from the lung depends on migratory langerin^{+} CD11b^{-} but not plasmacytoid dendritic cells. J Exp Med 205: 1621–1634.
28. Ingulli E, Funatake C, Jacovetty EL, Zanetti M (2009) Cutting edge: antigen presentation to CD8 T cells after influenza A virus infection. J Immunol 182: 29–33.
29. Belz G, Smith C, Kleinert L, Reading P, Brooks A, et al. (2004) Distinct migrating and nonmigrating dendritic cell populations are involved in MHC class I-restricted antigen presentation after lung infection with virus. Proceedings of the National Academy of Sciences of the United States of America 101: 8670–8675.
30. Fear VS, Burchell JT, Lai SP, Wikstrom ME, Blank F, et al. (2011) Restricted aeroallergen access to airway mucosal dendritic cells in vivo limits allergen-specific CD4^{+} T cell proliferation during the induction of inhalation tolerance. J Immunol 187: 4561–4570.
31. Bozanich EM, Gualano RC, Zosky GR, Larcombe AN, Turner DJ, et al. (2008) Acute Influenza A infection induces bronchial hyper-responsiveness in mice. Respir Physiol Neurobiol 162: 190–196.
32. Eyles JL, Roberts AW, Metcalf D, Wicks IP (2006) Granulocyte colony-stimulating factor and neutrophils forgotten mediators of inflammatory disease. Nat Clin Pract Rheumatol 2: 500–510.
33. Narasaraju T, Yang E, Samy RP, Ng HH, Poh WP, et al. (2011) Excessive neutrophils and neutrophil extracellular traps contribute to acute lung injury of influenza pneumonitis. Am J Pathol 179: 199–210.
34. Snelgrove R, Goulding J, Didierlaurent A, Lyonga D, Vekaria S, et al. (2008) A critical function for CD200 in lung immune homeostasis and the severity of influenza infection. Nature immunology 9: 1074–1083.
35. Sterk P (1993) Virus-induced airway hyperresponsiveness in man. The European respiratory journal 6: 894–902.
36. Yoo J-K, Kim T, Hufford M, Braciale T (2013) Viral infection of the lung: Host response and sequelae. The Journal of allergy and clinical immunology 132: 1263–1276.
37. Legge KL, Braciale TJ (2003) Accelerated migration of respiratory dendritic cells to the regional lymph nodes is limited to the early phase of pulmonary infection. Immunity 18: 265–277.
38. Lin KL, Suzuki Y, Nakano H, Ramsburg E, Gunn MD (2008) CCR2^{+} monocyte-derived dendritic cells and exudate macrophages produce influenza-induced pulmonary immune pathology and mortality. J Immunol 180: 2562–2572.
39. Brimnes MK, Bonifaz L, Steinman RM, Moran TM (2003) Influenza Virus-induced Dendritic Cell Maturation Is Associated with the Induction of Strong T Cell Immunity to a Coadministered, Normally Nonimmunogenic Protein. J Exp Med 198: 133–144.
40. Dahl M, Dabbagh K, Liggitt D, Kim S, Lewis D (2004) Viral-induced T helper type 1 responses enhance allergic disease by effects on lung dendritic cells. Nature immunology 5: 337–343.
41. Suzuki S, Suzuki Y, Yamamoto N, Matsumoto Y, Shirai A, et al. (1998) Influenza A virus infection increases IgE production and airway responsiveness in aerosolized antigen-exposed mice. The Journal of allergy and clinical immunology 102: 732–740.
42. Ichinohe T, Lee HK, Ogura Y, Flavell R, Iwasaki A (2009) Inflammasome recognition of influenza virus is essential for adaptive immune responses. J Exp Med 206: 79–87.
43. Bilyk N, Holt PG (1993) Inhibition of the immunosuppressive activity of resident pulmonary alveolar macrophages by granulocyte/macrophage colony-stimulating factor. J Exp Med 177: 1773–1777.
44. Julia V, Hessel E, Malherbe L, Glaichenhaus N, O'Garra A, et al. (2002) A restricted subset of dendritic cells captures airborne antigens and remains able to activate specific T cells long after antigen exposure. Immunity 16: 271–283.
45. Southam DS, Dolovich M, O'Byrne PM, Inman MD (2002) Distribution of intranasal instillations in mice: effects of volume, time, body position, and anesthesia. Am J Physiol Lung Cell Mol Physiol 282: L833–839.
46. Zosky GR, von Garnier C, Stumbles PA, Holt PG, Sly PD, et al. (2004) The pattern of methacholine responsiveness in mice is dependent on antigen challenge dose. Respir Res 5: 15.
47. Cull V, Bartlett E, James C (2002) Type I interferon gene therapy protects against cytomegalovirus-induced myocarditis. Immunology 106: 428–437.
48. Hantos Z, Collins RA, Turner DJ, Janosi TZ, Sly PD (2003) Tracking of airway and tissue mechanics during TLC maneuvers in mice. J Appl Physiol 95: 1695–1705.
49. Hantos Z, Daroczy B, Suki B, Nagy S, Fredberg JJ (1992) Input impedance and peripheral inhomogeneity of dog lungs. J Appl Physiol 72: 168–178.
50. Stumbles P, Strickland D, Wikstrom M, Thomas J, von Garnier C, et al. (2010) Identification and isolation of rodent respiratory tract dendritic cells. Methods in molecular biology.pp. 249–312.
51. Wikstrom ME, Batanero E, Smith M, Thomas JA, von Garnier C, et al. (2006) Influence of mucosal adjuvants on antigen passage and CD4^{+} T cell activation during the primary response to airborne allergen. J Immunol 177: 913–924.

13

CD26/DPP4 Cell-Surface Expression in Bat Cells Correlates with Bat Cell Susceptibility to Middle East Respiratory Syndrome Coronavirus (MERS-CoV) Infection and Evolution of Persistent Infection

Yíngyún Caì[1], Shuǐqìng Yú[1], Elena N. Postnikova[1], Steven Mazur[1], John G. Bernbaum[1], Robin Burk[1], Téngfēi Zhāng[1], Sheli R. Radoshitzky[2], Marcel A. Müller[3], Ingo Jordan[4], Laura Bollinger[1], Lisa E. Hensley[1], Peter B. Jahrling[1], Jens H. Kuhn[1]*

1 Integrated Research Facility at Fort Detrick, National Institute of Allergy and Infectious Diseases, National Institutes of Health, Fort Detrick, Frederick, Maryland, United States of America, **2** United States Army Medical Research Institute of Infectious Diseases, Fort Detrick, Frederick, Maryland, United States of America, **3** Institute of Virology, University of Bonn Medical Centre, Bonn, Germany, **4** ProBioGen AG, Berlin, Germany

Abstract

Middle East respiratory syndrome coronavirus (MERS-CoV) is a recently isolated betacoronavirus identified as the etiologic agent of a frequently fatal disease in Western Asia, Middle East respiratory syndrome. Attempts to identify the natural reservoirs of MERS-CoV have focused in part on dromedaries. Bats are also suspected to be reservoirs based on frequent detection of other betacoronaviruses in these mammals. For this study, ten distinct cell lines derived from bats of divergent species were exposed to MERS-CoV. Plaque assays, immunofluorescence assays, and transmission electron microscopy confirmed that six bat cell lines can be productively infected. We found that the susceptibility or resistance of these bat cell lines directly correlates with the presence or absence of cell surface-expressed CD26/DPP4, the functional human receptor for MERS-CoV. Human anti-CD26/DPP4 antibodies inhibited infection of susceptible bat cells in a dose-dependent manner. Overexpression of human CD26/DPP4 receptor conferred MERS-CoV susceptibility to resistant bat cell lines. Finally, sequential passage of MERS-CoV in permissive bat cells established persistent infection with concomitant downregulation of CD26/DPP4 surface expression. Together, these results imply that bats indeed could be among the MERS-CoV host spectrum, and that cellular restriction of MERS-CoV is determined by CD26/DPP4 expression rather than by downstream restriction factors.

Editor: Krzysztof Pyrc, Faculty of Biochemistry Biophysics and Biotechnology, Jagiellonian University, Poland

Funding: YC, SY, ENP, SM, RB, TZ, LB, and JHK performed this work for the US Department of Health and Human Services under contract number HHSN272200700016I (Battelle Memorial Institute). RB was supported by the Hartmut Hoffmann-Berling International Graduate School of Molecular & Cellular Biology (HBIGS), Heidelberg, Germany. The funders had no role in study design, data collection and analysis, decision to publish, or preparation of the manuscript.

Competing Interests: Dr. Ingo Jordan is employed by ProBioGen and is an author on patent application WO 2009/109377 A1 covering also the R05T and R06E cell lines. Both cell lines are freely available for research without restrictions.

* Email: kuhnjens@mail.nih.gov

Introduction

In 2012, a novel human coronavirus causing frequently fatal disease emerged in Western Asia [1] and was named "Middle East respiratory syndrome coronavirus (MERS-CoV)" [2]. As of June 11, 2014, MERS-CoV caused 699 laboratory-confirmed human infections in 21 countries, including 209 deaths (proportion of fatal cases ≈29.9%) [3]. Increasing evidence points to dromedaries (*Camelus dromedarius*) as an intermediate reservoir contributing to the emergence of Middle East respiratory syndrome (MERS) in humans. Several seroepidemiology studies have found MERS-CoV-neutralizing antibodies in dromedaries from Egypt, Jordan, Oman, and Saudi Arabia [4–9]. More recently, coronaviral genomes detected in nasal swabs obtained from dromedaries proved to be identical to genomes of human MERS-CoV isolates [4,5,9]. One such genome was detected in a patient who had been caring for a sick dromedary and directly from that animal [10]. In addition, MERS-CoV was directly isolated from a dromedary in Qatar [11].

The source of dromedary MERS-CoV infection remains to be elucidated, but it is not unlikely that they serve only as intermediary hosts [12]. Bats have been proposed as additional MERS-CoV hosts. This hypothesis is based on the fact that several betacoronaviruses related to MERS-CoV (e.g., severe acute respiratory syndrome-like coronaviruses, Tylonycteris bat coronavirus HKU4, Pipistrellus bat coronavirus HKU5) are known to infect bats in Africa, Europe, and Asia [1,13–16]. In addition, MERS-CoV genome fragments encoding parts of the RNA-dependent RNA polymerase were detected in one Egyptian tomb bat (*Taphozous perforates*) living close to a MERS-CoV-infected patient [14]. Finally, a novel coronavirus (NeoCoV) closely related to MERS-CoV was discovered in cape serotines (*Neoromicia capensis*) in South Africa [12]. Therefore, bats could possibly maintain MERS-CoV in nature and may occasionally infect dromedaries and thereby may infect humans similar to the bats-horse-human or bats-pig-human transmission cycle observed for henipaviruses [17,18].

Recently, CD26, also known as dipeptidyl peptidase 4 (DPP4) was identified as the human MERS-CoV cell entry receptor [19] and also as a receptor for Tylonycteris bat coronavirus HKU4 [20,21]. CD26/DPP4 receptor is conserved among different mammals (e.g., bats, dromedaries, humans), and the possibly broad species tropism of MERS-CoV may partly be the result of this conservation [19,22].

To further evaluate the hypothesis that bats may be implicated in transmission of the virus, we inoculated ten cell lines from phylogenetically diverse bats living in geographically distinct areas with MERS-CoV. Six bat cell lines were productively infected. The susceptibility or resistance of the ten cell lines to MERS-CoV infection directly correlated with the absence or presence of naturally expressed CD26/DPP4 on the cells surface. Anti-human CD26/DPP4 antibodies reduced MERS-CoV yield in susceptible bat cell cultures in a dose-dependent manner. Similar to other studies using MERS-CoV-resistant (non-bat) cell lines transfected with CD26/DPP4 [19], expression of human CD26/DPP4 in resistant bat cells rendered these cell lines susceptible to infection. Finally, we demonstrate that persistent MERS-CoV infections can be established in permissive bat cell lines after sequential virus passage, leading to downregulation of natural CD26/DPP4 cell-surface expression. Together, our data indicate that the host cell tropism of MERS-CoV may largely depend on the expression of suitable CD26/DPP4 orthologs, and that bats cannot be excluded as MERS-CoV reservoirs at this point in time.

Materials and Methods

Cell lines

Huh-7 (a kind gift from Hideki Ebihara, Rocky Mountain Laboratory, Hamilton, MT), Vero E6 (ATCC, #CRL-1568, Manassas, VA), and Vero (ATCC, #CCL-81) cells were grown in Dulbecco's modified Eagle's medium (DMEM) supplemented with 10% heat-inactivated fetal bovine serum (FBS, Sigma-Aldrich, St. Louis, MO). The bat cell lines used in this study are described in Table 1. R05T, R06E, and HypNi/1.1 cell lines were grown in DMEM/F-12 (Lonza, Walkersville, MD) supplemented with 10% FBS. All others bat cell lines were maintained in DMEM supplemented with 10% FBS. All cells were incubated at 37°C in a humidified 5% CO_2 atmosphere.

Virus propagation

Middle East respiratory syndrome coronavirus isolate HCoV-EMC/2012 (MERS-CoV/EMC) was kindly provided by the Department of Viroscience Lab, Erasmus University Medical Center, Rotterdam, NL. MERS-CoV isolate Hu/Jordan-N3/2012 (MERS-CoV/Jor) was kindly provided by Drs. Kanta Subbarao (National Institutes of Health, Bethesda, MD) and Gabriel Defang (Naval Medical Research Unit-3, Cairo, EG). Both viruses were propagated in Vero E6 cells at a multiplicity of infection (MOI) of 0.01 in DMEM supplemented with 2% FBS. The viruses were titrated on Vero cells by plaque assay.

Infection of bat cell lines

Bat cell lines were seeded in collagen-coated 24-well plates (Becton Dickinson Labware, Bedford, MA) at 2×10^5 cells/well. One day later, media were removed, and cells were washed once with DMEM without FBS (0% DMEM). Cells were then exposed to MERS-CoV/EMC or MERS-CoV/Jor at an MOI of 1. After 1 h of incubation at 37°C, viral inocula were removed and cells were washed once with 0% DMEM and then supplemented with DMEM containing 2% FBS (2% DMEM). At 1, 3, or 5 days post-exposure, supernatants were harvested and cleared of cellular debris by centrifugation.

Plaque assay

MERS-CoV particle yields were quantified by plaque assay [23]. Briefly, confluent monolayers of Vero cells in 6-well plates were exposed to serial dilutions of MERS-CoV, incubated at 37°C for 1 h under gentle rocking every 15 min, followed by removal of inocula and addition of a 0.8% tragacanth overlay (Sigma-Aldrich, St. Louis, MO). Infected cells were then incubated at 37°C for 72 h. The tragacanth overlay was removed, and the cells were stained with 2% crystal violet (Sigma-Aldrich) in 10% neutral buffered formalin (NBF, Fisher Scientific, Kalamazoo, MI). Plaques were enumerated manually.

CD26/DPP4 antibody inhibition assay

RoNi/7.1 or Huh-7 cells were incubated with different concentrations (0, 1.25, 2.5, 5, 10, 20 μg/ml) of goat anti-human CD26/DPP4 antibody (R&D Systems, Minneapolis, MN) or control goat IgG antibody at 37°C for 1 h. Antibody-treated cells were exposed to MERS-CoV/EMC at an MOI of 1 at 37°C for 1 h in the presence of antibodies. Virus-antibody inocula were then removed, cells were washed in 0% DMEM, fresh DMEM (2% FBS) was added, supernatants were harvested 24 h post-exposure, and viral yields were determined by plaque assay. At the same time, plates were fixed with 10% NBF and then stained with rabbit polyclonal anti-MERS-CoV spike protein antibody (Sino Biological, Beijing, China) followed by secondary Alexa Fluor 488-conjugated goat anti-rabbit IgG antibody (Life Technologies, Carlsbad, CA). Hoechst 33342 dye was used to stain nuclei. The percentage of infected cells was measured and analyzed using the Operetta high content imaging system (PerkinElmer Waltham, MA) and analysis software (Harmony 3.1).

Flow cytometry

Bat cells were washed with phosphate-buffered saline (PBS) and then dissociated with cell dissociation buffer (Life Technologies). Cells were spun down, washed, and resuspended in 4% paraformaldehyde for fixation. Cells were stained with goat anti-human CD26/DPP4 antibody followed by Alex Fluor 488-conjugated rabbit anti-goat IgG antibody. As a control, the cells were stained with the same concentration of isotype control goat IgG antibody followed by the same secondary antibody. Samples were collected using an LSR Fortessa flow cytometer (BD Biosciences, San Jose, CA). FlowJo software version 9.7.5 (TreeStar, Ashland, OR) was used to analyze the data.

Transmission electron microscopy

Confluent bat cells were inoculated with MERS-CoV/EMC at an MOI of 1 for 1 h at 37°C. After viral inocula were removed, cells were washed once with 0% DMEM and then supplemented with 2% DMEM. Media were removed 24 h later, and electron microscopy grade fixative, 2.5% glutaraldehyde (E.M. Sciences, Warrington, PA) in Millonig's sodium phosphate buffer (Tousimis

Table 1. Origin of tested bat cell lines.

Bat cell line [reference]	Origin	Type of bat	Geographic distribution of bat (according to http://www.iucnredlist.org)
EidNi/41.3 [35]	African straw-colored fruit bat (*Eidolon helvum*) adult kidney	pteropid (frugivorous)	Angola; Benin; Botswana; Burkina Faso; Burundi; Cameroon; Central African Republic; Chad; Côte d'Ivoire; Democratic Republic of the Congo; Equatorial Guinea; Ethiopia; Gabon; Gambia; Ghana; Guinea; Guinea-Bissau; Kenya; Lesotho; Liberia; Malawi; Mali; Mauritania; Mozambique; Namibia; Niger; Nigeria; Republic of Congo; Rwanda; Sao Tomé and Principe; **Saudi Arabia**[a]; Senegal; Sierra Leone; South Africa; South Sudan; Sudan; Swaziland; Tanzania; Togo; Uganda; **Yemen**; Zambia; Zimbabwe
EpoNi/22.1 [36]	Büttikofer's epauletted fruit bat (*Epomops buettikoferi*) adult kidney	pteropid (frugivorous)	Côte d'Ivoire; Ghana; Guinea; Guinea-Bissau; Liberia; Nigeria; Senegal; Sierra Leone
HypLu/45.1 [36]	hammer-headed fruit bat (*Hypsignathus monstrosus*) fetal lung	pteropid (frugivorous)	Angola; Benin; Burkina Faso; Cameroon; Central African Republic; Côte d'Ivoire; Democratic Republic of the Congo; Equatorial Guinea; Ethiopia; Gabon; Ghana; Guinea; Guinea-Bissau; Kenya; Liberia; Nigeria; Republic of the Congo; Sierra Leone; South Sudan; Togo; Uganda
HypNi/1.1 [36]	hammer-headed fruit bat (*Hypsignathus monstrosus*) fetal kidney	pteropid (frugivorous)	See HypLu/45.1
PESU-B5L [37]	eastern pipistrelle (*Pipistrellus subflavus*) adult lung	vespertilionid (insectivorous)	Belize; Canada; Guatemala; Honduras; Mexico; United States
R05T [38]	Egyptian rousette (*Rousettus aegyptiacus*) embryo	pteropid (frugivorous)	Angola; Burundi; Cameroon; Côte d'Ivoire; Cyprus; Democratic Republic of the Congo; **Egypt**; Equatorial Guinea; Eritrea; Ethiopia; Gabon; Gambia; Ghana; Guinea; **Iran**; Israel; **Jordan**; Kenya; **Lebanon**; Lesotho; Liberia; Libya; Malawi; Mozambique; Nigeria; **Oman**; Pakistan; Republic of the Congo; Rwanda; Sao Tomé and Principe; **Saudi Arabia**; Senegal; Sierra Leone; South Africa; South Sudan; Sudan; Syrian Arab Republic; Tanzania; Togo; Turkey; Uganda; **United Arab Emirates**; **Yemen**; Zambia; Zimbabwe
R06E [38]	Egyptian rousette (*Rousettus aegyptiacus*) embryo	pteropid (frugivorous)	See R05T
RoNi/7.1 [36]	Egyptian rousette (*Rousettus aegyptiacus*) adult kidney	pteropid (frugivorous)	See R05T
RoNi/7.2 - subclone of RoNi/7 used in [39]	Egyptian rousette (*Rousettus aegyptiacus*) adult kidney	pteropid (frugivorous)	See R05T
Tb1Lu [ATCC (#CCL-88)]	Brazilian free-tailed bat (*Tadarida brasiliensis*) adult lung	molossid (insectivorous)	Anguilla; Antigua and Barbuda; Argentina; Aruba; Barbados; Bolivia; Bonaire, Sint Eustatius and Saba; Brazil; Chile; Colombia; Costa Rica; Cuba; Dominica; Dominican Republic; Ecuador; El Salvador; French Guiana; Grenada; Guadeloupe; Guatemala; Guyana; Haiti; Honduras; Jamaica; Martinique; Mexico; Montserrat; Panama; Peru; Puerto Rico; Saint Kitts and Nevis; Saint Lucia; Saint Martin (French part); Saint Vincent and the Grenadines; Sint Maarten (Dutch part); Suriname; Trinidad and Tobago; United States; Venezuela; Virgin Islands

[a]Western Asian and Northern African countries in which MERS cases have been documented are printed in bold.

Research, Rockville, MD), was added directly to the dishes. After 10 min, bat cells were scraped off the dishes with a cell scraper, collected into 15-ml tubes, and immediately centrifuged at 500×*g* for 20 min. To complete fixation, cells were kept in fixative for 24 h at 4°C and were post-fixed in 1% osmium tetroxide (Electron Microscopy Sciences, Hatfield, PA). Post-fixed cells were stained *en bloc* with 2% uranyl acetate, dehydrated in a series of graded ethanols, and infiltrated and embedded in Spurr plastic resin (Electron Microscopy Sciences). A Leica EM UC7 ultramicrotome (Leica Microsystems, Buffalo Grove, IL) was used to section the embedded blocks into ultra-thin sections (60–80 nm). These sections were collected, mounted on 200-mesh copper grids (Electron Microscopy Sciences), and contrasted with Reynold's lead citrate. A FEI G2 Tecnai transmission electron microscope (FEI, Hillsboro, OR), operating at 80 kV, was used to examine and image the grids.

CD26 overexpression experiments

MERS-CoV-resistant PESU-B5L, R05T, R06E, or Tb1Lu or MERS-CoV-susceptible EidNi/41.3, EpoNi/22.1, HypLu/45.1, HypNi/1.1, RoNi/7.1, RoNi/7.2, or Vero E6 cells were transfected with a plasmid expressing human CD26/DPP4 (pCMV-xL-hDPP4, Origene Technologies, Rockville, MD) or control plasmid pcDNA3.1+ (Life Technologies) by Effectene (Qiagen, Frederick, MD) or Lipofectamine 3000 (Life Technologies) according to the manufacturer's instruction. At 24 h or 48 h post transfection, cells were washed once with 0% DMEM and then inoculated with MERS-CoV/EMC at an MOI of 3. Bat cells were incubated at 37°C for 1 h with gently rocking of the plates every 15 min. At 1 h after exposure, cells were washed twice with 0% DMEM, and 0.5 ml of 2% DMEM was added. At 24 h post-exposure, supernatants were harvested for virus yield determination. Plates were fixed with 10% NBF. Plates were stained with goat anti-human CD26/DPP4 followed by Alexa Fluor 594-conjugated donkey anti-goat IgG antibody and/or polyclonal rabbit anti-MERS-CoV spike protein antibody followed by Alex

Fluor 488-conjugated chicken anti-rabbit IgG antibody (Life Technologies). Images were acquired using the Operetta high content imaging system.

Establishment of persistent MERS-CoV infection

EidNi/41.3, EpoNi/22.1, HypLu/45.1, HypNi/1.1, RoNi/7.1, RoNi/7.2, or Vero E6 cells in 75 cm^2 flasks were infected with MERS-CoV/EMC or MERS-CoV/Jor at an MOI of 1. After 7 days, supernatants were harvested for virus yield analysis by plaque assay, and the cells were subcultured at a 1:10 dilution in new flasks. Subsequently, the infected cells were passaged at a 1:10 dilution weekly for a total of nine passages. From each passage, supernatants were harvested, and virus yields were determined by plaque assay.

Western blot analysis

EidNi/41.3 cells (non-infected or persistently infected with MERS-CoV, day 63) were washed with PBS and lysed in cell lysis buffer (Cell Signaling, Danvers, MA) according to the manufacturer's instruction. Equivalent amounts of total cellular lysates were resolved in 4% to 12% bis-tris gradient gels (Life Technologies) and then dry-transferred to polyvinylidene difluoride (PVDF) membranes (Life Technologies) by using the iBlot gel transfer system (Life Technologies). After blocking in 5% nonfat milk powder in PBS with 0.1% Tween (Sigma-Aldrich), membranes were incubated overnight with goat anti-human CD26/DPP4 antibody (1:500) or anti β-actin antibody (1:500, Abcam, Cambridge, MA), followed by incubation with appropriate horseradish peroxidase-conjugated secondary antibodies (Sigma-Aldrich). Signals were detected by SuperSignal West Femto chemiluminescent substrate (Thermo Fisher Scientific, Rockford, IL), and images were acquired using a Syngene G: Box Chemiluminescence imaging system (Syngene, Frederick, MD).

Results

Six of ten tested bat cell lines are susceptible to MERS-CoV infection

As bats could be a potential reservoir for MERS-CoV, we tested the susceptibility of ten diverse bat cells lines to infection with MERS-CoV/EMC or MERS-CoV/Jor at an MOI of 1. Viral titers in cell culture supernatants were determined by plaque assay on days 0, 1, 3, and 5 post-exposure of MERS-CoV. Six out of ten cell lines (EidNi/41.3, EpoNi/22.1, HypLu/45.1, HypNi/1.1, RoNi/7.1, and RoNi/7.2) propagated MERS-CoV (Figure 1A, 1B). In some cell lines (e.g., RoNi/7.2, EidNi/41.3) virus yields reached those observed in positive control (Vero E6) cells. PESU-B5L, R05T, R06E, and Tb1Lu cell lines did not support productive MERS-CoV virus infection (Figure 1A, 1B).

These results were also confirmed by immunofluorescence assay (IFA) in cell lines inoculated with MERS-CoV/EMC (Figure 1C) or MERS-CoV/Jor (Figure 1D). Infected cells were detected by MERS-CoV spike protein IFA. Representative images were picked from those taken on day 1 or day 3 post-exposure, as cytopathic viral effects diminished immunofluorescence in some cell lines (e.g., EidNi/41.3, RoNi/7.1, RoNi/7.2 cells, Figure 1C). Images of bat cells (day 1 post-exposure) inoculated with MERS-CoV/EMC taken by a transmission electron microscope (TEM, Figure 1E) show intracellularly budding virions in the endoplasmic reticulum-Golgi intermediate compartment (ERGIC), as well as double membrane vesicles (DMVs).

Cell-surface expression of CD26/DPP4 on bat cells

To evaluate whether CD26/DPP4 expression is related to susceptibility of bat cells to MERS-CoV infection, surface expression of CD26/DPP4 was analyzed in ten bat cell lines by flow cytometry using a polyclonal anti-human CD26/DPP4 antibody. None of the four MERS-CoV-resistant cell lines tested in this study (PESU-B5L, R05T, R06E, and Tb1Lu) were recognized by anti-human CD26/DPP4 antibody in this assay, whereas all susceptible bat cells (EidNi/41.3, EpoNi/22.1, HypLu/45.1, HypNi/1.1, RoNi/7.1, and RoNi/7.2) tested positive for CD26/DPP4 expression (Figure 2).

Anti-human CD26/DPP4 antibody inhibits MERS-CoV infection in bat cells

To confirm the role of CD26/DPP4 in MERS-CoV bat cell entry, RoNi/7.1 cells or control human Huh-7 cells were incubated with increasing concentrations of a monoclonal anti-human CD26/DPP4 antibody and subsequently exposed to MERS-CoV/EMC. CD26/DPP4 antibody treatment reduced MERS-CoV particle production in both RoNi/7.1 cells and Huh-7 cells, as evidenced by a dose-dependent reduction in viral yield in plaque assays (Figure 3A). Immunofluorescent images of infected cells stained against MERS-CoV spike protein confirm these results (Figure 3B). Thus, CD26/DPP4 plays a crucial role in MERS-CoV cell entry into bat cells.

Expression of human CD26/DPP4 confers MERS-CoV susceptibility to otherwise resistant bat cells

To test the hypothesis whether CD26/DPP4 alone determines bat cell susceptibility to MERS-CoV infection, we transfected MERS-CoV-resistant bat cell lines (PESU-B5L, R05T, R06E, TblLu) with a human CD26/DPP4 expression plasmid and then inoculated the cells with MERS-CoV. Transient expression of human CD26/DPP4 in these bat cell lines supported MERS-CoV replication as evidenced by increased viral yields compared to those measured in the same cell line transfected with empty control plasmid (Figure 4A). These results were confirmed by IFA using the same cells stained against MERS-CoV spike protein or CD26/DPP4 (Figure 4B). The merged immunofluorescent images clearly indicate the colocalization of MERS-CoV spike protein and CD26/DPP4 (Figure 4C). Thus, the restriction of MERS-CoV infection in the resistant bat cell lines may be determined by the absence of CD26/DPP4. Overexpression of human CD26/DPP4 in already susceptible bat cell lines led to an increase in virus yield in some bat cell lines (EpoNi/22.1, HypLu/45.1, RoNi/7.1, RoNi/7.2) or to a decrease in virus yield in other susceptible bat cell lines (EiD/41.3, HypNi/1.1, Figure 4D).

Persistent MERS-CoV infection induces downregulation of bat cell CD26/DPP4 expression

Persistent subclinical infection in a mammalian host reservoir is a hallmark of numerous zoonotic viruses. To investigate whether MERS-CoV can establish persistent infections in bats on the cellular level, we infected susceptible bat cell lines (i.e., EidNi/41.3, EpoNi/22.1, HypLu/45.1, HypNi/1.1, RoNi/7.1, RoNi/7.2) with MERS-CoV/EMC or MERS-CoV/Jor, and serially passaged these cells weekly for a total of 9 weeks (63 days). Persistent infection, as indicated by viral yields determined by plaque assay, was achieved in EidNi/41.3, EpoNi/22.1, HypNi/1.1, and HypLu/45.1 cell lines, control Vero E6 cells inoculated with MERS-CoV/EMC (Figure 5A), and EidNi/41.3 and EpoNi/22.1 cell lines inoculated with MERS-CoV/Jor (Figure 5B). Immunofluorescent images taken on day 33 after staining

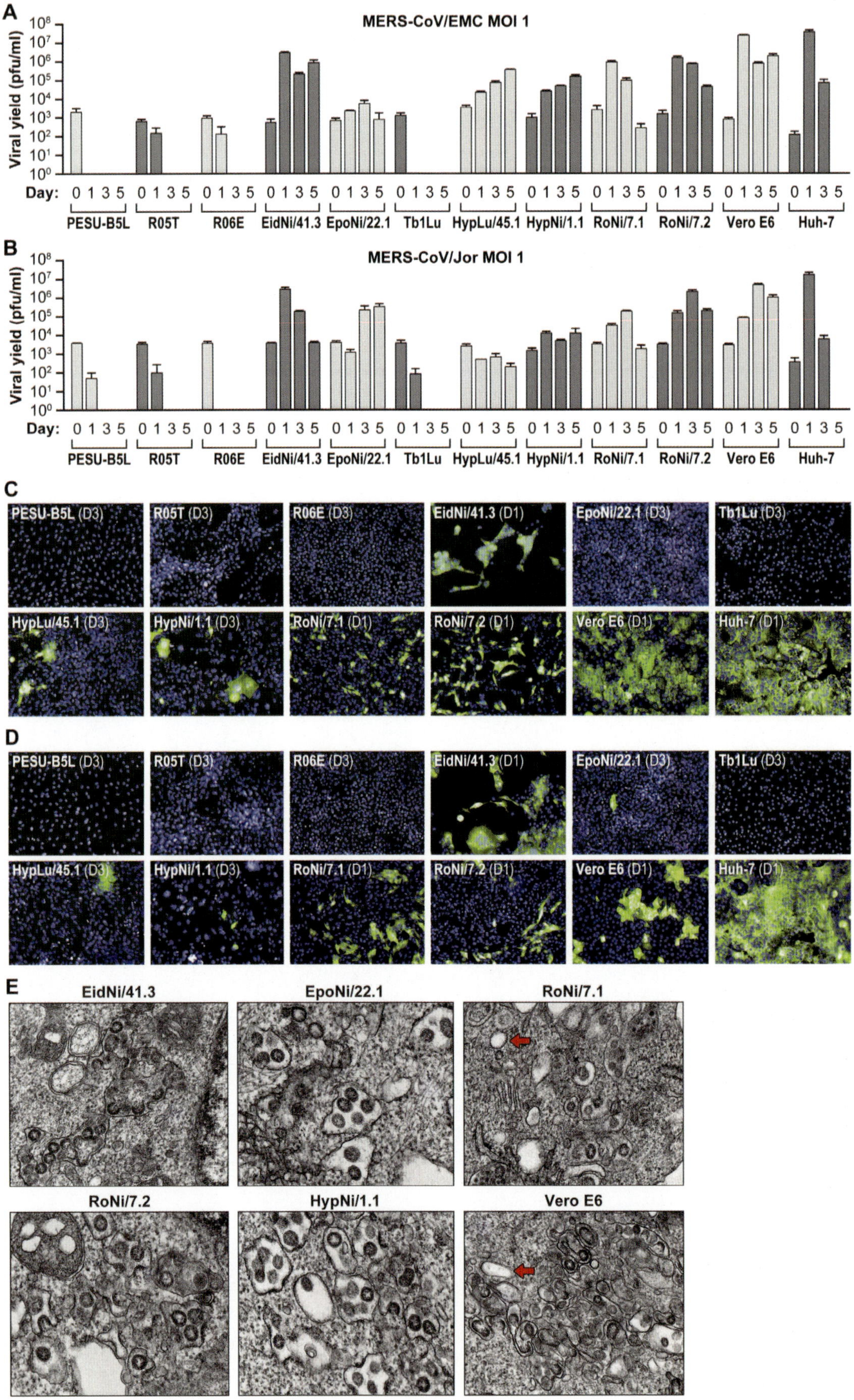
A
MERS-CoV/EMC MOI 1
Viral yield (pfu/ml)
Day: 0 1 3 5
PESU-B5L
R05T
R06E
EidNi/41.3
EpoNi/22.1
Tb1Lu
HypLu/45.1
HypNi/1.1
RoNi/7.1
RoNi/7.2
Vero E6
Huh-7
B
MERS-CoV/Jor MOI 1
C
D
E
EidNi/41.3
EpoNi/22.1
RoNi/7.1
RoNi/7.2
HypNi/1.1
Vero E6

Figure 1. Six of ten tested bat cell lines are susceptible to MERS-CoV infection. (A and B) Ten different bat cell lines were exposed to MERS-CoV/EMC (A) or MERS-CoV/Jor (B) at an MOI of 1. Supernatants were harvested at days 0, 1, 3, and 5 after virus exposure, and virus yields were determined by plaque assay on Vero cells. Error bars indicate the standard deviation of triplicate samples. (C and D) Same experiment: immunofluorescence assay (IFA) images of bat cell lines exposed to MERS-CoV/EMC (C) or MERS-CoV/Jor. (D) 1 (D1) or 3 (D3) days after virus exposure and stained against MERS-CoV spike protein (green). (E) Same experiment: TEM images of bat cells infected with MERS-CoV/EMC at day 1 after virus exposure. Red arrows point at double-membrane vesicles (DMVs) typical of coronavirus infections.

against MERS-CoV spike protein also confirm persistent infection in the same cell lines (Figure 5C, 5D). Intracellular viral particles, virion budding, and virion egress from EidNi/41.3 and EpoNi/22.1 cells and control Vero E6 cells are clearly visible on TEM images acquired at day 56 post-exposure (Figure 5E).

Flow cytometry was used to determine CD26/DPP4 cell-surface expression in EidNi/41.3 and control Vero E6 cells before virus exposure and at study endpoint (day 63) by incubation with an antibody against human CD26/DPP4 (Figure 5F). Prior to exposure of EidNi/41.3 cells to MERS-CoV, CD26/DPP4 expression (red line) was higher than that observed for isotypic IgG control (black line), confirming CD26/DPP4 cell-surface expression as shown previously (Figure 2). At day 63, CD26/DPP4 expression was nearly absent in EidNi/41.3 cells. At the same time point in control Vero E6 cells, CD26/DPP4 expression was decreased but still detected in cells inoculated with MERS-CoV/EMC, whereas surface expression of CD26/DPP4 could barely be detected in cells inoculated with MERS-CoV/Jor. Western blot analysis of EidNi/41.3 cells persistently infected with either MERS-CoV/EMC or MERS-CoV/Jor (day 63) also demonstrated no or minimal expression of CD26/DPP4 (Figure 5G).

Discussion

In vitro studies revealed that MERS-CoV can infect cell lines derived from nonhuman primates, civets, rabbits, goats, cows, sheep, chickens, and pigs, but not cell lines derived from cats, dogs, hamsters, or mice [22,24,25]. In this study, we explored the potential of bats to be a reservoir for MERS-CoV infection [13–15] by evaluating MERS-CoV infection in bat cell lines. We expanded the number of bat cell lines that are now known to be susceptible to MERS-CoV and identified several bat cell lines that are resistant to infection (Figure 1). These bat cell lines are derived from bats living in geographically disparate areas. Interestingly, bat cell lines that were susceptible to MERS-CoV infection (EidNi/41.3, EpoNi/22.1, HypLu/45.1, HypNi/1.1, RoNi/7.1, and RoNi/7.2) originated from bats found in Western Asia and

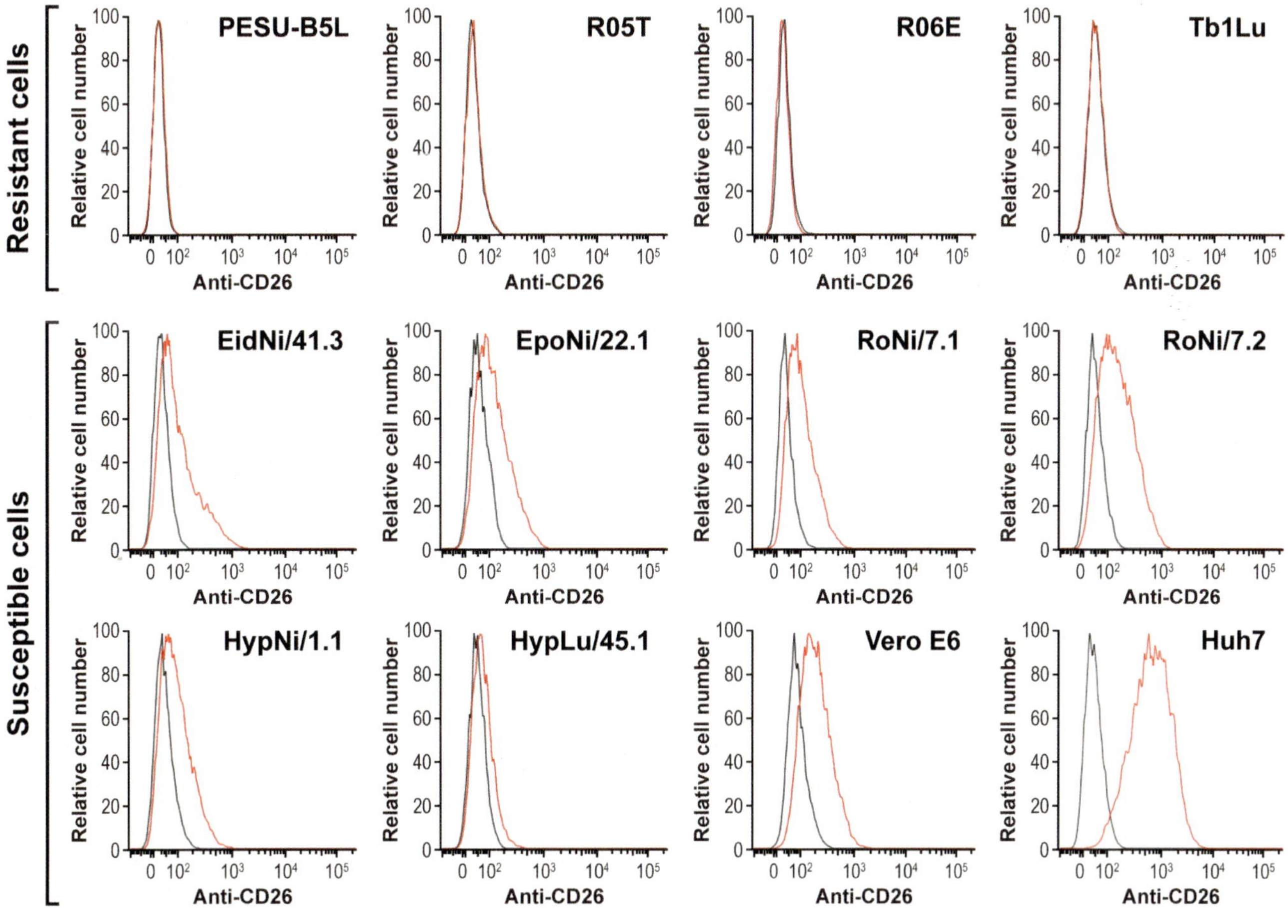

Figure 2. Cell-surface expression of CD26/DPP4 on bat cells. Cells of different bat cell lines were analyzed by flow cytometry after staining with goat anti-human DPP4/CD26 antibody (red line) or control antibody (black lines).

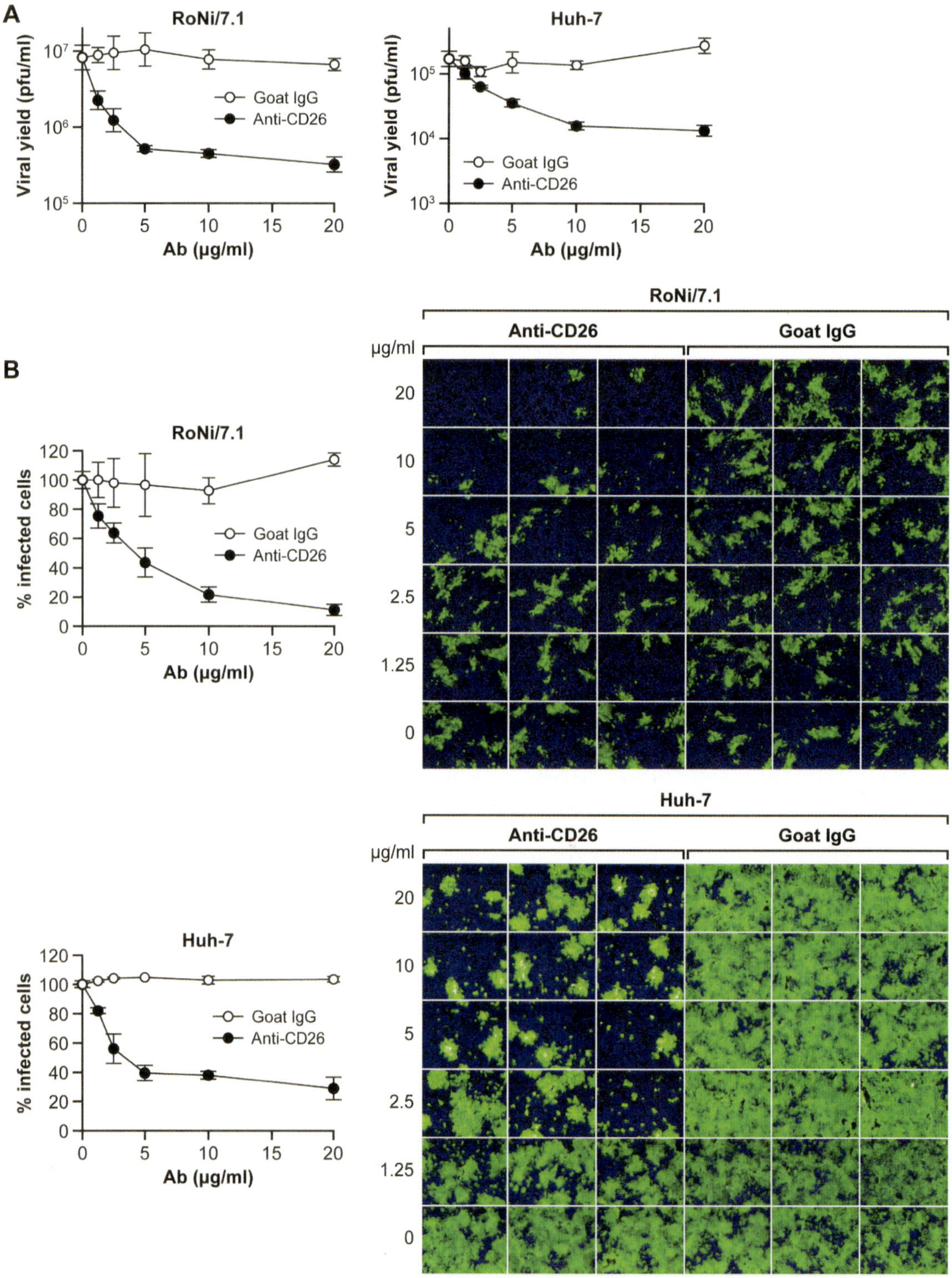

Figure 3. Anti-human CD26/DPP4 antibody inhibits MERS-CoV infection of bat cells. RoNi/7.1 or Huh-7 cells (control) were treated with increasing concentrations (0, 1.25, 2.5, 5, 10, and 20 μg/ml) of anti-human CD26/DPP4 antibody or control antibody and then exposed to MERS-CoV/EMC at an MOI of 1. (A) After 24 h, viral yields in supernatants were determined by plaque assay. (B) Cellular infection was determined by immunofluorescence assay (IFA) with an anti-MERS-CoV spike protein antibody (green). (B left) The percentage of infected cells was analyzed by high content imaging. (B right) Representative IFA images. Error bars indicate the standard deviation of triplicate samples.

Northern Africa. In these geographic areas, domestic and wild dromedaries can be found and natural human MERS-CoV infections are recorded (Table 1).

CD26/DPP4 is the cellular receptor for MERS-CoV [19]. This evolutionary conserved dimeric ectopeptidase is differentially expressed in various tissues but may not be the sole determinant for susceptibility at the organism level [25]. Importantly, cellular

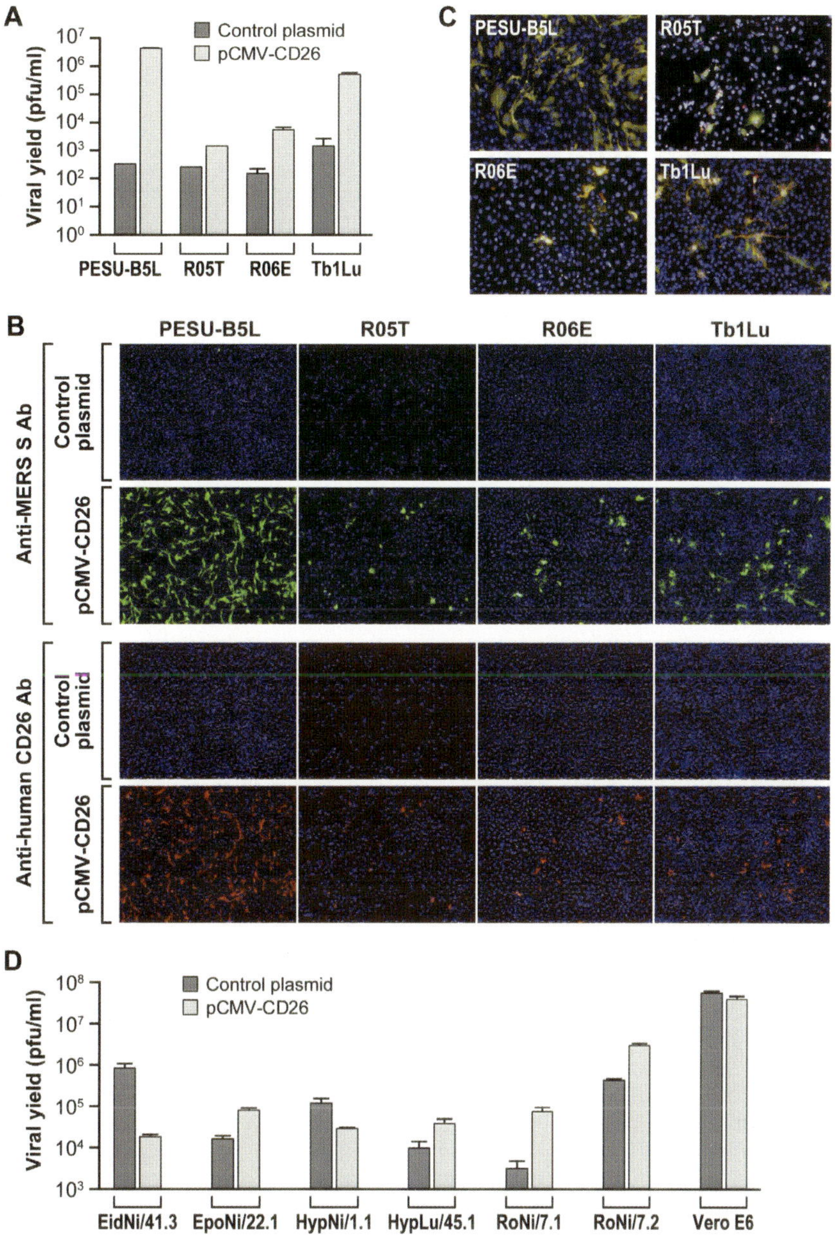

Figure 4. Expression of human CD26/DPP4 confers MERS-CoV susceptibility to otherwise resistant bat cells. (A) Viral yields from MERS-CoV-resistant PESU-B5L, R05T, R06E, and Tb1Lu bat cells. Cells were transfected with a plasmid expressing human CD26/DPP4 or empty control plasmid and exposed 48 h later to MERS-CoV/EMC at an MOI of 3. Supernatants were harvested at 24 h after virus exposure for quantification of virus yields by plaque assay. (B) Same experiment: representative immunofluorescence assay (IFA) images of cells stained with anti-MERS-CoV spike protein antibody (green, top) or anti-human CD26/DPP4 antibody (red, bottom). (C) Merged IFA images demonstrate colocalization of MERS-CoV spike protein and CD26/DPP4. (D). Viral yields from MERS-CoV-susceptible bat cells transfected with a plasmid expressing human CD26/DPP4 or empty control plasmid using procedures identical to resistant cells in (A) except that cells were exposed to virus 24 h after transfection. Error bars indicate the standard deviation of duplicate samples.

susceptibility to MERS-CoV infection not only depends on the expression of CD26/DPP4, but also on its sequence. For instance, five amino-acid variations in the MERS-CoV-binding domain of hamster, ferret, and mouse CD26/DPP4 compared to human CD26/DPP4 have been linked to the resistance of hamster, ferret, and mouse cell lines to MERS-CoV infection [22]. Our study confirms the role of CD26/DPP4 as receptor for two divergent MERS-CoV isolates and correlates its presence or absence on the surface of bat cells directly with bat cell susceptibility or resistance to productive MERS-CoV infection (Figures 2 and 3). Bat cells that tested negative for CD26/DPP4 expression by flow cytometry using the polyclonal anti-human CD26/DPP4 antibody may possibly express a CD26/DPP4 ortholog that is not recognized by this antibody. Although the cells were derived from bats of different geographic origins, they could be rendered permissive by ectopic expression of human CD26/DPP4 (Figure 4A–C).

Overexpression of human CD26/DPP4 in already MERS-CoV-susceptible bat cell lines led to an increase in virus yield in

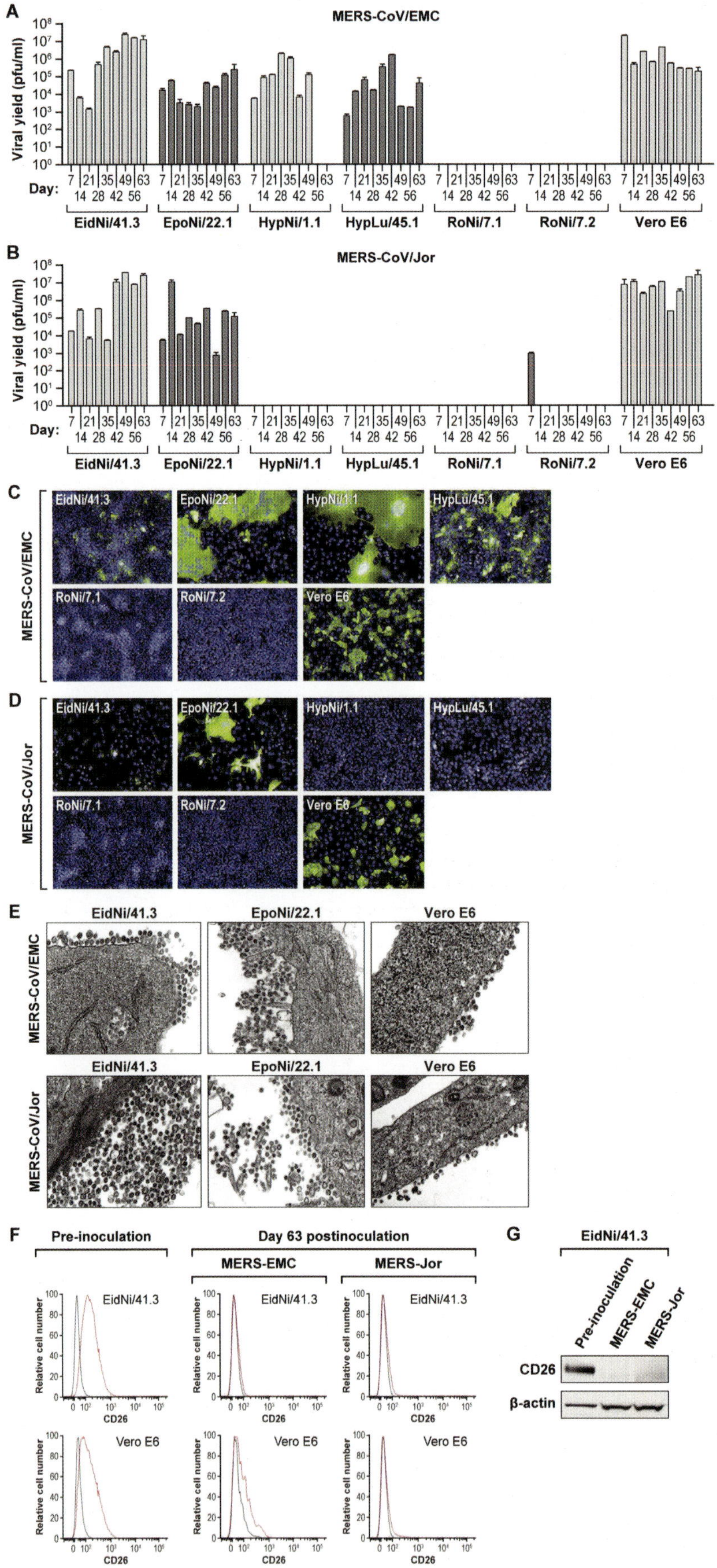
A
MERS-CoV/EMC
Viral yield (pfu/ml)
Day:
EidNi/41.3
EpoNi/22.1
HypNi/1.1
HypLu/45.1
RoNi/7.1
RoNi/7.2
Vero E6
B
MERS-CoV/Jor
C
MERS-CoV/EMC
D
MERS-CoV/Jor
E
F
Pre-inoculation
Day 63 postinoculation
MERS-EMC
MERS-Jor
Relative cell number
CD26
G
EidNi/41.3
Pre-inoculation
MERS-EMC
MERS-Jor
CD26
β-actin

Figure 5. Persistent MERS-CoV infection of bat cells induces downregulation of bat cell CD26/DPP4 expression. Bat cell lines susceptible to infection were infected with MERS-CoV/EMC (A) or MERS-CoV/Jor (B) at an MOI of 1. After 7 days, supernatants were harvested for virus yield analysis by plaque assay, and the cells were subcultured at a 1:10 dilution in new flasks. Subsequently, the persistently infected cells were passaged at a 1:10 dilution weekly. Error bars indicate the standard deviation of duplicate samples. (C and D) Same experiment: immunofluorescence assay (IFA) images of bat cells persistently infected with MERS-CoV/EMC (C) or MERS-CoV/Jor (D) at day +33 stained with anti-MERS-CoV spike protein antibody (green). (E) Same experiment: TEM images of bat cells persistently infected with MERS-CoV/EMC at day 56. (F) Flow cytometry data of CD26/DPP4 surface expression (red line: anti-human CD26-/DPP4 antibody; black line: control antibody) in persistently infected cells. (G) CD26/DPP4 expression in persistently infected EidNi/41.3 cells (day 63) as detected by western blot.

some bat cell lines and to a decrease in virus yield in others (Figure 4D). We hypothesize that this variation may be due to differences in the number of bat CD26/DPP4 molecules on the cell-surface of each bat cell. For instance, overexpression of human CD26/DPP4 in a bat cell line with naturally high bat CD26/DPP4 surface expression may not have an effect on virion entry efficiency since all virions already find enough binding partners in the untransfected cell. Vice versa, if a bat cell line expresses little CD26/DPP4, finding a binding partner would present a bottleneck for MERS-CoV virions, and overexpression of human CD26/DPP4 might overcome this bottleneck and thereby increase virus yield. Second, we hypothesize that overexpression of human CD26/DPP4 may interfere with transport and/or functionality of certain bat CD26/DPP4 orthologs due to heterodimerization and consequent structural changes.

Our results indicate that, at least on the cellular level, presence or absence of functional CD26/DPP4 with a suitable MERS-CoV-binding domain is a major determinant for MERS-CoV cellular tropism in bats. In addition to potential differences in the MERS-CoV-binding domain of distinct bat CD26/DPP4 orthologs, presence or absence of yet-to-be-identified co-receptors and bat species-specific cellular factors acting downstream of virion adsorption and fusion may further influence to what extent a productive infection can be established. However, these considerations alone are not sufficient to pinpoint bats as epidemiologically relevant MERS-CoV hosts, as the immune system at the level of the organism may interfere with infection prior to cell entry or lead to rapid viral clearance.

One characteristic of natural virus host reservoirs is that hosts frequently are persistently infected with virus in the absence of clinical signs. Continuous transmission of viruses from such a reservoir to other animals, including humans, is a hallmark of zoonoses and explains repeated introduction of viruses into susceptible animal populations [26]. A number of zoonotic viruses are known to persistently and subclinically infect rodents (e.g., arenaviruses, hantaviruses) or bats (henipaviruses), which then directly or indirectly infect humans [17,27–31]. Among the betacoronaviruses, the group of coronaviruses including MERS-CoV, murine coronavirus and severe acute respiratory syndrome (SARS)-related coronaviruses that are related to MERS-CoV, are known to cause persistent infection in their mammalian hosts [16,32]. During persistent SARS-CoV infection in Vero E6 cells and also during acute infection in laboratory mice, the SARS-CoV entry receptor, angiotensin converting enzyme 2 (ACE2), is downregulated [33,34]. ACE2 downregulation contributes to the severity of lung pathology of SARS [34].

In this study, we established persistent infection (up to 63 days post-exposure) in EidNi/41.3, EpoNi/22.1, HypNi/1.1, and HypLu/45.1 bat and control Vero E6 cells using MERS-CoV/EMC, and in EidNi/41.3 and EpoNi/22.1 bat and control Vero E6 cells using MERS-CoV/Jor. Interestingly, sequencing of the receptor-binding domain of MERS-CoV/EMC- and MERS-CoV/Jor-containing samples taken on day 63 from persistently infected EidNi/41.3 and Vero E6 cells did not reveal any amino-acid changes compared to the wild-type/reference sequences (GenBank: JX869059.2 and KC776174.1, respectively; data not shown). Similar to SARS-CoV-induced ACE2 downregulation, persistent MERS-CoV infection in bat cell lines and Vero E6 cells was associated with downregulation of CD26/DPP4 (Figure 5). The observation that cultures continued to release significant virion amounts on day 63 post-inoculation, but also exhibited low to absent CD26/DPP4 cell-surface expression, is consistent with receptor downregulation as one mechanism for persistent infection with MERS-CoV in our experiments. Virus carryover between cell/virus passages probably did not influence these results as excreted viruses should be unable to re-infect cells in the absence of CD26/DPP4 receptor. The mechanism of CD26/DPP4 downregulation upon persistent MERS-CoV infection requires further study. Western blot-based examination of lysates of persistently infected cells at day 63 indicate that CD26/DPP4 is either not expressed anymore or is very efficiently degraded (Figure 5G).

The reason for the observed differences in establishing persistent infection in these cell lines among the two different MERS-CoV isolates is unclear, but may have epizootiological significance and needs to be examined in future studies.

Our results are consistent with the suggested role of bats in MERS-CoV transmission. If CD26/DPP4-positive cells of bats become infected with MERS-CoV and if subsequently the receptor surface expression is downregulated as we observe in our experiments, a persistent infection could be established. Such animals may provide a reservoir that continuously sheds infectious virus, possibly transmitting the virus to other mammals, such as dromedaries. Further evaluation is needed to determine whether downregulation of CD26/DPP4 is a general hallmark of persistent MERS-CoV infection in animal models of MERS and whether the receptor influences pathogenesis in a manner similar to that seen with ACE2 downregulation in persistent SARS-CoV infection.

Acknowledgments

We would like to thank Eric Donaldson (FDA) for providing PESU-B5L cells. We are grateful to our colleague, Jiro Wada (IRF-Frederick), for assisting us with the preparation of figures. The content of this publication does not necessarily reflect the views or policies of the US Department of the Army, the US Department of Defense, the US Department of Health and Human Services, or of the institutions and companies affiliated with the authors.

Author Contributions

Conceived and designed the experiments: YC ENP JGB SRR LEH PBJ JHK. Performed the experiments: YC SY ENP SM JGB RB TZ. Analyzed the data: YC ENP SRR MAM IJ LB JHK. Contributed reagents/materials/analysis tools: MAM IJ SRR. Wrote the paper: YC RB SRR MAM IJ LB JHK.

References

1. Zaki AM, van Boheemen S, Bestebroer TM, Osterhaus AD, Fouchier RA (2012) Isolation of a novel coronavirus from a man with pneumonia in Saudi Arabia. N Engl J Med 367: 1814–1820.
2. de Groot RJ, Baker SC, Baric RS, Brown CS, Drosten C, et al. (2013) Middle East respiratory syndrome coronavirus (MERS-CoV): announcement of the Coronavirus Study Group. J Virol 87: 7790–7792.
3. World Health Organization (2014) Middle East respiratory syndrome coronavirus (MERS-CoV) summary and literature update – as of 11 June 2014. (MERS-CoV summary update; 16). Available at: http://www.who.int/csr/disease/coronavirus_infections/archive_updates/en/. Accessed October 14, 2014.
4. Briese T, Mishra N, Jain K, Zalmout IS, Jabado OJ, et al. (2014) Middle East respiratory syndrome coronavirus quasispecies that include homologues of human isolates revealed through whole-genome analysis and virus cultured from dromedary camels in Saudi Arabia. MBio 5: e01146–01114.
5. Haagmans BL, Al Dhahiry SH, Reusken CB, Raj VS, Galiano M, et al. (2014) Middle East respiratory syndrome coronavirus in dromedary camels: an outbreak investigation. Lancet Infect Dis 14: 140–145.
6. Perera RA, Wang P, Gomaa MR, El-Shesheny R, Kandeil A, et al. (2013) Seroepidemiology for MERS coronavirus using microneutralisation and pseudoparticle virus neutralisation assays reveal a high prevalence of antibody in dromedary camels in Egypt, June 2013. Euro Surveill 18: pii = 20574.
7. Reusken CB, Ababneh M, Raj VS, Meyer B, Eljarah A, et al. (2013) Middle East Respiratory Syndrome coronavirus (MERS-CoV) serology in major livestock species in an affected region in Jordan, June to September 2013. Euro Surveill 18: 20662.
8. Nowotny N, Kolodziejek J (2014) Middle East respiratory syndrome coronavirus (MERS-CoV) in dromedary camels, Oman, 2013. Euro Surveill 19: 20781.
9. Alagaili AN, Briese T, Mishra N, Kapoor V, Sameroff SC, et al. (2014) Middle East respiratory syndrome coronavirus infection in dromedary camels in Saudi Arabia. MBio 5: e00884–00814.
10. Azhar EI, El-Kafrawy SA, Farraj SA, Hassan AM, Al-Saeed MS, et al. (2014) Evidence for camel-to-human transmission of MERS Coronavirus. N Engl J Med 370: 2499–2505.
11. Raj VS, Farag EA, Reusken CB, Lamers MM, Pas SD, et al. (2014) Isolation of MERS coronavirus from a dromedary camel, Qatar, 2014. Emerg Infect Dis 20: 1339–1342.
12. Corman VM, Ithete NL, Richards LR, Schoeman MC, Preiser W, et al. (2014) Rooting the phylogenetic tree of middle East respiratory syndrome coronavirus by characterization of a conspecific virus from an African bat. J Virol 88: 11297–11303.
13. Annan A, Baldwin HJ, Corman VM, Klose SM, Owusu M, et al. (2013) Human betacoronavirus 2c EMC/2012-related viruses in bats, Ghana and Europe. Emerg Infect Dis 19: 456–459.
14. Memish ZA, Mishra N, Olival KJ, Fagbo SF, Kapoor V, et al. (2013) Middle East respiratory syndrome coronavirus in bats, Saudi Arabia. Emerg Infect Dis 19: 1819–1823.
15. Ithete NL, Stoffberg S, Corman VM, Cottontail VM, Richards LR, et al. (2013) Close relative of human Middle East respiratory syndrome coronavirus in bat, South Africa. Emerg Infect Dis 19: 1697–1699.
16. Palacios G, Jabado O, Renwick N, Briese T, Lipkin WI (2005) Severe acute respiratory syndrome coronavirus persistence in Vero cells. Chin Med J (Engl) 118: 451–459.
17. Pulliam JR, Epstein JH, Dushoff J, Rahman SA, Bunning M, et al. (2012) Agricultural intensification, priming for persistence and the emergence of Nipah virus: a lethal bat-borne zoonosis. J R Soc Interface 9: 89–101.
18. Plowright RK, Foley P, Field HE, Dobson AP, Foley JE, et al. (2011) Urban habituation, ecological connectivity and epidemic dampening: the emergence of Hendra virus from flying foxes (Pteropus spp.). Proc Biol Sci 278: 3703–3712.
19. Ohnuma K, Haagmans BL, Hatano R, Raj VS, Mou H, et al. (2013) Inhibition of Middle East respiratory syndrome coronavirus infection by anti-CD26 monoclonal antibody. J Virol 87: 13892–13899.
20. Wang Q, Qi J, Yuan Y, Xuan Y, Han P, et al. (2014) Bat origins of MERS-CoV supported by bat coronavirus HKU4 usage of human Receptor CD26. Cell Host Microbe 16: 328–337.
21. Yang Y, Du L, Liu C, Wang L, Ma C, et al. (2014) Receptor usage and cell entry of bat coronavirus HKU4 provide insight into bat-to-human transmission of MERS coronavirus. Proc Natl Acad Sci U S A 111: 12516–12521.
22. van Doremalen N, Miazgowicz K, Shauna Milne-Price S, Bushmaker T, Robertson S, et al. (2014) Host species restriction of Middle East respiratory syndrome coronavirus through its receptor dipeptidyl peptidase 4. J Virol 88: 9220–9232. doi: 9210.1128/JVI.00676-00614.
23. Dobos P (1976) Use of gum tragacanth overlay, applied at room temperature, in the plaque assay of fish and other animal viruses. J Clin Microbiol 3: 373–375.
24. Chan JF, Chan KH, Choi GK, To KK, Tse H, et al. (2013) Differential cell line susceptibility to the emerging novel human betacoronavirus 2c EMC/2012: implications for disease pathogenesis and clinical manifestation. J Infect Dis 207: 1743–1752.
25. de Wit E, Prescott J, Baseler L, Bushmaker T, Thomas T, et al. (2013) The Middle East respiratory syndrome coronavirus (MERS-CoV) does not replicate in Syrian hamsters. PLoS One 8: e69127.
26. Nishiura H, Hoye B, Klaassen M, Bauer S, Heesterbeek H (2009) How to find natural reservoir hosts from endemic prevalence in a multi-host population: a case study of influenza in waterfowl. Epidemics 1: 118–128.
27. Traub E (1936) Persistence of lymphocytic choriomeningitis virus in immune animals and its relation to immunity. Journal of Experimental Medicine 63: 847–862.
28. Goyens J, Reijniers J, Borremans B, Leirs H (2013) Density thresholds for Mopeia virus invasion and persistence in its host Mastomys natalensis. J Theor Biol 317: 55–61.
29. Klein SL, Calisher CH (2007) Emergence and persistence of hantaviruses. Curr Top Microbiol Immunol 315: 217–252.
30. de Oliveira RC, Guterres A, Fernandes J, D'Andrea PS, Bonvicino CR, et al. (2014) Hantavirus reservoirs: current status with an emphasis on data from Brazil. Viruses 6: 1929–1973.
31. Wang HH, Kung NY, Grant WE, Scanlan JC, Field HE (2013) Recrudescent infection supports hendra virus persistence in Australian flying-fox populations. PLoS One 8: e80430.
32. Baric RS, Sullivan E, Hensley L, Yount B, Chen W (1999) Persistent infection promotes cross-species transmissibility of mouse hepatitis virus. J Virol 73: 638–649.
33. Mizutani T, Fukushi S, Saijo M, Kurane I, Morikawa S (2005) JNK and PI3k/Akt signaling pathways are required for establishing persistent SARS-CoV infection in Vero E6 cells. Biochim Biophys Acta 1741: 4–10.
34. Kuba K, Imai Y, Rao S, Gao H, Guo F, et al. (2005) A crucial role of angiotensin converting enzyme 2 (ACE2) in SARS coronavirus-induced lung injury. Nat Med 11: 875–879.
35. Biesold SE, Ritz D, Gloza-Rausch F, Wollny R, Drexler JF, et al. (2011) Type I interferon reaction to viral infection in interferon-competent, immortalized cell lines from the African fruit bat Eidolon helvum. PLoS One 6: e28131.
36. Kuhl A, Hoffmann M, Muller MA, Munster VJ, Gnirss K, et al. (2011) Comparative analysis of Ebola virus glycoprotein interactions with human and bat cells. J Infect Dis 204 Suppl 3: S840–849.
37. Huynh J, Li S, Yount B, Smith A, Sturges L, et al. (2012) Evidence supporting a zoonotic origin of human coronavirus strain NL63. J Virol 86: 12816–12825.
38. Jordan I, Horn D, Oehmke S, Leendertz FH, Sandig V (2009) Cell lines from the Egyptian fruit bat are permissive for modified vaccinia Ankara. Virus Res 145: 54–62.
39. Hoffmann M, Muller MA, Drexler JF, Glende J, Erdt M, et al. (2013) Differential sensitivity of bat cells to infection by enveloped RNA viruses: coronaviruses, paramyxoviruses, filoviruses, and influenza viruses. PLoS One 8: e72942.

14

Reduced Mucosal Associated Invariant T-Cells Are Associated with Increased Disease Severity and *Pseudomonas aeruginosa* Infection in Cystic Fibrosis

Daniel J. Smith[1,2,4]*, Geoffrey R. Hill[3], Scott C. Bell[1,2,5], David W. Reid[1,2,4]

1 Department of Thoracic Medicine, The Prince Charles Hospital, Brisbane, Queensland, Australia, **2** School of Medicine, University of Queensland, Brisbane, Queensland, Australia, **3** Bone Marrow Transplant Laboratory, QIMR Berghofer Medical Research Institute, Brisbane, Queensland, Australia, **4** Infection and Inflammation Laboratory, QIMR Berghofer Medical Research Institute, Brisbane, Queensland, Australia, **5** Queensland Children's Medical Research Institute, Royal Children's Hospital, Brisbane, Queensland, Australia

Abstract

Background: Primary defects in host immune responses have been hypothesised to contribute towards an inability of subjects with cystic fibrosis (CF) to effectively clear pulmonary infections. Innate T-lymphocytes provide rapid pathogen-specific responses prior to the development of classical MHC class I and II restricted T-cell responses and are essential to the initial control of pulmonary infection. We aimed to examine the relationship between peripheral blood lymphocyte phenotype and clinical outcomes in adults with CF.

Methods: We studied 41 subjects with CF and 22, age matched, non-smoking healthy control subjects. Lymphocytes were extracted from peripheral blood samples and phenotyped by flow-cytometry. Lymphocyte phenotype was correlated with sputum microbiology and clinical parameters.

Results: In comparison to healthy control subjects, mucosal associated invariant T (MAIT)-lymphocytes were significantly reduced in the peripheral blood of subjects with CF (1.1% versus 2.0% of T-lymphocytes, $P = 0.002$). MAIT cell concentration was lowest in CF subjects infected with *P. aeruginosa* and in subjects receiving treatment for a pulmonary exacerbation. Furthermore a reduced MAIT cell concentration correlated with severity of lung disease.

Conclusion: Reduced numbers of MAIT cells in subjects with CF were associated with *P. aeruginosa* pulmonary infection, pulmonary exacerbations and more severe lung disease. These findings provide the impetus for future studies examining the utility of MAIT cells in immunotherapies and vaccine development. Longitudinal studies of MAIT cells as biomarkers of CF pulmonary infection are awaited.

Editor: Johan K. Sandberg, Karolinska Institutet, Sweden

Funding: Internal funding was received from QIMR Berghofer Medical Research Institute. The institute had no role in decision to publish the manuscript.

Competing Interests: The authors have declared that no competing interests exist.

* Email: daniel.smith@health.qld.gov.au

Introduction

Cystic fibrosis (CF) pulmonary disease is typified by a vicious cycle of bacterial infection and exuberant, but ineffective host immune response [1]. The inability of the intense inflammatory response to clear infection has led to speculation that intrinsic immune defects may contribute to the persistence of pathogens in CF [2]. At the level of the airway lumen, the cellular immune response is dominated by activated neutrophils. However, in contrast, airway epithelial biopsies demonstrate a profound T lymphocyte (T-cell) infiltrate, supporting an important role for adaptive immune responses in the orchestration of a sustained inflammatory response [3].

To date, studies of peripheral, adaptive immune responses in CF have largely focused on the classic dichotomy of T-helper (Th)-1 and Th-2 responses [4]. These early studies suggested a skew towards a Th2 in most CF subjects with *P. aeruginosa* infection, which resulted in increased pulmonary inflammation and disease progression [4–6]. The activation of the "classical" adaptive immune response involves antigen recognition, followed by T-cell recruitment and clonal expansion at the site of infection. Consequently, there is a time lag between the host's recognition of the presence of a pathogen and the development of an effective, adaptive immune response. In recent times, an increasing number of unconventional "innate" T-cell populations have been described (including γ/δ, semi-invariant natural killer (iNKT) and M3-restricted T-cells), which are capable of mounting a more immediate response to pathogens than was previously thought possible. Mucosal associated invariant T (MAIT) cells are a recently described sub-class of innate T-cells, which can be differentiated from other T-cells by the presence of an evolutionary conserved T-cell receptor (TCR)

(Vα7.2−Jα33). MAIT cells recognise bacterial and fungal metabolites presented on the major histocompatibility complex (MHC) related protein-1 (MR1) (including the common CF pathogens *Pseudomonas aeruginosa* and *Staphylococcus aureus*), but not viruses [7,8]. These "innate" T-cell populations provide rapid pathogen-specific responses prior to the development of classical MHC class I and II restricted T-cell responses and importantly may also provide a sustained cytokine response in chronic infection [9,10].

To date, there is limited knowledge of how changes in circulating lymphocyte populations may relate to pulmonary infection in CF [11]. In this study we performed extensive phenotyping of peripheral blood mononuclear cell populations (PBMCs) obtained from subjects with CF and compared these profiles to those in healthy, age matched, controls. Our particular focus was on the correlation of γ/δ and MAIT innate T-cell values with clinical and microbiological parameters.

Methods

Participants and sample collection

Forty-one subjects with CF attending the Adult CF Centre, The Prince Charles Hospital, Queensland, Australia and 22 age-matched, non-smoking, healthy control subjects each supplied a single venous blood sample.

In subjects with CF, total white cell count (WCC), C-reactive protein (CRP) and clinical demographics including, age, CF genotype, lung function, body mass index, pulmonary exacerbation frequency and pulmonary pathogens (based on standard sputum microbiological testing) were recorded. Longitudinal rate of decline in forced expiratory volume in one second (FEV_1) was determined in CF subjects by means of linear regression analysis (limited to subjects with at least five FEV_1 measurements recorded over a minimum surveillance period of 2 years).

To explore the effect of pulmonary exacerbations on lymphocyte concentrations a sub-set of 13 "stable" CF subjects (stable respiratory symptoms and a CRP <5 mg L^{-1} at time of blood collection) were compared to eight CF subjects in whom blood was collected within 72 hours of admission to hospital for the intravenous antibiotic treatment of a "pulmonary exacerbation", defined as increased respiratory symptoms (cough, sputum volume or purulence, dyspnoea) (Figure S1 in File S1).

Ethics approval was obtained from The Prince Charles Hospital, Queensland, Australia, Human Research and Ethics Committee (HREC/11/QPCH/36 and HREC2008:2885) and all subjects provided written, informed consent.

Separation and storage of peripheral blood mononuclear cells (PBMCs)

Twelve millilitres of venous blood was collected into lithium heparinised tubes and separated into plasma and cellular components. The cellular component was re-suspended in RPMI (Gibco)+2% heat inactivated Foetal Calf Serum (HiFCS) and PBMCs separated by means of Histopaque 1.077 (Sigma-Aldrich) density gradient separation, as per the manufacturer's protocol.

Table 1. Subject demographics.

	Healthy Controls	Cystic Fibrosis	P value
Sex (Female:Male)	11:11	17:24	0.5
Age (years)	26 (25–32)	28 (22–32)	0.9
BMI (kg/metre^2)	24.6 (21.4–28.3)	23.5 (20.5–25.8)	0.3
FEV_1 (Litres)	4.1 (3.5–4.7)	2.2 (1.4–2.5)	<0.001
FEV_1% Predicted (%)	110 (101–120)	58 (37–75)	<0.001
FVC (Litres)	4.9 (4.4–5.7)	3.1 (2.6–4.1)	<0.001
FVC % Predicted (%)	107 (95–112)	76 (58–84)	<0.001
CFTR Genotype			
F508del Homozygotes		20	
F508del Heterozygotes		18	
Other mutations		3	
Sputum Microbiology*			
Pseudomonas aeruginosa		36	
Staphylococcus aureus		12	
Aspergillus fumigatus		5	
Haemophilus influenzae		4	
Stenotrophomonas maltophilia		3	
Chryseobacterium indologenes		2	
Scedosporium apiospermum		2	
Mycobacterium intracellulare		1	
Burkholderia gladioli		1	
Achromobacter xylosoxidans		1	
Methicillin resistant *S. aureus*		1	

Data presented as median (interquartile range).
*Summary data, subjects may have had more than one pathogen isolated in sputum, individual microbiological data available in Table S1 in File S2.

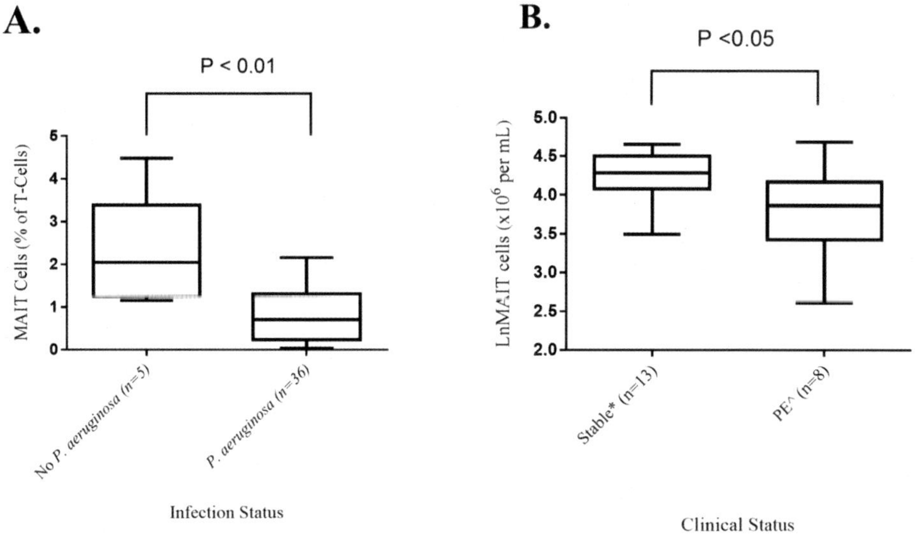

Figure 1. MAIT Cell percentage in CF subjects based on A. Presence of *P. aeruginosa* in sputum cultures, B. Clinical status. PE: pulmonary exacerbations, *two and ^one not infected with *P. aeruginosa*, between group differences determined by Mann-Whitney U test.

Following separation, PBMCs were washed twice, re-suspended in RPMI and 15% dimethyl sulfoxide (DMSO), gradually frozen to −80°C and transferred to storage in liquid nitrogen for later batch analysis (concentration 5–20×10^6 cells/ml).

Flow Cytometry

PBMCs were rewarmed and re-suspended by drop-wise addition of 10 ml of RPMI+2%HiFCS, washed twice and re-suspended in phosphate buffered saline (PBS) with 1% HiFCS (FACS buffer). A cell count was performed and the volume adjusted to obtain a cell concentration of 10×10^6 cells/ml.

One hundred micro-litre aliquots of cells were incubated with each of two antibody staining panels as follows:

Panel 1 [adapted from [12]]: FITC anti-human CD16, Pacific Blue anti-human CD14, APC anti-human CD1c, Alexa Fluor700 anti-human CD3, APC/Cy7 anti-human HLA-DR, PE/Cy7 anti-human CD56, PE/Cy7 anti-human CD20, Anti-CD8 antibody – PE Texas (Abcam) and V500 anti-CD4 (BD biosciences) were added to 100 μL of cells and incubated in the dark for 15 minutes. Cells were washed twice in 1 ml of FACS buffer and fixation was performed by incubation with 500 μl of Cytofix (BD biosciences) for 10 minutes. Finally, samples were washed and suspended in 300 μl of FACS buffer.

Table 2. Comparison of lymphocyte sub-sets between CF and healthy control subjects.

Lymphocyte Population (size gated, CD14−)	CF (n = 41)	Non-CF (n = 22)	P-Value
T-Cells (CD3+CD16−)	**72.6 (68.1–79.6)**	**74.9 (67.9–79.0)**	0.6
CD4+CD8−	65.2 (56.1–70.5)	65.1 (59.9–71.4)	0.6
CD8+CD4−	25.7 (21.1–32.5)	27.4 (22.7–32.8)	0.6
MAIT Cells (CD161+, TCR Va7.2+)	1.1 (0.4–1.9)	2.0 (1.4–3.1)	**0.002**
γ/δ T-cells (TCR γ/δ+)	10.4 (6.5–13.4)	6.4 (4.6–9.4)	**0.012**
CD4+CD8+	0.3 (0.2–1.0)	0.4 (0.3–1.7)	0.1
CD4−CD8−*	2.1 (0.9–3.3)	1.6 (1.1–2.3)	0.3
B-Cells (CD3−CD16−CD20+HLA-DR+)	**9.5 (4.9–14.3)**	**4.8 (3.9–8.7)**	0.1
Non-Resting (CD1c−)	64.6 (57.0–74.4)	71.6 (60.5–75.1)	0.5
Resting (CD1c+)	35.0 (24.8–43.	28.1 (25.0–38.3)	0.4
NK-Cells (CD3−)	**9.5 (6.9–12.2)**	**13.1 (8.0–18.0)**	**0.013**
CD16+CD56dim HLA-DR−	75.1 (61.0–86.7)	88.0 (84.7–92.6)	**0.001**
CD16−CD56+HLA-DR−	8.9 (6.1–13.2)	6.1 (4.5–9.1)	**0.016**
CD16−CD56+HLA-DR+	14.4 (5.1–24.1)	4.3 (2.7–9.2)	**0.005**
CD3+CD16+	**2.2 (1.1–3.8)**	**1.8 (1.1–3.6)**	0.7
Contaminants/Undefined	**3.7 (3.0–5.2)**	**2.4 (1.9–3.9)**	**0.013**

*After exclusion of MAIT and γ/δ T-cells. Values expressed as percentage of parent population, Median (interquartile range). Significance of between group differences determined by Mann-Whitney U test.

A.

	LnMAIT Cell Concentration (cells per mL)	γ/δ T-Cell Concentration (cells per mL)
FEV_1% predicted	r = 0.47 p = 0.003	r = 0.35 p = 0.030
FEV_1% predicted decline per year	r = 0.28 p = 0.10	r = 0.31 p = 0.06
FVC% predicted	r = 0.43 p = 0.006	r = 0.33 p = 0.042
Body Mass Index (kg/m²)	r = 0.12 P = 0.48	r = -0.03 P = 0.86
C-reactive protein (mg/L)	r = -0.39 p = 0.021	r = -0.44 p = 0.008

B.

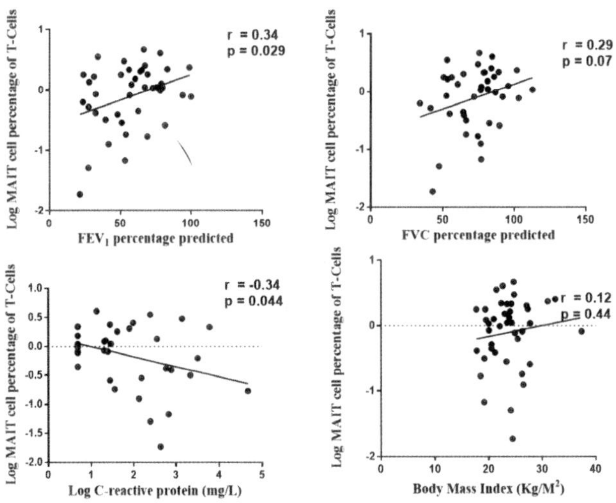

Figure 2. Relationship between MAIT and γ/δ T-cell counts and percentages with lung function. A. Pearson's Correlation co-efficient (r) and significance value (p) of MAIT and γ/δ T-cells and B. Correlation plots for MAIT Cell expressed as percentage of T-cell population, with FEV_1 and FVC % predicted, C-reactive protein and body mass index. MAIT: Mucosal invariant T-Lymphocytes, γ/δ T-Cell: Gamma-Delta T-lymphocytes, FEV_1: Forced expiratory volume in one second, FVC: Forced vital capacity.

Table 3. Lymphocyte sub-set phenotypes in CF subjects based on the presence of *P. aeruginosa* infection compared to healthy control subjects.

	CF, No *P. aeruginosa* (n = 5)	**CF, *P. aeruginosa* infection (n = 36)**	**P-Value^**	**Non-CF (n = 22)**	**P-Value$**
Sex (Female:Male)	3:2	14:22	0.4	11:11	1.0
Age (years)	23.3 (18.4–41.7)	28 (24.5–32.6)	0.8	26 (25–32)	0.5
BMI (kg/metre²)	24.7 (19.9–31.7)	23.4 (20.5–25.3)	0.5	24.6 (21.4–28.3)	0.8
FEV_1% Predicted (%)	72.4 (59.1–88.8)	63.6 (43.4–80.1)	0.3	110 (101–120)	**0.001**
FVC % Predicted (%)	83.9 (68.1–95.9)	79.3 (71.1–88.7)	0.5	107 (95–112)	**0.012**
Lymphocyte Population (size gated, CD14−)					
T-Cells (CD3+CD16−)	**68.2 (63.4–76.8)**	**72.9 (68.3–81.3)**	0.4	**74.9 (67.9–79.0)**	0.3
CD4+CD8−	64.4 (49.6–70.0)	65.2 (56.9–70.5)	0.6	65.1 (59.9–71.4)	0.5
CD8+CD4−	26.2 (22.8–38.8)	25.1 (20.5–33.1)	0.6	27.4 (22.7–32.8)	0.9
MAIT Cells (CD161+, TCR Va7.2+)	2.4 (1.4–3.6)	1.0 (0.3–1.8)	**0.023**	2.0 (1.4–3.1)	1.0
γ/δ T-cells (TCR γ/δ+)	8.0 (6.0–16.0)	10.5 (6.6–13.4)	0.7	6.4 (4.6–9.4)	0.2
CD4+CD8+	0.2 (0.2–0.2)	0.3 (0.2–1.1)	**0.014**	0.4 (0.3–1.7)	**0.004**
CD4−CD8−*	3.1 (1.6–4.1)	2.1 (0.7–2.8)	0.2	1.6 (1.1–2.3)	0.1
B-Cells (CD3−CD16−CD20+HLA-DR+)	**17.2 (14.0–20.9)**	**8.5 (3.6–13.0)**	**0.002**	**4.8 (3.9–8.7)**	**0.003**
Non-Resting (CD1c−)	74.5 (69.1–79.0)	64.1 (55.5–73.7)	0.1	71.6 (60.5–75.1)	0.1
Resting (CD1c+)	24.9 (20.3–30.5)	35.9 (25.3–43.9)	0.1	28.1 (25.0–38.3)	0.1
NK-Cells (CD3−)	**9.6 (4.6–10.9)**	**9.5 (7.8–12.5)**	**0.5**	**13.1 (8.0–18.0)**	**0.039**
CD16+CD56dim HLA-DR−	69.2 (48.5–80.9)	76.1 (63.8–88.1)	0.2	88.0 (84.7–92.6)	**0.006**
CD16−CD56+HLA-DR−	10.9 (7.1–14.5)	8.5 (6.1–13.3)	0.5	6.1 (4.5–9.1)	**0.1**
CD16−CD56+HLA-DR+	21.4 (10.8–37.4)	14.2 (4.5–23.8)	0.2	4.3 (2.7–9.2)	**0.006**
CD3+CD16+	**2.0 (0.9–2.6)**	**2.5 (1.0–4.2)**	0.4	**1.8 (1.1–3.6)**	0.9
Contaminants/Undefined	**1.8 (1.6–3.5)**	**3.7 (3.1–5.4)**	0.017	**2.4 (1.9–3.9)**	**0.4**

^CF No *P. aeruginosa versus* CF *P. aeruginosa* infection. $CF No *P. aeruginosa versus* Non-CF. *After exclusion of MAIT and γ/δ T-cells. Values expressed as percentage of parent population, Median (interquartile range). Significance of between group differences determined by Mann-Whitney U test.

Table 4. Lymphocyte sub-sets in CF subjects based on clinical stability and compared to healthy control subjects.

	CF, Pulmonary exacerbation (n = 8)	CF, Stable (n = 13)	P-Value^	Non-CF (n = 22)	P-Value$
Sex (Female:Male)	1:7	8:5	**0.027**	11:11	0.5
Age (years)	32.2 (30.1–39.1)	22.7 (20.5–26.9)	**0.001**	26 (25–32)	**0.010**
BMI (kg/metre^2)	24.6 (23.5–26.0)	23.0 (21.5–27.0)	0.4	24.6 (21.4–28.3)	0.7
FEV_1% Predicted (%)	49.7 (40.3–68.5)	83.2 (74.1–88.8)	**0.001**	110 (101–120)	**<0.001**
FVC % Predicted (%)	74.6 (71.2–79.3)	90.0 (85.9–96.4)	**0.001**	107 (95–112)	**0.001**
Lymphocyte Population (size gated, CD14−)					
T-Cells (CD3+CD16−)	**71.6 (68.1–82.3)**	**71.3 (67.1–77.1)**	0.6	**74.9 (67.9–79.0)**	0.3
CD4+CD8−	65.9 (52.2–76.2)	58.3 (55.3–68.9)	0.5	65.1 (59.9–71.4)	0.1
CD8+CD4−	23.8 (16.4–37.8)	29.2 (23.6–35.3)	0.3	27.4 (22.7–32.8)	0.7
MAIT Cells (CD161+, TCR Va7.2+)	1.1 (0.3–2.1)	1.1 (0.9–1.9)	0.7	2.0 (1.4–3.1)	**0.018**
γ/δ T-cells (TCR γ/δ+)	11.1 (7.1–16.5)	10.5 (6.4–13.6)	0.8	6.4 (4.6–9.4)	**0.017**
CD4+CD8+	0.2 (0.2–1.0)	0.2 (0.2–0.3)	0.5	0.4 (0.3–1.7)	**0.010**
CD4−CD8−*	2.6 (1.4–3.5)	2.2 (1.3–3.4)	0.6	1.6 (1.1–2.3)	0.1
B-Cells (CD3−CD16−CD20+HLA-DR+)	**9.6 (2.5–14.0)**	**13.1 (8.5–16.7)**	0.3	**4.8 (3.9–8.7)**	**0.001**
Non-Resting (CD1c−)	73.4. (65.5–79.9)	70.4 (59.9–79.9)	0.8	71.6 (60.5–75.1)	0.7
Resting (CD1c+)	25.6 (19.9–34.1)	29.3 (18.1–40.1)	0.8	28.1 (25.0–38.3)	0.7
NK-Cells (CD3−)	**10.1 (5.9–12.6)**	**9.6 (5.4–11.8)**	0.7	**13.1 (8.0–18.0)**	**0.020**
CD16+CD56dim HLA-DR−	70.7 (52.9–83.7)	69.2 (55.3–80.5)	0.9	88.0 (84.7–92.6)	**<0.001**
CD16−CD56+HLA-DR−	9.9 (8.6–12.6)	8.0 (6.7–13.3)	0.6	6.1 (4.5–9.1)	**0.026**
CD16−CD56+HLA-DR+	19.4 (5.8–37.2)	21.4 (13.2–30.6)	0.8	4.3 (2.7–9.2)	**<0.001**
CD3+CD16+	**2.0 (1.2–4.0)**	**2.5 (1.1–4.2)**	1.0	**1.8 (1.1–3.6)**	0.7
Contaminants/Undefined	**3.6 (3.1–4.2)**	**3.5 (2.5–4.1)**	0.6	**2.4 (1.9–3.9)**	**0.4**

^CF pulmonary exacerbation *versus* CF stable, $CF stable *versus* Non-CF. *After exclusion of MAIT and γ/δ T-cells. Values expressed as percentage of parent population, Median (interquartile range). Significance of between group differences determined by Mann-Whitney U test.

Panel 2: Surface staining was performed by incubation with V500 anti-CD4, FITC anti-TCR Va7.2, PerCP/Cy5.5 anti-CD161, APC/Cy7 anti-CD3, PE anti-TCR γ/δ, PE Texas red Anti-CD8 for 15 minutes at room temperature in the dark. Cells were washed twice in 1 ml of FACS buffer, fixed and resuspended in 300 μl of buffer solution.

Unless stated otherwise, antibodies were obtained for Biolegend, San Diego. Antibody titration was performed to optimise antibody-cell concentration prior to testing.

Sample analysis was performed on a Fortessa IV flow cytometer (BD Biosciences). A lymphocyte gate was set based on forward and side scatter properties and a minimum of 50,000 gated events were capture for each sample.

MAIT cells were defined as $CD3^{+}/CD4^{-}/CD8^{+}$or−/$CD161^{+}$/TCR $Va7.2^{+}$ [13].

For subjects with CF, automated haemocytometer, absolute lymphocyte counts were obtained and T-cell sub-types were considered as both, absolute numbers of cells per mL of blood and percentage of the whole T-cell population.

Data analysis was performed using Flowjo version 7.6 (Treestar), representative gating plots are available in Figure S2 in File S1.

Statistical Analysis

Statistical analysis was performed using PASW, version 18 (SPSS Inc. Chicago IL, USA) and Graph-pad Prism, version 6. Between group differences in PBMC populations were examined using student's t-test or Mann-Whitney U test. Shapiro-Wilk test and q-q plots were used to determine normal distribution of continuous variables. Non-normally distributed continuous variables (WCC, CRP, MAIT cell absolute count and percentage, B-cell count, NKT-cell and NK-cell percentage) were natural logarithm transformed and Pearson's correlation used to determine relationships between variables. A p-value<0.05 was considered to represent statistical significance.

Results

The characteristics of subjects with CF and healthy controls are provided in Table 1. Thirty-six of the 41 subjects with CF had chronic pulmonary infection with *P. aeruginosa* (either in isolation or in combination with another CF respiratory pathogen) on routine microbiological cultures. The remaining five subjects did not have *P. aeruginosa* infection on current, or previous sputum cultures (Table S1 in File S1 for complete sputum microbiological data).

A greater number of subjects in the pulmonary exacerbation group were male, these subjects were also older, with more severe lung disease, when compared to the stable subjects.

Comparison of lymphocyte sub-sets between groups, demonstrated a reduction in the percentage of MAIT cells in subjects with CF, compared to healthy controls (median 1.1% versus 2.0%, p = 0.002), with an accompanying increase in the percentage of γ/δ T-cells (median 10.4% versus 6.4%, p = 0.012). CF subjects also displayed reduced percentages of NK-cells (median 9.5% versus

13.1%, p = 0.013). The percentage of cells in all of the other major lymphocyte sub-sets was similar between groups (Table 2).

Relationship between MAIT cells, microbiological and clinical parameters in subjects with CF

Absolute MAIT cell concentrations and the proportion of T-cells that were MAIT cells (MAIT cell percentage), in the five subjects without *P. aeruginosa* infection were significantly higher than in patients with chronic *P. aeruginosa* infection (Table 3 and Figure 1A). MAIT cell percentages in subjects not infected with *P. aeruginosa* were similar to healthy controls subjects. No difference was seen in the MAIT cell percentage of subjects with a *P. aeruginosa* infection, based on their co-pathogen (Figure S3 in File S1).

Absolute blood MAIT cell counts in the sub-group of stable CF subjects were higher, when compared to subjects sampled early in the course of treatment for a pulmonary exacerbation (Figure 1B). However, the MAIT cell percentage was similar between stable and pulmonary exacerbation subjects (Table 4).

Absolute MAIT cell count and MAIT cell percentage correlated positively with FEV_1 and FVC percentage predicted. A weak relationship was seen between increased rate of FEV_1 decline and MAIT cells counts, but this did not reach statistical significance (Figure 2).

MAIT cell percentage and absolute MAIT cell concentrations were inversely correlated with CRP ($r = -0.34$, $p = 0.044$ and $r = -0.39$, $p = 0.021$, respectively), however, there was no relationship between MAIT cells and total WCC.

Relationship between γ/δ T-cells, microbiological and clinical parameters in subjects with CF

Absolute γ/δ T-cell counts correlated with FEV_1 and FVC percentage predicted values. A trend toward more rapid rate of lung function decline in FEV_1 was seen in subjects with lower γ/δ T-cells numbers (Figure 2A). No relationship between γ/δ T-cells when expressed as a percentage of total T-cells and lung function parameters was observed (Figure 2B).

γ/δ T-cell percentage and absolute cell number were inversely correlated with CRP ($r = -0.44$, $p = 0.008$) and absolute γ/δ T-cell number was higher in stable CF subjects compared to subjects experiencing a pulmonary exacerbation (Figure S4 in File S1).

There was no relationship between γ/δ T-cell counts or percentages and absolute WCC or profile of infection with *P. aeruginosa* (Table 3).

Relationship between other lymphocyte sub-subset and clinical parameter

Absolute blood lymphocyte count was positively correlated with FEV_1 and FVC (litres and percentage predicted), however, no relationship was seen between absolute WCC and the percentage of the major lymphocyte sub-sets (T-cells, B-cells, NK-cells, CD3+/CD16+ cells) or lung function (Table S2 in File S1).

Total lymphocyte count was decreased in CF subjects being treated for a pulmonary exacerbation.

B-cell percentage was higher in subjects not infected with *P. aeruginosa*, compared to CF subjects with chronic *P. aeruginosa* infection and healthy controls. There was a trend towards lower B-cell percentages in CF subjects during a pulmonary exacerbation compared to stable CF patients (Figure S5A and B in File S1).

Discussion

In this study we demonstrate for the first time that the peripheral blood of subjects with CF is characterized by a relative lymphopenia and major reductions in circulating MAIT cells and to a lesser extent an increase in γ/δ T-cells compared to normal healthy controls, consistent with both quantitative and qualitative differences in innate T-cell immunity in CF. Importantly, lung disease severity, systemic inflammation, clinical status and the presence or absence of chronic *P. aeruginosa* infection were all significantly related to the number of circulating MAIT cells in peripheral blood.

The reduction in absolute lymphocyte counts as lung disease severity increases in the current study is consistent with a single previous study of peripheral blood lymphocytes in children with CF [11]. Similar to this earlier study, a reduction in the percentage of NK-cells was also seen in subjects with CF, however, in contrast, no difference in the percentage of CD4+ T cells was seen and the percentages of other major lymphocyte subsets were similar between CF subjects and healthy control subjects [11]. NK-cells represent an innate, cytotoxic subset of lymphocyte which primarily respond to viral infections and tumour cells [14]. In addition, NK cells provide critical support to the eradication of bacterial pulmonary infection (including *P. aeruginosa*), principally through the generation of Th2 cytokines and IFN-γ [15,16].

A higher percentage of B-cells was seen in CF subjects not infected with *P. aeruginosa* and a trend towards lower concentrations in subjects who were undergoing treatment for an acute pulmonary exacerbation. B-cells are critical for pulmonary protection against encapsulated bacteria and B-cells cultured *in vitro* respond to the mucoid exopolysaccharide of *P. aeruginosa* [17]. Further longitudinal studies are required to delineate the role of B-cells during acute pulmonary exacerbations and to determine whether changes in circulating numbers can be attributed to peripheral destruction, tissue sequestration or transformation to plasma cells.

The association between MAIT cells counts and *P. aeruginosa* infection, severe lung function impairment, increased systemic inflammation and acute pulmonary exacerbations in subjects with CF may suggest that MAIT cell deficiency is associated with susceptibility to pulmonary infection in CF. However, the sub-group of CF subjects undergoing a pulmonary exacerbation may have been biased towards a lower MAIT cell concentration, as more subjects in this sub-group were male and in general they had poorer baseline lung function [18]. Furthermore, these data are cross-sectional and do not inform on whether low MAIT cell numbers contribute to *P. aeruginosa* colonisation and disease progression, or whether low numbers simply reflect depletion of MAIT cells in the circulation, because of recruitment to the airway mucosa.

MAIT cells provide a pivotal link between the innate and adaptive immune responses. The semi-invariant T-cell receptor on MAIT cells recognises metabolite derivatives of pathogens (e.g. vitamin B (riboflavin and folic acid)) presented combined to MR-1 [19]. Activated MAIT cells produce high concentrations of pro-inflammatory interleukin (IL)-17 [20], which invokes a potent cascade of cytokines and chemokines (e.g. IL-8 and G-CSF) that promote neutrophil migration into the airways. Interleukin-17 is involved in neutrophil recruitment in CF and high concentrations have been described in sputum and bronchoalveolar lavage fluid of subjects with CF infected with *P. aeruginosa* and also in those patients with severe disease [21–23].

Mouse models demonstrate MAIT cell recruitment into the lungs at a very early stage of bacterial infection and sustained

MAIT cell responsiveness during the late stages of infection contributes towards an ongoing cytokine response [10]. In mice with selective MAIT cell deficiency the immune response was ineffective in controlling pulmonary infection [10].

Whilst we provide the first description of circulating MAIT cells in CF, understanding of the role of MAIT cells in human disease is limited. A reduction in the proportion of circulating MAIT cells has been reported in subjects with human immunodeficiency virus (HIV), *Mycobacterium tuberculosis* (MTB) and other severe pulmonary infections, and sepsis [7,8,24–26]. In HIV infection, blood MAIT cells concentrations decrease progressively from time of infection, however, MAIT cell density remains relatively preserved in rectal mucosa, suggesting possible preferential recruitment and thus loss from the circulating pool [27,28]. Similarly, MTB reactive MAIT cells are enriched in lung lymph of healthy people when compared to matched blood samples [29]. Collectively, the results of these earlier studies and our current work suggest that although blood MAIT cell counts may not reflect tissue concentrations, they may still prove to be a useful, surrogate biomarker of the immune response within the lung [30]. We demonstrate a strong, inverse relationship between MAIT cell counts and CRP and the specificity of MAIT cell responsiveness to bacterial and fungal infections, offers the potential for improved specificity compared to CRP, which will respond to both viruses and non-infective sources of systemic inflammation [31]. Further mechanistic studies of MAIT cells in CF, including assessment in the actual airway will provide novel insights into their role in innate and adaptive immunity in the CF lung, including whether effective vaccines can be developed that boost MAIT cell function to allow eradication of key bacterial pathogens.

γ/δ T-cells represent a minor population of circulating T-cells, which has the capacity to expand rapidly in response to bacterial infection [32]. γ/δ T-and MAIT cells share many similarities; they both produce IL-17 and preferentially migrate to mucosal surfaces from the circulation [33]. In murine pulmonary infection models, γ/δ T-cells rapidly accumulate in the lung, in response to a range bacterial pathogens, where they facilitate the influx of neutrophils and subsequent bacterial clearance [32]. The small increase in the proportion of γ/δ T-cells in the blood of CF subjects in the current study is consistent with findings of a single previous study in CF [34]. However, the relationship between γ/δ T-cells and clinical parameters in CF subjects were only significant when absolute γ/δ T-cell concentrations were considered and these relationships may simply reflect changes in the absolute numbers of T-cells, rather than any implying any specific role for γ/δ T-cell in pathology.

Our current study has several limitations. Firstly, cross-sectional data collection, does not inform whether a causal relationships exists between lymphocytes subsets and clinical parameters. Furthermore, the limited number of patients included in the analysis of stable disease *versus* pulmonary exacerbation, and inclusion of only five patients not infected with *P. aeruginosa* means type I statistical errors are possible. Longitudinal studies which collect blood samples from the same subject before and after the acquisition of *P. aeruginosa,* or during a pulmonary exacerbation and again during a period of stable disease are required. Finally, blood lymphocyte population may not reflect airway populations and studies which correlate lymphocyte concentrations in airway biopsies to those in the blood are anticipated.

Conclusion

In summary, we describe important differences in the proportions of circulating MAIT and γ/δ T-cell in adult patients with CF, compared to healthy control subjects. Reduced numbers of MAIT cells were associated with *P. aeruginosa* pulmonary infection and more severe lung disease. Our findings provide the impetus for future studies examining the utility of MAIT cells in immunotherapies and vaccine development, and longitudinal studies of MAIT cells as biomarkers of CF pulmonary infection.

Supporting Information

File S1 Tables S1, S2, and Figures S1–S5. Table S1 in File S1. Sputum microbiology of CF subjects. Table S2 in File S1. Relationship between White cell count and lymphocyte subsets, and C-reactive protein, body mass index and lung function. Figure S1 in File S1 Flow diagram of subjects include in sub-group analysis. Figure S2 in File S1 Representative flow-cytometry gating plots. Figure S3 in File S1. MAIT cell percentage in CF subjects with *Pseudomonas aeruginosa* and a co-pathogen in sputum culture. Figure S4 in File S1. Comparison of γ/δ T-cell counts in stable subjects and subjects undergoing antibiotic treatment for a pulmonary exacerbation. Figure S5 in File S1. Comparison of lymphocyte counts and percentage of lymphocyte sub-sets between A. Stable and pulmonary exacerbations B. *P. aeruginosa* infected and non-infected CF subjects.

File S2 Individual Subject Raw Data.

Author Contributions

Conceived and designed the experiments: DS DR GH SB. Performed the experiments: DS. Analyzed the data: DS. Contributed reagents/materials/analysis tools: DS DR GH. Contributed to the writing of the manuscript: DS DR GH SB.

References

1. Elizur A, Cannon CL, Ferkol TW (2008) Airway inflammation in cystic fibrosis. Chest 133: 489–495.
2. Ratner D, Mueller C (2012) Immune responses in Cystic Fibrosis; are they intrinsically defective? Am J Respir Cell Mol Biol.
3. Regamey N, Tsartsali L, Hilliard TN, Fuchs O, Tan HL, et al. (2012) Distinct patterns of inflammation in the airway lumen and bronchial mucosa of children with cystic fibrosis. Thorax 67: 164–170.
4. Moser C, Jensen PO (2011) Adaptive Immune Responses and Biofilm Infections. Biofilm Infections: 201–214.
5. Hartl D, Griese M, Kappler M, Zissel G, Reinhardt D, et al. (2006) Pulmonary T(H)2 response in Pseudomonas aeruginosa-infected patients with cystic fibrosis. J Allergy Clin Immunol 117: 204–211.
6. Moser C, Kjaergaard S, Pressler T, Kharazmi A, Koch C, et al. (2000) The immune response to chronic Pseudomonas aeruginosa lung infection in cystic fibrosis patients is predominantly of the Th2 type. APMIS 108: 329–335.
7. Gold MC, Lewinsohn DM (2013) Co-dependents: MR1-restricted MAIT cells and their antimicrobial function. Nat Rev Microbiol 11: 14–19.
8. Le Bourhis L, Martin E, Peguillet I, Guihot A, Froux N, et al. (2010) Antimicrobial activity of mucosal-associated invariant T cells. Nat Immunol 11: 701–708.
9. Lanier LL (2013) Shades of grey–the blurring view of innate and adaptive immunity. Nat Rev Immunol 13: 73–74.
10. Meierovics A, Yankelevich WJ, Cowley SC (2013) MAIT cells are critical for optimal mucosal immune responses during in vivo pulmonary bacterial infection. Proc Natl Acad Sci U S A 110: E3119–3128.
11. Hausler M, Schweizer K, Biesterfel S, Opladen T, Heimann G (2002) Peripheral decrease and pulmonary homing of CD4+CD45RO+ helper memory T cells in cystic fibrosis. Respir Med 96: 87–94.
12. Autissier P, Soulas C, Burdo TH, Williams KC (2010) Evaluation of a 12-color flow cytometry panel to study lymphocyte, monocyte, and dendritic cell subsets in humans. Cytometry A 77: 410–419.
13. Martin E, Treiner E, Duban L, Guerri L, Laude H, et al. (2009) Stepwise development of MAIT cells in mouse and human. PLoS Biol 7: e54.
14. Hamerman JA, Ogasawara K, Lanier LL (2005) NK cells in innate immunity. Curr Opin Immunol 17: 29–35.

15. Culley FJ (2009) Natural killer cells in infection and inflammation of the lung. Immunology 128: 151–163.
16. Wesselkamper SC, Eppert BL, Motz GT, Lau GW, Hassett DJ, et al. (2008) NKG2D is critical for NK cell activation in host defense against Pseudomonas aeruginosa respiratory infection. J Immunol 181: 5481–5489.
17. Daley L, Pier GB, Liporace JD, Eardley DD (1985) Polyclonal B cell stimulation and interleukin 1 induction by the mucoid exopolysaccharide of Pseudomonas aeruginosa associated with cystic fibrosis. J Immunol 134: 3089–3093.
18. Novak J, Dobrovolny J, Novakova L, Kozak T (2014) The decrease in number and change in phenotype of mucosal-associated invariant T cells in the elderly and differences in males and females of reproductive age. Scand J Immunol.
19. Lopez-Sagaseta J, Dulberger CL, McFedries A, Cushman M, Saghatelian A, et al. (2013) MAIT recognition of a stimulatory bacterial antigen bound to MR1. J Immunol 191: 5268–5277.
20. Dusseaux M, Martin E, Serriari N, Peguillet I, Premel V, et al. (2011) Human MAIT cells are xenobiotic-resistant, tissue-targeted, CD161hi IL-17-secreting T cells. Blood 117: 1250–1259.
21. McAllister F, Henry A, Kreindler JL, Dubin PJ, Ulrich L, et al. (2005) Role of IL-17A, IL-17F, and the IL-17 receptor in regulating growth-related oncogene-alpha and granulocyte colony-stimulating factor in bronchial epithelium: implications for airway inflammation in cystic fibrosis. J Immunol 175: 404–412.
22. Tan HL, Regamey N, Brown S, Bush A, Lloyd CM, et al. (2011) The Th17 pathway in cystic fibrosis lung disease. Am J Respir Crit Care Med 184: 252–258.
23. Tiringer K, Treis A, Fucik P, Gona M, Gruber S, et al. (2013) A Th17- and Th2-skewed cytokine profile in cystic fibrosis lungs represents a potential risk factor for Pseudomonas aeruginosa infection. Am J Respir Crit Care Med 187: 621–629.
24. Grimaldi D, Le Bourhis L, Sauneuf B, Dechartres A, Rousseau C, et al. (2014) Specific MAIT cell behaviour among innate-like T lymphocytes in critically ill patients with severe infections. Intensive Care Med 40: 192–201.
25. Wong EB, Akilimali NA, Govender P, Sullivan ZA, Cosgrove C, et al. (2013) Low levels of peripheral CD161++CD8+ mucosal associated invariant T (MAIT) cells are found in HIV and HIV/TB co-infection. PLoS One 8: e83474.
26. Jiang J, Wang X, An H, Yang B, Cao Z, et al. (2014) Mucosal-associated Invariant T-Cell Function Is Modulated by Programmed Death-1 Signaling in Patients with Active Tuberculosis. Am J Respir Crit Care Med 190: 329–339.
27. Cosgrove C, Ussher JE, Rauch A, Gartner K, Kurioka A, et al. (2013) Early and nonreversible decrease of CD161++/MAIT cells in HIV infection. Blood 121: 951–961.
28. Leeansyah E, Ganesh A, Quigley MF, Sonnerborg A, Andersson J, et al. (2013) Activation, exhaustion, and persistent decline of the antimicrobial MR1-restricted MAIT-cell population in chronic HIV-1 infection. Blood 121: 1124–1135.
29. Gold MC, Cerri S, Smyk-Pearson S, Cansler ME, Vogt TM, et al. (2010) Human mucosal associated invariant T cells detect bacterially infected cells. PLoS Biol 8: e1000407.
30. Shoki AH, Mayer-Hamblett N, Wilcox PG, Sin DD, Quon BS (2013) Systematic review of blood biomarkers in cystic fibrosis pulmonary exacerbations. Chest 144: 1659–1670.
31. Levy H, Kalish LA, Huntington I, Weller N, Gerard C, et al. (2007) Inflammatory markers of lung disease in adult patients with cystic fibrosis. Pediatr Pulmonol 42: 256–262.
32. Ito M, Kojiro N, Ikeda T, Ito T, Funada J, et al. (1992) Increased proportions of peripheral blood gamma delta T cells in patients with pulmonary tuberculosis. Chest 102: 195–197.
33. Sutton CE, Mielke LA, Mills KH (2012) IL-17-producing gammadelta T cells and innate lymphoid cells. Eur J Immunol 42: 2221–2231.
34. Raga S, Julia MR, Crespi C, Figuerola J, Martinez N, et al. (2003) Gammadelta T lymphocytes from cystic fibrosis patients and healthy donors are high TNF-alpha and IFN-gamma-producers in response to Pseudomonas aeruginosa. Respir Res 4: 9.

15

An AGM Model for Changes in Complement during Pregnancy: Neutralization of Influenza Virus by Serum Is Diminished in Late Third Trimester

Anne E. Mayer*, Griffith D. Parks

Department of Microbiology and Immunology, Wake Forest School of Medicine, Winston-Salem, NC 27101, United States of America

Abstract

Pregnant women in the third trimester are at increased risk of severe influenza disease relative to the general population, though mechanisms behind this are not completely understood. The immune response to influenza infection employs both complement (C′) and antibody (Ab). The relative contributions of these components to the anti-viral response are difficult to dissect because most humans have pre-existing influenza-specific Abs. We developed the African green monkey (AGM) as a tractable nonhuman primate model to study changes in systemic innate immunity to influenza during pregnancy. Because the AGMs were influenza-naïve, we were able to examine the role of C′ in influenza virus neutralization using serum from non-pregnant animals before and after influenza infection. We determined that serum from naïve AGMs neutralized influenza via C′, while post-infection neutralization did not require C′, suggesting an Ab-mediated mechanism. The latter mimicked neutralization using human serum. Further, we found that *ex vivo* neutralization of influenza with both naïve and influenza-immune AGM serum occurred by virus particle aggregation and lysis, with immune serum lysing virus at a much higher rate than naïve serum. We hypothesized that the anti-influenza C′ response would diminish late in AGM pregnancy, corresponding with the time when pregnant women suffer increased influenza severity. We found that influenza neutralization capacity is significantly diminished in serum collected late in the third trimester. Strikingly, we found that circulating levels of C3, C3a, and C4 are diminished late in gestation relative to nonpregnant animals, and while neutralization capacity and serum C3a return to normal shortly after parturition, C3 and C4 levels do not. This AGM model system will enable further studies of the role of physiologic and hormonal changes in downregulating C′-mediated anti-viral immunity during pregnancy, and it will permit the identification of therapeutic targets to improve outcomes of influenza virus infection in pregnant women.

Editor: Ilhem Messaoudi, University of California Riverside, United States of America

Funding: This work was supported by National Institutes of Health www.nih.gov AI083253 (GDP), AI101675 (GDP), NCI CCSG P30CA012197 (flow cytometry and imaging core), RR019963/OD010965 (animal resources), T32 OD010957 (AEM). The funders had no role in study design, data collection and analysis, decision to publish, or preparation of the manuscript.

Competing Interests: The authors have declared that no competing interests exist.

* Email: anmayer@wakehealth.edu

Introduction

Pregnancy is a unique physiologic state that is essential for the survival of all mammalian species. It requires the maternal immune system to perform the seemingly contradictory roles of tolerance to accept the fetus (as an alloantigen) and protection of the mother and fetus from infection and inflammatory insults. Pregnancy has historically been characterized as a state of immune suppression [1]; however, this description oversimplifies the complex physiologic requirements of the progression from implantation and placentation, to rapid fetal growth and development, to preparation for delivery [2]. These distinct phases of pregnancy have different physiologic needs and are accompanied by highly regulated hormone alterations, shifting profiles of energy expenditure, and a changing immunological milieu [3,4]. Given these unique alterations, it stands to reason that pregnant women experience a distinct range of immunological challenges [2,5,6]. Together, this raises the clinically relevant question of how the innate immune response to viruses is altered during pregnancy [7].

Influenza virus infection is associated with a disproportionately high burden of disease in pregnant women around the world, during both pandemics and seasonal outbreaks [3,8,9]. During the 2009 H1N1 pandemic, for example, pregnant women were at ten-times the risk of severe infection relative to non-pregnant women [9]. There has been extensive documentation of pregnant women infected with influenza virus suffering disproportionately severe respiratory disease and the public health impact of this phenomenon [10–12]. These severe influenza virus infections are most common late in pregnancy [9,10,13] and may lead to serious outcomes such as low gestational weight, preterm birth, and infant failure to thrive, even in the absence of fetal infection [9,14,15]. These effects pose significant public health challenges and are of great economic cost worldwide.

Though complement (C′) has been traditionally regarded as playing an important role in protection from bacterial infections, it also plays a significant role in the innate response to a number of viruses including VSV, mumps, measles, Newcastle disease, parainfluenza viruses, and influenza virus [16–21]. The C′ cascade has unique and essential roles in early responses to infection such as direct virus neutralization, induction of chemotaxis, enhancement of phagocytosis, immune complex clearance, and lysis of infected cells [22]. Specifically, C′ is essential for effective clearance of influenza virus [21,23,24]. For example, C3−/− mice are highly susceptible to influenza virus infection—with increased virus titers and delayed clearance relative to WT mice [23].

While natural antibodies (nAbs) play an important role in eliciting an effective immune response against primary infections with influenza virus [24,25], natural IgM (nIgM) does not effectively neutralize influenza virus in the absence of C′ [21]. This also holds true for other types of low affinity Abs, such as cross-reactive Abs [26,27]. Further, it has been shown that C′ can fix Ab to mediate opsonization or membrane attack, via the classical pathway. From a clinical context, seasonal influenza epidemics are comprised of disease among individuals previously infected with closely related strains in prior seasons; this indicates that cross-reactive Abs are often not adequate to protect healthy adults, even in the presence of normal C′. In fact, the role that cross-reactive Ab plays in protecting a patient from a new influenza virus infection is highly strain-dependent [28]. We hypothesize that differences in C′ between pregnant women and other healthy adult populations contribute to the increased disease severity seen in the pregnant population. Here we developed a model that enabled us to identify the unique and non-redundant roles of C′ in influenza virus neutralization with influenza-naïve serum.

While C′ effects indirectly enhance the downstream immune response (e.g. by increasing phagocytosis and acting as chemoattractants for innate immune cell types), we have more recently come to appreciate that the C′ system can also directly regulate humoral immunity and T cell functions [29–31]. Therefore, alterations in C′ levels and/or function have the potential for broader effects on the whole immune response to a pathogen. The role of C′ in increased severity of influenza during pregnancy, however, has not been previously explored.

C′ activation is correlated with poor pregnancy outcomes such as pre-eclampsia and preterm birth, leading to the proposal that C′ inhibition is an "absolute requirement" of normal pregnancy [32]. It has been proposed that C′ activation during pregnancy leads to a pro-inflammatory, pro-coagulant, and tissue damaging environment surrounding the fetus [33]. For example, high levels of anaphylatoxins, such as C5a, induce the release of potent anti-angiogenic factors, which sequester growth factors that are essential for normal placental development and healthy pregnancy [34–36]. However, these studies seem at odds with a number of reports that C′ is activated during pregnancy [37–39]. Such disparities may reflect the difficulties inherent in performing longitudinal studies in pregnant women. Further, to our knowledge, no analysis of functional C′ activity against pathogens has been performed using samples from pregnant women. Thus, the question of how C′ functions against pathogens such as influenza virus during pregnancy remains unresolved.

Human studies pose significant obstacles to addressing this experimental question because of differences in anti-influenza virus antibody levels among subjects, which confounds the analysis of the role of C′ in neutralization [40,41]. Thus, we sought to identify an influenza-naïve pregnancy model system that closely mimics the pregnancy physiology of women. Mice are the most common animal model used in pregnancy studies because they are relatively inexpensive, are reared in an easily controlled environment, and their short gestation period enables rapid experiments and large sample sizes. However, murine reproductive physiology differs greatly from that of humans [42,43]. The African green monkey (AGM) is a strikingly suitable model for studies of reproductive physiology, with many characteristics in common with humans (Table 1). For example, AGMs have cycle types, hormone levels, and pregnancy physiology very similar to those of humans. Additionally, while AGM fetal development occurs in a similar fashion as humans, the 5.5-month AGM gestation period is slightly compressed and more accessible than that of humans. For this study, the Wake Forest University Primate Center (WFUPC) Vervet Research Colony (VRC) served as a source for groups of pregnant and control female AGMs. Access to the VRC enabled us to perform longitudinal sampling during and after pregnancy.

Here, we demonstrate the utility of this novel AGM model system by determining how C′ levels and the capacity for C′-mediated virus neutralization change during pregnancy. We found that late in third trimester (T3), pregnant animals have significantly diminished circulating C′ factors and decreased capacity to neutralize influenza virus. Our data support a model whereby these late T3 C′ reductions, which may be essential to permit the maintenance of healthy pregnancy, could increase the severity of influenza disease.

Materials and Methods

Cells, viruses, and serum

Monolayer cultures of MDBK cells [44] were grown in Dulbecco's modified Eagle medium (DMEM) supplemented with 10% heat-inactivated fetal bovine serum (FBS), penicillin (100 units/ml), streptomycin (100 ug/ml) and 2 mM L-Glutamine. U937 cells (ATCC, Manassas, VA) were grown in RPMI supplemented as above. Influenza A virus engineered to encode GFP as a fusion protein with the viral NS1 protein was the kind gift of Adolfo Garcia-Sastre [45] and was grown in 10 day old embryonated chicken eggs as described previously [46]. The properties of individual normal human sera (NHS) from healthy donors has been described previously [20]. Commercially available pooled human sera was from Complement Technology, Inc. (Tyler, TX).

Ethics statements and animal husbandry

Individual NHS samples were collected following approval of the Wake Forest University IRB under human protocol number BG04–504 and written consent of the individuals. AGM studies were carried out in strict accordance with the recommendations in the Guide for the Care and Use of Laboratory Animals of the National Institutes of Health. The protocols were approved by the Wake Forest University Animal Care and Use Committee (A13–023; A13–027) and utilized animals from the Vervet Research Colony (VRC) of the Wake Forest University Primate Center (WFPC). At the time of the study, the colony consisted of 486 animals in their second to eighth generation in captivity. All animals were colony-born and were of known age. Regular procedures revolve around the tri-annual TB testing program, during which time every animal in the colony is captured, sedated, physically examined, and tested for TB, and (if female) given a reproductive ultrasound. In addition, an appropriate environmental enrichment SOP for the influenza infection project (A13–023) was approved by the Wake Forest University Nonhuman Primate Environmental Enrichment Committee. This included, but was not limited to: pair-housing the majority of the time, but single-housed temporarily for experimental requirements; monkeys

Table 1. Reproductive comparisons across species.

	Mouse[a]	Human[b]	AGM[c]
Gestation Length	18–20 days	~280 days	~155 days
Number of Offspring per Parturition	6–8	1–2	1–2
Hormone Sources During Pregnancy	Corpus luteum is source of progesterone; systemic progesterone withdrawal prior to parturition	Corpus luteum initial source; placenta after eighth week	Placenta is source of progesterone
Structure of Female Reproductive Tract	Duplex (two separate uterine horns)	Simplex (single cavity) uterus	Simplex uterine cavity similar to human
Cycling Estrogen Levels	~100 pg/ml (estrous peak)	~400 pg/ml (preovulatory peak)	~500 pg/ml (preovulatory peak)
Cycle Type	Estrous (4–5 d)	Menstrual (28 d)	Menstrual (31 d)
Age at Onset of Puberty	6 w	10–11 y	3 y

[a]See reference [76].
[b]See reference [77].
[c]See reference [78–84].

located to have auditory, visual, and olfactory stimulation from other monkeys in the room; and monkeys received species-appropriate toys and manipulate, which were rotated regularly. All experimental procedures were performed only with sedated animals and appropriate analgesia was administered. Steps were taken to ameliorate suffering and improve animal welfare in accordance with the recommendations of the Weatherall report (2006). Pregnant, postpartum, and control animals for the pregnancy portion of this work were housed in large maternal social groups with indoor/outdoor housing and equipment for normal physical activity. All animals were fed the Purina #5038 normal protein monkey chow diet *ad libitum*. Food was removed the night before procedures requiring sedation and/or anesthesia. Animals in this project were fully under the care of veterinarians at the WFU School of Medicine in accordance with the standards incorporated in The Guide to the Care and Use of Laboratory Animals (2011).

Animal infection

Healthy 18–22 yo African Green monkeys (*Chlorocebus aethiops*) were sedated with ketamine, and placed in a dorsal position before receiving 8×10^9 50% Egg Infective Dose (EID_{50}) of purified H1N1 influenza strain A/Puerto Rico/8/1934 (PR8) delivered in 2 ml sterile PBS. One ml was delivered to the trachea and 0.5 ml was delivered to each nostril. Femoral blood was collected at the days pi indicated in the figure legends and allowed to clot for 45 min at 37°C. The clot was retracted and serum was separated by centrifugation, aliquoted and stored at −80°C. Complement inactivated serum was prepared by heating inactivation (HI) of normal AGM serum (NAGS) at 56°C for 30 min.

Pregnant animals

Fifty-nine AGMs in the VRC were identified as pregnant between January and May 2012 and used in this study. Control animals were selected at random from the VRC during two dates overlapping with collection dates for pregnant animals. The animals used in the study are described in Table 2. We used third trimester and postpartum samples from a longitudinal sampling scheme that involved tracking and sampling of each animal two to three times during pregnancy, once within 5–10 days following parturition at check-in (PC), and once two to six months postpartum (PP). Repeated blood samples from the pregnant animals in the breeding colony were obtained during TB testing dates, following sedation and ultrasound confirmation of pregnancy status. Briefly, during the 2012 breeding season, femoral vein blood samples were collected from each pregnant animal during the regularly scheduled TB testing in January, May, and September. We faced the challenge of having no *a priori* knowledge of conception dates for females in the VRC colony. Ultrasound was used to estimate the gestational age of the fetus based on fetal head circumference [47]. Additional dates were scheduled in April and July 2012 for blood draws, physical exams, and ultrasounds to confirm healthy gestation. Serum was isolated and stored as described above. Samples used in C′ ELISAs and neutralization experiments were categorized based on the gestation date when the sample was collected.

Serum neutralization assays

PR8 neutralization experiments were performed by treating 5 PFU of PR8-GFP with normal or HI human or AGM sera diluted in RPMI (in a total volume of 100 μl), as indicated in the figure legends for 45 min at 37°C. U937 cells (2×10^5) were added, and the mixtures were analyzed 48 h later for GFP expression. This extended incubation period allowed for high sensitivity and detection of small differences in neutralization capacity across serum samples. The effective dose 50 (ED_{50}) was developed as a measure representative of neutralization capacity for serum samples collected from pregnant and postpartum animals. Neutralization assays were carried out using different dilutions of sera, as described above. For each dilution (1:40, 1:80, 1:160, and 1:320) of each serum sample, the percent neutralization was calculated using the following equation:

$$\%\ \text{neutralization}_{(NAGS)} = [1- (\%GFP^{+}_{(NAGS)})/(\%GFP^{+}_{(No\ serum)})]*100$$

This number was plotted on the y-axis against the corresponding serum dilution on the x-axis, and a logistic regression was performed over the whole series, as shown in Results. In this fashion, a logistic regression was performed for samples from each animal, and the ED_{50} was determined by calculating the amount of serum required to achieve a y-value of 50% neutralization.

Electron microscopy

Electron microscopy (EM) analysis of sucrose gradient-purified PR8 was carried out as previously described [20]. Briefly, 5 μl of a 1:5 dilution of PR8 (13.8 μg of PR8) was incubated with 5 μl of a 1:5 dilution of AGM serum at 37°C for the time period indicated

Table 2. Characteristics of AGM pregnant and control samples.

	Pregnant	Controls
Total number of animals	53 (+6 prior to sampling)	24
Age range	3.3–17 years	5–20 years
% primiparous	18.9%	N/A
% with history of poor outcomes[a]	22.6%	N/A
% with 2012 poor outcome[b]	16.9%	N/A
T1[c]	13 (11.8%)[d]	N/A
T2[c]	37 (33.6%)[d]	N/A
T3[c]	60[e] (54.5%)[d]	N/A
Parturition check-in[c]	58	N/A
2–6 mo post partum[c]	54	N/A

[a]Percent of animals that have had stillbirths, aborted fetuses, or infant mortality less than 6 months old in pregnancies prior to 2012.
[b]Same as a, but during 2012 breeding season when samples were collected.
[c]Number of animals (percent of animals in parentheses) for which we collected a sample during Trimester 1 (<55 days), Trimester 2 (55–110 days), Trimester 3 (>110 days), at parturition check-in (5–10 days after parturtion), and 2–6 months postpartum.
[d]Number in parentheses indicates percent of total pregnancy samples collected during indicated trimester.
[e]7 animals (60–53 = 7) were sampled twice during T3.

in the figure legend. Zero min incubations were performed on ice. After the indicated time, mixtures were placed on Formvar carbon-coated 200-mesh gold grids (EM Sciences, PA) and incubated in a humidified chamber for 10 min before fixing with 2.5% glutaraldehyde. Samples were negatively stained with 2% phospho-tungstic acid and analyzed with a Technai transmission electron microscope.

Western blotting

Western blotting was performed as described previously [48]. Specifically, either 1:50, 1:250, and 1:500 dilutions of each NHS and NAGS samples (for species comparison) or 1:200 and 1:400 dilutions of each pregnancy NAGS sample (for quantification) were electrophoresed and transferred to a nitrocellulose blot which was probed with goat anti-human C3 primary Ab at a 1:2000 dilution (Calbiochem), followed by HRP-conjugated donkey anti-goat at a dilution of 1:4000. Quantities of AGM C3 were determined relative to 50 ng, 100 ng, and 200 ng samples of purified human C3 (Complement Technology, Inc., Tyler, TX) using a Kodak Image Station 4000R and Carestream MI software (Molecular Imaging System Carestream, Health Inc.).

ELISA

MaxiSorp 96-well ELISA plates (Nalge Nunc International, Penfield, NY) were coated with 100 µl of diluted serum (1:32,000 for C3; 1:16,000 for C3a; 1:6000 for C4), or with dilutions of purified C3, C3a or C4 human standards (all from Complement Technology). Plates were incubated at 4°C overnight, washed three times with PBS/Tween (0.2%), and wells were blocked with 200 µl of PBS containing 5% milk for 1 hr at 37°C. 100 µl of diluted primary goat anti-human C3 (1:2000), rabbit anti-human C3a (1:5000) or goat anti-human C4 (1:2000) (all from Calbiochem) was added to each well and incubated for 1 h at room temperature (RT). Wells were washed five times with PBS/Tween before incubation at RT for 1 h with 100 µl per well of HRP-conjugated donkey anti-goat (1:20,000 for C3 and C4) or goat anti-rabbit IgG (1:50,000 for C3a) (Jackson ImmunoResearch Laboratories, PA) followed by development with substrate TMB (tetramethylbenzidine dihydrochloride, Sigma). The absorbance was determined at 450 nm on a ELx800 plate Absorbance Microplate Reader (Bio Tek Instruments, Inc., Vermont).

Statistics

Graphpad Prism and was used to perform all analyses. The Shapiro-Wilk normality test was performed on each group. Based on these findings, two-tailed unpaired t-tests were performed on log-transformed neutralization percentages for comparisons between NAGS and NHS and between naïve and immune sample dates, as well as to compare C3 β-chain concentrations between control and T3 groups. In the comparison of Control vs T3 % serum for PR8 ED_{50}, the T3 distribution did not pass the Shapiro-Wilk normality test, so the Mann-Whitney compare ranks two-tailed non-parametric test was used. A one-way ANOVA and Tukey correction for multiple comparisons was used for comparisons of greater than two categories. Mean and SD are shown as measures of dispersion for each group tested in every figure. p-values represented as: * $p<0.05$; ** $p<0.001$; *** $p<0.0001$.

Results

Comparison of C′ concentrations in human and AGM sera

To our knowledge, direct quantitative comparisons of serum C3 concentrations in humans and AGMs have not been previously published. To verify relevance of the AGM model for human C′ studies, three dilutions of NAGS (Fig. 1, lanes 4–6) or NHS (Fig. 1, lanes 7–9) were analyzed by western blot for C3 levels. While there were slight differences in mobility of C3 α- and C3 β–chains between species, these data strongly suggest that human (Hu) and AGM serum C′ proteins are expressed at similar levels.

Comparison of human versus AGM sera for C′-mediated neutralization of influenza virus

A highly sensitive functional assay was developed for comparing the capacity of human and AGM serum to neutralize influenza virus *in vitro*. In this assay, dilutions of normal or heat inactivated (HI) human or AGM sera were mixed with a recombinant influenza virus PR8 that was engineered to express GFP as a

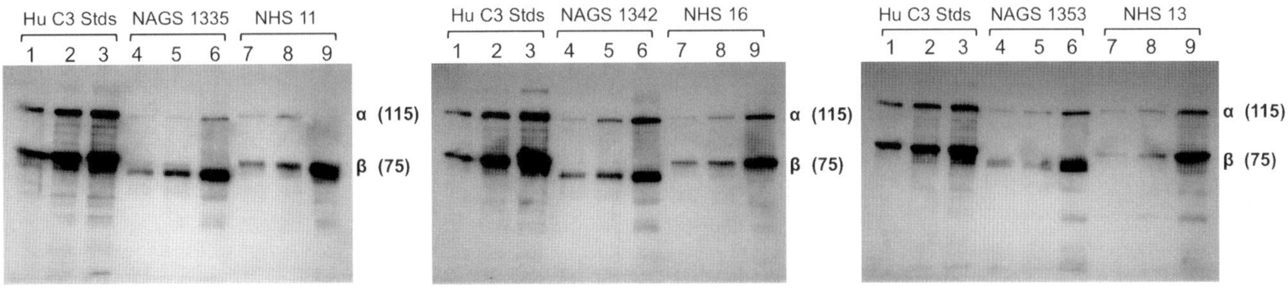

Figure 1. Comparison of C3 concentrations in NHS and NAGS. NAGS and NHS were used to compare C3 concentrations by western blot, relative to purified Hu C3 controls. Controls of 50 ng, 100 ng, and 200 ng are in lanes 1, 2, and 3, respectively, on each of the three blots. 1:500, 1:250, and 1:50 dilutions of NAGS are in lanes 4, 5, and 6, respectively and of NHS are in lanes 7, 8, and 9, respectively. One NAGS donor and one NHS donor were on each blot, as indicated in the figure by NAGS or NHS number. C3 β- and C3 α-chain and their MW in kilodaltons are indicated on each blot.

fusion protein with the viral NS-1 protein [45]. After 40 min at 37°C, samples were used to infect U937 human monocytes. 48 h post-infection (pi) the percent GFP+ cells was determined by flow cytometry. As shown in Fig. 2, Panel A, virus in the absence of serum resulted in ~23% of cells being infected. When virus was treated with a 1:40 dilution of HI AGM serum (Fig. 2, Panel C), there was no reduction in infectivity. However, following treatment with a 1:40 dilution of NAGS, only 2% of the cells were infected (Fig. 2, Panel D). This loss of infectivity with NAGS but not with HI AGM serum indicates that neutralization was dependent on intact C′ pathways. Further, PR8-GFP neutralization by NAGS was dose dependent, as treatment with 1:80, 1:160, and 1:320 dilutions of serum resulted in 9.7, 16.5, and 23.7% of cells being infected, respectively (Fig. 2, Panels E, F, G). When expressed as a percent of infected cells seen in the no-serum-treated control, diluted NAGS showed a dose dependent neutralization of PR8-GFP with 1:40, 1:80, 1:160, and 1:320 serum dilutions corresponding with 9.3%, 41.9, 71.0, and 102.2% of cells infected, respectively (Fig. 2, Panel H).

We hypothesized that neutralization of PR8-GFP with normal human serum (NHS) would occur in the absence of C′ due to pre-existing anti-influenza Abs, while NAGS neutralization would be C′-dependent because there are no circulating influenza viruses in the WFPC AGM colony. To test this hypothesis, we compared the capacity of NHS and NAGS to neutralize PR8-GFP using the flow cytometry assay described above. We found that neutralization of PR8-GFP by both pooled NHS and pooled NAGS is concentration dependent (Fig. 3A). However, NHS neutralized PR8-GFP more efficiently than NAGS—only 22% of the maximum infectivity was observed when treated with a 1:160 dilution of NHS, while there was maximum infectivity following treatment with a 1:160 dilution of NAGS (Fig. 3A). Importantly, we found that HI Hu serum neutralized PR8-GFP, but HI AGM serum did not (Fig. 3A). This indicates that influenza neutralization by pooled NHS can occur in a C′-independent fashion, while influenza neutralization with pooled NAGS requires C′.

To determine the variability in individual animals in the VRC, PR8 neutralization assays were performed using HI and NAGS samples. Results from four representative samples are shown in Fig. 3B. All animals showed dose-dependent anti-PR8 neutralization capacity. As expected, every HI serum sample tested lacked the capacity for PR8-GFP neutralization in the absence of C′ activity (Fig. 3B, cross-hatched bars), suggesting that these animals have no pre-existing anti-PR8 Abs. We also found that all of the animals tested had low variability of C′-mediated neutralization over the NAGS dilution series tested (Fig. 3B, data not shown). This demonstrates that NAGS does not have the pre-existing capacity to neutralize influenza virus in a C′-independent fashion.

In contrast, NHS samples are highly variable in this regard, likely due to variable previous exposure to any given strain of influenza virus. To demonstrate this, we performed the same influenza virus neutralization assay using NHS from three human subjects (Fig. 3C). Each of the three subjects demonstrated a different possible outcome. First, NHS #6 demonstrates the poorest neutralization of the three samples, where neutralization with a 1:40 dilution of NHS or HI serum yields the highest percent of cells infected compared to the other to human samples. NHS #3 demonstrates improved neutralization, with a lower percent of cells infected after treatment with 1:40 NHS than NHS #6 (Fig. 3C). Lastly, NHS #9 demonstrated a neutralization profile indicative of strain-specific Ab neutralization of influenza virus. While there was a dose-dependent effect of NHS #9 on viral neutralization, there was also C′-independent neutralization occurring, as indicated by 0.7% of cells infected by virus when treated with HI serum. This variability in Hu serum neutralization capacity makes it impossible to dissect the specific role of C′ during pregnancy using samples from Hu subjects.

Comparison of PR8 neutralization by AGM pre- and post-immunization sera

To test the importance of neutralizing C′ in PR8-naïve versus PR8-immune animals, we inoculated two adult, non-pregnant AGMs with PR8 by a combined intra-nasal and intra-tracheal routes and collected serum samples from each animal at 14 d post-inoculation. In an identical experimental set up, we used real time PCR on tracheal washes collected two days after AGM inoculation with PR8 to confirm that PR8 replication can occur in the AGM respiratory tract (data not shown).

The capacity of sera to neutralize PR8 was tested using the PR8-GFP flow cytometry assay described above. As shown in Fig. 4, pre-immune sera showed dose-dependent neutralization of PR8-GFP and no neutralization was seen with HI sera. Interestingly, post-immune sera (normal and HI) were better at neutralizing PR8 than any Hu serum sample tested, as evidenced by complete neutralization of PR8-GFP out to a 1:640 dilution (Fig. 4). The finding that PR8 was neutralized by HI post- but not pre-immune sera demonstrated that C′ is less important for *ex vivo* influenza neutralization after AGMs have been exposed to influenza virus.

C′-mediated virus neutralization can proceed by aggregation and/or lysis (Johnson, 2008). To determine the mechanism of virus neutralization by pre-immune AGM sera, we mixed PR8 and NAGS for various lengths of time and examined the virus

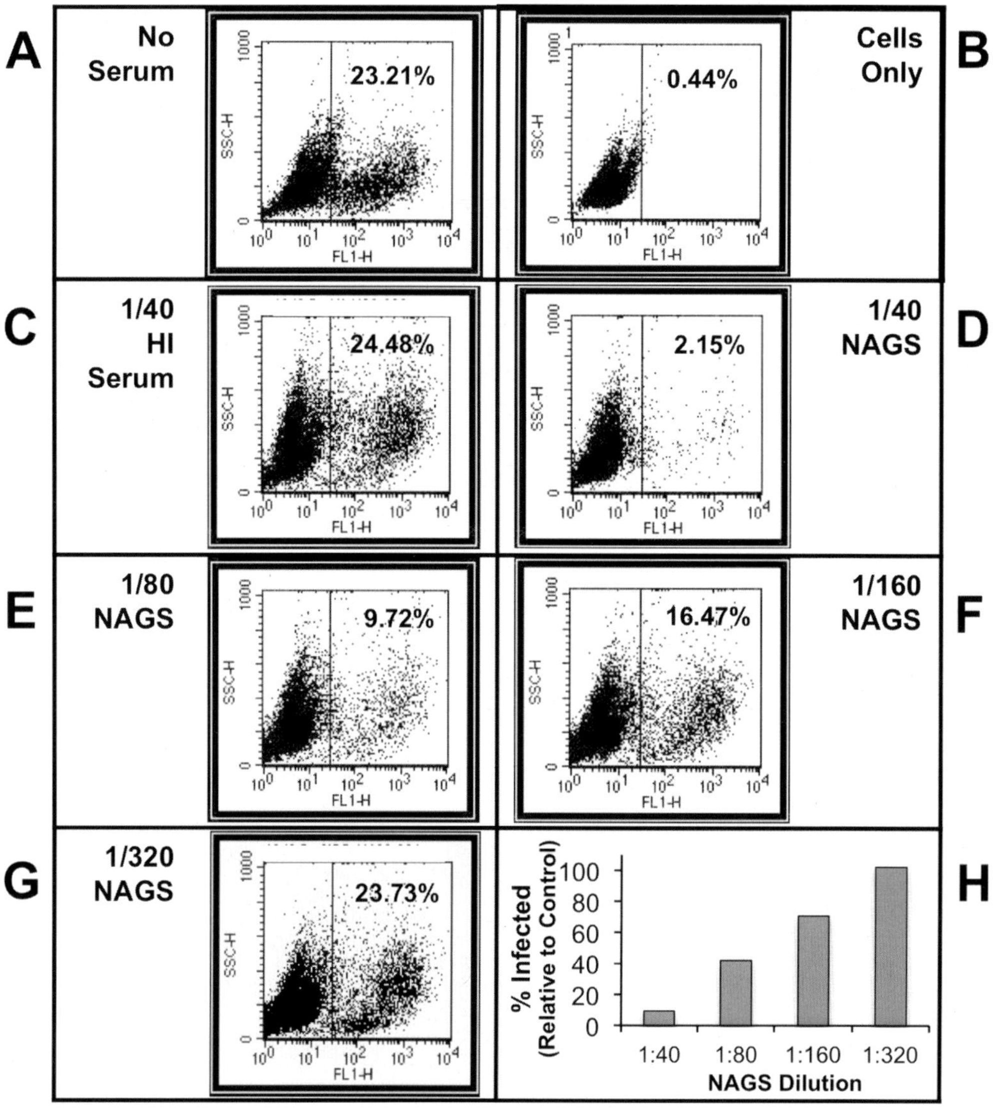

Figure 2. Flow cytometry-based PR8-GFP neutralization assay. PR8-GFP was mixed with a range of NAGS dilutions for 40 min at 37°C, and then used to infect U937 cells for 48 hr. Flow cytometry was used to determine the percentage of the cell population that was positive for GFP expression. Controls were: (A) Virus with no serum; (B) Cells only—no serum and no virus; (C) Virus plus 1:40 HI AGM serum. AGM serum dilutions used to treat virus were: (D) 1:40 NAGS; (E) 1:80 NAGS; (F) 1:160 NAGS; (G) 1:320 NAGS. (H) Percent of cells that were GFP-positive following neutralization with indicated dilutions of NAGS from one example animal, expressed relative to that found for the no serum control.

structures by electron microscopy (EM) (Fig. 5). The PR8-serum mixture was kept on ice at time 0 to limit enzyme-driven C′ activity. Incubation with pre-immune serum resulted in intact, single virus particles at time 0 (Fig. 5A). After 5 min at 37°C, these pre-immune mixtures induced the formation of small, scattered aggregates of virus particles (Fig. 5A). By 30 min there were very few single virus particles apparent, but rather mid-sized aggregates, containing some lysed virus particles (Fig. 5A). Notably, after 30 min, treatment with HI pre-immune serum appeared to have no effect on virus morphology, as EM demonstrated scattered single, whole virus particles, similar to those visualized on the time 0 EM (Fig. 5A). These data indicate that C′-mediated neutralization of influenza virus with pre-immune sera proceeds through aggregation with only limited lysis at the dilution used.

In contrast, incubation with post-immune serum induced small virus particle aggregates as early as time 0 (Fig. 5B) and larger aggregates of lysed virus particles by 5 min, as evidenced by extensive nucleocapsid leakage (Fig. 5C, arrows). By 30 min there were no intact individual virus particles on the EM grid, rather they appeared only as scattered lysed virus particle debris (Fig. 5B). HI post-immune serum resulted in small virus particle aggregates but no lysis, similar to that seen on the time 0 grid (Fig. 5B). In summary, as compared with pre-immune serum, post-immune serum neutralization of PR8 involved rapid formation of large aggregates and substantial viral lysis. In the absence of active C′ (HI), post-immune serum resulted in virus particle aggregation without lysis. Thus, post-immune serum achieves neutralizing effects on virus in the absence of C′, while this was not the case with pre-immune serum.

Decreased C′ neutralization capacity late in pregnancy

We sought to apply the above C′-mediated neutralization assays to the question of how C′ neutralization capacity changes during

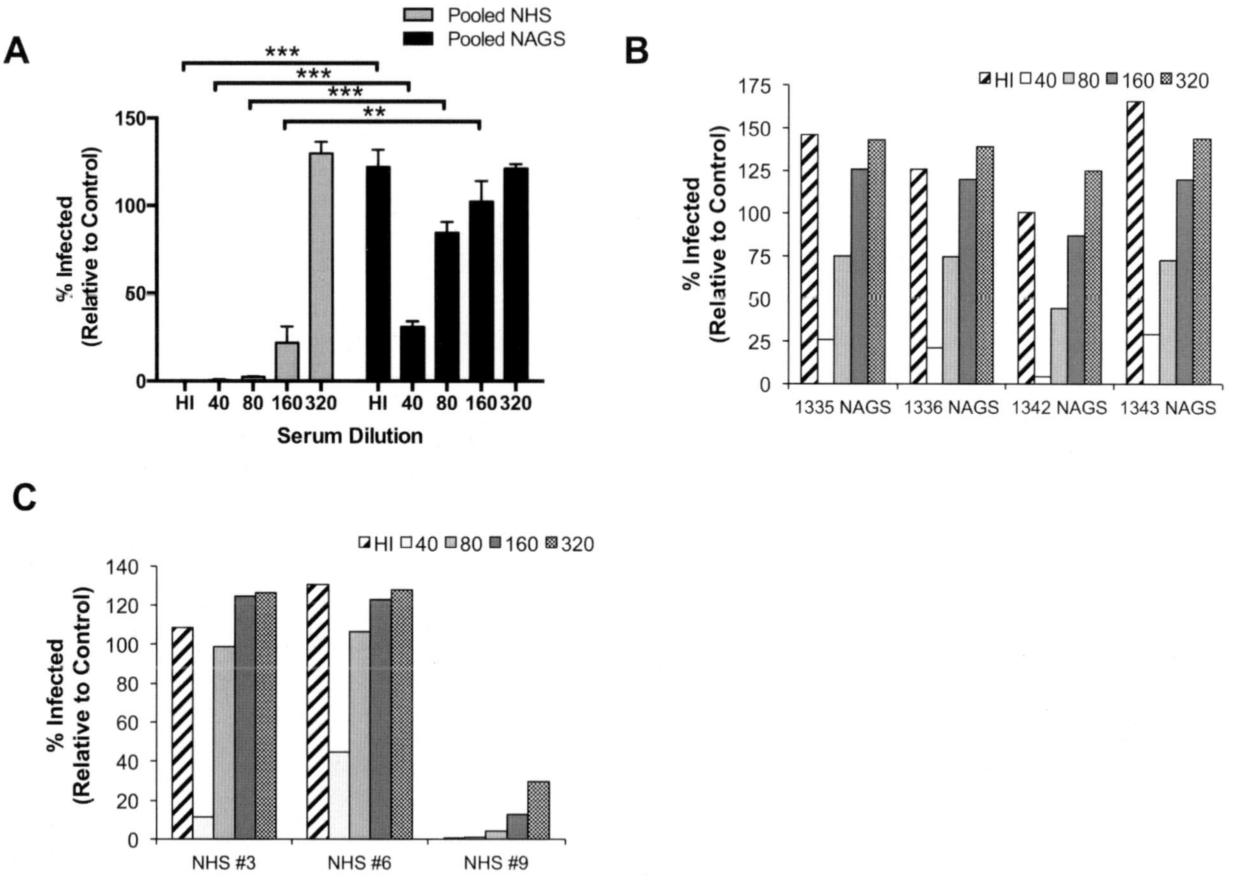

Figure 3. Comparison of C′-dependent neutralization of parainfluenza and influenza viruses by NHS and NAGS. (A) Influenza neutralization. PR8-GFP was incubated with the indicated fold dilutions of pooled Hu or AGM HI sera or varying dilutions of pooled NHS or NAGS for infection of U937 cells and analyzed as described in Fig. 2 (pooled samples are comprised of 4 individuals, Hu or AGM). Bars indicate mean of percent infected over triplicate experiments plus SD. ** $p<0.001$; *** $p<0.0001$ based on t-tests on log-transformed percentages for matching serum treatments for NHS and NAGS; treatments with no differences shown were not significantly different. (B) Variability in PR8 neutralization among samples from individual AGMs. PR8-GFP was incubated with the indicated fold dilutions of NAGS from four representative AGMs and analyzed as described in (A). There was no significant difference among animals based on a one-way ANOVA of log-transformed neutralization percentages. (C) Variability in PR8 neutralization among samples from individual Hus. Performed as in panel B, but with three individual Hus. Based on a one-way ANOVA of log transformed neutralization percentages, Hu subjects were significantly different from one another; $p=0.0045$.

pregnancy. Serum samples were collected from 53 different animals at various time points during pregnancy and postpartum. As shown in Table 2, regardless of when during gestation an animal was identified as pregnant, it was most likely that we would capture a T3 sample using our sampling scheme. This late gestation bias in our sampling worked well for this particular study, as pregnant women are most susceptible to influenza late in pregnancy. For this reason, we chose to focus on samples from this group for our experiments.

We tested the neutralization capacity of AGM sera collected at various times during pregnancy using the method described in Fig. 2. We quantified the percent of virus neutralized for a range of dilutions of sera and performed a logistic regression over the dilution series. For each animal at each pregnancy sampling date, we calculated the serum dilution that would be required to achieve 50% neutralization, or the *effective dose 50* (ED_{50}). As shown for the two examples in Fig. 6A, a higher ED_{50} (i.e. where dashed line "a" crosses the x-axis for the grey series) indicates a poorer capacity to neutralize, and a lower ED_{50} (i.e. where dashed line "b" crosses the x-axis for the black series) indicates a better capacity to neutralize. The ED_{50} was determined for 34 serum samples collected from pregnant animals during their T3 and for 20 control (nonpregnant) females. For each serum sample, HI samples did not neutralize PR8-GFP (data not shown). As demonstrated by Fig. 6B, serum from T3 animals had significantly decreased capacity to neutralize PR8-GFP, as evidenced by the finding that ~1.5 times the T3 serum was required to neutralize PR8-GFP compared to control animals.

We took advantage of our large sample size and full range of gestation dates and binned the T3 samples into smaller trimester tertiles (Fig. 6C). By comparing ED_{50} over early, mid, and late T3, we found that neutralization capacity is diminished in late T3 ($p<0.05$), but there is no significant difference between control sera and early or mid T3 sera (Fig. 6C). To determine how long after parturition this reduced neutralization capacity persisted, neutralization capacity at parturition check-in (PC, 5–10 days after parturition) and postpartum (PP, 2–6 months after parturition) was tested for the animals for which we had late T3 samples. Remarkably, we found that anti-influenza C′ neutralization capacity returned to control levels as early as 5–10 days postpartum (PC samples, Fig. 6D), and remained at control levels 2–6 months postpartum—that is, throughout and beyond lactation—(PP samples, Fig. 6D), which was the end of our study period. Further, the trend of decreased ED_{50} from late T3 to PC

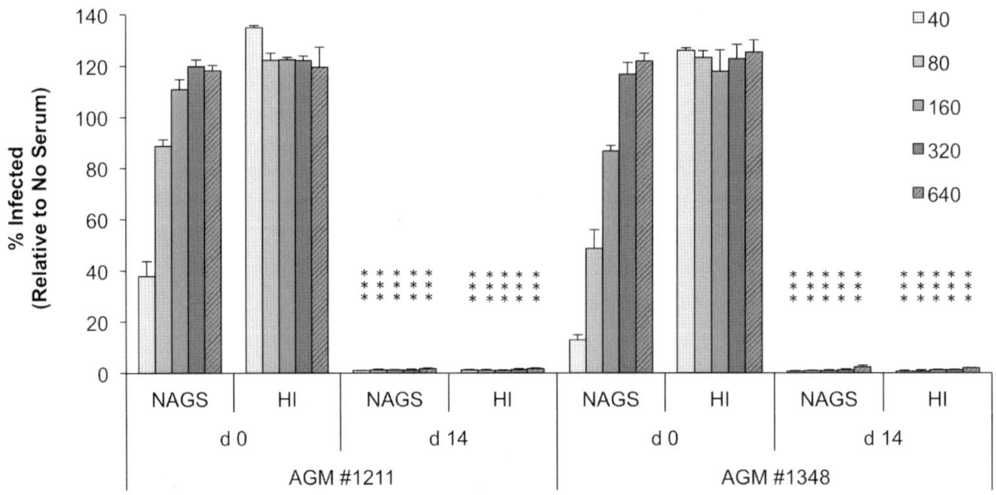

Figure 4. Effect of HI on the neutralization capacity of pre- and post-immune sera from AGM experimentally infected with PR8. Two AGMs were inoculated with PR8 as described in the Materials and Methods. Pre-immune sera (d 0) and sera collected at d 14 post-infection were tested at the indicated fold dilutions for *in vitro* neutralization of PR8-GFP as described in Fig. 2. Results are expressed as the mean plus SD from triplicate experiments to determine the percentage of GFP-positive cells compared to *in vitro* control infections (which lacked serum treatment). *** $p<0.0001$ as compared to matching serum treatment for the same animal at day 0 (shown on day 14 values) based on t-tests on log transformed neutralization percentages.

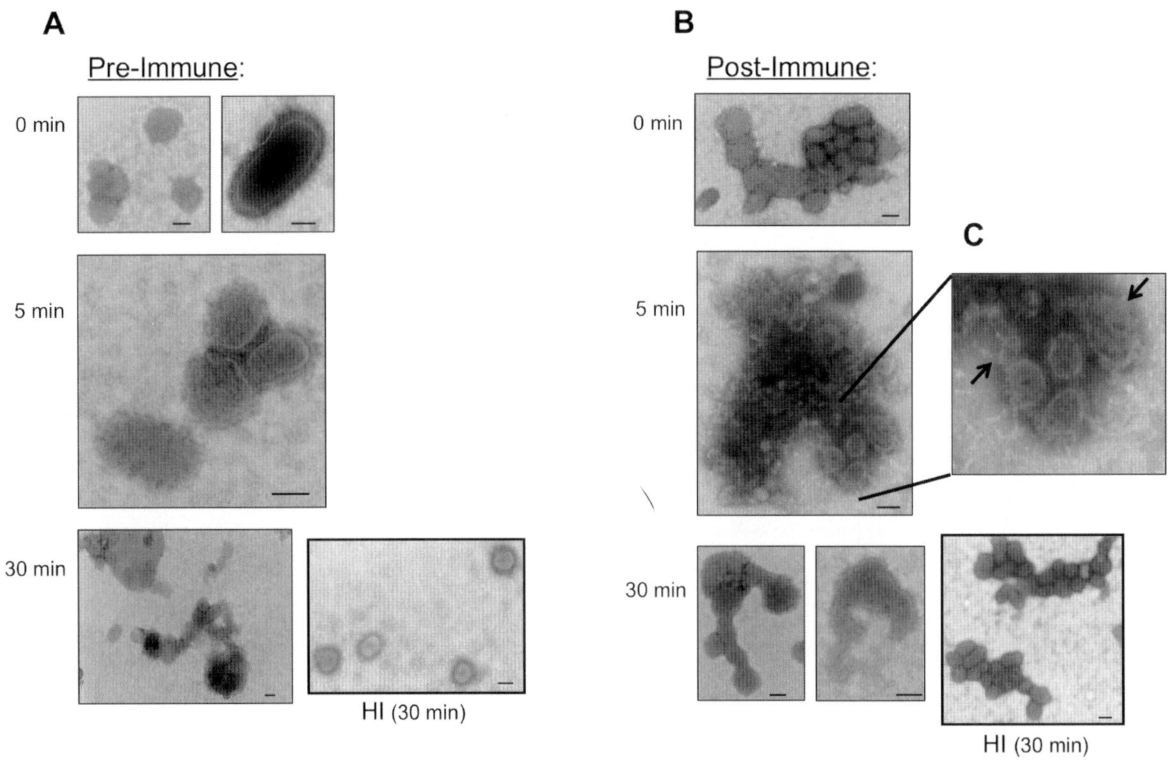

Figure 5. EM visualization of PR8 neutralization mechanism and kinetics by pre-immune, post-immune, and HI AGM sera. Sucrose-purified PR8 was incubated with a 1:20 dilution of normal or HI (A) pre-immune or (B) post-immune AGM serum at 37°C for 0, 5, or 30 min, as indicated. These mixtures were fixed and negatively stained on a carbon-coated mesh grid and analyzed by EM. (C) Zoom of indicated area of post-immune 5 min time point with arrows indicating nucleocapsid leakage from lysed virus particles. Bar indicates 100 nm in each image, and magnification is as follows: (A) 0 min- 68,000x; 5 min- 68,000x; 30 min- 49,000× (B) 0 min- 49,000x; 5 min- 49,000x; 30 min- 49,000× (left); 98,000× (right).

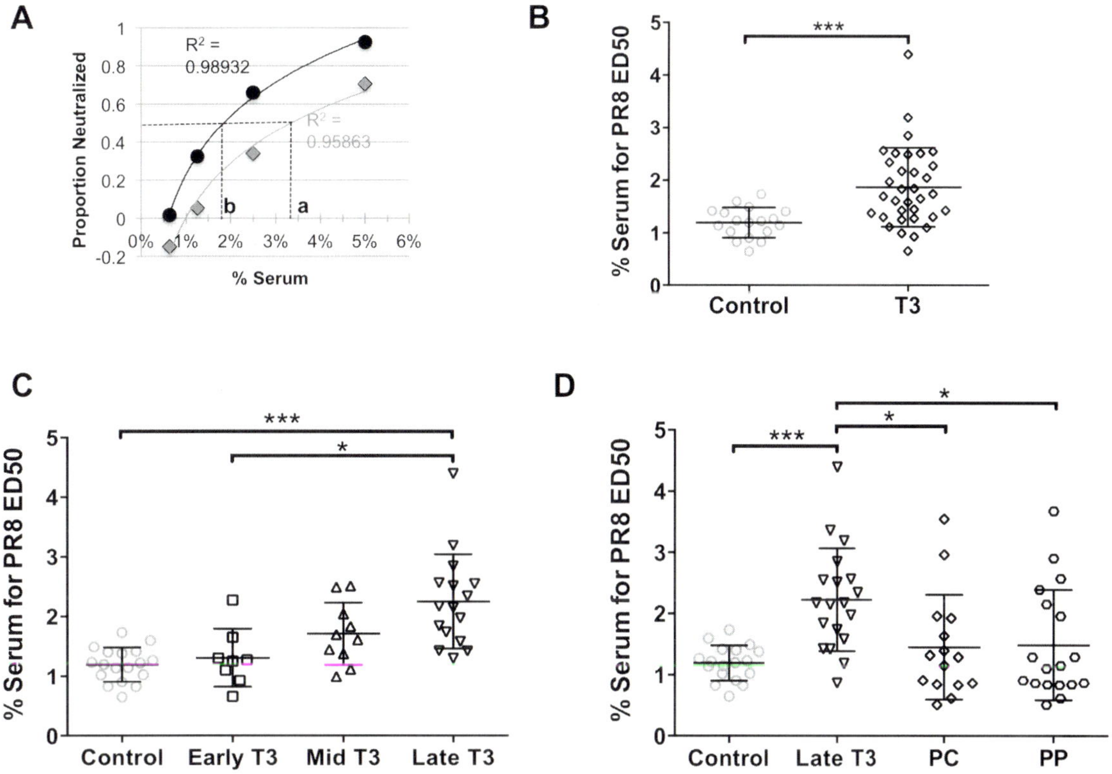

Figure 6. Capacity of T3 and postpartum serum C′ to neutralize PR8-GFP. C′ neutralization capacity was quantified as a function of the serum concentration effective in achieving 50% neutralization (ED_{50}) for each animal. (A) Logistic regressions for two example animals, where dashed line crossing the x-axis (a or b) represents the ED50 for each animal; R^2 is the coefficient of determination as an indication of how well the data points fit the regression model. ED50s were determined for AGMs at a range of gestation and postpartum dates: (B) T3 = 110–165 days; Shapiro-Wilks normality test indicated T3 population was not normally distributed; difference between T3 and control group tested with Mann-Whitney compare ranks two-tailed non-parametric test. (C) Early T3 = 110–128 days, Mid T3 = 129–146 days, Late T3 = 147–165 days gestation; (D) PC = parturition check-in, 5–10 days after parturition; PP = postpartum, 2–6 months after parturition. Differences among groups in panels C and D were tested with one-way ANOVA with Tukey correction for multiple comparisons. Lines within data point distribution represent mean +/− SD in panels B–D; * $p<0.05$; ** $p<0.001$; *** $p<0.0001$.

persisted when it was analyzed on an individual basis, utilizing our longitudinal sampling scheme (Fig. S1A). Likewise, there was no significant change in individual ED_{50} from PC to PP (Fig. S1B).

Pregnant AGMs have decreased levels of serum C′ factors in late T3

One possible mechanism to explain the above decreased neutralization capacity in T3 is that there is a corresponding decrease in levels of C′ factors. To test this, C′ factor concentrations were quantified in the same serum samples as those used to determine ED_{50}. Western blot analysis was used to determine circulating concentrations of AGM C3 β-chain, because this is the non-cleaved portion of C3 that remains intact regardless of activation state. Levels of AGM C3 β-chain were compared to the C3-β band associated with known quantities of human C3 (Fig. 7A). In accordance with decreased neutralization capacity shown above, there was a decrease in C3-β concentration in serum from T3 animals (Fig. 7B). When C3 β-chain concentrations were examined across early, mid, and late T3, we found that C3 β-chain concentrations were significantly decreased in samples from both mid and late T3 (Fig. 7C).

As an alternative approach, we developed ELISAs to quantify levels of C′ factors in AGM sera relative to purified human C′ standards. As shown in Fig. 7D, serum C3 concentrations were significantly reduced in late T3, consistent with the western blotting results above, and C3 concentration remained low up to 6 mos postpartum. Similarly, C4 concentrations were decreased in late T3 and remained low in PC and PP samples (Fig. 7E). As with C3 and C4, serum levels of the anaphylatoxin C3a were significantly decreased in late T3 (Fig. 7F). In contrast, however, C3a levels were increased in PC and PP samples (Fig. 7F), correlating with decreased ED_{50} (i.e. increased neutralization capacity) at those time points (Fig. 6D).

Our AGM sampling system enabled us to analyze large numbers of samples from animals over the whole course of the third trimester of the 5.5-month long gestation period, and to track individual animals longitudinally. As an example of this, one pregnant animal was sampled as part of a control group of (non-pregnant) animals one year later. The T3 C′ profile for this animal was compared to her "control" C′ profile as an example of an individual who fits the trends we established for the pregnant population (Fig. S2). This animal had reduced serum neutralization capacity, C3, C3a, and C4 in late T3 relative to one year later when she was a normally cycling, non-pregnant and non-lactating female in the VRC (Fig. S2).

Discussion

In this study we tested the hypothesis that anti-viral C′ function is altered during pregnancy. To address this, we developed the

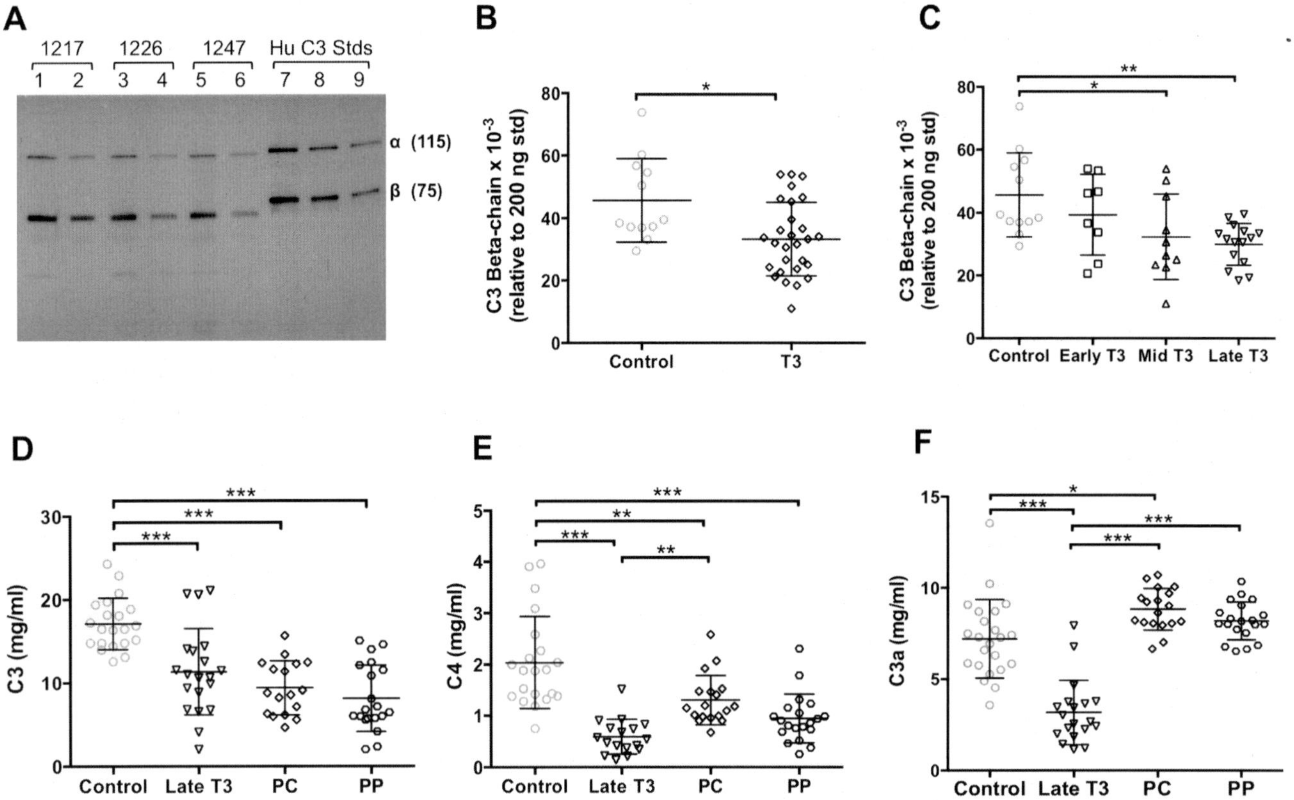

Figure 7. C′ factor quantification in T3 and postpartum AGMs. AGM serum C3 β-chain was quantified by western blot relative to purified Hu C3 standards. (A) Representative western blot with 1:200 (lanes 1, 3, and 5) and 1:400 (lanes 2, 4, and 6) serum dilutions shown sequentially for each of three different animals (1217, 1246, and 1247). Standards of 200 ng, 100 ng, and 50 ng of human C3 are in lanes 7, 8, and 9, respectively. (B) Quantification of serum C3 β-chain in T3 vs control animals, based on C3 β-chain band associated with 200 ng of standard Hu C3; difference between groups tested with unpaired two-tailed t-test. (C) Quantification of serum C3 β-chain across T3 tertiles (times defined in legend for Fig. 6C). ELISAs were used to quantify (D) C3, (E) C4, and (F) C3a, relative to purified human standards for each protein, during late T3 and at postpartum timepoints, as defined in the legend for Fig. 6D. Differences among groups in panels C–F were tested with one-way ANOVA with Tukey correction for multiple comparisons. Lines within data point distribution represent mean +/− SD in panels B–F; * $p<0.05$; ** $p<0.001$; *** $p<0.0001$.

AGM as a model for studies of C′ neutralization of influenza virus. The AGMs did not have detectable influenza virus neutralizing Abs, and therefore were most likely influenza-naïve. However, serum from influenza virus-naive AGMs neutralized PR8 through C′-dependent pathways by way of virus aggregation with limited lysis. Importantly, we showed that late in the third trimester of pregnancy, AGMs have significantly decreased serum C3, C3a, C4 and reduced influenza virus neutralization capacity relative to control animals. Taken together, our results demonstrate a late-pregnancy decrease in circulating C′ factors, which coincides with decreased C′-dependent neutralization of influenza virus—effects that correlate with the timing when pregnant women suffer severe influenza virus infections. This study is the first to demonstrate the effects of pregnancy on the C′ response to a human pathogen.

The role of C′ in protection from influenza virus infections is often overlooked. However, Jayasekera, *et al.* (2007) demonstrated that nIgM and C′ in mouse serum work together to neutralize influenza virus by forming coated viral aggregates, though nIgM or C′ alone were each insufficient to neutralize influenza virus. Our results suggest that if AGMs have circulating anti-influenza virus IgM, it also requires C′ to effectively neutralize influenza virus. This is based on our finding that sera from naïve animals neutralized influenza virus, but not when it was HI. Also similar to what Jayasekera, *et al.* demonstrated with naïve mouse sera neutralization, our studies found that PR8 formed aggregates with limited lysis in the presence of naïve AGM serum, but neither aggregation nor lysis was detected with HI sera.

Many aspects of an influenza virus infection are dramatically altered by the absence of C′ [23]. $C3^{-/-}$ mice have delayed viral clearance and increased lung viral titers relative to WT mice, as well as reduced T cell priming in lung-draining lymph nodes and subsequent decreases in effector T cell number and function in the lungs. This suggests that if humans also display the decreased C′ levels and neutralization capacity that we observed late in AGM pregnancy, these changes may play a significant role in the increased burden of influenza illness suffered by women in late pregnancy. Additionally, C′ alterations may be an initiating and/or additive factor in other known pregnancy immune alterations, such as decreased Ig titers and a Th2 shift [2,3,49–52]. By extension, the role of C′ in other pregnancy infections associated with severe T3 disease such as measles, varicella-zoster, and hepatitis E virus, should be further explored [13].

Regulation of C′, and especially down-regulation of C′-mediated effects at the placental-maternal interface, is thought to be essential for fetal survival [53–55]. Deficiency in the rodent specific membrane-bound C′ inhibitory protein, Crry, led to mortality in 76% of neonates by 9.5 days post-coitus (dpc) and universal neonatal mortality by 16.5 dpc [56]. When mice lacked both *Crry* and *C3* genes, however, gestational viability was completely rescued, demonstrating that absence of C′ regulation directly results in neonatal death in mice [56]. Despite the clear importance of C′ in pregnancy maintenance, changes in the C′ system during human pregnancy are not completely understood.

A small number of studies have addressed changes in C′ levels during human pregnancy. One study indicated that pregnant women have increased plasma levels of the anaphylatoxins C3a, C4a, and C5a [39]. However, inflammatory effects of the anaphylatoxins were not measured, uncleaved C′ factors were not quantitated, and the pregnant women sampled were not synchronized in gestation date. Thus, time-dependent effects on C′-function may not have been evident. One of the only studies of longitudinal effects of pregnancy on C′ demonstrated a drop in serum C3 early in pregnancy, with a return to control or slightly elevated levels by second (T2) and third trimester (T3); this same study showed no difference in pathogen-independent C′-mediated hemolysis during these phases of pregnancy [37]. Lastly, a small study [38] found no significant changes in plasma C3 and C4 in individuals over the course of T3, though plasma C3 levels trended downward over the course of T3 in the study samples as a whole. This study, however, included no comparisons to samples from non-pregnant controls [38]. Most importantly, none of these prior studies used functional readouts for C′ control of infection. Thus, though past human studies have generated somewhat inconsistent results, the accepted paradigm is that pregnancy is, paradoxically, a state of C′ activation [37–39,57].

There are several possible reasons why our findings may seem divergent from this model. First, it is possible that C′ regulation during AGM pregnancy is distinct from that during human pregnancy. We speculate that this is improbable given the high level of genetic relatedness between humans and old world monkeys and that the C′ system is highly evolutionarily conserved. More likely, the differences in study design and readouts between human studies and our work may present different aspects of complex C′ regulation during pregnancy.

We found decreased neutralization capacity and serum C′ protein concentrations in late T3 of AGM pregnancy. Studies indicating increased levels of C′ proteins during human pregnancy have largely focused on mid-T1 to mid-T3 [37,39,57]. Even so, several studies have shown trends of decreasing C3 and/or C4 late in pregnancy, which support our finding, albeit with a small number of samples that precludes conclusive analysis [37,38,57].

Comparing our findings to those of previous studies may also be problematic due to different sample preparations used in each study [37–39,57]. Specifically, there are inconsistencies in use of plasma versus serum, which differ in their handling of coagulation factors, as well conditions for sample preparation (i.e clotting time and preparation temperatures). There are known interactions between coagulation factors and C′ factors C3, C4, and C5, which may lead to spurious activation of the C′ system [58,59]. In addition, it is thought that pregnant women are in a hypercoagulable state due to increased levels of procoagulants and decreased levels of coagulation inhibitors [60]. Thus, the effect of coagulation factors, some of which remain in plasma but not serum, on C′ may be different for pregnant and nonpregnant women. In particular, this has the potential to skew concentrations of C′ activation products, such as C3a, C4a, and C5a. Finally, no prior human studies have examined functional response of pregnancy serum C′ to a pathogen. In this way, our finding here with neutralization of influenza may be a more clinically relevant readout than those previously reported.

C′ activation in the absence of infections would seem to be in direct conflict with physiologic needs of both the mother and the fetus during pregnancy, since C′ activation can promote inflammation, cell lysis, and anti-angiogenesis [33,35]. Thus, while C′ plays a key role in protecting both the mother and fetus from potential infection [32], excessive C′ activation due to infection can contribute to disease pathogenesis and be very dangerous to the fetus, particularly late in pregnancy [61,62]. The evolutionary balance between protecting the mother and fetus from infection, and protecting the fetus from the effects of C′ activation, might be expected to be tipped towards the latter as pregnancy progresses. Late in pregnancy, the mother has invested substantial energy resources into the fetus, and the fetus has a more developed immune system that is better equipped to respond to infection independently. Therefore, it might be most beneficial for the maternal C′ system to be down-regulated late in gestation. Our findings support this hypothesis, since we observed decreased C′ factors, decreased C3a anaphylatoxin (potentially secondary to decreased C3), and, most notably, decreased effectiveness in influenza virus neutralization late in T3.

Decreased influenza virus neutralization capacity in late T3 is the most striking and impactful finding from our study. Such changes, even at the magnitude of the 1.5- to 2.5-fold decreases we observed, have the potential to significantly alter clinical outcomes in at least three ways. First, complement is exceedingly potent—small amounts of C′ proteins can have large neutralizing effects on virus particles. Second, C′ activation products result in a sequestering effect and therefore contribute directly to vascular leakage, which enables serum proteins (including C′ proteins) to access sites of injury, such as infected lung tissue, at disproportionately high concentrations [63,64]. Finally, the C′ cascade both self-amplifies and upregulates downstream immune responses, thus small changes can have exponentially larger downstream effects. In combination with our finding that, when in linear range, 2-fold dilutions of serum and its C′ factors can result in 3-times the number of PR8-GFP infected cells (Fig. 3B), the characteristics of the C′ system described here indicate that small changes in C′ concentrations and neutralization capacity can have both large (and amplifying) immediate effects on the severity of the viral infection, as well as alter the potency of the adaptive immune response.

Though small changes in C′ are widely accepted to have large effects on response to infection [65], to our knowledge the magnitude of this effect has not been previously reported. For similar reasons, it is impossible to interpret the variation in neutralization capacity seen within individuals during the postpartum period we tested (Fig. S1). While there were not significant changes across the whole group, individual changes during this time may result in changes in severity of viral infection at the individual level. Future studies using our pregnant AGM model could provide the first natural system in which the effects of small changes in C′ during viral infection are quantified.

One possible mechanism for decreased virus neutralization capacity late in T3 is dilution of C′ factors (and therefore diminished neutralization capacity) due to the 40–50% increase in blood volume that occurs during pregnancy [66]. In humans, return to normal blood volume occurs within approximately two weeks after birth [67], while other blood elements (such as RBC volume) return to normal over the course of 8 weeks after birth [68]. Yet we observed no difference in C′ neutralization capacity between PC (5–10 days postpartum) and PP (2–6 months postpartum) samples, and C3 and C4 remained lower than in control animals at both of these time points. This indicates that the decreased C′ factors and neutralization capacity that we observed late in pregnancy are regulated by means beyond simple blood dilution. During pregnancy, capacity to neutralize influenza virus may be diminished because there are fewer circulating C′ factors, but functional activity of circulating C′ factors could also be downregulated. Likewise, neutralization capacity may improve postpartum, despite low C′ factors, if C′ potency improves. An alternative explanation might be that nIgM plays a larger role in neutralization postpartum than it does during pregnancy—also possibly due to increased concentration or potency.

Interestingly, in contrast to low postpartum C3 and C4 levels, we observed increased postpartum C3a levels. This finding might be explained by one or a combination of the following: 1) C′ is highly activated postpartum, causing cleavage of C3 and an abundance of the anaphylatoxin C3a in serum; 2) new C3 and C4 are not being produced adequately to replace C3/C4 depleted during C′ activation, possibly due to loss during lactation [69]; 3) C3a clearance is reduced due to decreased expression of C3a receptors or inhibition of other downstream events. Regardless of the mechanism, C′ factors, and therefore C′ activity and C′ neutralization capacity, appear to be tightly regulated in a temporal and complex fashion during pregnancy. This regulation undergoes drastic alterations at the time of parturition, as demonstrated by changes in neutralization capacity and C3a by 5–10 days after parturition (Fig. 6D and 7F).

One possible mechanism by which C′ alterations might occur during pregnancy and postpartum is through changes in sex hormones such as progesterone and estrogen. Both of these sex hormones peak during pregnancy at 20–30 times normal peak cycling levels; at parturition they return precipitously to normal levels. Prior work has shown that estrogen administered at pregnancy concentrations to non-pregnant mice is sufficient to recreate the abrogated innate immune response to influenza virus infection observed in pregnant mice [70]. However, C′ levels and C′ function were not examined in this study. Interestingly, there is a known estrogen response element (ERE) in the promoter of C3 [71], thus providing one possible mechanism by which sex hormones could alter C′ levels and its capacity to respond to viral infection. Given that female AGM cycling hormone levels match those of humans, the AGM model would be ideal to address these questions.

NHPs are increasingly appreciated as strong model systems for examining influenza virus pathogenesis and immune response [72,73]. NHPs infected with influenza virus exhibit clinical signs similar to those of humans including fever, malaise, nasal discharge, and cough; additionally, virus replication can be detected in the nasal passages and respiratory tract [74,75]. They are particularly valuable experimentally because captive NHPs in research colonies are generally influenza-naïve. While many previous NHP influenza virus studies have utilized macaques, there is no strongly established nonhuman primate model for reproductive physiology or immunity during pregnancy. That is a novel aspect of our work. Cycling, sexual and mating behavior, and the absence of a true "breeding season" make the AGM a more comprehensive model for human reproductive physiology than the macaque provides for this developing field. Finally, we have access to a robust AGM breeding colony, which can serve as a precious resource for addressing such questions.

Thus, pregnant AGMs model the scenario where pregnant women are infected with an emergent seasonal or pandemic influenza strain. This is a valuable system for studying the effects of changes in C′-mediated neutralization during an experimental primary infection or vaccination scenario, or with differing primary and secondary infections to study the role of C′ in cross protection. Though many reagents and laboratory methods have been developed specifically for macaques, AGM-specific reagents are less common. Thus, our work also exemplifies the process of optimization of existing reagents for a different NHP species. However, the AGM genome has been sequenced and is in the process of being annotated. Because of this, it is likely that in the near future, an increasing number of AGM-specific reagents may be developed.

Likewise, longitudinal approaches afforded by NHP colonies could be particularly useful for studies of infant mortality, stillbirth, aborted pregnancy, and other poor pregnancy outcomes. For example, the findings reported here could be used as a baseline for comparing C′ function in AGM pregnancies with poor outcomes (i.e. stillbirth, aborted fetus), rather than simple serum or plasma protein measurements that do not consistently correlate with pregnancy outcomes [36,38]. AGM breeding colonies have poor pregnancy outcomes at rates approximating those among humans, and they provide access for tracking, assessment, and follow-up studies in these circumstances. Further, due to the multi-generational nature of breeding colonies, alterations in innate immune response among certain animals and lineages could be traceable to genetic differences. As genome-wide association studies (GWAS) become increasingly accessible and more commonly performed, we may be able to identify clinically relevant single nucleotide polymorphisms (SNPs) in genes for C3 or other C′ factors. In future studies, the AGM model system we have developed will enable us to both determine the role of physiologic and hormonal changes in downregulating C′-mediated immunity during pregnancy and permit the identification of therapeutic targets to improve viral infection outcome in pregnant women.

Supporting Information

Figure S1 Changes in capacity of serum C′ to neutralize PR8-GFP for individual animals over time. Serum anti-PR8-GFP ED_{50} was quantified, as described in legend to Fig. 6, and tracked for 14 individual animals over time (A) from late T3 to PC and (B) from PC to PP. Solid lines represent negative slopes and dotted lines represent positive slopes in ED_{50} over time with animal numbers indicated in panels A and B. (C) Table of information about the 14 animals that were tracked over time in A and B; no correlation found between changes in ED_{50} and the pregnancy traits listed here. Two-tailed Wilcoxon matched-pairs signed rank test was performed for A and B, where * $p<0.05$, no difference shown indicates no significant difference over individual pairs.

Figure S2 C′ neutralization capacity and serum C′ factors in one AGM during T3 and one year after pregnancy. Neutralization capacity (A) and serum C3, C3a, and C4 concentrations (B) for AGM 1375 late in T3 (black bars) were compared to one year later when 1375 was a non-pregnant female "control" (grey bars). n = 1 animal; bars represent mean and SD of technical triplicates.

Acknowledgments

We thank Ken Grant for help with electron microscopy, Matt Jorgensen, Tara Chavanne, Glicerio Ignacio, Tyler Aycock, and Maria Blevins for expertise in animal work, David Ornelles for biostatistics consultation, and acknowledge the excellent technical assistance of Ellen Young and John Johnson. This work was supported by NIH grants AI083253 (GDP) and AI101675 (GDP), and by the flow cytometry core and imaging core of the WFUCCC (NCI CCSG P30CA012197). Animal resources were supported by NIH grant RR019963/OD010965 (Kaplan). AEM is supported by NIH Training Award Grant T32 OD010957.

Author Contributions

Conceived and designed the experiments: AEM GDP. Performed the experiments: AEM GDP. Analyzed the data: AEM GDP. Contributed reagents/materials/analysis tools: AEM GDP. Wrote the paper: AEM GDP.

References

1. Billington WD (2003) The immunological problem of pregnancy: 50 years with the hope of progress. A tribute to Peter Medawar. J Reprod Immunol 60: 1–11.
2. Mor G, Cardenas I (2010) The immune system in pregnancy: a unique complexity. Am J Reprod Immunol 63: 425–433.
3. Pazos M, Sperling RS, Moran TM, Kraus TA (2012) The influence of pregnancy on systemic immunity. Immunol Res 54: 254–261.
4. Robinson DP, Klein SL (2012) Pregnancy and pregnancy-associated hormones alter immune responses and disease pathogenesis. Horm Behav 62: 263–271.
5. Arck PC, Hecher K (2013) Fetomaternal immune cross-talk and its consequences for maternal and offspring's health. Nat Med 19: 548–556.
6. Kourtis AP, Read JS, Jamieson DJ (2014) Pregnancy and infection. N Engl J Med 370: 2211–2218.
7. Kraus TA, Engel SM, Sperling RS, Kellerman L, Lo Y, et al. (2012) Characterizing the pregnancy immune phenotype: results of the viral immunity and pregnancy (VIP) study. J Clin Immunol 32: 300–311.
8. Taubenberger JK, Morens DM (2006) 1918 Influenza: the mother of all pandemics. Emerg Infect Dis 12: 15–22.
9. Neuzil KM, Reed GW, Mitchel EF, Simonsen L, Griffin MR (1998) Impact of influenza on acute cardiopulmonary hospitalizations in pregnant women. Am J Epidemiol 148: 1094–1102.
10. Cox S, Posner SF, McPheeters M, Jamieson DJ, Kourtis AP, et al. (2006) Hospitalizations with respiratory illness among pregnant women during influenza season. Obstet Gynecol 107: 1315–1322.
11. Freeman DW, Barno A (1959) Deaths from Asian influenza associated with pregnancy. Am J Obstet Gynecol 78: 1172–1175.
12. Oluyomi-Obi T, Avery L, Schneider C, Kumar A, Lapinsky S, et al. (2010) Perinatal and maternal outcomes in critically ill obstetrics patients with pandemic H1N1 Influenza A. J Obstet Gynaecol Can 32: 443–447, 448–452.
13. Sappenfield E, Jamieson DJ, Kourtis AP (2013) Pregnancy and susceptibility to infectious diseases. Infect Dis Obstet Gynecol 2013: 752852.
14. Doyle TJ, Goodin K, Hamilton JJ (2013) Maternal and neonatal outcomes among pregnant women with 2009 pandemic influenza A(H1N1) illness in Florida, 2009–2010: a population-based cohort study. PLoS One 8: e79040.
15. Dodds L, McNeil SA, Fell DB, Allen VM, Coombs A, et al. (2007) Impact of influenza exposure on rates of hospital admissions and physician visits because of respiratory illness among pregnant women. CMAJ 176: 463–468.
16. Ochsenbein AF, Pinschewer DD, Odermatt B, Carroll MC, Hengartner H, et al. (1999) Protective T cell-independent antiviral antibody responses are dependent on complement. J Exp Med 190: 1165–1174.
17. Devaux P, Christiansen D, Plumet S, Gerlier D (2004) Cell surface activation of the alternative complement pathway by the fusion protein of measles virus. J Gen Virol 85: 1665–1673.
18. Hirsch RL, Wolinsky JS, Winkelstein JA (1986) Activation of the alternative complement pathway by mumps infected cells: relationship to viral neuraminidase activity. Arch Virol 87: 181–190.
19. Welsh RM (1977) Host cell modification of lymphocytic choriomeningitis virus and Newcastle disease virus altering viral inactivation by human complement. J Immunol 118: 348–354.
20. Johnson JB, Capraro GA, Parks GD (2008) Differential mechanisms of complement-mediated neutralization of the closely related paramyxoviruses simian virus 5 and mumps virus. Virology 376: 112–123.
21. Jayasekera JP, Moseman EA, Carroll MC (2007) Natural antibody and complement mediate neutralization of influenza virus in the absence of prior immunity. J Virol 81: 3487–3494.
22. Ricklin D, Hajishengallis G, Yang K, Lambris JD (2010) Complement: a key system for immune surveillance and homeostasis. Nat Immunol 11: 785–797.
23. Kopf M, Abel B, Gallimore A, Carroll M, Bachmann MF (2002) Complement component C3 promotes T-cell priming and lung migration to control acute influenza virus infection. Nat Med 8: 373–378.
24. Fernandez Gonzalez S, Jayasekera JP, Carroll MC (2008) Complement and natural antibody are required in the long-term memory response to influenza virus. Vaccine 26 Suppl 8: I86–93.
25. Ohshima N, Iba Y, Kubota-Koketsu R, Asano Y, Okuno Y, et al. (2011) Naturally occurring antibodies in humans can neutralize a variety of influenza virus strains, including H3, H1, H2, and H5. J Virol 85: 11048–11057.
26. Vogt MR, Dowd KA, Engle M, Tesh RB, Johnson S, et al. (2011) Poorly neutralizing cross-reactive antibodies against the fusion loop of West Nile virus envelope protein protect in vivo via Fcgamma receptor and complement-dependent effector mechanisms. J Virol 85: 11567–11580.
27. Terajima M, Cruz J, Co MD, Lee JH, Kaur K, et al. (2011) Complement-dependent lysis of influenza a virus-infected cells by broadly cross-reactive human monoclonal antibodies. J Virol 85: 13463–13467.
28. Monsalvo AC, Batalle JP, Lopez MF, Krause JC, Klemenc J, et al. (2011) Severe pandemic 2009 H1N1 influenza disease due to pathogenic immune complexes. Nat Med 17: 195–199.
29. Carroll MC, Isenman DE (2012) Regulation of humoral immunity by complement. Immunity 37: 199–207.
30. Ghannam A, Fauquert JL, Thomas C, Kemper C, Drouet C (2014) Human complement C3 deficiency: Th1 induction requires T cell-derived complement C3a and CD46 activation. Mol Immunol 58: 98–107.
31. Liszewski MK, Kolev M, Le Friec G, Leung M, Bertram PG, et al. (2013) Intracellular complement activation sustains T cell homeostasis and mediates effector differentiation. Immunity 39: 1143–1157.
32. Girardi G, Prohaszka Z, Bulla R, Tedesco F, Scherjon S (2011) Complement activation in animal and human pregnancies as a model for immunological recognition. Mol Immunol 48: 1621–1630.
33. Denny KJ, Woodruff TM, Taylor SM, Callaway LK (2013) Complement in pregnancy: a delicate balance. Am J Reprod Immunol 69: 3–11.
34. Ahmed A (2011) New insights into the etiology of preeclampsia: identification of key elusive factors for the vascular complications. Thromb Res 127 Suppl 3: S72–75.
35. Girardi G, Yarilin D, Thurman JM, Holers VM, Salmon JE (2006) Complement activation induces dysregulation of angiogenic factors and causes fetal rejection and growth restriction. J Exp Med 203: 2165–2175.
36. Denny KJ, Coulthard LG, Finnell RH, Callaway LK, Taylor SM, et al. (2013) Elevated complement factor C5a in maternal and umbilical cord plasma in preeclampsia. J Reprod Immunol 97: 211–216.
37. Baines MG, Millar KG, Mills P (1974) Studies of complement levels in normal human pregnancy. Obstet Gynecol 43: 806–810.
38. Kovar IZ, Riches PG (1988) C3 and C4 complement components and acute phase proteins in late pregnancy and parturition. J Clin Pathol 41: 650–652.
39. Richani K, Soto E, Romero R, Espinoza J, Chaiworapongsa T, et al. (2005) Normal pregnancy is characterized by systemic activation of the complement system. J Matern Fetal Neonatal Med 17: 239–245.
40. Ross TM, Lin CJ, Nowalk MP, Huang HH, Spencer SM, et al. (2014) Influence of pre-existing hemagglutination inhibition titers against historical influenza strains on antibody response to inactivated trivalent influenza vaccine in adults 50-80 years of age. Hum Vaccin Immunother 10.
41. Palese P, Wang TT (2011) Why do influenza virus subtypes die out? A hypothesis. MBio 2.
42. Elovitz MA, Mrinalini C (2004) Animal models of preterm birth. Trends Endocrinol Metab 15: 479–487.
43. Lee KY, DeMayo FJ (2004) Animal models of implantation. Reproduction 128: 679–695.
44. Paterson RG, Leser GP, Shaughnessy MA, Lamb RA (1995) The paramyxovirus SV5 V protein binds two atoms of zinc and is a structural component of virions. Virology 208: 121–131.
45. Manicassamy B, Manicassamy S, Belicha-Villanueva A, Pisanelli G, Pulendran B, et al. (2010) Analysis of in vivo dynamics of influenza virus infection in mice using a GFP reporter virus. Proc Natl Acad Sci U S A 107: 11531–11536.
46. Klimov A, Balish A, Veguilla V, Sun H, Schiffer J, et al. (2012) Influenza virus titration, antigenic characterization, and serological methods for antibody detection. Methods Mol Biol 865: 25–51.
47. Nyland TG, Hill DE, Hendrickx AG, Farver TB, McGahan JP, et al. (1984) Ultrasonic assessment of fetal growth in the nonhuman primate (Macaca mulatta). J Clin Ultrasound 12: 387–395.
48. Parks GD, Alexander-Miller MA (2002) High avidity cytotoxic T lymphocytes to a foreign antigen are efficiently activated following immunization with a recombinant paramyxovirus, simian virus 5. J Gen Virol 83: 1167–1172.
49. Jamieson DJ, Theiler RN, Rasmussen SA (2006) Emerging infections and pregnancy. Emerg Infect Dis 12: 1638–1643.
50. Wilder RL (1998) Hormones, pregnancy, and autoimmune diseases. Ann N Y Acad Sci 840: 45–50.
51. Ostensen M, Villiger PM (2002) Immunology of pregnancy-pregnancy as a remission inducing agent in rheumatoid arthritis. Transpl Immunol 9: 155–160.
52. Benster B, Wood EJ (1970) Immunoglobulin levels in normal pregnancy and pregnancy complicated by hypertension. J Obstet Gynaecol Br Commonw 77: 518–522.
53. Francis J, Rai R, Sebire NJ, El-Gaddal S, Fernandes MS, et al. (2006) Impaired expression of endometrial differentiation markers and complement regulatory proteins in patients with recurrent pregnancy loss associated with antiphospholipid syndrome. Mol Hum Reprod 12: 435–442.
54. Pacheco LD, Hankins GD, Costantine MM, Anderson GD, Pawelczyk E, et al. (2011) The role of human decay-accelerating factor in the pathogenesis of preterm labor. Am J Perinatol 28: 565–570.

55. Liszewski MK, Farries TC, Lublin DM, Rooney IA, Atkinson JP (1996) Control of the complement system. Adv Immunol 61: 201–283.
56. Xu C, Mao D, Holers VM, Palanca B, Cheng AM, et al. (2000) A critical role for murine complement regulator crry in fetomaternal tolerance. Science 287: 498–501.
57. Gallery ED, Raftos J, Gyory AZ, Wells JV (1981) A prospective study of serum complement (C3 and C4) levels in normal human pregnancy: effect of the development of pregnancy-associated hypertension. Aust N Z J Med 11: 243–245.
58. Oikonomopoulou K, Ricklin D, Ward PA, Lambris JD (2012) Interactions between coagulation and complement—their role in inflammation. Semin Immunopathol 34: 151-165.
59. Amara U, Flierl MA, Rittirsch D, Klos A, Chen H, et al. (2010) Molecular intercommunication between the complement and coagulation systems. J Immunol 185: 5628–5636.
60. Cerneca F, Ricci G, Simeone R, Malisano M, Alberico S, et al. (1997) Coagulation and fibrinolysis changes in normal pregnancy. Increased levels of procoagulants and reduced levels of inhibitors during pregnancy induce a hypercoagulable state, combined with a reactive fibrinolysis. Eur J Obstet Gynecol Reprod Biol 73: 31–36.
61. Conroy AL, McDonald CR, Silver KL, Liles WC, Kain KC (2011) Complement activation: a critical mediator of adverse fetal outcomes in placental malaria? Trends Parasitol 27: 294–299.
62. Holmberg V, Onkamo P, Lahtela E, Lahermo P, Bedu-Addo G, et al. (2012) Mutations of complement lectin pathway genes MBL2 and MASP2 associated with placental malaria. Malar J 11: 61.
63. Bolger MS, Ross DS, Jiang H, Frank MM, Ghio AJ, et al. (2007) Complement levels and activity in the normal and LPS-injured lung. Am J Physiol Lung Cell Mol Physiol 292: L748–759.
64. Bossi F, Fischetti F, Pellis V, Bulla R, Ferrero E, et al. (2004) Platelet-activating factor and kinin-dependent vascular leakage as a novel functional activity of the soluble terminal complement complex. J Immunol 173: 6921–6927.
65. Murphy K (2011) Janeway's Immunobiology: Garland Science.
66. Hytten F (1985) Blood volume changes in normal pregnancy. Clin Haematol 14: 601–612.
67. Simpson KC (2001) AHWONN's Perinatal nursing. Philadelphia: Lippincott.
68. Bowes WK (2002) Postpartum care. In: Gabbe S, Niebyl, J, Simpson, J., editor.Obstetrics: Normal and problem pregnancies. 4th ed. New York: Churchill Livingstone.
69. Lewis-Jones DI, Lewis-Jones MS, Connolly RC, Lloyd DC, West CR (1985) The influence of parity, age and maturity of pregnancy on antimicrobial proteins in human milk. Acta Paediatr Scand 74: 655–659.
70. Pazos MA, Kraus TA, Munoz-Fontela C, Moran TM (2012) Estrogen mediates innate and adaptive immune alterations to influenza infection in pregnant mice. PLoS One 7: e40502.
71. Fan JD, Wagner BL, McDonnell DP (1996) Identification of the sequences within the human complement 3 promoter required for estrogen responsiveness provides insight into the mechanism of tamoxifen mixed agonist activity. Mol Endocrinol 10: 1605–1616.
72. Moncla LH, Ross TM, Dinis JM, Weinfurter JT, Mortimer TD, et al. (2013) A novel nonhuman primate model for influenza transmission. PLoS One 8: e78750.
73. Baskin C (2013) The role and contributions of systems biology to the non-human primate model of influenza pathogenesis and vaccinology. Curr Top Microbiol Immunol 363: 69–85.
74. Berendt RF (1974) Simian model for the evaluation of immunity to influenza. Infect Immun 9: 101–105.
75. Bodewes R, Rimmelzwaan GF, Osterhaus AD (2010) Animal models for the preclinical evaluation of candidate influenza vaccines. Expert Rev Vaccines 9: 59–72.
76. (1966) Biology of the Laboratory Mouse. New York: Dover Publications, Inc.
77. Jones REL, Lopez K (2013) Human Reproductive Biology: Academic Press.
78. Carroll RL, Mah K, Fanton JW, Maginnis GN, Brenner RM, et al. (2007) Assessment of menstruation in the vervet (Cercopithecus aethiops). Am J Primatol 69: 901–916.
79. Hess DL, Hendrickx AG, Stabenfeldt GH (1979) Reproductive and hormonal patterns in the African green monkey (Cercopithecus aethiops). J Med Primatol 8: 273–281.
80. Koritnik DR, Wood LL, Shandilya LN, Rudel LL (1984) Lipids, lipoproteins, and endocrine profiles during pregnancy in the African green monkey (Cercopithecus aethiops). Metabolism 33: 840–844.
81. Kundu MC, May MC, Chosich J, Bradford AP, Lasley B, et al. (2013) Assessment of luteal function in the vervet monkey as a means to develop a model for obesity-related reproductive phenotype. Syst Biol Reprod Med 59: 74–81.
82. Stephens SM, Pau FK, Yalcinkaya TM, May MC, Berga SL, et al. (2013) Assessing the pulsatility of luteinizing hormone in female vervet monkeys (Chlorocebus aethiops sabaeus). Comp Med 63: 432–438.
83. Else JG, Eley RM, Wangula C, Worthman C, Lequin RM (1986) Reproduction in the vervet monkey (Cercopithecus aethiops): II. Annual menstrual patterns and seasonality. American Journal of Primatology 11: 333–342.
84. Eley RM, Tarara RP, Worthman CM, Else JG (1989) Reproduction in the vervet monkey (Cercopithecus aethiops): III. The menstrual cycle. American Journal of Primatology 17: 1–10.

Specificity and Effector Functions of Human RSV-Specific IgG from Bovine Milk

Gerco den Hartog[¤1,2], Shamir Jacobino[1], Louis Bont[1,3], Linda Cox[4], Laurien H. Ulfman[5], Jeanette H. W. Leusen[1*9], R. J. Joost van Neerven[2,59]

1 Laboratory of Translational Immunology, Immunotherapy group, UMC Utrecht, Utrecht, The Netherlands, **2** Cell Biology and Immunology, Wageningen University, Wageningen, The Netherlands, **3** Department of Pediatrics, UMC Utrecht, Utrecht, The Netherlands, **4** Bioceros, Utrecht, The Netherlands, **5** FrieslandCampina, Amersfoort, The Netherlands

Abstract

Background: Respiratory syncytial virus (RSV) infection is the second most important cause of death in the first year of life, and early RSV infections are associated with the development of asthma. Breastfeeding and serum IgG have been shown to protect against RSV infection. Yet, many infants depend on bovine milk-based nutrition, which at present lacks intact immunoglobulins.

Objective: To investigate whether IgG purified from bovine milk (bIgG) can modulate immune responses against human RSV.

Methods: ELISAs were performed to analyse binding of bIgG to human respiratory pathogens. bIgG or hRSV was coated to plates to assess dose-dependent binding of bIgG to human Fcγ receptors (FcγR) or bIgG-mediated binding of myeloid cells to hRSV respectively. *S. Epidermidis* and RSV were used to test bIgG-mediated binding and internalisation of pathogens by myeloid cells. Finally, the ability of bIgG to neutralise infection of HEp2 cells by hRSV was evaluated.

Results: bIgG recognised human RSV, influenza haemagglutinin and *Haemophilus influenza.* bIgG bound to FcγRII on neutrophils, monocytes and macrophages, but not to FcγRI and FcγRIII, and could bind simultaneously to hRSV and human FcγRII on neutrophils. In addition, human neutrophils and dendritic cells internalised pathogens that were opsonised with bIgG. Finally, bIgG could prevent infection of HEp2 cells by hRSV.

Conclusions: The data presented here show that bIgG binds to hRSV and other human respiratory pathogens and induces effector functions through binding to human FcγRII on phagocytes. Thus bovine IgG may contribute to immune protection against RSV.

Editor: Stephania A. Cormier, University of Tennessee Health Science Center, United States of America

Funding: The study was funded by FrieslandCampina (www.frieslandcampina.com). The funder provided support in the form of salaries for authors LU and RJJvN, but FrieslandCampina did not have any additional role in the study design, data collection and analysis, decision to publish, or preparation of the manuscript. The salary for author LC was provided by Bioceros. Bioceros did not have any additional role in the study design, data collection and analysis, decision to publish, or preparation of the manuscript. The specific roles of these authors are articulated in the 'author contributions' section.

Competing Interests: The authors LU and RJJvN are employees of FrieslandCampina, whose company funded this study. A patent application based in part on this work has been filed (but has not been published yet) by FrieslandCampina. (Ruminant antibodies in defense against infections in humans, number 13199606.8-1358 – LU, JL, and RJJvN coinventors) RJJvN, JL and LU will not receive financial benefit from the patent. The author LC is an employee of Bioceros. There are no further patents, products in development or marketed products to declare.

* Email: jleusen@umcutrecht.nl

9 These authors contributed equally to this work.

¤ Current address: Division of Gastroenterology, University of California San Diego, La Jolla, California, United States of America

Introduction

Respiratory syncytial virus (RSV) infection is a major cause of death in the first year of life, with especially high mortality rates in African and Asian countries [1,2,3]. Upper respiratory tract infections (URTI) with RSV generally cause relatively mild disease that does not require treatment. These infections can progress, however, into lower respiratory tract infections (LRTI) and cause severe disease, especially in pre-mature infants. RSV can also cause recurrent infection of the upper respiratory tract.

An important complication of upper respiratory infections is middle ear inflammation and-related deafness [4,5], and RSV infections are associated with the development of asthma at a later age [6,7,8].

Other common causes for respiratory tract infections are *Haemophilus influenzae* type b (Hib), *parainfluenza virus, rhinovirus* and *influenza virus* [9,10,11].

Protective immunity against respiratory pathogens like influenza and RSV is mediated by IgG and IgA [12,13,14,15,16]. RSV-specific serum IgG levels in neonates are inversely associated with increased prevalence of RSV infections [17,18], and breastfeeding reduces the incidence and severity of RSV infection [19,20]. In addition, the levels of anti-influenza IgA in breast milk correlates with decreased frequency of respiratory illness with fever [16]. These findings indicate that pathogen-specific antibodies are crucial for protection against respiratory infections, and that orally ingested immunoglobulins (like breastmilk-derived IgA) may contribute to immunity to airway infections.

Human and bovine milk contain high levels of immunoglobulins, which are important for protecting the infant from infections with bacteria and viruses [21,22]. Cross-species activity between human and bovine immune-related milk proteins has been reported before [23,24], and cow's milk contains bovine IgG (bIgG) that binds to gastrointestinal pathogens that also infect humans, such as *Shigella flexneri, Escherichia coli, Clostridium difficile, Streptococcus mutants, Cryptosporidium parvum, Helicobacter pylori,* and rotavirus [25].

At present there is, however, no information on binding of bovine IgG to human respiratory viruses.

Most infant nutrition is bovine milk-based, but lacks intact bIgG as a result of heat treatment during processing. To investigate if bIgG would be a useful ingredient in these formulas, the aim of the present study was to investigate the specificity and functional relevance of bIgG against RSV and other human respiratory pathogens, the ability of bIgG to bind to human Fcγ receptors, and the induction of effector functions in human myeloid cells.

Materials and Methods

Bovine milk samples and preparation of bIgG

bIgG was purified from commercially available bovine colostrum (Colostrum 35% IgG, Reflex Nutrition, Bristol, UK) using an AFFI-T^{TM} column (Kem-en-Tec) followed by a protein G column (5 ml; Amersham). bIgG was eluted with 0.1 M glycine-HCl pH 2.7 elution buffer and neutralised with 1 M Tris-HCl pH 9.0, followed by dialysation against PBS and sterilisation (0.2 μm filter). Fresh milk and colostrum samples were supplied by FrieslandCampina (the Netherlands).

Detection of pathogen-specific IgG

Maxisorb ELISA-plates (Nunc) were coated with 0.5–2 μg/ml pathogen antigens, derived from human vaccines (Influvac 2012/2013 (0.5 μg/ml), Abbott Biologicals), Act-HIB (Sanofi pasteur MSD (0.5 μg/ml)), DTP (1/200, Nederland vaccine instituut), or 25 μl inactivated RSV A2 or rhinovirus (kindly provided by Prof. S Johnston, Imperial College London, UK). Plates were blocked with 0.5% gelatine/PBS, washed (0.05% tween-20/PBS), and samples were added and titrated. Plates were washed four times and 1/2000 HRP-conjugated sheep anti bovine IgG1 (Abd Serotec, Kidlington, UK) or 1/6000 anti-human IgG (Jackson ImmunoResearch, West Grove, PA, USA) were used as detector antibody. Plates were washed extensively and developed with TMB and read at 450 nm. For inhibition ELISAs purified IgG from human plasma (Intravenous Immunoglobulin, pooled from >1000 donors, or IVIg) (Sanquin blood supply, The Netherlands) or bIgG equivalent to 167 μg/ml was pre-incubated at room temperature with twice the amount used for coating of hRSV or vaccine. Binding to F protein of bRSV was analysed by a commercial ELISA, according to the manufacturer's descriptions (Bio-X Diagnostics, Jemelle, Belgium).

Generation of RSV extracts

RSV A2 was added to HEp2 cells (IMDM with L-glutamin, HEPES and 1% FSC) and incubated for six days. Cells were lysed (0.5% NP-40) [26]) and used for ELISAs.

Also PEG-precipitated RSV lysate was prepared. Slowly ice cold 50% PEG6000 in 150 mM NaCl, 1 mM EDTA and 6.1 g/L Tris was added to RSV-infected Hep2 cells while stirring (end concentration PEG was 10%). The mixture was stirred at 4°C for three hours. The PEG-precipitated virus mixture was centrifuged (30 min, 4000 rpm at 4°C). Supernatant was removed and the pellet taken up in 10% sucrose and stored in N2.

Isolation and culture of human myeloid cells

Ethical approval of the use of blood samples was obtained from the institutional review boards the 'Medical Ethical Committee' of the UMC Utrecht, The Netherlands and Sanquin Blood Supply, The Netherlands. Review and approval was obtained prior to the experiments were conducted and are in accordance with the declaration of Helsinki. Donors provided written informed consent and the blood samples were used anonymously. Blood was obtained at the UMC Utrecht (collected in heparin vacutainers (BD Biosciences) or buffy coats (Sanquin blood supply, The Netherlands) were diluted 1:1 in PBS. Diluted blood was layered on top of a Histopaque-ficoll gradient and centrifuged for 25 min, 1500 rpm, slow acceleration and without brake. PBMCs and PMNs were harvested and washed in RPMI. Red blood cells were lysed with ammonium buffer (pH 7, UMC Utrecht pharmacy) for 10 minutes on ice.

Monocytes were purified using CD14 microbeads (Myltenyi biotec, Bergisch Gladbach, Germany), according the manufacturers prescriptions, with the following modifications: cells were incubated in half the volume of MACS buffer and CD14 beads, and incubated for 30 minutes on a roller at 4°C. Monocytes were cultured in RPMI containing 10% FCS. For differentiation to macrophages, monocytes were cultured overnight in the presence of 10 ng/ml IFN-γ (Peprotech, Rocky Hill, NJ, USA). Monocyte-derived DCs (moDC) were differentiated for five days under the influence of 50 ng/ml GM-CSF (Peprotech).

Binding of bIgG to cells expressing FcγR

96 wells maxisorb plates (Nunc) were coated with Ig in 0.1 M $NaHPO_4$, pH 9 overnight (4°C). Cells were incubated with 5 μM calcein AM (Invitrogen) in PBS (PMNs were labelled in HEPES [27]) for 30 min at 37°C (PMNs for 20 min), washed with RPMI containing 0.2% gelatin. $1.5*10^5$ calcein-labelled cells were added, centrifuged (500 rpm, 5 min) and allowed to attach for 45 min at 37°C (10 min for PMN) in RPMI containing 0.2% gelatin. Initial fluorescence and fluorescence after several washing steps was recorded (excitation 485 nm, emission 527 nm, ThermoFisher Scientific Fluoroskan Ascent FL). For FcγR-specific inhibition of binding of calcein-labelled cells 2 or 5 μg/ml Fab fragments of clone 3G8 (FcγRIII) or IV.3 (FcγRII) were used. Stable FcγRI-transfected IIA1.6 cells were previously shown to bind to human IgG but not bIgG and were therefore not included in this study [28].

Pathogen-specific Ig cell-binding assay

96 wells maxisorb plates were coated with PEG-precipitated RSV at 4°C overnight. Plates were washed (PBS) and blocked with 1% gelatine/PBS (1 hour 37°C) and washing three times (PBS-

tween). Bovine or human IgG (or buffer) was allowed to bind to RSV for 3 hours at room temperature. Plates were washed 3 times followed by washing once with RPMI containing 0.2% gelatine. The assay was continued as described under 'Binding of IgG to human FcγR'.

FcγR-mediated internalisation assay

$8*10^5$ CFU/ml FITC-labelled *S. epidermidis* was incubated with 20 µl of varying concentrations of IVIg or bIgG overnight at 4°C. Twenty µl of pre-cooled cells ($1.5*10^5$) were added and incubated with the bacteria on ice for 30 min. Plates were washed and incubated at 37°C or 4°C (45 min. macrophages, 20 min moDCs) in 150 µl RPMI. Cells were washed and stained with 1/200 biotinylated anti FITC antibodies (Southern Biotec), followed by washing and 1/100 streptavidin APC (eBiosciences). Cells were washed and fixed with 1% PFA/PBS and analysed on FACS Canto II. All washing steps were performed three times with ice-cold FACS buffer and a cooled centrifuge at 1500 rpm for 5 minutes.

GFP-RSV internalisation assay

Renilla-GFP RSV (1*10^5 plaque forming units (PFU)) was pre-incubated for 1 hour at 37°C with 40 µl RPMI (10% FCS and 1% pen/strep) in the presence or absence of antibodies and then cooled for 15 min on ice. Pre-cooled PMN (1.5*10^5 cells) and 40 µl RSV-Ig mixture was added and allowed to bind for 15 min in 96-wells plates. Plates were washed and incubated for 15 min at 37°C in pre-warmed RPMI. After washing, cells were treated with trypsin for 10 min on ice to remove extracellular RSV. Cells were incubated twice (30 sec) with acid medium (RPMI pH 2.5, 0.1% FCS) to remove FcR bound RSV-Ig, with a 1 min centrifugation step (1500 rpm) in between and afterwards. Finally, cells were washed and fixed with 1% PFA in PBS and GFP expression was analysed by flow cytometry.

RSV neutralisation assay

HEp2 cells (5*10^4 cells) cultured in IMDM (10% FCS, 1% pen/strep) were seeded overnight in flat-bottom 96-wells plates. Renilla-GFP RSV (1*10^5 PFU) was pre-incubated for 1 hour at 37°C with 100 µl medium (1% FCS) in the presence or absence of antibodies and then added to the cells. Cells were trypsinised after 18–24 hour incubation and GFP expression was analysed by flow cytometry.

Results

Binding of bIgG to human respiratory tract pathogens

To study binding of purified human plasma IgG (IVIg) and bovine colostrum IgG (bIgG) to human RSV (hRSV) lysate of HEp2 cells (control) or RSV infected HEp2 cells was coated to an ELISA plate. Dose-dependent binding of bIgG to RSV (>2 SD above background) was observed at concentrations starting at 1.8 µg/ml (Figure 1A).

IVIg and bIgG also bound to flu and Hib antigens (Figure 1A). Pathogen-specific bIgG could be detected at levels up to 11 µg/ml. Compared to bIgG, less IVIg was required to detect the pathogens. Binding of bIgG to rhinovirus was only detectable at very high IgG levels (data not shown). hRSV, HIB and influvac-specific IgG could also be detected in pooled bovine milk samples (not shown).

To test the specificity of the bIgG-binding to human respiratory pathogens, inhibition ELISAs were performed. These experiments confirmed the specificity of the binding of bIgG to RSV, influenza and Hib (Figure 1B). However, binding of bIgG to flu could also be partly inhibited by Hib, suggesting the presence of cross reactive epitopes.

Binding of bIgG to human FcγRs

To study binding of bIgG to human FcγRs, monocytes were incubated overnight in the presence or absence of IFN-γ to enhance FcγR expression, and exposed to plate-bound bIgG. Human monocytes of 5 out of 5 donors bound to immobilised bIgG, as well as to IVIg, which was increased by pre-incubating the cells with IFN-γ (Figure 2A). Binding of monocytes to bIgG was dose-dependent and comparable or slightly lower compared to human IVIg (Figure 2B).

Also binding of PMN to bIgG was evaluated. PMNs of 4/5 donors bound to IVIg as well as to bIgG (Figure 2C).

To identify which receptor was involved in binding of PMN to bIgG, unstimulated PMN which lack FcγRI [29], were incubated with FcγRII (Fab)- and FcγRIII (F(ab)2)-specific blocking mAb prior to addition of the cells to the Ig-coated plates (Figure 2C). Pre-incubation with FcγRII-blocking Fabs reduced binding of PMN to bIgG of all three donors tested. Binding of PMN in both the presence and absence of FcγRII-specific Fabs was comparable for IVIg and bIgG, although some donor-specific differences were observed. Pre-incubation of PMN with FcγRIII-specific Fabs resulted in slightly decreased binding of IVIg, but not of bIgG.

Binding of macrophages and PMN to RSV-specific Ig

To study whether human phagocytes can bind to bIgG that has captured RSV, an experiment was performed requiring bIgG to simultaneously bind to RSV immobilised on a plate and human macrophages (Figure 3A). Binding of cells to RSV-specific IVIg or bIgG was dose-dependent and lost when IgG was (boiled prior to addition to the plate). No binding was observed when plates were coated with gelatin instead of RSV (data not shown). Bovine RSV-specific IgG was also able to bind simultaneously to RSV and PMN (Figure 3B).

Next, PMN were pre-incubated with anti FcγRII and/or anti FcγRIII Fabs prior to addition to RSV-bound Ig. Pre-incubation of PMN with anti FcγRII, but not anti FcγRIII Fabs, reduced binding of PMN to RSV-specific IVIg and bIgG (Figure 3B). Pre-incubation of Ig with RSV completely inhibited cell-binding, confirming that cell-binding in this assay is indeed RSV-specific.

bIgG induces FcγR-mediated phagocytosis

In addition to extracellular binding of pathogens, internalisation is required for efficient clearance of pathogens and efficient induction of memory T cells. FITC-labelled bacteria (*S. epidermidis*) were used as model for bIgG-mediated internalisation of pathogens by macrophages and moDCs. To discriminate between extracellular bound bacteria and internalised bacteria, APC-conjugated antibodies recognising FITC were used.

Medium, *S. epidermidis* left non-opsonised or opsonised with different concentrations of IVIg or bIgG were added to macrophages. Cells were allowed to bind to bacteria at 4°C, washed and incubated at 37°C (allowing internalisation) or 4°C (allowing binding, but not internalisation) for 45 minutes. Subsequently, cells were stained with APC anti FITC. Both IVIg and bIgG enhanced the binding of bacteria to macrophages, indicated by increased percentages of cells that are FITC positive (Figures 4A and B). Also internalisation ($FITC^+APC^-$) of bacteria was enhanced by IVIg and bIgG. The increased binding and internalisation was dose-dependent, and only observed for cells incubated at 37°C.

Similarly, bIgG enhanced internalisation of *S. epidermidis* by moDCs of three other donors (Figure 4C). These data show that

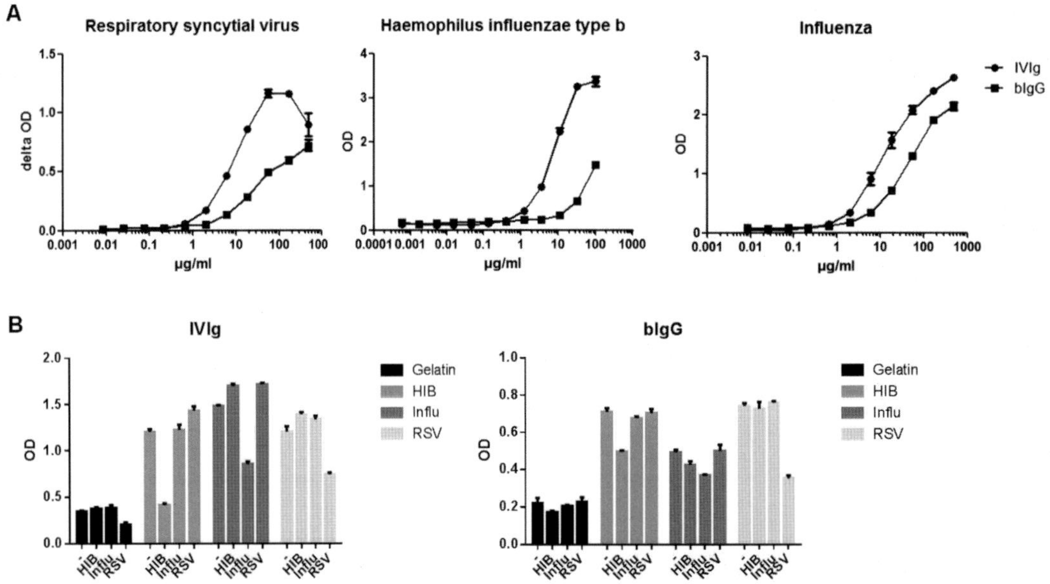

Figure 1. bIgG binds to human airway pathogens. A) RSV, influenza or *Haemophilus influenzae* type b was coated in ELISA plates and human (IVIg) or bovine (bIg) IgG was added in different concentrations (x-axes in µg/ml). Mean OD or delta OD (RSV) values and S.E.M. are shown of triplicate measurements. **B**) Inhibition of binding of IVIg (left) or bIg (right) to vaccines by pre-incubating the Ig-samples (167 µg/ml) with the antigen. Horizontal text below graphs indicates vaccine used for coating, whereas diagonal text indicates the vaccine used for pre-incubation; '−' indicates pre-incubation with medium. Mean and S.E.M. of triplicate measurements are shown.

bIgG is able to enhance binding as well as internalisation of pathogens by human immune cells.

Binding and internalisation of soluble hRSV by human PMNs

PMN, like macrophages, play a crucial role in the elimination of opsonised pathogens. To investigate whether pathogen-opsonisation by bIgG can enhance internalisation by human PMNs GFP-labelled hRSV was opsonised with bIgG. In the absence of antibodies little internalisation of hRSV by human PMN was observed, measured as the percentage of GFP positive cells by flow cytometry (Figure 5). By contrast, pre-incubation of hRSV with both IVIg and bIgG resulted in a dose-dependent increase of hRSV internalisation. While IVIg was more effective than bIgG at the two highest concentrations tested, bIgG was particularly more effective at lower concentrations.

Neutralisation of HEp2 infection by RSV

Pre-term birth children receive intravenous palivizumab to prevent RSV infection [30]. The F-protein epitope recognised by palivizumab seems to be conserved between human and bovine RSV as palivizumab also recognises the F protein of bovine RSV (data not shown). Therefore, like palivizumab, bIgG might be able to prevent infection with hRSV. To this aim GFP-renilla-RSV was pre-incubated with bIgG, IVIg or palivizumab and added to HEp2 cells. After 18–24 hours incubation, cells were harvested and analysed for GFP expression by flow cytometry. Both IVIg and bIgG dose-dependently neutralised RSV, although 6.4 times more bIgG compared to IVIg was needed to inhibit HEp2 cell infection by RSV (IC50: 64 and 10 µg/ml, respectively) (Figure 6B).

Discussion

Pathogen-specific immunoglobulins are supplied to newborns through breastfeeding. These immunoglobulins help to protect the neonate against infections by pathogenic bacteria and viruses. Neonates, especially those born pre-maturely, are relatively vulnerable to pathogenic infections in the respiratory tract [2]. We aimed to study whether intact bovine milk-derived immunoglobulins can modulate immune responses to respiratory pathogens. The data presented here show that bIgG recognises several pathogens that are known to cause infections in the respiratory tract of infants. In addition, bIgG bound to human FcγRII, and enhance phagocytosis of pathogens by human myeloid immune cells. Bovine IgG was shown to bind to human RSV, and could even prevent infection of HEp2 cells by human RSV *in vitro*.

Cows are susceptible to pathogens like bovine RSV, and transfer bovine RSV-specific antibodies into colostrum and mature milk after delivery [31,32]. Those observations suggest that cow's indeed seem to develop neutralising antibodies against bRSV, that cross-react with hRSV. It is relevant to note that even though significant levels of bIgG specific for human respiratory pathogens were detected, the cows were not immunised against human pathogens. However, it is common practice to vaccinate calves against bovine RSV around weaning when the maternal-derived IgG levels are decreasing. Our data suggest that for RSV, protecting the calf against bRSV through immunisation may give rise to milk that has the potential to be protective against bovine as well as human RSV.

bIgG was also able to neutralise infection of HEp2 cells with hRSV. Compared to palivizumab, a humanized anti-RSV therapeutic mAb, and IV-Ig, a significantly higher concentration of bIgG was required for neutralisation of infection of HEp2 cells by hRSV. Palivizumab is often given prophylactically and therefore is present at the moment when hRSV is encountered by the neonate. Direct neutralization of hRSV by orally deposited bIgG on mucosal surfaces is possible, but not very likely. Activated

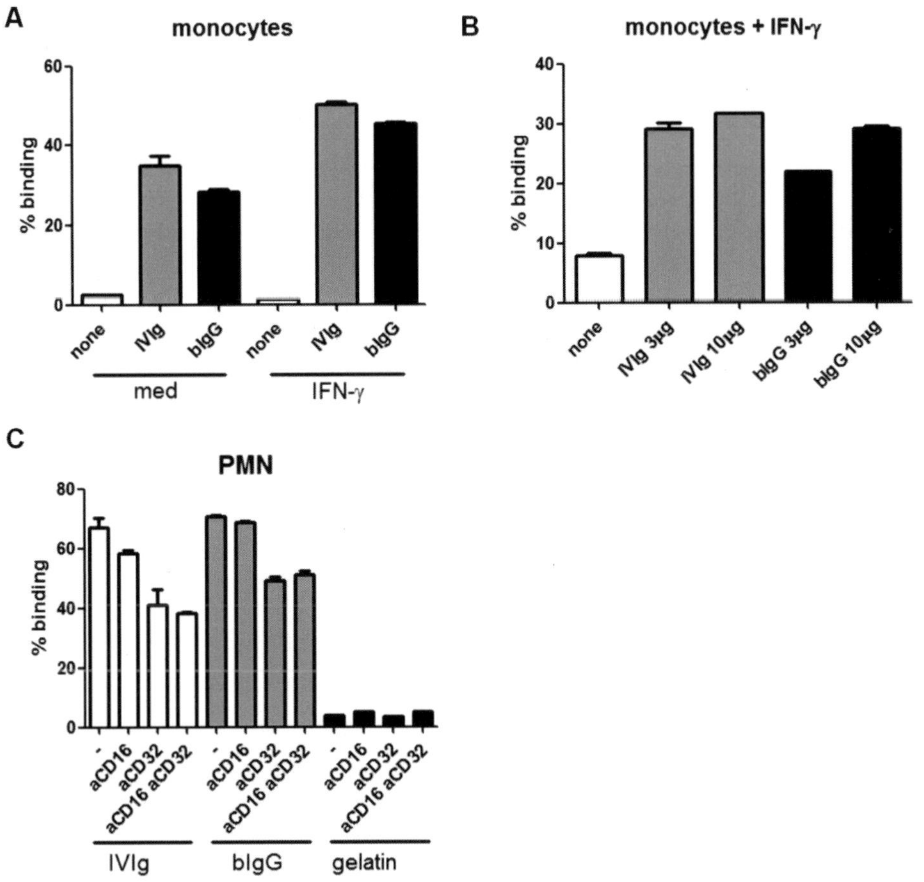

Figure 2. bIgG binds to human FcγRII. A) IgG was immobilised on 96 wells ELISA plates. Monocytes were incubated overnight in the absence or presence of 10 ng/ml IFN-γ. **B)** Different concentrations of IgG were coated and IFN-γ stimulated monocytes were added. **C)** Binding of PMNs to 10 μg/ml human (IVIg) and bovine IgG (bIg). PMNs were incubated for 10 minutes in the absence (-) or presence of 3 μg/ml Fabs recognizing FcγRIII (CD16) or FcγRII (CD32). As negative control, plates were coated with gelatin (none) instead of Ig. Binding of bIgG by monocytes and PMNs was observed for three different donors. For all panels binding of cells after five washes is shown and expressed as percentage of initial. Mean and S.E.M. is shown of triplicate measurements.

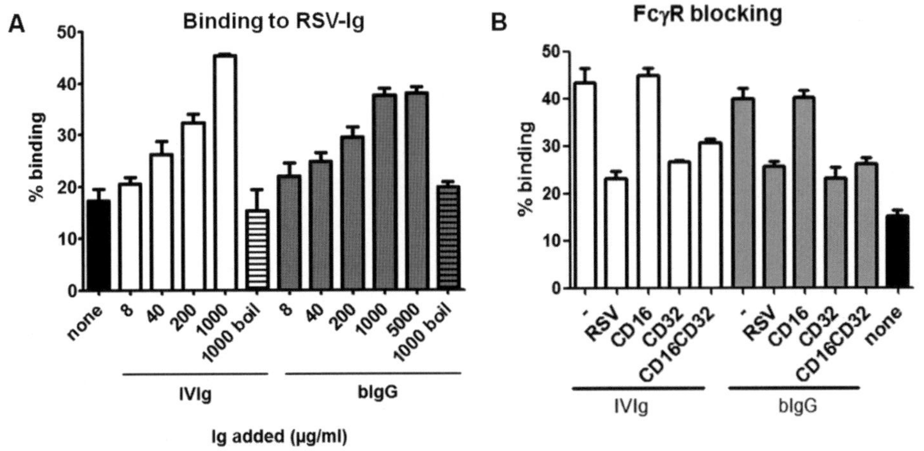

Figure 3. Bovine IgG simultaneously binds to human RSV and human FcγRII. Plates were coated with PEG-precipitated RSV, grown in HEp2 cells. **A)** Varying concentrations of human (IVIg) or bovine (bIgG) Ig were added, followed by incubation with calcein-labelled macrophages. A representative example of four donors tested is shown. No binding of cells was observed when Ig was inactivated prior to addition to the plate, or when Ig was added to gelatine coated plates (data not shown). **B)** 1000 μg/ml IVIg or bIgG was added to RSV-coated plates. PMNs were pre-incubated with medium, and/or anti FcγRII (CD32) or FcγRIII (CD16) Fabs. Independent experiments were performed with three donors. Graphs show mean and S.E.M. of triplicate measurements.

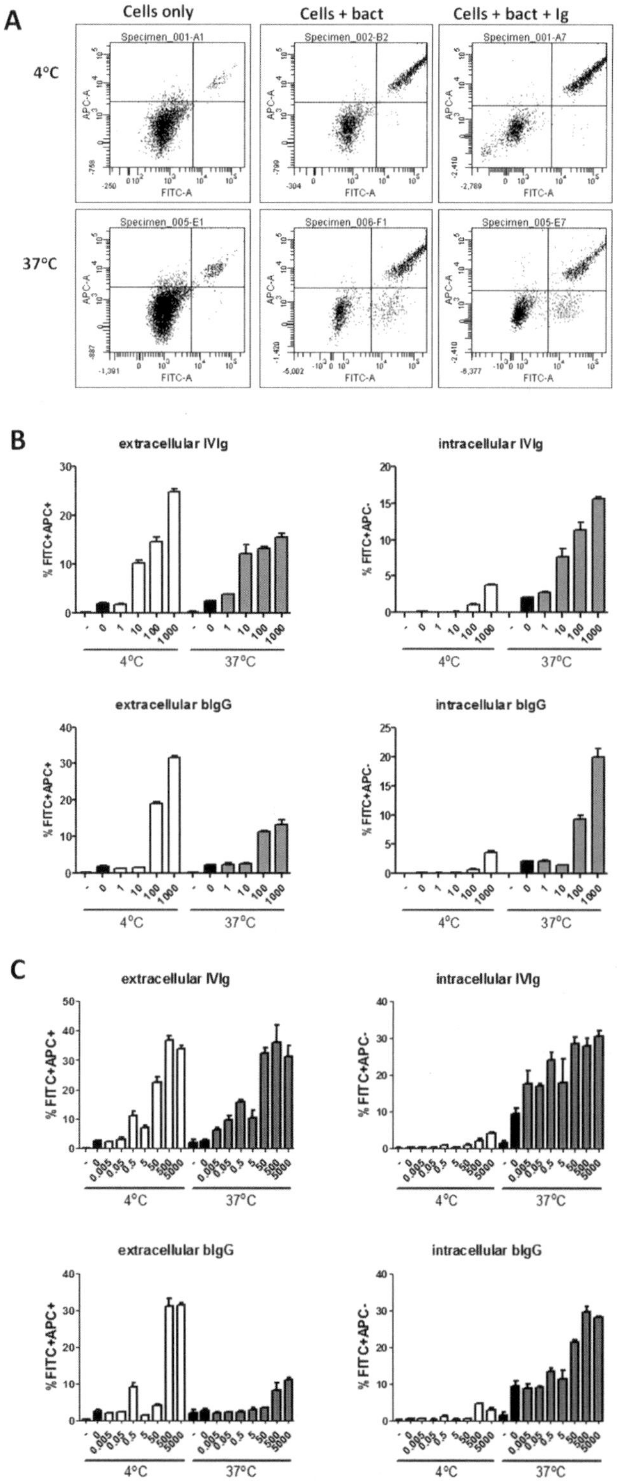

Figure 4. bIg-mediated binding and phagocytosis of *S. epidermidis* by IFN-γ-stimulated monocytes and GM-CSF-differentiated moDCs. FITC-labelled bacteria were opsonised or not with human (IVIg) or bovine (bIgG) IgG. Subsequently cells were allowed to bind to opsonised bacteria and incubated at 4°C (negative control) or 37°C degrees and stained with APC-conjugated antibodies recognizing FITC. Extracellular bacteria were defined as FITC+APC+ and intracellular bacteria as FITC+APC−. Extracellular bacteria can be observed at both 4°C and 37°C incubated cells, whereas intracellular bacteria are only present in cells incubated at 37°C. A) Example of FACS dot plot and gating strategy. B and C) Percentage of IFN-γ conditioned monocytes (B) and moDCs (C) with extracellular (left) and intracellular (right) bacteria of IVIg (top) and bIgG (bottom) incubated at 4°C or 37°C (indicated at x-axes). Black bars indicate medium (-) or bacteria alone without Ig (0). X-axes show μg/ml Ig used for opsonisation of bacteria. Mean and S.E.M. of triplicate measurements are shown of one out of three donors tested.

T and B cells recirculate throughout the body and home to different tissues. Tissue specific homing explains why oral administration of antigen-specific IgG leads to increased presence of memory T and B cells in other organs like the lungs and the breasts [33,34,35,36,37]. Likewise, passive oral vaccination has been shown to induce active immune responses in the gastro-intestinal (GI) tract, but also in the upper airways and in breast tissue [38]. Therefore, bIgG consumption may induce adaptive immunity against respiratory pathogens in a similar manner. Dietary bIgG encounters swallowed respiratory pathogens in the GI tract or in the tonsillar crypts in Waldeyer's ring, forming immune-complexes that efficiently bind to DCs in the tissue [39,40].

As bIgG can bind to RSV, this may lead to viral uptake through FcγR-mediated phagocytosis and, therefore, may facilitate an enhanced T-cell response through binding to FcγRII, as reported by Gosselin for human IgG [41]. The interaction of bIgG with hFcγRII and internalisation of bIgG immune-complexes has been observed for multiple donors, indicating it is a robust phenomenon (Table S1).

As shown in Figure 3, bIgG could bind simultaneously to hRSV and FcγRII on human innate immune cells, and moDCs could internalise bIgG-coated hRSV, which is needed for antigen presentation. This confirms earlier findings that demonstrated binding of bIgG to human FcγRII expressed on myeloid cells [42]. Cross-linking of FcγRII by DCs causes NFκB activation and

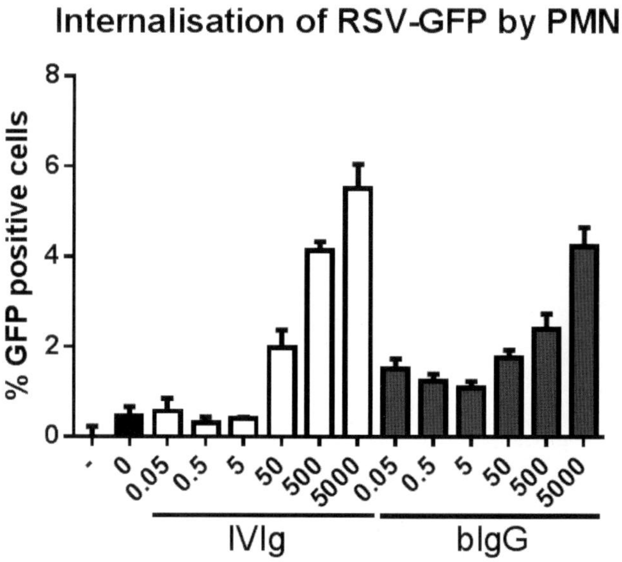

Figure 5. Bovine Ig enhances internalisation of hRSV by hPMN. GFP-renilla expressing RSV was pre-incubated with medium in the presence or absence of IVIg or bIgG and allowed to bind to PMN at 4°C. Subsequently, cells were incubated at 37°C and thereafter treated with trypsin and acid to remove extracellular RSV. Cells were then washed and analysed by flow cytometry for the percentage of GFP+ cells. GFP+ cells were tested in the absence of RSV (–), in the presence of RSV but absence of Ig (0) and in the presence of IVIg or bIgG (μg/ml). Mean and S.E.M. of triplicate measurements of one out of five donors tested are shown.

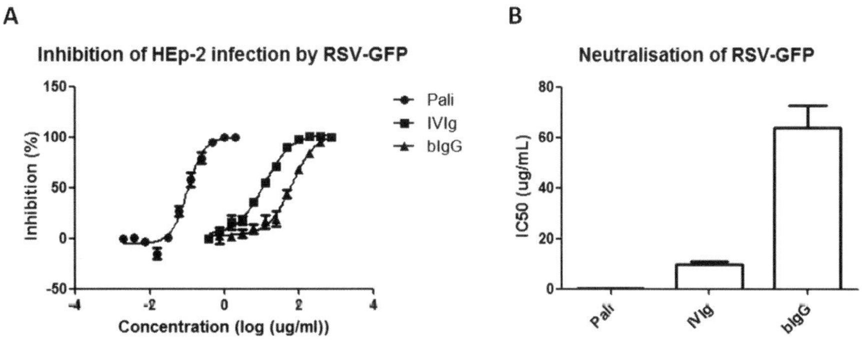

Figure 6. Neutralisation of infection of HEp-2 cells by human RSV. A) 5*10^4 HEp-2 cells were seeded overnight in flat bottom 96-wells plates and infected the next day with 1*10^5 PFU RSV-GFP which was pre-incubated with different concentrations of bovine (bIgG) or human (IVIg) IgG or monoclonal F-protein-specific palivizumab. GFP intensity was determined by flow cytometry as a measure for HEp2 cell infection by RSV-GFP. For the calculation of the inhibition percentage the MFI of uninfected cells was set to 100% and the MFI of infected cells without Ab incubation to 0%. Mean and S.E.M. of three independent experiments is shown. **B**) IC50 values for neutralisation of RSV-GFP by palivizumab, IVIg and bIgG are shown.

maturation of DCs [39]. FcγRII-mediated antigen uptake and presentation, as well as DC maturation is crucial for activation and differentiation of T cells. As a result bIgG may facilitate adaptive T cell responses. This can thus result in long-lasting protection against airway pathogens via the T-cell dependent induction of pathogen-specific (IgA) antibodies in the upper airways.

Our current findings are based on various in vitro assays and require in vivo studies to show formally demonstrate that like Ig from breast milk, bIgG can assist the development of immune memory responses. Another aspect that needs further study is how effective bIgG is in inducing protective immunity in immunocompromised individuals, like children suffering from recurrent asthma caused by viral infections, and in newborns in whom the immune system has not yet matured. Therefore, inclusion of intact bIgG in infant nutrition may contribute to the induction of adaptive immunity against airway infections. Interestingly, several epidemiological studies have linked the consumption of milk to a reduced incidence of asthma [43,44,45,46]. This effect was later shown to be associated with the consumption of raw milk, and the detectability of intact milk proteins [47]. As RSV infections may predispose infants to develop asthma at a later age [6,7,8], we would like to speculate that there is a possibility that the effect we describe here for RSV-specific bovine antibodies may contribute to the effect of raw milk consumption on asthma development.

Although nutritional intervention studies are needed to formally demonstrate if dietary bIgG can contribute to protection against respiratory pathogens, and possibly also against the development of asthma, the *in vitro* data reported here support this concept.

Author Contributions

Conceived and designed the experiments: GdH LB LU JHWL RJJvN. Performed the experiments: GdH SJ LC. Analyzed the data: GdH SJ JL LU LC RJJvN. Contributed reagents/materials/analysis tools: JHWL. Contributed to the writing of the manuscript: GdH JHWL RJJvN.

References

1. Black RE, Morris SS, Bryce J (2003) Where and why are 10 million children dying every year? The Lancet 361: 2226–2234.
2. Nair H, Nokes DJ, Gessner BD, Dherani M, Madhi SA, et al. (2010) Global burden of acute lower respiratory infections due to respiratory syncytial virus in young children: a systematic review and meta-analysis. The Lancet 375: 1545–1555.
3. Lozano R, Naghavi M, Foreman K, Lim S, Shibuya K, et al. (2012) Global and regional mortality from 235 causes of death for 20 age groups in 1990 and 2010: a systematic analysis for the Global Burden of Disease Study 2010. The Lancet 380: 2095–2128.
4. Pitkäranta A, Virolainen A, Jero J, Arruda E, Hayden FG (1998) Detection of Rhinovirus, Respiratory Syncytial Virus, and Coronavirus Infections in Acute Otitis Media by Reverse Transcriptase Polymerase Chain Reaction. Pediatrics 102: 291–295.
5. Ruuskanen O, Arola M, Putto-Laurila A, Mertsola J, Meurman O, et al. (1989) Acute otitis media and respiratory virus infections. The Pediatric Infectious Disease Journal 8: 94–99.
6. Régnier SA, Huels J (2013) Association Between Respiratory Syncytial Virus Hospitalizations in Infants and Respiratory Sequelae: Systematic Review and Meta-analysis. The Pediatric Infectious Disease Journal 32: 820–826 810.1097/INF.1090b1013e31829061e31829068.
7. Mohapatra SS, Boyapalle S (2008) Epidemiologic, Experimental, and Clinical Links between Respiratory Syncytial Virus Infection and Asthma. Clinical Microbiology Reviews 21: 495–504.
8. Pérez-Yarza EG, Moreno A, Lázaro P, Mejías A, Ramilo O (2007) The Association Between Respiratory Syncytial Virus Infection and the Development of Childhood Asthma: A Systematic Review of the Literature. The Pediatric Infectious Disease Journal 26: 733–739 710.1097/INF.1090b1013e3180618c3180642.
9. Rudan I, Boschi-Pinto C, Biloglav Z, Mulholland K, Campbell H (2008) Epidemiology and etiology of childhood pneumonia. Bulletin of the World Health Organization 86: 408–416B.
10. Watt JP, Wolfson LJ, O'Brien KL, Henkle E, Deloria-Knoll M, et al. (2009) Burden of disease caused by Haemophilus influenzae type b in children younger than 5 years: global estimates. Lancet (London, England) 374: 903–911.
11. Bezerra PGM, Britto MCA, Correia JB, Duarte MdCMB, Fonceca AM, et al. (2011) Viral and Atypical Bacterial Detection in Acute Respiratory Infection in Children Under Five Years. PLoS ONE 6: e18928.
12. Walsh E, Falsey AR (2004) Humoral and Mucosal Immunity in Protection from Natural Respiratory Syncytial Virus Infection in Adults. Journal of Infectious Diseases 190: 373–378.
13. Palladino G, Mozdzanowska K, Washko G, Gerhard W (1995) Virus-neutralizing antibodies of immunoglobulin G (IgG) but not of IgM or IgA isotypes can cure influenza virus pneumonia in SCID mice. Journal of Virology 69: 2075–2081.
14. Cox RJ, Brokstad KA, Ogra P (2004) Influenza Virus: Immunity and Vaccination Strategies. Comparison of the Immune Response to Inactivated and Live, Attenuated Influenza Vaccines. Scandinavian Journal of Immunology 59: 1–15.
15. Cox RJ, Brokstad KA, Zuckerman MA, Wood JM, Haaheim LR, et al. (1994) An early humoral immune response in peripheral blood following parenteral inactivated influenza vaccination. Vaccine 12: 993–999.

16. Schlaudecker EP, Steinhoff MC, Omer SB, McNeal MM, Roy E, et al. (2013) IgA and Neutralizing Antibodies to Influenza A Virus in Human Milk: A Randomized Trial of Antenatal Influenza Immunization. PLoS ONE 8: e70867.
17. Ochola R, Sande C, Fegan G, Scott PD, Medley GF, et al. (2009) The Level and Duration of RSV-Specific Maternal IgG in Infants in Kilifi Kenya. PLoS ONE 4: e8088.
18. Ogilvie MM, Santhire Vathenen A, Radford M, Codd J, Key S (1981) Maternal antibody and respiratory syncytial virus infection in infancy. Journal of medical virology 7: 263–271.
19. Nishimura T, Suzue J, Kaji H (2009) Breastfeeding reduces the severity of respiratory syncytial virus infection among young infants: A multi-center prospective study. Pediatrics International 51: 812–816.
20. Oddy WH (2004) A Review of the Effects of Breastfeeding on Respiratory Infections, Atopy, and Childhood Asthma. Journal of Asthma 41: 605–621.
21. Harris NL, Spoerri I, Schopfer JF, Nembrini C, Merky P, et al. (2006) Mechanisms of Neonatal Mucosal Antibody Protection. J Immunol 177: 6256–6262.
22. Hilpert H, Briissow H, Mietens C, Sidoti J, Lerner L, et al. (1987) Use of Bovine Milk Concentrate Containing Antibody to Rotavirus to Treat Rotavirus Gastroenteritis in Infants. Journal of Infectious Diseases 156: 158–166.
23. den Hartog G, Savelkoul HFJ, Schoemaker R, Tijhaar E, Westphal AH, et al. (2011) Modulation of Human Immune Responses by Bovine Interleukin-10. PLoS ONE 6: e18188.
24. van Neerven RJJ, Knol EF, Heck JML, Savelkoul HFJ (2012) Which factors in raw cow's milk contribute to protection against allergies? Journal of Allergy and Clinical Immunology 130: 853–858.
25. Korhonen H, Marnila P, Gill H (2000) Bovine milk antibodies for health. British Journal of Nutrition 84: 135–146.
26. Wilson SD, Roberts K, Hammond K, Ayres JG, Cane PA (2000) Estimation of incidence of respiratory syncytial virus infection in schoolchildren using salivary antibodies. Journal of medical virology 61: 81–84.
27. Koenderman L, van der Linden JA, Honing H, Ulfman LH (2010) Integrins on neutrophils are dispensable for migration into three-dimensional fibrin gels. Thrombosis & Haemostasis 104: 599.
28. van der Poel CE, Karssemeijer RA, Boross P, van der Linden JA, Blokland M, et al. (2010) Cytokine-induced immune complex binding to the high-affinity IgG receptor, FcγRI, in the presence of monomeric IgG. Blood 116: 5327–5333.
29. Anderson CL, Shen L, Eicher DM, Wewers MD, Gill JK (1990) Phagocytosis mediated by three distinct Fc gamma receptor classes on human leukocytes. The Journal of Experimental Medicine 171: 1333–1345.
30. Blanken MO, Rovers MM, Molenaar JM, Winkler-Seinstra PL, Meijer A, et al. (2013) Respiratory Syncytial Virus and Recurrent Wheeze in Healthy Preterm Infants. New England Journal of Medicine 368: 1791–1799.
31. Poel WHM, Kramps JA, Middel WGJ, Oirschot JT, Brand A (1993) Dynamics of bovine respiratory syncytial virus infections: a longitudinal epidemiological study in dairy herds. Archives of Virology 133: 309–321.
32. Elvander M (1996) Severe respiratory disease in dairy cows caused by infection with bovine respiratory syncytial virus. Veterinary Record 138: 101–105.
33. Ebina T, Sato A, Umezu K, Ishida N, Ohyama S, et al. (1985) Prevention of rotavirus infection by oral administration of cow colostrum containing antihumanrotavirus antibody. Medical microbiology and immunology 174: 177–185.
34. Dullaers M, Li D, Xue Y, Ni L, Gayet I, et al. (2009) A T Cell-Dependent Mechanism for the Induction of Human Mucosal Homing Immunoglobulin A-Secreting Plasmablasts. Immunity 30: 120–129.
35. Mora JR, von Andrian UH (2006) T-cell homing specificity and plasticity: new concepts and future challenges. Trends in Immunology 27: 235–243.
36. Mora JR, von Andrian UH (2009) Role of retinoic acid in the imprinting of gut-homing IgA-secreting cells. Seminars in Immunology 21: 28–35.
37. Stevens SK, Weissman IL, Butcher EC (1982) Differences in the migration of B and T lymphocytes: organ-selective localization in vivo and the role of lymphocyte-endothelial cell recognition. The journal of immunology 128: 844–851.
38. Maijó M, Miró L, Polo J, Campbell J, Russell L, et al. (2012) Dietary Plasma Proteins Modulate the Adaptive Immune Response in Mice with Acute Lung Inflammation. The Journal of Nutrition 142: 264–270.
39. Bánki Z, Kacani L, Müllauer B, Wilflingseder D, Obermoser G, et al. (2003) Cross-Linking of CD32 Induces Maturation of Human Monocyte-Derived Dendritic Cells Via NF-κB Signaling Pathway. The journal of immunology 170: 3963–3970.
40. Esposito-Farese ME, Sautès C, de la Salle H, Latour S, Bieber T, et al. (1995) Membrane and soluble Fc gamma RII/III modulate the antigen-presenting capacity of murine dendritic epidermal Langerhans cells for IgG-complexed antigens. The journal of immunology 155: 1725–1736.
41. Gosselin EJ, Wardwell K, Gosselin DR, Alter N, Fisher JL, et al. (1992) Enhanced antigen presentation using human Fc gamma receptor (monocyte/macrophage)-specific immunogens. The journal of immunology 149: 3477–3481.
42. Kramski M, Lichtfuss GF, Navis M, Isitman G, Wren L, et al. (2012) Anti-HIV-1 antibody-dependent cellular cytotoxicity mediated by hyperimmune bovine colostrum IgG. European Journal of Immunology 42: n/a-n/a.
43. Riedler J, Braun-Fahrländer C, Eder W, Schreuer M, Waser M, et al. (2001) Exposure to farming in early life and development of asthma and allergy: a cross-sectional survey. The Lancet 358: 1129–1133.
44. Perkin MR, Strachan DP (2006) Which aspects of the farming lifestyle explain the inverse association with childhood allergy? Journal of Allergy and Clinical Immunology 117: 1374–1381.
45. Waser M, Michels KB, Bieli C, Flöistrup H, Pershagen G, et al. (2007) Inverse association of farm milk consumption with asthma and allergy in rural and suburban populations across Europe. Clinical & Experimental Allergy 37: 661–670.
46. Ege MJ, Frei R, Bieli C, Schram-Bijkerk D, Waser M, et al. (2007) Not all farming environments protect against the development of asthma and wheeze in children. Journal of Allergy and Clinical Immunology 119: 1140–1147.
47. Loss G, Apprich S, Waser M, Kneifel W, Genuneit J, et al. (2011) The protective effect of farm milk consumption on childhood asthma and atopy: The GABRIELA study. Journal of Allergy and Clinical Immunology 128: 766–773. e764.

17

Enterovirus 71 Induces Mitochondrial Reactive Oxygen Species Generation That is Required for Efficient Replication

Mei-Ling Cheng[1,2,3], Shiue-Fen Weng[4], Chih-Hao Kuo[4], Hung-Yao Ho[2,4,5]*

1 Department of Biomedical Sciences, College of Medicine, Chang Gung University, Tao-Yuan, Taiwan, **2** Healthy Aging Research Center, Chang Gung University, Tao-Yuan, Taiwan, **3** Metabolomics Core Laboratory, Chang Gung University, Tao-Yuan, Taiwan, **4** Department of Medical Biotechnology and Laboratory Science, College of Medicine, Chang Gung University, Tao-Yuan, Taiwan, **5** Office of Research and Development, Chang Gung Memorial Hospital, Tao-Yuan, Taiwan

Abstract

Redox homeostasis is an important host factor determining the outcome of infectious disease. Enterovirus 71 (EV71) infection has become an important endemic disease in Southeast Asia and China. We have previously shown that oxidative stress promotes viral replication, and progeny virus induces oxidative stress in host cells. The detailed mechanism for reactive oxygen species (ROS) generation in infected cells remains elusive. In the current study, we demonstrate that mitochondria were a major ROS source in EV71-infected cells. Mitochondria in productively infected cells underwent morphologic changes and exhibited functional anomalies, such as a decrease in mitochondrial electrochemical potential $\Delta\Psi_m$ and an increase in oligomycin-insensitive oxygen consumption. Respiratory control ratio of mitochondria from infected cells was significantly lower than that of normal cells. The total adenine nucleotide pool and ATP content of EV71-infected cells significantly diminished. However, there appeared to be a compensatory increase in mitochondrial mass. Treatment with mito-TEMPO reduced eIF2α phosphorylation and viral replication, suggesting that mitochondrial ROS act to promote viral replication. It is plausible that EV71 infection induces mitochondrial ROS generation, which is essential to viral replication, at the sacrifice of efficient energy production, and that infected cells up-regulate biogenesis of mitochondria to compensate for their functional defect.

Editor: Hsin-Chih Lai, Chang-Gung University, Taiwan

Funding: This project is supported by grants from Chang Gung University (CMRPD190443, CMRPD1A0562, CMRPD1C0751, CMRPD1A0563, CMRPD1A0521, CMRPD1A0522, CMRPD391683, CMRPD1C0441, and CMRPD1C0761), National Science Council of Taiwan (NSC99-2320-B-182-021-MY3 and NSC101-2320-B-182-024-MY3), and the Ministry of Education of Taiwan (EMRPD1C0271 and EMRPD1D0241). The funders had no role in study design, data collection and analysis, decision to publish, or preparation of the manuscript.

Competing Interests: The authors have declared that no competing interests exist.

* Email: hoh01@mail.cgu.edu.tw

Introduction

Enterovirus 71 (EV71), a member of the family *Picornaviridae*, is a non-enveloped RNA virus [1]. Since its identification in 1969 [2], episodes of EV71 outbreak occurred periodically throughout the world [3–6]. Clinical manifestation of EV71 infection includes febrile illness, acute respiratory disease, hand-foot-and-mouth disease, herpangia, myocarditis, aseptic meningitis, acute flaccid paralysis, brainstem and/or cerebellar encephalitis, Guillain-Barre syndrome, or combinations of these clinical features [7,8]. Though hand-foot-and-mouth disease is a benign disease, the neurologic and systemic complications are more severe [9]. Children aged below 5 years are susceptible to development of permanent neurologic sequelae, or even succumb to such complications [10]. To date, the largest epidemic of EV71 occurred in China in 2008 and 2009. Nearly 490000 cases, of which 126 deaths occurred, were reported; over a million cases of hand-foot-and-mouth disease were reported in 2009 [4,5]. EV71 infection recurs every 2 or 3 years in Asia-Pacific region.

It is evident that redox environment is a factor affecting host-microbe interactions. The susceptibility of host cells to HIV, coxsackievirus and influenza virus is affected by redox microenvironment [11–15]. We have recently found that increased oxidative stress in host cells enhances EV71 infection [16]. It is intriguing that viral infection can itself induce oxidative stress in host cells. Increased superoxide production has been observed in pneumonia caused by influenza A virus [17]. Herpes simplex virus (HSV) infection of microglia cells elicits oxidative stress, which probably causes the neurotoxicity [18]. Rhinovirus and respiratory syncytial virus induce ROS production in fibroblasts and epithelial cells [19,20]. We have recently found that EV71 infection can lead to increased reactive oxygen species (ROS) generation [16]. However, the mechanism for ROS production in EV71-infected cells remains elusive.

Mitochondria are important organelle for cellular energy metabolism, and have been recently implicated in responses of host cell to viral infection. They lie at the crossroad of metabolism, redox homeostasis, apoptosis, and innate immune signaling, and probably form a multi-functional signaling platform termed mitoxosome [21]. Mitochondria-associated adaptors such as MAVS are involved in modulation of innate immunity [22]. Additionally, intermembrane space proteins, such as cytochrome c and Smac/DIABLO, and outer mitochondrial membrane proteins, such as Bcl-2, are involved in initiation and regulation of apoptosis [23,24]. Viral infection is associated with changes in mitochondrial functions. Hepatitis C virus (HCV)-infected cells have impaired oxidative phosphorylation and increased ROS generation [25,26]. Expression of HCV protein represses mitochondrial membrane potential and mitochondrial coupling efficiency, and leads to increased ROS production [27]. Likewise, expression of human immunodeficiency virus (HIV) Tat protein, hepatitis B virus X protein, severe acute respiratory syndrome (SARS) coronavirus non-structural protein 10 results in mitochondrial depolarization [28–30]. These proteins are known to induce oxidative stress [30–32]. It is currently unknown whether EV71-induced oxidative stress is associated with mitochondrial dysfunction.

In the present study, we investigated the mechanistic aspect of ROS generation induced by EV71 infection. We examined the changes in mitochondria in EV71-infected cells. Our findings show that EV71 infection induces mitochondrial dysfunction and anomalous changes in their morphology and subcellular distribution. These mitochondria represent the sites of ROS generation. Such changes are associated with altered cellular energy metabolism. Mitochondrial ROS are essential to viral replication process. The increase in mitochondrial mass in infected cells may compensate for energy deficit caused by abnormal mitochondria.

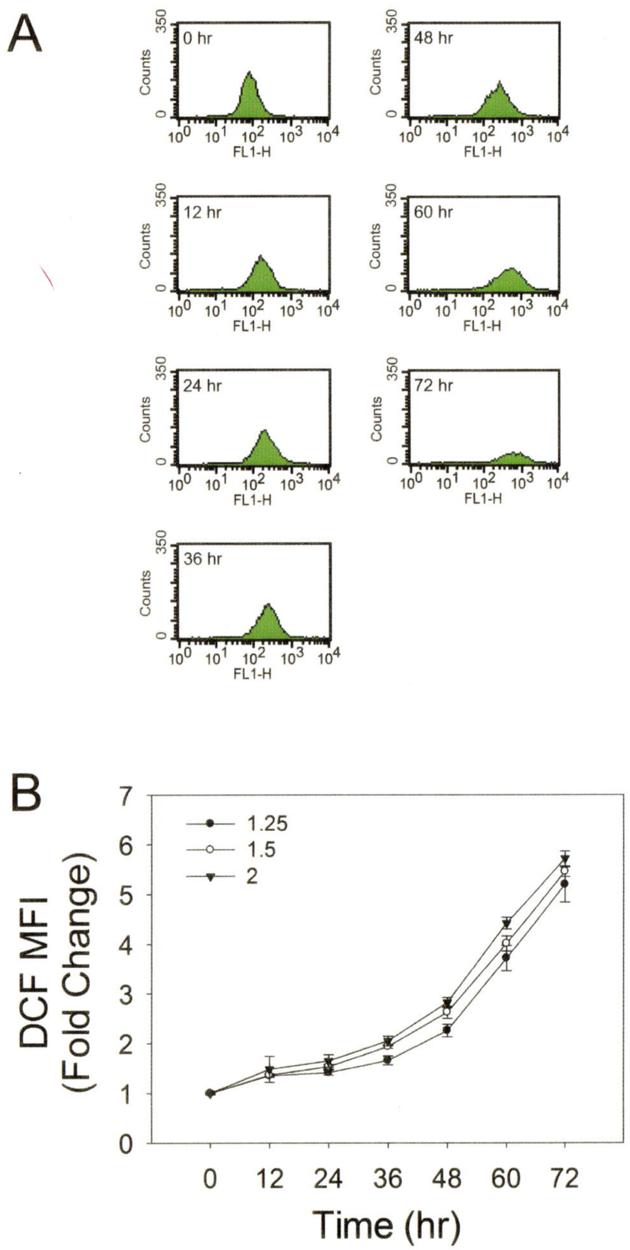

Figure 1. EV71 infection induces ROS in neural cells in a time-dependent manner. SF268 cells were infected with EV71 at m.o.i. of 1.25, 1.5 and 2 for 0, 12, 24, 36, 48, 60 and 72 hr, and were subject to H_2DCFDA staining and flow cytometric analysis. (A) Representative histograms of cell counts (*counts*) vs. DCF fluorescence (*FL1-H*) for cells infected at an m.o.i. of 1.25 at indicated times are shown. (B) The mean fluorescence intensity (MFI) of DCF of infected cells is expressed as fold change relative to that of uninfected cells. The results are presented as mean±SD of three separate experiments.

Materials and Methods

Cell culture and virological techniques

SF268 glioblastoma cells (National Cancer Institute Center for Cancer Research ID: 59) were cultured in Dulbecco's modified Eagle's medium (DMEM) supplemented with 10% fetal calf serum (FCS), 2 mM glutamine, 2 mM non-essential amino acids, 100 U/ml penicillin, 0.1 mg/ml streptomycin, and 0.25 µg/ml amphotericin at 37°C in a humidified atmosphere of 5% CO_2 [33,34]. EV71 (BrCr strain; ATCC VR784) was propagated in Vero cells as described previously [16]. Vero cells (ATCC CCL-81) were cultured in modified Eagle's medium (MEM) supplemented with 10% FCS, 100 U/ml penicillin, 0.1 mg/ml streptomycin and 0.25 µg/ml amphotericin in an atmosphere of 5% CO_2 at 37°C. Quantitative PCR analysis of the copy number of EV71 genomic DNA was performed as described previously [16].

Detection of ROS and $\Delta\Psi_m$ by confocal microscopy

Visualization of ROS generation was performed by confocal microscopy as described previously [35]. The fluorescence of dichlorofluorescein (DCF) is derived from oxidation of its fluorogenic precursor [35]. In brief, cells were grown in glass-bottomed culture dish, and infected with virus at m.o.i. of 1.25. The infected cells were stained with 100 nM MitoTracker Red and 5 µM H_2DCFDA for 20 min at 37°C. and counterstained with with 5 µg/ml of Hoechst 33342. The specimens were examined with Zeiss LSM 510 Meta system (Carl Zeiss MicroImaging GmbH, Heidelberg, Germany). Confocal fluorescence images of labeled cells were acquired using Plan-Apochromat 100×1.40 NA oil immersion objective. To scan for DCF signal, we used the 488 nm excitation line of argon laser, beam splitter (HFT 405/488/561/633/KP720), and an emission window set at 505–550 nm. To scan for MitoTracker Red signal, we used the 561 nm excitation line of DPSS laser and an emission window set at 575–615 nm. For scanning of Hoechst dye, we used 405 nm excitation line of diode laser and an emission an emission window set at 420–480 nm. To scan for Hoechst dye signal, we used the 405 nm excitation line of diode laser and an emission an emission window set at 420–480 nm. We analyzed all images using Zeiss Zen software package (Carl Zeiss MicroImaging GmbH, Heidelberg, Germany).

Confocal microscopic analysis of $\Delta\Psi_m$ was performed as described previously [36]. The mitochondrial membrane potential was determined using the cationic, lipophilic dye JC-1 (5,5′,6,6′-tetrachloro-1,1′,3,3′-tetraethylbenz- imidazolocarbocyanine io-

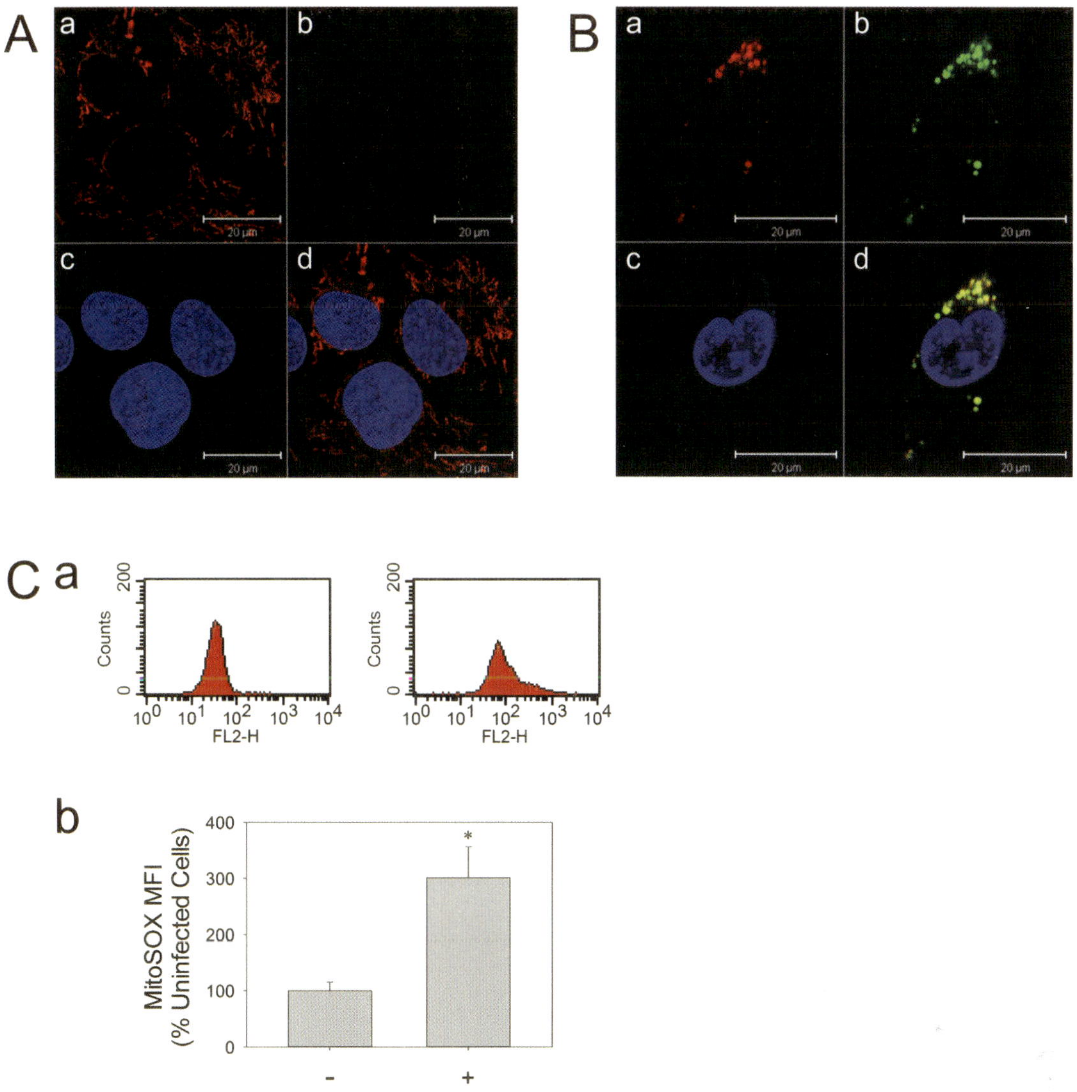

Figure 2. EV71 infection causes mitochondrial ROS production. (A) SF268 cells were mock- (A) or infected with (B) EV71 at an m.o.i. of 1.25 for 54 hr, and were subject to H_2DCFDA and Mitotracker Red staining and confocal microscopic examination. The MitoSOX-stained mitochondria (a), DCF-stained ROS generation sites (b), and Hoechst 33342-stained nuclei (c) are shown. The corresponding images are overlaid (d). The photographs shown here are representative of three experiments. Scale bar, 20 μm. (C) SF268 cells were mock- or infected with EV71 at an m.o.i. of 1.25 for 48 hr, and were subject to MitoSOX Red staining and flow cytometric analysis. (a) Representative histograms of cell counts (*counts*) vs. MitoSOX fluorescence (*FL2-H*) for un- (*left panel*) and infected cells (*right panel*) are shown. (b) The mean fluorescence intensity (MFI) of MitoSOX of mock- (−) and infected (+) cells is expressed as the percentage of that of uninfected cells. The results are presented as mean±SD, n = 3. *$p<0.05$ vs. uninfected cells.

dide) (Invitrogen, CA, USA). JC-1 monomers emit at 527 nm, and J-aggregates emit at 590 nm. Infected cells were loaded with 0.5 μM of JC-1 in culture medium at 37°C for 60 min, and counterstained with 5 μg/ml of Hoechst 33342 prior to examination with Leica TCS SP2 MP system (Leica Microsystems, Mannheim, Germany). Confocal fluorescence images of JC-1 labeled cells were obtained using HCX PL-APO CS 100×1.40 NA oil immersion objective. To scan for signal of JC-1 monomeric form, we used the 488 nm excitation line of argon laser, triple-dichroic beam splitter (TD 488/543/633) and an emission window set at 500–540 nm. To scan for signal of JC-1 aggregated form, we used the 543 nm excitation line of He-Ne laser, triple-dichroic beam splitter (TD 488/543/633) and an emission window set at 580–620 nm. To scan for Hoechst dye signal, we employed a fiber coupling system equipped with a Ti:Sapphire laser (model Millenia/Tsunami; Spectra-Physics; Mountain View, CA, USA), and selected the wavelength of 800 nm for illumination. Image analysis was performed with Leica LCS software packages.

Cytometric analysis of ROS, mitochondrial mass, and $\Delta\Psi_m$

ROS formation was analyzed quantitatively by cytometric analysis. In brief, infected cells were loaded with 2 μM MitoSOX red or 5 μM H_2DCFDA for 20 min at 37°C, washed twice with PBS, and trypsinized for flow cytometric analysis as previously described [37]. The mean fluorescence intensity (MFI) of the fluorescence of oxidized MitoSOX red or MFI of DCF fluorescence was quantified using CellQuest Pro software (Becton Dickinson, CA, USA). Likewise, for determination of mitochon-

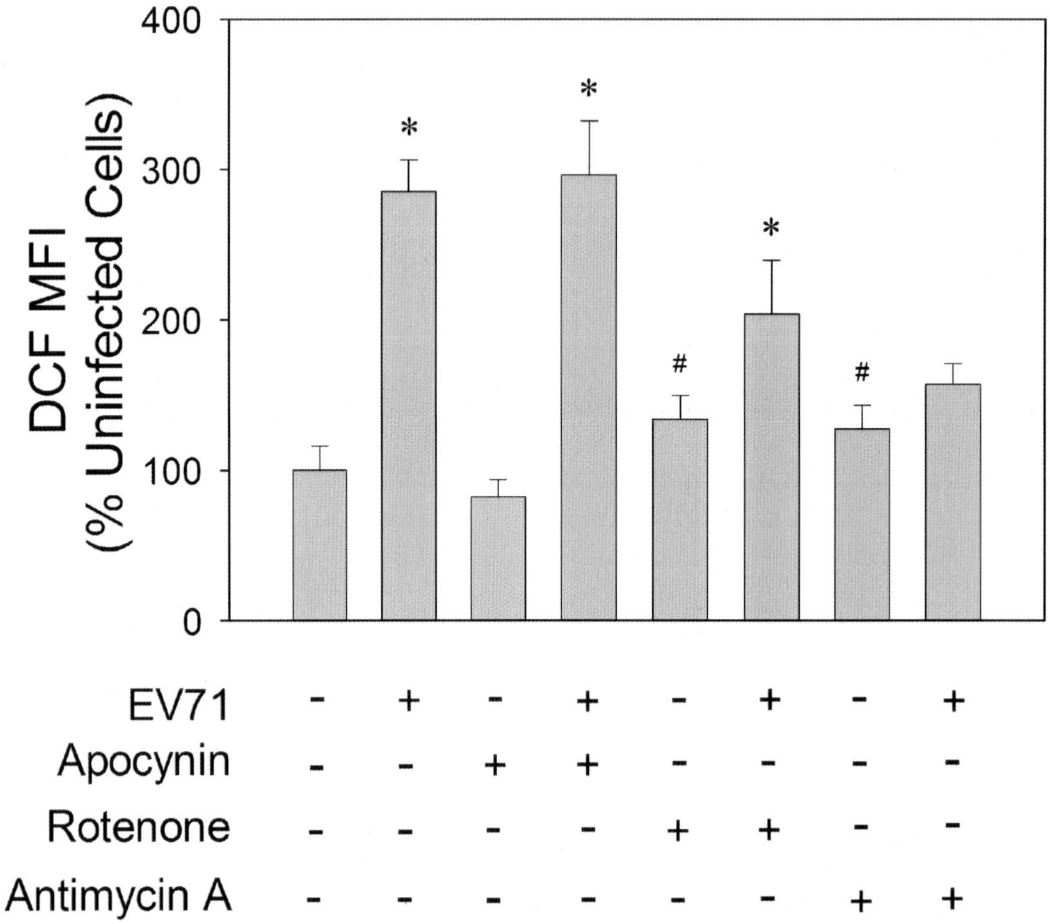

Figure 3. Mitochondrial electron transport-dependent ROS generation. SF268 cells were mock- or infected with EV71 at an m.o.i. of 1.25, and treated without or with apocyanin, rotenone or antimycin A. Forty-eight hours later, cells were stained with H_2DCFDA and analyzed by flow cytometry. The MFI of DCF of infected cells is expressed as the percentage of that of uninfected cells. The results are presented as mean±SD, n = 3. *p<0.05 vs. untreated, uninfected cells; #p<0.05, drug-treated vs. untreated cells.

drial mass, cells were stained with 100 nM Mitotracker Red 580FM (Invitrogen, CA, USA), and analyzed according to manufacturer's instruction. MFI was quantified using CellQuest Pro software. For analysis of $\Delta\Psi_m$, infected cells were loaded with 0.5 μM JC-1 as described above. The cell monolayer was washed three times with PBS, and trypsinized for cytometric analysis. Cells were analyzed for JC-1 monomer fluorescence (FL1 channel) and J-aggregate fluorescence (FL2 channel) with CELLQuest software. The ratio of the mean fluorescence intensity of FL2 channel to that of FL1 channel was calculated.

Measurement of oxygen consumption

SF268 cells were infected with EV71 at m.o.i. of 1.25 for indicated times, washed twice with PBS, and trypsinized. The cells were pelleted, and then resuspended in respiration buffer (20 mM NaKPO4 (pH 7.2), 65 mM KCl, 125 mM sucrose, 2 mM $MgCl_2$). The cell suspension was transferred to the respiratory chamber of Mitocell equipped with Clark-type electrode, which was connected to Strathkelvin 928 6-Channel Oxygen System (Strathkelvin Instruments, Glasgow, UK). Oxygen consumption rate was monitored. In some experiments, oligomycin was added to cell suspension at 2 μg/ml. Data are expressed as μg O_2 per 5×10^5 cells per min. For data normalization with respect to mitochondrial mass, the oxygen consumption rate was normalized to mitochondrial mass determined by Mitotracker Red 580FM Staining as described above. Data are expressed as μg O_2 per mitochondrial mass unit (MMU) per min. A similar approach for determination of oxygen consumption rate per unit of mitochondrial mass was previously described [38].

Isolation of mitochondria and measurement of respiratory control ratio (RCR)

Cells were infected with EV71 at m.o.i. of 1.25, washed twice with PBS, and scrapped in ice-cold SHE buffer (0.25 M sucrose, 1 mM EGTA, 3 mM HEPES). The cells were homogenized. The homogenate was centrifuged at 1000×g at 4°C for 10 min, and subsequently centrifuged at 10000×g at 4°C for 10 min. Finally, the mitochondrial pellet was suspended in a suitable volume of SHE buffer.

For measurement of oxygen consumption of mitochondrial preparation, 0.5 mg of mitochondria was added to 300 μl of assay buffer (20 mM K_2HPO_4/KH_2PO_4 (pH 7.2), 125 mM sucrose, 65 mM KCl, 2 mM $MgCl_2$), and transferred to the Mitocell chamber equipped with Clark-type electrode. Malate and glutamate were added to chamber at the final concentration of 5 mM. ADP was added at a concentration of 0.5 mM to stimulate oxygen consumption. The respiratory control ratio (RCR) is defined as rate of ADP-stimulated state 3 oxygen consumption

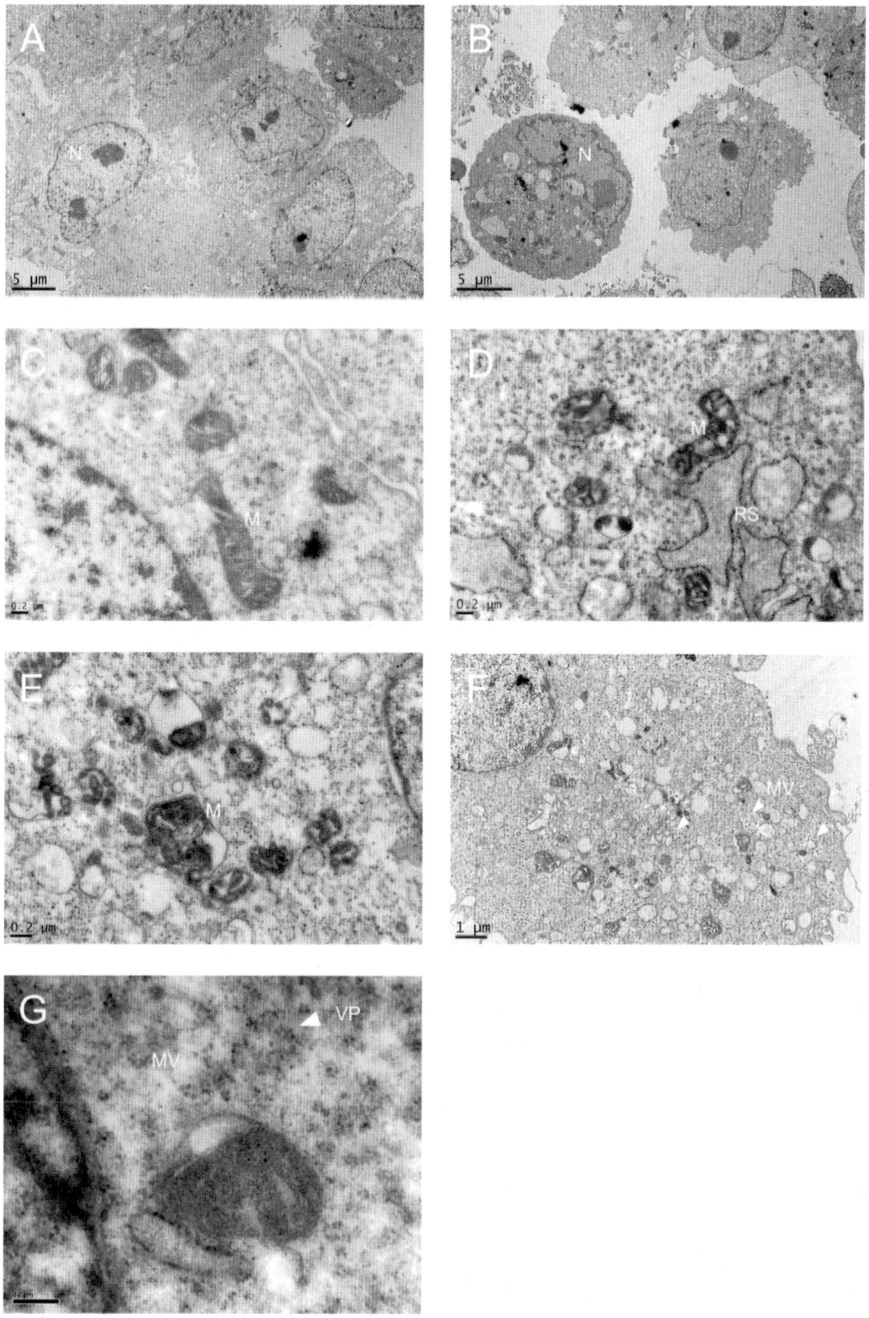

Figure 4. EV71 infection results in morphological changes in mitochondria. SF268 cells were mock- (A & C) or infected with (B, D–G) EV71 at an m.o.i. of 1.25 for 48 hr, and processed for electron microscopic examination. The mock-infected cells had typical nucleus (N) and mitochondria (M). In EV71-infected cells, a number of mitochondria underwent changes in morphology, characterized by deranged cristae (D & E). The developing viral replication site (RS) was lined with ribosomes and was in proximity to mitochondria (D). Numerous single or double membrane-bound vesicles (MV) developed in EV71-infected cells, and some contained virus particles (VP). For A & B, bar represents 5 µm; for F, bar represents 1 µm; for C, D, E & G, bar represents 0.2 µm.

divided by the rate of oxygen consumption (State 4_o) determined in the presence of 2 µg/ml oligomycin [39]. The state 4o is a specific indicator of mitochondrial proton movement being limited by leakiness of inner mitochondrial membrane to proton. RCR was calculated as state 3 oxygen consumption rate divided by that of state 4_o.

Transmission electron microscopy

The transmission electron microscopy was performed as previously described with slight modifications [40]. Briefly stated, the infected cells were washed three times with PBS; trypsinized; placed in a BEEM capsule; and centrifuged to form a pellet with a size of 0.5–1 mm^3. The pellet was fixed with fresh 2.5% glutaraldehyde/PBS at 4°C for 2 hr. After fixation, it was rinsed with PBS thrice for 10 min each. One ml of 1% OsO_4 was added

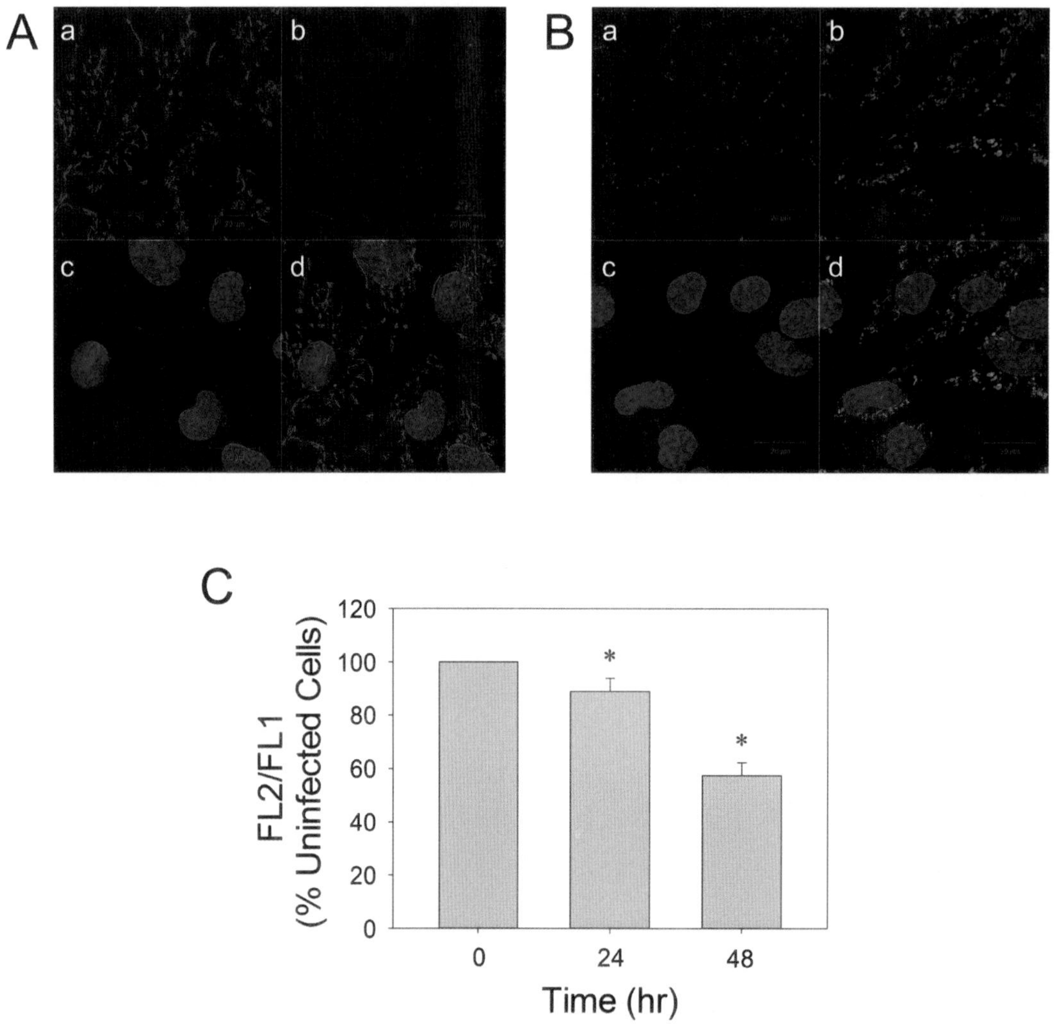

Figure 5. EV71 infection causes decline in $\Delta\Psi_m$. SF268 cells were mock- (A) or infected with (B) EV71 at an m.o.i. of 1.25 for 48 hr. Cell were stained with JC-1 and Hoechst 33342 dyes, and examined by confocal microscopy. Intracellular distribution of JC-1 J-aggregate (a) and monomer (b) is indicative of $\Delta\Psi_m$ in cells. Nuclei of these cells are shown (c). The corresponding images are overlaid (d). The photographs shown here are representative of three experiments. Scale bar, 20 μm. (C) SF268 cells were mock- or infected with EV71 at an m.o.i. of 1.25 for indicated times, and were subject to JC-1 staining and flow cytometric analysis. The ratio of MRI of FL2 channel to that of FL1 channel (FL2/FL1) was calculated, and is expressed relative to that of uninfected cells. Results are mean ± SD, n = 3. *$p<0.05$ vs. uninfected cells.

to the cell pellet for 1 hr. The pellet was washed with PBS thrice for 10 min each, and then with 50% ethanol thrice for 10 min each. The specimen was then stained *en bloc* with 0.5% uranyl acetate/50% ethanol at 4°C overnight. It was dehydrated in ethanol with graded concentrations (70%, 80%, 90%, 95%, 100%, 100%, 100%, 100%) for 15 min each. The specimen was successively infiltrated with ethanol/Spurr's resin (50%:50%), ethanol/Spurr's resin (25%:75%), and pure Spurr's resin overnight for each treatment. It was then heated at 70°C for 72 hr. Thin sections with thickness of 70 nm were obtained with the use of ultramicrotome, and picked on TEM grids. Sections were stained with 2% uranyl acetate for 30 min, followed by 6 min staining with 0.4% lead citrate. The sections were rinsed with water, blotted dry, and examined on a JEOL JEM-1230 electron microscope.

Determination of adenine nucleotides

Levels of ATP, ADP and AMP were determined using UPLC under conditions as previously described for measurement of nicotinamide nucleotides [41].

Western blotting and silver staining

SDS-PAGE and western blotting were performed as previously described [42]. The chemiluminescent signal was detected with X-ray film (Fujifilm, Japan). The silver staining was performed as previously described [43].

Results

EV71 induces mitochondrial ROS generation

Infection of neural SF268 cells with EV71 induces oxidative stress in time-dependent manner. The levels of ROS, as indicated by DCF fluorescence, in cells infected at multiplicity of infection (m.o.i.) of 2 were 3- and 6-fold that of uninfected control at 48 and 72 hr respectively (Figure 1). As mitochondria are major sites of

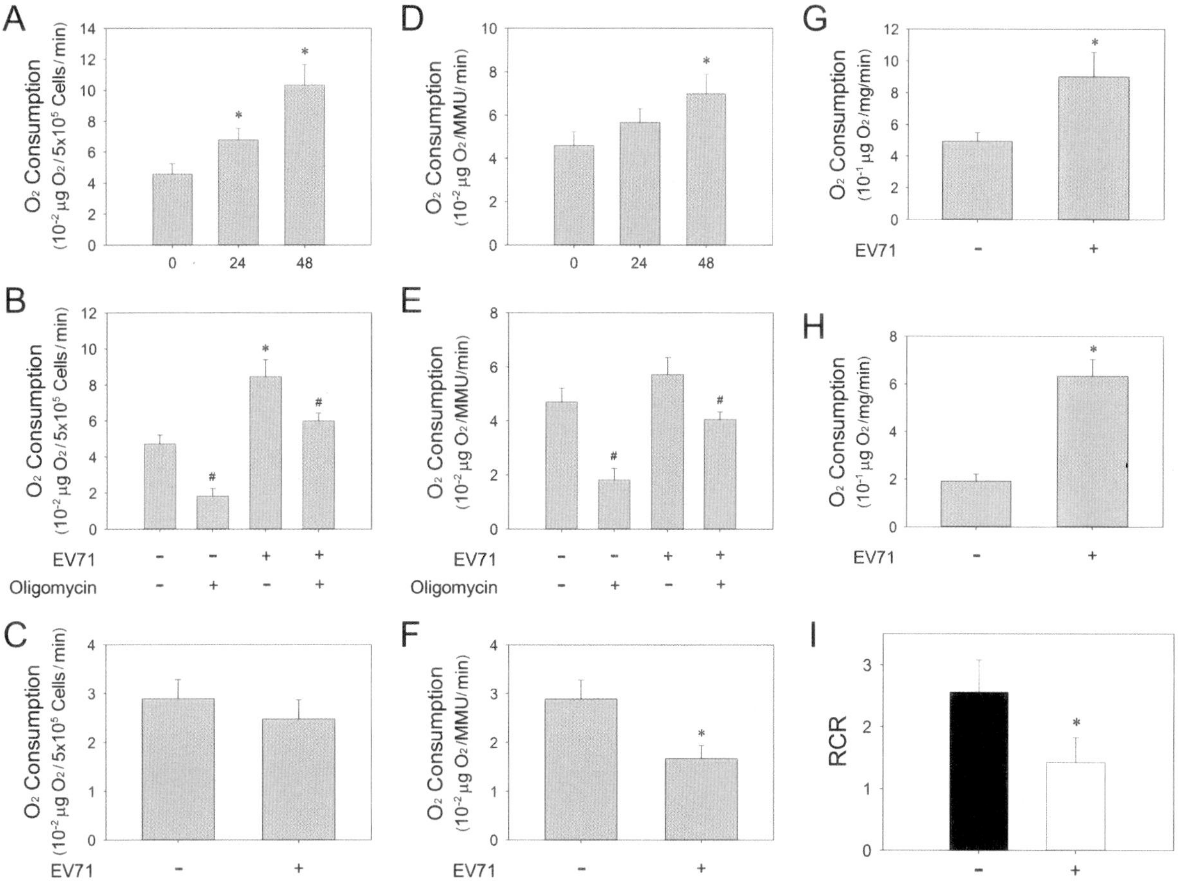

Figure 6. EV71 infection-induced oxygen consumption is associated with a reduction in respiratory efficiency. (A) SF268 cells were mock- or infected with EV71 at an m.o.i. of 1.25 for indicated times. Oxygen concentration was assayed with Clark oxygen electrode, and oxygen consumption rate (10^{-2} µg $O_2/5\times10^5$ cells/min) was calculated accordingly. Results are mean ± SD, n = 6. *p<0.05 vs. uninfected cells. (B) SF268 cells were mock- or infected with EV71 at an m.o.i. of 1.25, and were treated without or with oligomycin. Oxygen concentration was assayed with Clark oxygen electrode, and oxygen consumption rate (10^{-2} µg $O_2/5\times10^5$ cells/min) was calculated. Results are mean ± SD, n = 6. *p<0.05 vs. uninfected cells; #p<0.05, oligomycin-treated vs. untreated cells. (C) Oligomycin-sensitive oxygen consumption rate was calculated as the difference in the absence and presence of oligomycin. (D & E) The oxygen consumption was measured as described in (A) and (B). Data were normalized to the relative mitochondrial mass unit (MMU) of control and infected cells. Results are mean ± SD, n = 6. *p<0.05 vs. uninfected cells. (F) Oligomycin-sensitive oxygen consumption rate was calculated as described in (C), and normalized to the relative mitochondrial mass unit (MMU) of control and infected cells. (G–I) SF268 cells were mock- (−) or infected (+) with EV71 at an m.o.i. of 1.25 for 48 hr, and mitochondria were isolated and assayed for oxygen consumption rates (10^{-1} µg O_2/mg mitochondrial protein/min) during state 3 (G) and 4_o (H) respiration as described in *Materials and Methods*. RCRs were calculated accordingly, and are shown (I). Results are mean ± SD, n = 6. *p<0.05 vs. uninfected cells.

ROS generation, we test if EV71 induces ROS generation in mitochondria. The EV71 infected-SF268 cells were stained at 54 hr post-infection (p.i.) with Mitotracker Red and H_2DCFDA, and examined under confocal microscope. As expected, the DCF fluorescence increased in EV71-infected cell but not in the uninfected cells (Figures 2A & B). More important, the sites of ROS production coincided with mitochondria in EV71-infected cells (Figure 2B). It was consistent with staining of the infected cells with MitoSOX Red, a mitochondrion-specific probe for ROS (Figure 2C). The infected cells showed 3-fold increase in mitochondrial ROS generation. At infection time greater than 60 hr, the infected cells exhibited a great loss of viability. To study the host cell responses to viral infection, we focused on analyses of cells at early or mid-phase of infection in subsequent studies.

The mitochondrial production of ROS is validated by pharmacological approach. Treatment of EV71-infected cells with complex I inhibitor rotenone and complex III inhibitor antimycin A significantly inhibited ROS generation (Figure 3). Unlike respiratory complex inhibitors, treatment of cells with apocyanin, a NADPH oxidase (NOX) inhibitor, did not affect EV71-induced ROS generation. These findings suggest that NOX is not involved in ROS generation in infected SF268 cells, and that ROS is generated at a site of mitochondrial electron transport chain distal to complex III.

ROS production is associated with mitochondrial morphological anomalies

Increased ROS production is suggestive of mitochondrial anomalies. To test such possibility, we examined the subcellular structure of infected SF268 cells using electron microscope. Forty-eight hour after infection, numerous SF268 cells were rounded. A number of membrane bound vesicle appeared in cytoplasm (Figures 4B & F). In some cells, replication sites of EV71 developed from rough endoplasmic reticulum, and were characterized by the presence of ribosomes at its periphery and accumulation of mitochondria in its proximity (Figure 4D). Smooth membrane bound vesicles were also observed. The replication sites and the virus-induced membrane vesicles were

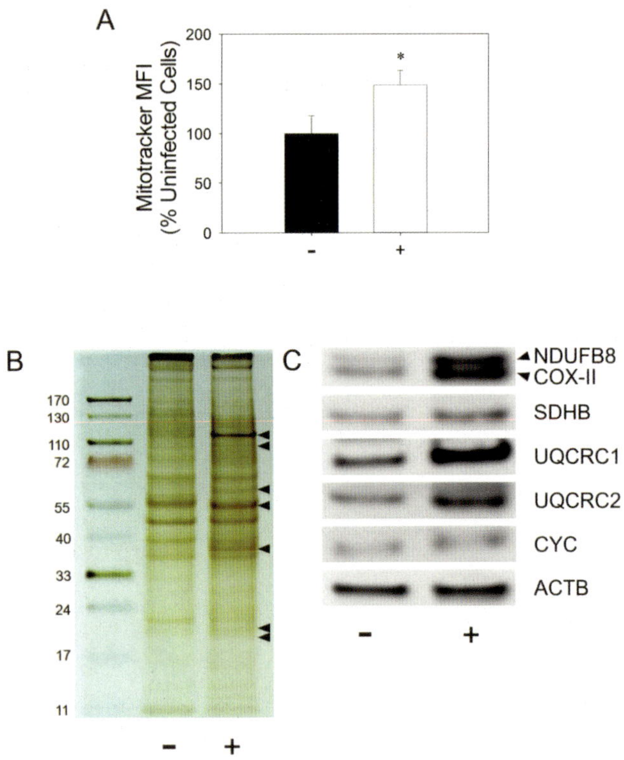

Figure 7. Mitochondrial mass increases and expression of mitochondrial proteins changes in response to EV71 infection. (A) SF268 cells were mock- (−) or infected (+) with EV71 at an m.o.i. of 1.25 for 48 hr, and were subject to Mitotracker dye staining and flow cytometric analysis as described in *Materials and Methods*. The MFI of the stained cells is expressed relative to that of control cells. Results are mean ± SD, n = 3. *p<0.05 vs. uninfected cells. (B & C) Cells were un- or infected under the similar condition, and mitochondria were isolated for SDS-PAGE electrophoresis and silver staining (B). In the silver-stained gel, the leftmost lane corresponds to protein markers with respective molecular weights indicated alongside the bands. (C) Cells similarly infected were harvested for western blotting with indicated antibodies. A representative experiment out of three is shown here.

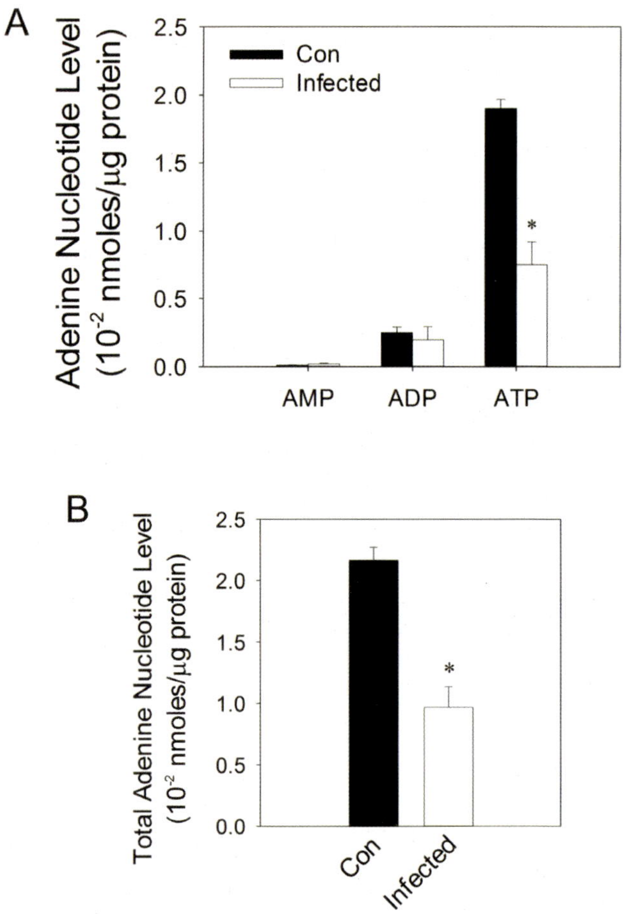

Figure 8. Levels of ATP, ADP and AMP in EV71-infected cells. SF268 cells were mock- (*Con*) or infected (*Infected*) with EV71 at an m.o.i. of 1.25 for 48 hr, and were harvested for UPLC-based analyses of ATP, ADP and AMP. These adenine nucleotides are normalized to cellular protein content. Levels of ATP, ADP and AMP (A) and total adenine nucleotides (B) are shown. Results are mean ± SD, n = 3. *p<0.05 vs. uninfected cells.

absent from the uninfected cells. A significant percentage of atypical mitochondria were observed. They were more electron-dense in infected cells as compared with control cells (Figure 4C & D). The crista arrangement in mitochondria of the infected cells became largely distorted (Figure 4D). The cristae were swollen and appeared as "holes" in electron micrograph. In some mitochondria, the crista structure was lost. The outer membrane was no longer closely apposed to the inner membrane, and the intermembrane space was enlarged (Figure 4E). Inner membrane was less conspicuous and even discontinuous in some mitochondria. These findings suggest that EV71 induces morphological anomalies in mitochondria.

EV71 causes decline in mitochondrial electrochemical potential $\Delta\Psi_m$

It is plausible that EV71 induces mitochondrial dysfunction in EV71-infected cells. A functional parameter of mitochondria is electrochemical potential $\Delta\Psi_m$. We studied $\Delta\Psi_m$ in infected cells using JC-1 staining. Mitochondria are heterogeneous in morphology, ranging from round, ovoid structure to long, interconnected structure. In uninfected cells, most mitochondria appeared red and represent energized mitochondria (Figure 5A). A large percentage of the energized mitochondria were elongated tubular or oblong structure. They formed a network distributed more evenly throughout cytoplasm. Upon infection, there were changes in mitochondria. Most mitochondria showed green fluorescence, and were depolarized or de-energized (Figure 5B). They appeared to cluster in the perinuclear region (Figures 2B & 5B). Some of mitochondria were swollen, and a majority of the remainder took a short ovoid form. Additionally, we applied a flow cytometric analysis to quantify $\Delta\Psi_m$ in infected cells. Infection of cells with EV71 causes about 10 and 40% reduction in $\Delta\Psi_m$ at 24 and 48 hr p.i., respectively. These findings suggest that EV71 infection induces significant drop in electrochemical potential.

EV71-induced ROS generation and reduction in $\Delta\Psi_m$ are associated with defective electron transport

It is likely that increase in ROS generation and reduction in $\Delta\Psi_m$ are causally related to anomalous electron transport. Amperometric method was applied to measure the oxygen consumption rate, which reflects the function of electron transport chain. As shown in Figure 6A, the oxygen consumption rate of SF268 cells increased after EV71 infection. The rate (normalized to cell number) was elevated about 2.3-fold at 48 hr p.i. However, the oligomycin-insensitive oxygen consumption (i.e. oxygen

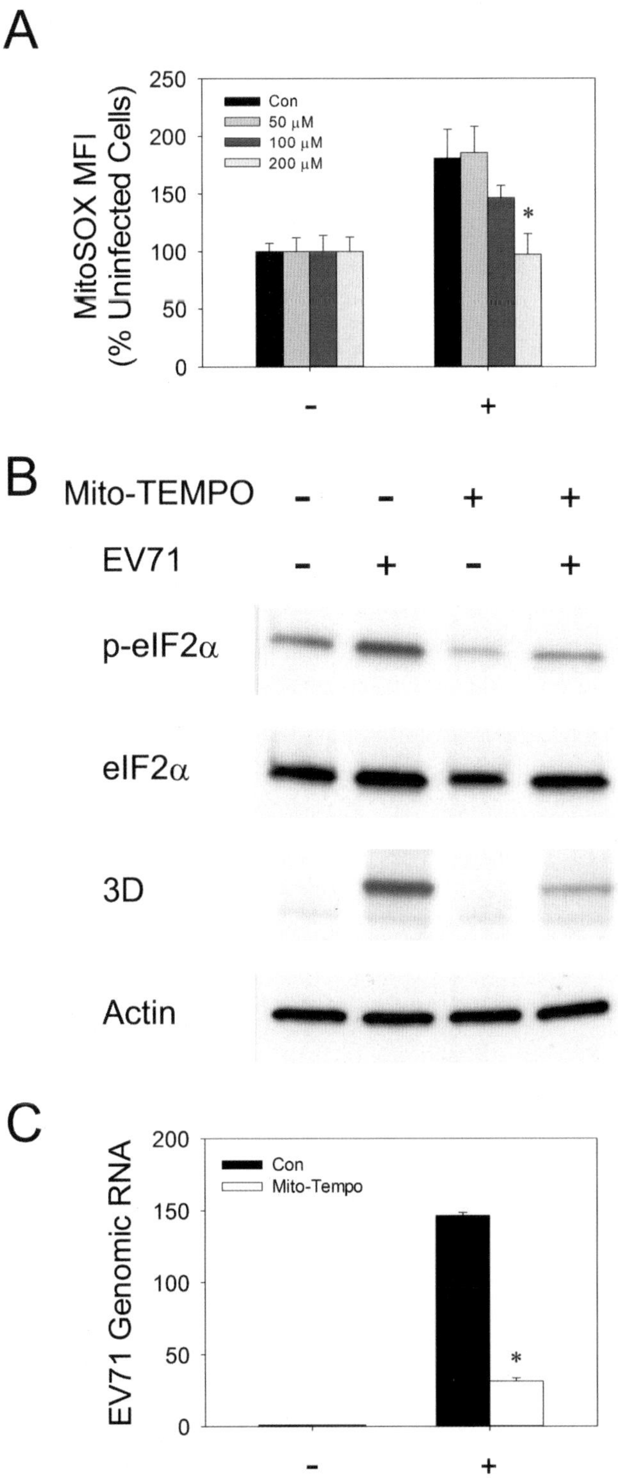

Figure 9. Mitochondrial ROS are essential to EV71 replication. (A) SF268 cells were mock- (−) or infected (+) with EV71 at an m.o.i. of 1.25, and treated without (*Con*) or with indicated concentrations of Mito-TEMPO. Forty-eight hours later, cells were subject to MitoSOX Red staining and flow cytometric analysis. The mean fluorescence intensity (MFI) of MitoSOX of mock- and infected cells is expressed as the percentage of that of uninfected cells. The results are presented as mean ± SD, n = 3. *$p<0.05$ vs. infected Con group. (B) SF268 cells were mock- or infected with EV71 at an m.o.i. of 1.25, and treated without or with 200 μM of Mito-TEMPO. Forty-eight hours later, cells were harvested for western blotting with antibodies to phosphorylated eIF2α and total eIF2α, viral protein 3D, and actin. A representative experiment out of three is shown here. (C) SF268 cells were mock- (−) or infected (+) with EV71 at an m.o.i. of 1.25, and treated without (*Con*) or with 200 μM of Mito-TEMPO. Forty-eight hours later, cells were analyzed for levels of EV71 genomic RNA. The results are presented as means ± SD n = 3. *$p<0.05$ vs. infected Con group.

consumption in the presence of oligomycin), which represents that unrelated to ATP synthesis, accounted for a large percentage of oxygen consumption in infected cells. Oligomycin-insensitive oxygen consumption rate was about 38% of total oxygen consumption in control cells, while it increased about 3.3-fold and was up to 70% of total oxygen consumption in infected cells (Figure 6B). Oligomycin-sensitive oxygen consumption rates (i.e. difference in rates of oxygen consumption measured in the absence and presence of oligomycin, which represents oxygen used for oxidative phosphorylation) of control and infected cells were not significantly different (Figure 6C). A different picture emerged when the oxygen consumption rates were normalized to the relative mitochondrial mass of control and infected cells (Figure 6D–F). The oligomycin-sensitive oxygen consumption rate of infected cells was 42% lower than that of control cells (Figure 6F). Furthermore, we measured state 3 and 4_o respiration of isolated mitochondria from control and EV71-infected cells (Figure 6G–I), and calculated the respective respiratory control ratio (RCR), which is considered an index of electron transport coupling. As shown in Figure 6I, it was 44% lower for mitochondria from infected cells than for those from control cells.

EV71 infection causes an increase in mitochondrial mass and alteration in protein expression

There appears to be a discrepancy between oxygen consumption rates normalized to cell number and mitochondrial mass. It is possible that EV71-infected cells have a compensatory increase in mitochondrial mass. To test such possibility, we stained control and infected cells with mitochondrion-specific dye, and analyzed them cytometrically for quantification of mitochondrial mass. As shown in Figure 7A, mitochondrial mass of EV71-infected cells at 48 hr p.i. was about 50% higher than that of control. It was accompanied by an increased expression of mitochondrial proteins. Figure 7B shows the silver-stained SDS-PAGE of mitochondrial preparations from control and infected cells. Intensities of a number of bands increased in infected cells, which is probably indicative of enhanced expression of mitochondrial proteins. Additionally, some proteins were differentially expressed in control and infected cells. Furthermore, we determined the expression of specific mitochondrial proteins using immunoblotting. Expression of such mitochondrial proteins as NADH dehydrogenase (ubiquinone) 1 β subcomplex 8 (NDUFB8), ubiquinol-cytochrome C reductase core protein I (UQCRC1), ubiquinol-cytochrome C reductase core protein II (UQCRC2), and cytochrome c oxidase II (COX-II) was elevated. Other proteins, for example succinate dehydrogenase complex subunit B iron sulfur protein (SDHB) and cytochrome C (CYC), remained largely unchanged in their expression. These findings suggest that EV71 infection induces mitochondrial proliferation and changes in expression of mitochondrial proteins.

Mitochondrial dysfunction is associated with anomalous metabolism of adenine nucleotides

It is possible that mitochondrial dysfunction affects ATP supply. We measured the levels of ATP, ADP and AMP in control and infected cells. As shown in Figure 8, intracellular level of ATP was reduced by about 60% in infected cells, while those of ADP and

AMP remained largely unchanged. Total adenine nucleotides decreased in infected cells. The energy charge ($\frac{[ATP]+\frac{1}{2}[ADP]}{[ATP]+[ADP]+[AMP]}$) of control and infected cells were 0.94 and 0.87, respectively. These findings suggest that EV71 infection results in lower energy status of infected cells.

Mitochondrial ROS generation is essential to EV71 replication

We have previously shown that ROS are conducive to viral replication. It is possible that mitochondrion-generated ROS act as signal to initiate molecular events associated with EV71 replication. We treated control and uninfected cells with mitochondrion-specific antioxidant mito-TEMPO, and studied its consequences on EV71 infection. To determine the optimal mito-TEMPO concentration for experiments, we treated control and EV71-infected cells with increasing concentrations of mito-TEMPO, and studied its effect on ROS generation. Mito-TEMPO reduced EV71-induced mitochondrial ROS generation in a dose-dependent manner (Figure 9A). At 200 μM, mito-TEMPO completely suppressed mitochondrial ROS production in infected cells. This concentration was used in subsequent experiments. It is known that phosphorylation of eIF2α signifies the initiation of viral protein synthesis during enteroviral infection [44,45]. We treated control and EV71-infected cells with 200 μM mito-TEMPO, and examined the effect of mito-TEMPO on eIF2α phosphorylation. As shown in Figure 9B, the level of eIF2α phosphorylation increased significantly in infected cells. Treatment with mito-TEMPO reduced both basal and EV71-induced eIF2α phosphorylation. It was associated with significant reduction in expression of viral 3D protein and viral replication (Figures 9B & C). At 48 hr p.i., the copy number of viral genome in cells treated with mito-TEMPO was about 80% lower than that of untreated cells (Figure 9C). These findings suggest that mitochondrial ROS are essential to EV71 replication.

Discussion

In the present study, we demonstrate that EV71 induces mitochondrial dysfunction and ROS generation, which acts to promote replication. There appears to be increases in mitochondrial mass, which probably represents a mechanism to compensate for mitochondrial defects.

EV71 induces generation of ROS, which in turn promotes viral replication [16]. The co-localization of fluorescence signals of Mitotracker Red and DCF as well as the increase in fluorescence of MitoSox Red in infected cells suggest that ROS generated in EV71-infected cells are of mitochondrial origin. Previous study has shown that EV71 activates Rac1-dependent NADPH oxidase [46]. The findings that treatment of infected cells with rotenone and antimycin A but not with apocyanin inhibited ROS generation are suggestive of ROS generation through inadvertent reaction between electron passing down electron transport chain and oxygen. Moreover, ROS appear to be generated at a point of electron transport chain downstream of complex III. For instance, cytochrome C can transfer electron directly to $p66^{Shc}$, a redox enzyme, to generate ROS [47]. The heme center of cytochrome C may also act to enhance ROS production [48].

The mechanism for EV71-induced ROS production is currently enigmatic. A number of viral proteins interact with mitochondria or their proteins, and causes mitochondrial dysfunction and ROS generation. For example, hepatitis B virus X protein (HBx) interacts with mitochondrial heat shock protein 60 and 70, and VDAC3 [29,49], and promotes oxidative stress [50]. HCV core protein binds to mitochondria and increases oxidative stress [51–53]. Influenza A virus PB1-F2 protein targets to mitochondria and induces their anomalies [54,55]. Our preliminary results have recently shown that EV71 proteins associate with mitochondria and elicit oxidative stress.

The functional significance of ROS in EV71 remains unclear. It is undisputable that ROS generation has functional consequence on viral infection. Rabies virus can induce oxidative stress in dorsal root ganglion neurons, which diminishes axonal growth [56]. Oxidative stress also promotes S-glutathionylation of cellular proteins, which regulates activities of various cellular proteins [57]. It has been shown that de-glutathionylation of interferon regulatory factor 3 is required for its efficient interaction with CBP and transactivation of interferon genes [58]. Treatment with mito-TEMPO that reduces mitochondrial ROS generation inhibits eIF2α phosphorylation, a hallmark event in EV71 infection. It is probable that ROS play a regulatory role in EV71 infection.

Mitochondria play a prominent role in energy metabolism. Electron transport through respiratory complexes and the resulting proton motive force are critical to oxidative phosphorylation. Virus-induced mitochondrial dysfunction is not specific for EV71 and can be observed for other viruses. In most cases, viral infection induces mitochondrial dysfunction, and reduction in proton motive force and cellular ATP content. Hepatitis C virus (HCV)-infected cells show mitochondrial dysfunction and decrease in $\Delta\Psi_m$ [59]. Infection of mouse neural cells with Sindbis virus causes mitochondrial dysfunction [60]. The lowered mitochondrial respiratory efficiency of EV71-infected cells is consistent with change in cristae. It has been recently shown that cristae shape affects the interaction between respiratory complexes and the respiratory efficiency [61]. Decrease in RCR is accompanied by decrease in $\Delta\Psi_m$. A drop in $\Delta\Psi_m$ causes a deficit in oxidative phosphorylation, which is indicated by decreases in energy charge and ATP/ADP ratio. Moreover, it has been recently shown that dissipation of proton motive force leads to defective MAVS signaling and hence crippled antiviral defense [62,63].

The subcellular distribution of mitochondria in EV71-infected cells changes after infection. After infection, the mitochondria are converted from the interconnecting tubular form to short ovoid form, and are clustered near nuclei. Perinuclear clustering of mitochondria has also been observed for HBV and HCV [64,65]. It is reasoned that re-distribution of mitochondria in infected cells serves the purpose either to meet the energy requirement of viral infection process or to cordon off mitochondria to prevent pro-apoptotic mediators.

Energy is needed for synthesis of viral protein and nucleic acid. Changes in metabolism in host cells have been implicated in viral pathogenesis [66]. The depletion of ATP during EV71 infection is attributed to its direct incorporation into newly synthesized viral genome, or to its involvement in energy-requiring processes. Decrease in RCR has much impact on cellular metabolism. To ensure the continual ATP supply to support viral replication process, the infected cells may put a strain on "shop-worn" but still working mitochondria for energy production, and may activate glycolytic pathway to meet such need. Our preliminary results have recently shown that glycolytic pathway may be enhanced in EV71-infected cells. The decrease in respiratory efficiency of mitochondria, together with the low ATP-generating efficiency of glycolysis, results in reduction in energy charge. Moreover, mitochondria are involved in biosynthesis of such biomolecules as lipids. Picornaviral replication machinery is assembled on membrane, which is probably derived from endoplasmic reticulum [67]. Such process depends on significant alteration of membrane lipids. Alteration of mitochondria during infection may shift the lipid metabolic reactions, such as phosphatidylserine decarboxylation, cytochrome P450-dependent steroid metabolism or acetyl-CoA/citrate metabolism, to fulfill the metabolic need associated with viral replication. It has been recently shown that poliovirus induces long chain acyl-CoA synthetase 3 activity [68], the mitochondrial outer membrane protein that regulates fatty acid import for formation of replication complex. It is envisaged that impaired mitochondria are functionally altered to sustain viral replication.

As mentioned in preceding paragraphs, functional alterations of mitochondria may play vital roles during EV71 infection. Mitochondria undergo adaptive changes to compensate for their reduced respiratory efficiency and diminished functions. A non-exclusive view is that different pools of mitochondria exist [69,70]. Some mitochondria may experience different extent of dysfunctional change. The damaged but still-functional mitochondria may undergo biogenesis and make up for the deficit in mitochondrial functions. The increases in mitochondrial mass may represent such adaptive response. It is not unprecedented that virus induces mitochondrial biogenesis. For instance, human cytomegalovirus infection causes biogenesis of mitochondria [71]. Accumulation of mitochondria in the vicinity of viral assembly factories in African swine fever virus-infected cells is accompanied by *de novo* synthesis of mitochondria mass [72]. Increased mitochondrial mass in EV71-infected cells is accompanied by differential increases in levels of mitochondrial proteins. Mitochondrial proteins, such as COX-II, are specifically elevated. Increase in level of COX-II is consistent with increase in its transcription [73]. Interestingly, levels of mitochondrial proteins are differentially changed during infection. It is speculative whether such differential changes in protein expression contribute to mitochondrial respiratory functions. It has been recently suggested that the respiratory chain complexes are not arranged simply in a linear order of enzymatic complexes. These complexes display different activities toward one another [74]. Subunits of respiratory complexes differ in their correlation between protein expression and enzymatic activity [75]. It is exemplified by the 8 kDa subunit of complex I, for which one-thirds of protein level correlates with 70% of complex I activity. It follows that differential increases in mitochondrial proteins can contribute to maintenance of respiratory functions.

Previous studies have shown that EV71 infection elicits apoptosis in SF268 cells [76]. Conspicuous apoptosis is detected at 72 hr post-infection. However, apoptosis is atypical in the sense that Bid is not cleaved in EV71-infected SF268 cells. tBid, the cleavage product of Bid, is involved in permeabilization of mitochondrial outer membrane [77]. It is currently unknown whether mitochondrial membrane permeabilization is involved in EV71-induced death of SF268 cells. It is likely that mitochondria in these cells differ in some ways from those of infected non-neural cells, which exhibit typical apoptosis. Moreover, our studies focus on the early or mid-phase of infection. It is conceivable that mitochondria can undergo biogenesis in SF268 cells at early or mid-phase of infection, whilst they experience destructive changes during the late phase of infection.

Vesicular structures in picornavirus-infected cells represent the site of replication. These membranous structures are thought to be derived from endoplasmic reticulum (ER). Synthesis of picornaviral protein can activate ER stress response. It has been recently shown that EV71 induces ER stress response and causes eIF2α phosphorylation through activation of PKR and PERK [44]. Phosphorylation of eIF2α suppresses cap-dependent translation, causing a shift in translation to that of internal ribosome-entry site (IRES)-containing cellular mRNA and enteroviral RNA [78]. Interestingly, ROS are implicated in activation of PKR and PERK [79–83], raising the possibility that mitochondrial ROS may play signaling role in the process.

Antioxidants may be used as therapeutic intervention of enteroviral infection. We have previously shown that *N*-acetylcysteine and epigallocatechin gallate can suppress EV71 replication [16,35]. The antiviral activities of epigallocatechin gallate and related compounds correlate with their antioxidative activities. The fact that mito-TEMPO has antiviral effect pinpoints mitochondrial ROS as target for therapeutic intervention.

Taken together, EV71 causes alterations in mitochondria to induce ROS generation. The mitochondrial ROS are essential to viral replication. The "dysfunction" of mitochondria, such as decline in respiratory functions, may represent virus-induced functional alterations, which are optimized for viral replication. Mitochondria may undergo adaptive or compensatory increase in mitochondrial mass to serve such purpose.

Author Contributions

Conceived and designed the experiments: HYH MLC. Performed the experiments: HYH MLC SFW CHK. Analyzed the data: HYH MLC. Contributed reagents/materials/analysis tools: HYH MLC. Contributed to the writing of the manuscript: HYH MLC.

References

1. Racaniello VR (2001) Picornaviridae: the viruses and their replication. In: Fields BN, Knipe DM, Howley PM, Griffin DE, editors. Fields' Virology. Philadelphia: Lippincott Williams & Wilkins. 685–722.
2. Schmidt NJ, Lennette EH, Ho HH (1974) An apparently new enterovirus isolated from patients with disease of the central nervous system. J Infect Dis 129: 304–309.
3. Ho M, Chen ER, Hsu KH, Twu SJ, Chen KT, et al. (1999) An epidemic of enterovirus 71 infection in Taiwan. Taiwan Enterovirus Epidemic Working Group. N Engl J Med 341: 929–935.
4. Yang F, Ren L, Xiong Z, Li J, Xiao Y, et al. (2009) Enterovirus 71 outbreak in the People's Republic of China in 2008. J Clin Microbiol 47: 2351–2352.
5. Yang F, Zhang T, Hu Y, Wang X, Du J, et al. (2011) Survey of enterovirus infections from hand, foot and mouth disease outbreak in China, 2009. Virol J 8: 508.
6. McMinn PC (2002) An overview of the evolution of enterovirus 71 and its clinical and public health significance. FEMS Microbiol Rev 26: 91–107.
7. Ishimaru Y, Nakano S, Yamaoka K, Takami S (1980) Outbreaks of hand, foot, and mouth disease by enterovirus 71. High incidence of complication disorders of central nervous system. Arch Dis Child 55: 583–588.
8. Lin TY, Chang LY, Hsia SH, Huang YC, Chiu CH, et al. (2002) The 1998 enterovirus 71 outbreak in Taiwan: pathogenesis and management. Clin Infect Dis 34 Suppl 2: S52–57.
9. Ooi MH, Wong SC, Lewthwaite P, Cardosa MJ, Solomon T (2010) Clinical features, diagnosis, and management of enterovirus 71. Lancet Neurol 9: 1097–1105.
10. Huang CC, Liu CC, Chang YC, Chen CY, Wang ST, et al. (1999) Neurologic complications in children with enterovirus 71 infection. N Engl J Med 341: 936–942.
11. Beck MA, Handy J, Levander OA (2000) The role of oxidative stress in viral infections. Ann N Y Acad Sci 917: 906–912.
12. Beck MA, Levander OA, Handy J (2003) Selenium deficiency and viral infection. J Nutr 133: 1463S–1467S.
13. Cai J, Chen Y, Seth S, Furukawa S, Compans RW, et al. (2003) Inhibition of influenza infection by glutathione. Free Radic Biol Med 34: 928–936.
14. Beck MA, Shi Q, Morris VC, Levander OA (2005) Benign coxsackievirus damages heart muscle in iron-loaded vitamin E-deficient mice. Free Radic Biol Med 38: 112–116.
15. Aquaro S, Muscoli C, Ranazzi A, Pollicita M, Granato T, et al. (2007) The contribution of peroxynitrite generation in HIV replication in human primary macrophages. Retrovirology 4: 76.
16. Ho HY, Cheng ML, Weng SF, Chang L, Yeh TT, et al. (2008) Glucose-6-phosphate dehydrogenase deficiency enhances enterovirus 71 infection. J Gen Virol 89: 2080–2089.

17. Oda T, Akaike T, Hamamoto T, Suzuki F, Hirano T, et al. (1989) Oxygen radicals in influenza-induced pathogenesis and treatment with pyran polymer-conjugated SOD. Science 244: 974–976.
18. Schachtele SJ, Hu S, Little MR, Lokensgard JR (2010) Herpes simplex virus induces neural oxidative damage via microglial cell Toll-like receptor-2. J Neuroinflammation 7: 35.
19. Kaul P, Biagioli MC, Singh I, Turner RB (2000) Rhinovirus-induced oxidative stress and interleukin-8 elaboration involves p47-phox but is independent of attachment to intercellular adhesion molecule-1 and viral replication. J Infect Dis 181: 1885–1890.
20. Mochizuki H, Todokoro M, Arakawa H (2009) RS virus-induced inflammation and the intracellular glutathione redox state in cultured human airway epithelial cells. Inflammation 32: 252–264.
21. Tal MC, Iwasaki A (2011) Mitoxosome: a mitochondrial platform for cross-talk between cellular stress and antiviral signaling. Immunol Rev 243: 215–234.
22. Ohta A, Nishiyama Y (2011) Mitochondria and viruses. Mitochondrion 11: 1–12.
23. Kuwana T, Newmeyer DD (2003) Bcl-2-family proteins and the role of mitochondria in apoptosis. Curr Opin Cell Biol 15: 691–699.
24. Brunelle JK, Letai A (2009) Control of mitochondrial apoptosis by the Bcl-2 family. J Cell Sci 122: 437–441.
25. Piccoli C, Quarato G, Ripoli M, D'Aprile A, Scrima R, et al. (2009) HCV infection induces mitochondrial bioenergetic unbalance: causes and effects. Biochim Biophys Acta 1787: 539–546.
26. Wang T, Weinman SA (2006) Causes and consequences of mitochondrial reactive oxygen species generation in hepatitis C. J Gastroenterol Hepatol 21 Suppl 3: S34–37.
27. Piccoli C, Scrima R, Quarato G, D'Aprile A, Ripoli M, et al. (2007) Hepatitis C virus protein expression causes calcium-mediated mitochondrial bioenergetic dysfunction and nitro-oxidative stress. Hepatology 46: 58–65.
28. Lecoeur H, Borgne-Sanchez A, Chaloin O, El-Khoury R, Brabant M, et al. (2012) HIV-1 Tat protein directly induces mitochondrial membrane permeabilization and inactivates cytochrome c oxidase. Cell Death Dis 3: e282.
29. Rahmani Z, Huh KW, Lasher R, Siddiqui A (2000) Hepatitis B virus X protein colocalizes to mitochondria with a human voltage-dependent anion channel, HVDAC3, and alters its transmembrane potential. J Virol 74: 2840–2846.
30. Li Q, Wang L, Dong C, Che Y, Jiang L, et al. (2005) The interaction of the SARS coronavirus non-structural protein 10 with the cellular oxido-reductase system causes an extensive cytopathic effect. J Clin Virol 34: 133–139.
31. Lachgar A, Sojic N, Arbault S, Bruce D, Sarasin A, et al. (1999) Amplification of the inflammatory cellular redox state by human immunodeficiency virus type 1-immunosuppressive tat and gp160 proteins. J Virol 73: 1447–1452.
32. Waris G, Huh KW, Siddiqui A (2001) Mitochondrially associated hepatitis B virus X protein constitutively activates transcription factors STAT-3 and NF-kappa B via oxidative stress. Mol Cell Biol 21: 7721–7730.
33. Rutka JT, Giblin JR, Dougherty DY, Liu HC, McCulloch JR, et al. (1987) Establishment and characterization of five cell lines derived from human malignant gliomas. Acta Neuropathol 75: 92–103.
34. Kornblith PL, Szypko PE (1978) Variations in response of human brain tumors to BCNU in vitro. J Neurosurg 48: 580–586.
35. Ho HY, Cheng ML, Weng SF, Leu YL, Chiu DT (2009) Antiviral effect of epigallocatechin gallate on enterovirus 71. J Agric Food Chem 57: 6140–6147.
36. Ho HY, Cheng ML, Chiu HY, Weng SF, Chiu DT (2008) Dehydroepiandrosterone induces growth arrest of hepatoma cells via alteration of mitochondrial gene expression and function. Int J Oncol 33: 969–977.
37. Cheng ML, Shiao MS, Chiu DT, Weng SF, Tang HY, et al. (2011) Biochemical disorders associated with antiproliferative effect of dehydroepiandrosterone in hepatoma cells as revealed by LC-based metabolomics. Biochem Pharmacol 82: 1549–1561.
38. Moran M, Rivera H, Sanchez-Arago M, Blazquez A, Merinero B, et al. (2010) Mitochondrial bioenergetics and dynamics interplay in complex I-deficient fibroblasts. Biochim Biophys Acta 1802: 443–453.
39. Kristian T, Hopkins IB, McKenna MC, Fiskum G (2006) Isolation of mitochondria with high respiratory control from primary cultures of neurons and astrocytes using nitrogen cavitation. J Neurosci Methods 152: 136–143.
40. Schrand AM, Schlager JJ, Dai L, Hussain SM (2010) Preparation of cells for assessing ultrastructural localization of nanoparticles with transmission electron microscopy. Nat Protoc 5: 744–757.
41. Cheng ML, Ho HY, Lin HY, Lai YC, Chiu DT (2013) Effective NET formation in neutrophils from individuals with G6PD Taiwan-Hakka is associated with enhanced NADP(+) biosynthesis. Free Radic Res 47: 699–709.
42. Lin CJ, Ho HY, Cheng ML, You TH, Yu JS, et al. (2010) Impaired dephosphorylation renders G6PD-knockdown HepG2 cells more susceptible to H(2)O(2)-induced apoptosis. Free Radic Biol Med 49: 361–373.
43. Shevchenko A, Wilm M, Vorm O, Mann M (1996) Mass spectrometric sequencing of proteins silver-stained polyacrylamide gels. Anal Chem 68: 850–858.
44. Jheng JR, Lau KS, Tang WF, Wu MS, Horng JT (2010) Endoplasmic reticulum stress is induced and modulated by enterovirus 71. Cell Microbiol 12: 796–813.
45. Hanson PJ, Zhang HM, Hemid MG, Ye X, Qiu Y, et al. (2013) Viral Replication Strategies: Manipulation of ER Stress Response Pathways and Promotion of IRES-Dependent Translation. In: Rosas-Acosta G, editor. Viral Replication. Croatia: Intech. 103–126.
46. Tung WH, Hsieh HL, Lee IT, Yang CM (2011) Enterovirus 71 induces integrin beta1/EGFR-Rac1-dependent oxidative stress in SK-N-SH cells: role of HO-1/CO in viral replication. J Cell Physiol 226: 3316–3329.
47. Giorgio M, Migliaccio E, Orsini F, Paolucci D, Moroni M, et al. (2005) Electron transfer between cytochrome c and p66Shc generates reactive oxygen species that trigger mitochondrial apoptosis. Cell 122: 221–233.
48. Akopova OV, Kolchinskaya LI, Nosar VI, Bouryi VA, Mankovska IN, et al. (2012) Cytochrome C as an amplifier of ROS release in mitochondria. Fiziol Zh 58: 3–12.
49. Zhang SM, Sun DC, Lou S, Bo XC, Lu Z, et al. (2005) HBx protein of hepatitis B virus (HBV) can form complex with mitochondrial HSP60 and HSP70. Arch Virol 150: 1579–1590.
50. Anand SK, Tikoo SK (2013) Viruses as modulators of mitochondrial functions. Adv Virol 2013: 738794.
51. Koike K (2007) Hepatitis C virus contributes to hepatocarcinogenesis by modulating metabolic and intracellular signaling pathways. J Gastroenterol Hepatol 22 Suppl 1: S108–111.
52. Paracha UZ, Fatima K, Alqahtani M, Chaudhary A, Abuzenadah A, et al. (2013) Oxidative stress and hepatitis C virus. Virol J 10: 251.
53. Schwer B, Ren S, Pietschmann T, Kartenbeck J, Kaehlcke K, et al. (2004) Targeting of hepatitis C virus core protein to mitochondria through a novel C-terminal localization motif. J Virol 78: 7958–7968.
54. Gibbs JS, Malide D, Hornung F, Bennink JR, Yewdell JW (2003) The influenza A virus PB1-F2 protein targets the inner mitochondrial membrane via a predicted basic amphipathic helix that disrupts mitochondrial function. J Virol 77: 7214–7224.
55. Yamada H, Chounan R, Higashi Y, Kurihara N, Kido H (2004) Mitochondrial targeting sequence of the influenza A virus PB1-F2 protein and its function in mitochondria. FEBS Lett 578: 331–336.
56. Jackson AC, Kammouni W, Fernyhough P (2011) Role of oxidative stress in rabies virus infection. Adv Virus Res 79: 127–138.
57. Grek CL, Zhang J, Manevich Y, Townsend DM, Tew KD (2013) Causes and consequences of cysteine S-glutathionylation. J Biol Chem 288: 26497–26504.
58. Prinarakis E, Chantzoura E, Thanos D, Spyrou G (2008) S-glutathionylation of IRF3 regulates IRF3-CBP interaction and activation of the IFN beta pathway. EMBO J 27: 865–875.
59. Quarato G, Scrima R, Agriesti F, Moradpour D, Capitanio N, et al. (2013) Targeting mitochondria in the infection strategy of the hepatitis C virus. Int J Biochem Cell Biol 45: 156–166.
60. Silva da Costa L, Pereira da Silva AP, Da Poian AT, El-Bacha T (2012) Mitochondrial bioenergetic alterations in mouse neuroblastoma cells infected with Sindbis virus: implications to viral replication and neuronal death. PLoS One 7: e33871.
61. Cogliati S, Frezza C, Soriano ME, Varanita T, Quintana-Cabrera R, et al. (2013) Mitochondrial cristae shape determines respiratory chain supercomplexes assembly and respiratory efficiency. Cell 155: 160–171.
62. Koshiba T, Yasukawa K, Yanagi Y, Kawabata S (2011) Mitochondrial membrane potential is required for MAVS-mediated antiviral signaling. Sci Signal 4: ra7.
63. Sasaki O, Yoshizumi T, Kuboyama M, Ishihara T, Suzuki E, et al. (2013) A structural perspective of the MAVS-regulatory mechanism on the mitochondrial outer membrane using bioluminescence resonance energy transfer. Biochim Biophys Acta 1833: 1017–1027.
64. Kim S, Kim HY, Lee S, Kim SW, Sohn S, et al. (2007) Hepatitis B virus x protein induces perinuclear mitochondrial clustering in microtubule- and Dynein-dependent manners. J Virol 81: 1714–1726.
65. Nomura-Takigawa Y, Nagano-Fujii M, Deng L, Kitazawa S, Ishido S, et al. (2006) Non-structural protein 4A of Hepatitis C virus accumulates on mitochondria and renders the cells prone to undergoing mitochondria-mediated apoptosis. J Gen Virol 87: 1935–1945.
66. El-Bacha T, Menezes MM, Azevedo e Silva MC, Sola-Penna M, Da Poian AT (2004) Mayaro virus infection alters glucose metabolism in cultured cells through activation of the enzyme 6-phosphofructo 1-kinase. Mol Cell Biochem 266: 191–198.
67. Miller S, Krijnse-Locker J (2008) Modification of intracellular membrane structures for virus replication. Nat Rev Microbiol 6: 363–374.
68. Nchoutmboube JA, Viktorova EG, Scott AJ, Ford LA, Pei Z, et al. (2013) Increased long chain acyl-Coa synthetase activity and fatty acid import is linked to membrane synthesis for development of picornavirus replication organelles. PLoS Pathog 9: e1003401.
69. Parekh AB (2003) Mitochondrial regulation of intracellular Ca2+ signaling: more than just simple Ca2+ buffers. News Physiol Sci 18: 252–256.
70. Hollander JM, Thapa D, Shepherd DL (2014) Physiological and Structural Differences in Spatially-Distinct Subpopulations of Cardiac Mitochondria: Influence of Pathologies. Am J Physiol Heart Circ Physiol.
71. Kaarbo M, Ager-Wick E, Osenbroch PO, Kilander A, Skinnes R, et al. (2011) Human cytomegalovirus infection increases mitochondrial biogenesis. Mitochondrion 11: 935–945.
72. Rojo G, Chamorro M, Salas ML, Vinuela E, Cuezva JM, et al. (1998) Migration of mitochondria to viral assembly sites in African swine fever virus-infected cells. J Virol 72: 7583–7588.
73. Shih SR, Stollar V, Lin JY, Chang SC, Chen GW, et al. (2004) Identification of genes involved in the host response to enterovirus 71 infection. J Neurovirol 10: 293–304.

74. Claus C, Schonefeld K, Hubner D, Chey S, Reibetanz U, et al. (2013) Activity increase in respiratory chain complexes by rubella virus with marginal induction of oxidative stress. J Virol 87: 8481–8492.
75. Rossignol R, Faustin B, Rocher C, Malgat M, Mazat JP, et al. (2003) Mitochondrial threshold effects. Biochem J 370: 751–762.
76. Chang SC, Lin JY, Lo LY, Li ML, Shih SR (2004) Diverse apoptotic pathways in enterovirus 71-infected cells. J Neurovirol 10: 338–349.
77. Korytowski W, Basova LV, Pilat A, Kernstock RM, Girotti AW (2011) Permeabilization of the mitochondrial outer membrane by Bax/truncated Bid (tBid) proteins as sensitized by cardiolipin hydroperoxide translocation: mechanistic implications for the intrinsic pathway of oxidative apoptosis. J Biol Chem 286: 26334–26343.
78. Harding HP, Calfon M, Urano F, Novoa I, Ron D (2002) Transcriptional and translational control in the Mammalian unfolded protein response. Annu Rev Cell Dev Biol 18: 575–599.
79. Liu ZW, Zhu HT, Chen KL, Dong X, Wei J, et al. (2013) Protein kinase RNA-like endoplasmic reticulum kinase (PERK) signaling pathway plays a major role in reactive oxygen species (ROS)-mediated endoplasmic reticulum stress-induced apoptosis in diabetic cardiomyopathy. Cardiovasc Diabetol 12: 158.
80. Verfaillie T, Rubio N, Garg AD, Bultynck G, Rizzuto R, et al. (2012) PERK is required at the ER-mitochondrial contact sites to convey apoptosis after ROS-based ER stress. Cell Death Differ 19: 1880–1891.
81. Joshi M, Kulkarni A, Pal JK (2013) Small molecule modulators of eukaryotic initiation factor 2alpha kinases, the key regulators of protein synthesis. Biochimie 95: 1980–1990.
82. Donnelly N, Gorman AM, Gupta S, Samali A (2013) The eIF2alpha kinases: their structures and functions. Cell Mol Life Sci 70: 3493–3511.
83. Ito T, Yang M, May WS (1999) RAX, a cellular activator for double-stranded RNA-dependent protein kinase during stress signaling. J Biol Chem 274: 15427–15432.

Bacterial Load of Pneumococcal Serotypes Correlates with Their Prevalence and Multiple Serotypes is Associated with Acute Respiratory Infections among Children Less Than 5 Years of Age

Bhim Gopal Dhoubhadel[1,5], Michio Yasunami[1], Hien Anh Thi Nguyen[2], Motoi Suzuki[1], Thu Huong Vu[2], Ai Thi Thuy Nguyen[3], Duc Anh Dang[2], Lay-Myint Yoshida[4]*, Koya Ariyoshi[1,5]

1 Department of Clinical Medicine, Institute of Tropical Medicine, Nagasaki University, Nagasaki, Japan, **2** Department of Bacteriology, National Institute of Hygiene and Epidemiology, Hanoi, Vietnam, **3** Department of Microbiology, Khanh Hoa General Hospital, NhaTrang, Vietnam, **4** Department of Pediatric Infectious Diseases, Institute of Tropical Medicine, Nagasaki University, Nagasaki, Japan, **5** Graduate School of Biomedical Sciences, Nagasaki University, Nagasaki, Japan

Abstract

Background: Among pneumococcal serotypes, some serotypes are more prevalent in the nasopharynx than others; determining factors for higher prevalence remain to be fully explored. As non-vaccine serotypes have emerged after the introduction of 7-valent conjugate vaccines, study of serotype specific epidemiology is in need. When two or more serotypes co-colonize, they evolve rapidly to defend host's immune responses; however, a clear association of co-colonization with a clinical outcome is lacking.

Methods: Children less than 5 years old who were admitted to hospital due to acute respiratory infections (ARI) (n = 595) and healthy children (n = 350) were recruited. Carriage of pneumococcus was determined by culture and lytA PCR in the nasopharyngeal samples. Serotype/serogroup detection and its quantification were done by the nanofluidic real time PCR system. Spearman's correlation and logistic regression were used to examine a correlation of serotype/serogroup specific bacterial load with its prevalence and an association of co-colonization with ARI respectively.

Results: Serotype/serogroup specific bacterial load was correlated with its prevalence, both in ARI cases (Spearman's rho = 0.44, n = 186; $P<0.0001$) and healthy children (Spearman's rho = 0.41, n = 115; $P<0.0001$). The prevalence of multiple serotypes was more common in ARI cases than in healthy children (18.5% vs 7.1%; aOR 2.92, 95% CI: 1.27–6.71; P = 0.01). The dominant serotype in the co-colonization had a 2 log10 higher bacterial load than the subdominant serotype, both in ARI cases ($P<0.001$) and healthy children ($P<0.05$).

Conclusions: High bacterial load in the nasopharynx may help transmit pneumococci among hosts, and increase the chance of successful acquisition and colonization. Co-colonization of multiple serotypes of pneumococci is linked with ARI, which infers the interactions of multiple serotypes may increase their pathogenicity; however, they may compete for growth in number.

Editor: Cristina Costa, University Hospital San Giovanni Battista di Torino, Italy

Funding: BGD received scholarship from the Government of Japan, Ministry of Education, Culture, Sports, Science, and Technology for Monbukagakusho (MEXT) scholarship. The study was funded by Japan Initiative for Global Research Network on Infectious Diseases (J-GRID) and Japan Science and Technology, Japan. The funders had no role in study design, data collection and analysis, decision to publish, or preparation of the manuscript.

Competing Interests: The authors have declared that no competing interests exist.

* Email: lmyoshi@nagasaki-u.ac.jp

Introduction

Streptococcus pneumoniae (pneumococcus) is a major cause of life threatening diseases including pneumonia, sepsis and meningitis in children worldwide [1]. Pneumococcus has distinct polysaccharide capsule which characterizes its more than 90 serotypes. It colonizes in the nasopharynx, which is the precursor for pneumococcal diseases and the source for transmission among people [2]. The emergence of non-vaccine serotypes (19A, 35B) after the introduction of 7-valent pneumococcal conjugate vaccine (PCV7) has become a concern for future epidemiology of pneumococcal diseases, and it highlights the need of serotype specific study of this common pathogen [3,4].

The prevalence of a serotype in the nasopharynx is inversely correlated with the invasiveness of the serotype [5]. Less invasive serotypes such as 6A, 6B, 19F, 23F tend to colonize more frequently and maintain the carriage for longer time; while the more invasive serotypes such as 1, 4, 5, 7F tend to colonize less frequently and maintain colonization for less duration [6,7]. The pneumococcal capsule, which is a major virulent factor, determines the serotype. It is found the thickness of the capsule positively correlates with the prevalence of the serotype/serogroup [8]. Furthermore, the capacity to grow of a serotype is correlated with its prevalence in an in vitro study [9]; however, it is unknown whether similar relationship exists in the natural niche in humans.

Co-colonization of multiple pneumococcal serotypes in the nasopharynx affects vaccine serotype replacement, carriage detection and pneumonia diagnosis [10]. Accurate determination of co-colonization and its role in pathogenesis are difficult to establish by using conventional serotyping method because of its low sensitivity and tedious laboratory work; therefore, a highly sensitive and specific molecular method is in need to detect multiple serotypes accurately and efficiently [11,12]. Although varied prevalence rates of co-colonization have been reported from different parts of the world [11–15], an epidemiological evidence of their association with a clinical outcome is lacking. Some epidemiological models have demonstrated that the serotypes compete among themselves for acquisition and persistence of colonization in the nasopharynx [16,17]; however, it is yet to be demonstrated quantitatively in humans.

In this study, we applied a highly sensitive and specific novel nanofluidic real time PCR system to identify serotypes/serogroups and quantify their bacterial load in nasopharyngeal samples of hospitalized acute respiratory infections (ARI) cases and healthy children. We aimed to assess the correlation of bacterial load of specific serotypes/serogroups with the prevalence and compare the prevalence of co-colonization of multiple serotypes between these two groups of children.

Methods

Study design

Acute respiratory infections (ARI) cases, as defined by World Health Organization (WHO), were recruited in the Department of Pediatrics, Khanh Hoa General Hospital, Nha Trang City, Vietnam from 07/04/2008 to 31/03/2009. The hospital has 750 beds, and is the only hospital that provides inpatient care for sick children in Nha Trang City. The participants were children under 5 years old from the study area, who were admitted to the pediatric ward during the study period with acute respiratory infections (ARI) defined by cough and/or difficulty in breathing (WHO). We also included healthy children to compare bacterial load and serotype distribution with ARI cases. Healthy children, who did not have fever, signs of respiratory infections or history of antibiotic intake in the month preceding the day of enrollment, were recruited from two communes in the study area. They were selected randomly during January 2008 from the under 5 years old children using the census data. Informed written consent was taken from the parents of the hospital admitted ARI cases and the healthy children. Details of the study site were described elsewhere [18].

Sample collection, storage and DNA extraction

A nasopharyngeal sample (NPS), (about 100 microliter in volume) was collected flexible dacron-tipped aluminum-shafted swabs (Copan, Brescia, Italy) from each participant according to the WHO protocol [19]. The samples were taken from ARI cases at the time of admission before they were treated with antibiotics. The samples were divided into two aliquots. One aliquot was sub-cultured onto 5% sheep blood agar and incubated overnight with 5% CO_2 at 37°C. Alpha hemolytic colonies with morphology suggestive of *S. pneumoniae* and positive Optochin test were considered potential *S. pneumoniae* isolates. The other aliquot was stored at −80°C. At a later stage DNA was extracted, following the protocol of QIAGEN kit for the Gram-positive bacteria, directly from the nasopharyngeal samples of the children from whom potential *S. pneumoniae* had been cultured. DNA was stored at -80°C, except for transportation to Nagasaki on dry ice, till used for the lytA PCR and the nanofluidic real time PCR system.

Identification of pneumococcus, its serotypes, quantification of bacterial load and definition of co-colonization of multiple serotypes

The DNA extract of the NPS from children with a potential *S. pneumoniae* culture positive isolate was analyzed by a lytA PCR that targeted the autolysin gene using the Light cycler II (Roche). Carriage of pneumococcus is defined as having positive lytA PCR NPS. The lytA positive samples were subjected to the nanofluidic real time PCR system for molecular serotyping. The nanofluidic real time PCR system can identify 50 serotypes in 29 groups, and it can detect minor population of multiple serotypes in co-colonization of pneumococci with the minimum level of detection of 30 to 300 copies. Total and specific serotype/serogroup bacterial loads were quantified using the standard curves. Details of the nanofluidic real time PCR system has been described elsewhere [20]. Samples positive for lytA and negative for all serotype/serogroup primer-pairs were grouped as non-typeable (NT). Co-colonization with multiple serotypes was defined as the presence of two or more serotypes/serogroups in a sample. In co-colonization the first serotype and second serotype were defined according to their bacterial loads; a serotype with the highest load was assigned as first serotype, with the second highest load as second serotype.

Statistical analysis

The data of pneumococcal loads, DNA copies, were changed into log10 scale. To compare the groups, Wilcoxon rank sum test was used for the continuous variables and Chi-square or Fisher exact test was used for categorical variables. Logistic regression was used to test the effects of pneumococcal load and co-colonization as risk factors for hospitalized children due to ARI. Odds ratios were adjusted for age, sex and daycare attendance. To test the correlation of bacterial load and prevalence of individual serotypes, Spearman's correlation was used. Analyses were performed using Stata v12.1 (StataCorp, College Station, Taxes, USA). The database for the analysis was submitted as (Table S1, S2).

Ethical approval

This study was approved by all the concerned research review boards: Nagasaki University Institutional Review Board Nagasaki, Japan; the National Institute of Hygiene and Epidemiology Scientific Review Committee, Hanoi and the Khanh Hoa Provincial Health Service Ethical Review Board, Nha Trang, Vietnam.

Results

Basic characteristics of ARI cases and healthy children

Among the hospital admitted ARI cases, 88.6% (527/595) were children less than 2 years old, proportion of male was 62% (369/595), and the median age was 10 months. Almost half, 45.5% of

ARI cases had history of antibiotic use before admission. The proportion of chest X-ray confirmed pneumonia among them was 22.8% (136/595). Among healthy children, 55.4% (194/350) were under 2 years of old, proportion of male was 52.6% (184/350), and the median age was 19 months.

Pneumococcal colonization and serotype distribution

Pneumococcal carriage rate was 32.6% (194/595) in ARI cases and 40% (140/350) in healthy children (figure 1). The proportion of typeable serotypes in ARI cases and healthy children were 95.9% (186/194) and 82.1% (115/140) respectively. Thirteen serotypes/serogroups of pneumococcus were detected in ARI cases and healthy children (figure 2). Serotypes/serogroups 19F, 6A/6B, 23F and 6C/6D were more prevalent in hospitalized ARI cases while serotypes/serogroups 14, 6A/6B, 19F, 15B/15C, 11 and non-typeables (NT) were common in healthy children. The proportion of serotypes/serogroups covered by pneumococcal conjugate vaccines: 7-valent (PCV7), 10-valent (PCV10) and 13-valent (PCV13) were approximately equal to one another, which was about 74% in ARI cases and 55% in healthy children (this was an approximate estimation as a serogroup was treated as a serotype as required).

Pneumococcal bacterial load

Higher bacterial load was associated with hospitalization due to ARI. The median bacterial load (total) was 6.61 log10/ml in ARI cases and 4.36 log10/ml in healthy children (OR = 9.96, 95%CI: 6.39–15.52; P<0.0001 and aOR = 9.07, 95%CI: 5.69–14.4; P< 0.0001). There was no difference in median bacterial load between males and females both in ARI cases (6.62 log10 in male Vs. 6.59 log10 in female; p-value: 0.76) and healthy children (4.36 log10 in male Vs. 4.32 log10 in female; p-value: 0.86). Bacterial loads of specific serotypes/serogroups were higher in ARI cases than healthy children in all detected serotypes (Figure 3). Serotypes 14, 19F, 23F, 6A/6B had higher median bacterial load than other serotypes in ARI cases while serotypes 14, 19F, 23A, 23F had higher load in healthy children. The bacterial load of serotype 6C/6D was found to be lower than other common serotypes in ARI cases.

Serotype/serogroup specific bacterial load was significantly higher in vaccine serotypes. When we compared the bacterial load of vaccine specific serotypes and non-vaccine serotypes, the load was higher in vaccine serotypes both in ARI cases: 6.61 log10 in vaccine serotypes and 5.51 log10 in non-vaccine serotypes (P< 0.0001), and in healthy children: 4.68 log10 in vaccine serotypes and 3.81 log10 in non-vaccine serotypes (P = 0.0001).

Correlation between bacterial load of serotypes and their prevalence

Serotype/serogroup specific bacterial load was positively correlated with serotype/serogroup prevalence. Serotype/serogroup specific bacterial load of individual NPS samples from ARI cases and healthy children were plotted against the prevalence of individual serotype/serogroup (i.e., proportion of the serotypes/serogroups in carriage positive samples). We found that the serotype/serogroup specific bacterial load had positive correlation with its prevalence, both in ARI cases (Spearman's rho = 0.44, n = 186, P<0.0001) and healthy children (Spearman's rho = 0.41, n = 115, P<0.0001) (Figure 4).

Co-colonization with multiple serotypes

Co-colonization of multiple serotypes of pneumococci was associated with ARI. Co-colonization of multiple-serotypes was detected in 18.5% (n = 36/194) in ARI cases and 7.1% (n = 10/140) in healthy children (OR 2.96, 95%CI 1.41–6.19; P = 0.004). When adjusted for age, sex and daycare, the adjusted odds ratio (aOR) was 2.92 (95%CI 1.27–6.71; P = 0.012). Co-colonization of serotypes 19F and 11, 19F and 15B/15C, 23F and 6A/6B

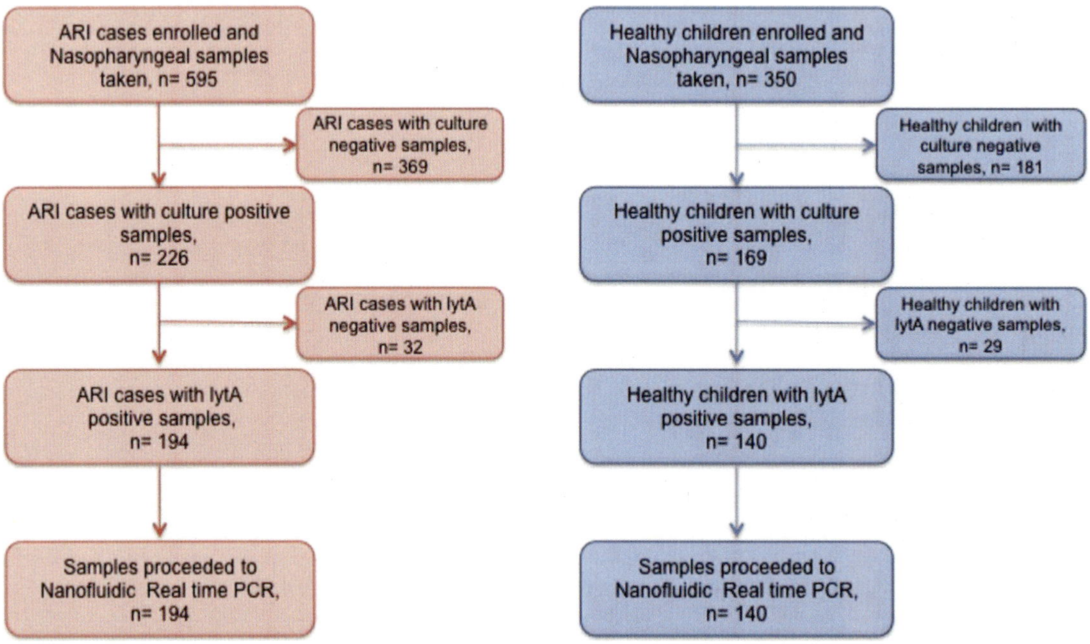

Figure 1. Participants recruited into the study, and their nasopharyngeal samples. Half of the aliquot of nasopharyngeal samples were cultured overnight in 5% sheep blood agar with 5% CO_2 at 37°C. DNA was extracted directly from the other half of the aliquot of the nasopharyngeal samples which yielded alpha hemolytic colonies and positive Optochin test. DNA was subjected to lytA PCR to confirm pneumococcus; and lytA positive samples were then processed for molecular serotyping in the nanofluidic real time PCR system.

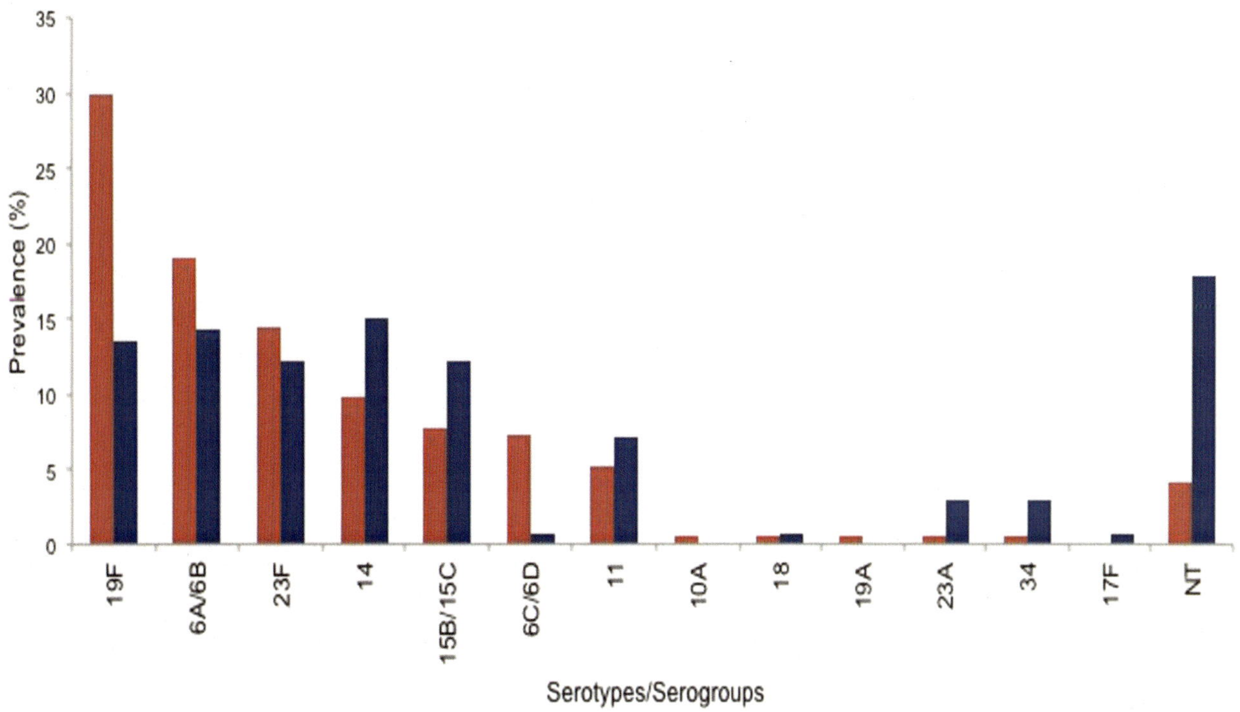

Figure 2. Distribution of serotypes/serogroups of pneumococcus in ARI cases and healthy children. Thirteen different serotypes/serogroups were detected; DNA samples which were positive for lytA (pneumococcus positive), but negative for tested 29 serotypes/serogroups were assigned as non-typeable (NT). Prevalence of each serotype/serogroup was calculated as proportion of total number of a serotype/serogroup to the total number of the lytA positive samples. Serotype/serogroup of ARI cases and healthy children were plotted in red and blue respectively. Proportion of serotype/serogroup covered by 13-valent conjugated vaccine (PCV13) was 74% in ARI cases and 55% in healthy children.

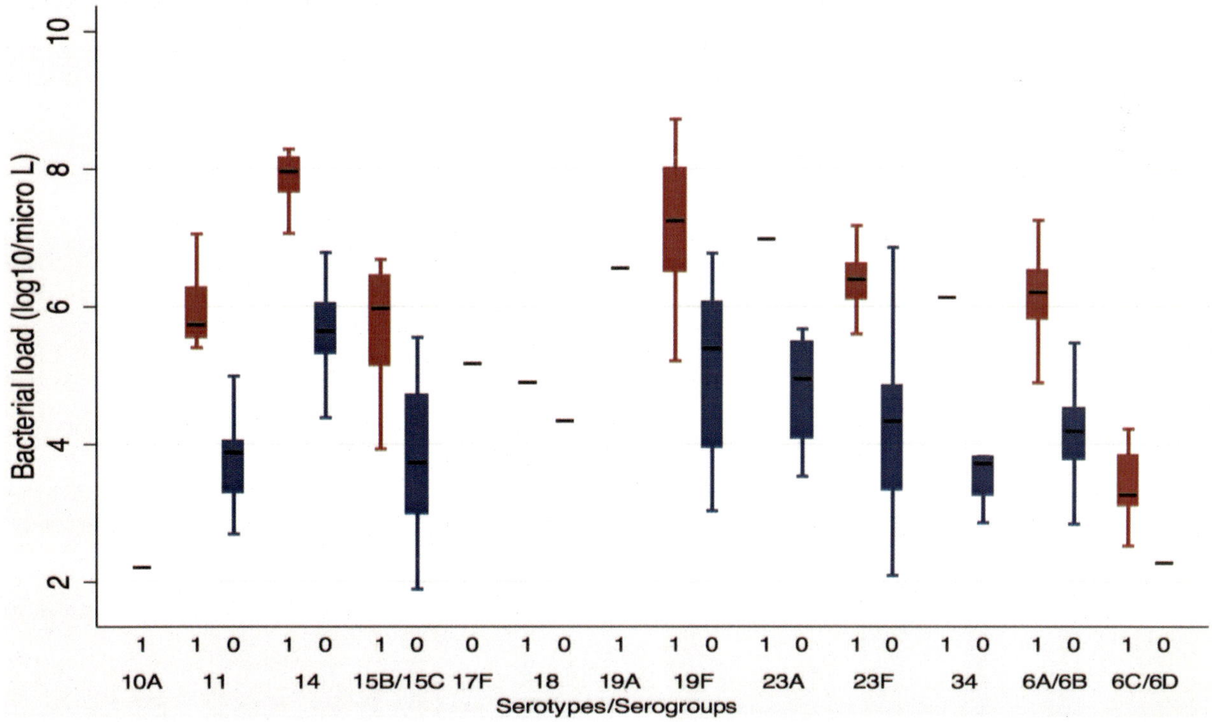

Figure 3. Bacterial load of specific serotypes/serogroups of pneumococcus in ARI cases and healthy children. Bacterial load of ARI cases (denoted by "1" in each serotype/serogroup) in red and healthy children (denoted by "0" in each serotype/serogroup) in blue, showed that the common serotypes 19F, 14, 23F, 6A/6B, 15B/15C had high bacterial load.

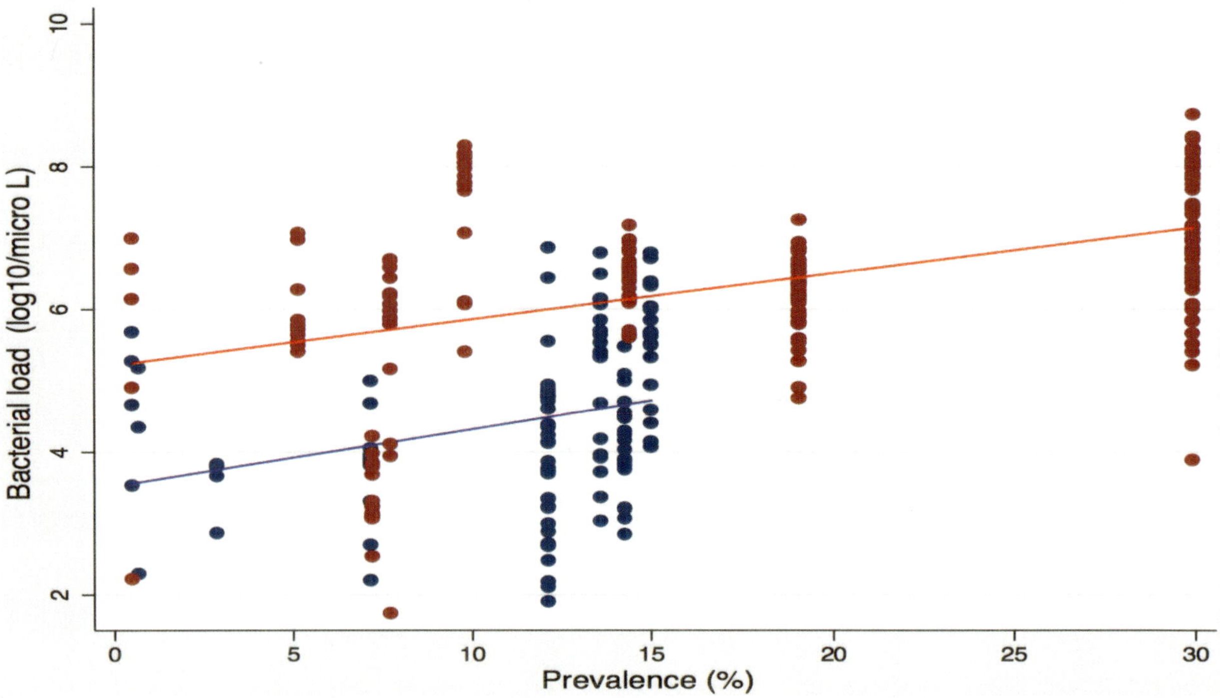

Figure 4. Relationship between bacterial load of specific serotypes/serogroups and their prevalence. Bacterial load of each of specific serotypes/serogroups was plotted against its prevalence. Both in ARI cases (red) and in healthy children (blue), a positive correlation was found. Each dot represents an ARI case or a healthy child in the plot, and the red and blue lines are the fitted values for ARI cases and healthy children respectively. Spearman's rho was 0.44 (n = 186; P<0.0001) and 0.41 (n = 115; P<0.0001) for ARI cases and healthy children respectively.

occurred more frequently in ARI cases. We observed none of the serotypes involved in co-colonization were 19A or 35B (Figure 5). Co-colonization of pneumococcus occurred in 18.56% (18/97) of ARI cases when pre-hospital antibiotics had been used and 38.71% (12/31) when no antibiotics were used (P = 0.002) [Unknown antibiotic status in 9.09% (6/66) of ARI cases]. The prevalence of co-colonization was found to be higher 32.5% (13/40) in age group of less than 6 months of age than 14.94% (23/154) in age group of 6 or more than 6 months of age in ARI cases (P = 0.01). But, we did not find any such difference in healthy children among these age groups, 0% (0/16) versus 7.04% (10/124) (P = 0.60).

One serotype/serogroup dominated the other serotype/serogroups in co-colonization. In co-colonization, the serotype/serogroup specific bacterial load was 2.45 log10 higher in the dominant serotypes than the subdominant serotypes in ARI cases, while it was 2.04 log10 higher in healthy children (Figure 6). The dominant serotype was a vaccine serotype in 100% (10/10) of co-colonization in healthy children (P = 0.003); while it was vaccine serotypes only in 72.22% (26/36) of co-colonization in ARI cases (P = 0.76). The median total bacterial load was higher, 4.81 log10 versus 4.31 log10 (P = 0.03), when co-colonization of multiple serotypes was present as compared to single serotype colonization in healthy children; however, no significant difference was found among them in ARI cases (6.65 log10 versus 6.58 log10, P = 0.59).

Discussion

Our data suggest two major findings. First, a positive correlation of serotype/serogroup specific bacterial load with prevalence of serotypes/serogroups, which may help to understand why some serotypes of pneumococcus are successful for colonization and maintenance of the carriage for longer time. The second finding, an association of co-colonization of multiple serotypes with acute respiratory infections in children may infer a role of multiple serotypes of pneumococci in pathogenesis of ARI in children. Both of these findings are novel in pneumococcal pathogenesis and epidemiology in humans.

It is known that the prevalence of serotypes is inversely correlated with their serotype specific invasiveness [5]. It is found that some serotypes/serogroups: 1, 4, 5, 7F are more invasive but less prevalent in the nasopharynx than other serotypes/serogroups: 6A, 6B, 19F, 23F, which are more prevalent but less invasive [5]. Contributing factors for this inverse relationship of prevalence and invasiveness remains to be fully explained. It is found that colonizing serotypes: 19F, 6A, 6B, 23F have higher serotype specific rates of acquisition of colonization and longer duration of carriage than invasive serotypes: 1, 4, 5, 7F in children [6,7]. This shows that the colonizing serotypes are more capable to colonize and maintain the carriage than invasive serotypes. In this regard, our finding of positive correlation of serotype/serogroup specific bacterial load with prevalence of serotype/serogroup may explain that the higher numbers of bacteria in the nasopharynx may help them to transmit from one host to other, so that they have higher chance of colonization, and their ability to grow in number may help to maintain the carriage for longer time against the normal mucosal clearance of the host.

Some in vitro studies show that serotype specific growth of pneumococcus is positively correlated with prevalence of the serotype [8,9]. Hathaway et al found that high carriage prevalence serotypes (6B, 9V, 19F, 23F) can produce their capsules that are less metabolically demanding, and they can grow even in nutritionally poor environment [9]. These in vitro findings match with our in vivo findings of high bacterial load of common

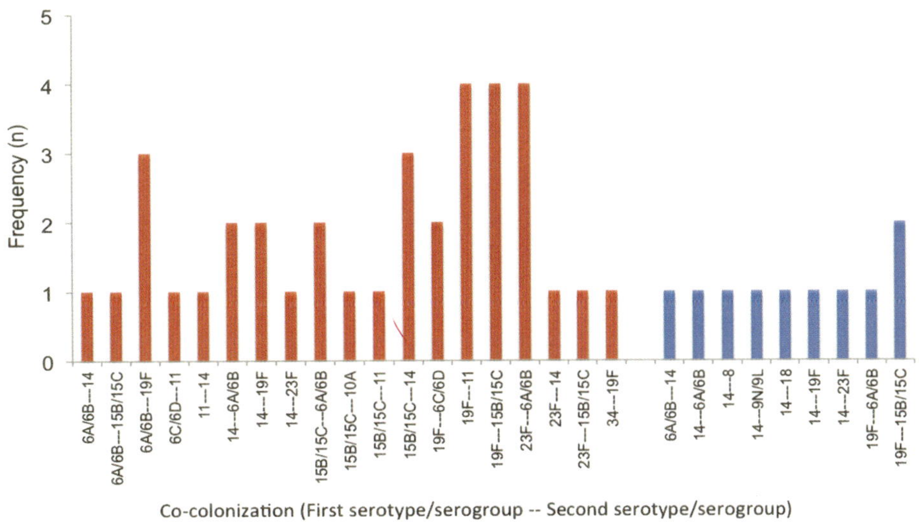

Figure 5. Distribution of co-colonization of multiple serotypes of pneumococcus. In ARI cases (red) co-colonization was detected in 36 samples out of 194 lytA positive samples (18.5%), while in healthy children (blue) it was detected in 10 samples out of 140 (7.1%) lytA positive samples. The odds ratio, adjusted for age, sex and daycare, was 2.92 (95%CI 1.27–6.71; P = 0.012). The serotypes/serogroups were positioned first and second according to their bacterial load.

serotypes/serogroups and their correlation with prevalence. Less prevalent but more invasive serotypes are characterized by poor growth, longer lag phase in bacterial growth [21], thinner capsule size and more prone to be killed by neutrophils than high prevalence serotypes [8].

We found the occurrence of co-colonization with multiple serotypes of pneumococcus was twice as common in hospitalized ARI cases as in healthy children. This is the first time to our knowledge that such an association of co-colonization of multiple serotypes of pneumococci with ARI is reported. Although prevalence of co-colonization has been reported to occur from 1.3% to 39% in children by using different methods in various settings [11–15], none has reported an association with a clinical outcome. Non-vaccine serotypes such as 19A and 35B, which have emerged after the introduction of PCV7 vaccine [3,4], were not detected in co-colonization both in ARI cases and healthy children in our study. Although the number of children with co-colonization was relatively small, our data discourage the

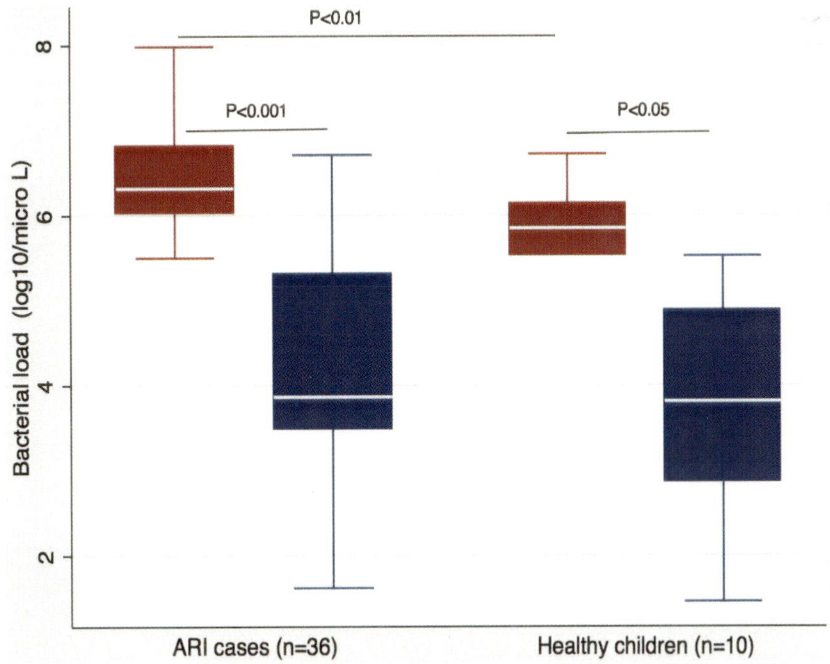

Figure 6. Dominance of one serotype/serogroup over the other in co-colonization of multiple serotypes/serogroups. Among two serotypes/serogroups present in a co-colonization, one serotype/serogroup (red) was found to be dominant by having 100 folds (2 log10) higher bacterial load than the other subdominant (blue) serotype/serogroup both in ARI cases and healthy children.

"unmasking phenomena" for emergence of non-vaccine serotypes [22]. The potential role of co-colonization in the emergence of 19A due to serotype replacement is partly explained by capsule switching phenomenon at the capsular locus by recombination [23,24]. As pneumococcus is highly recombinogenic and transformable bacteria, probability is high for genetic exchange when two or more pneumococcal serotypes inhabit at the same time in the nasopharynx [10]. This is true for evolution of not only vaccine-escape serotypes but also for the antibiotic resistant serotypes [24]. When multiple serotypes co-colonize, the genetic reservoir expands so called "Supragenome" will advance the microevolution of the pathogen and allow continued survival by evasion of serotype-specific immune response and adaptation by genetic change, which is demonstrated by the co-colonization of penicillin sensitive and penicillin resistance pneumococci at the same time [25]. Besides, it is found that in mouse model, pneumococci form a biofilm in the nasopharynx when multiple strains are present. The transformation efficiency becomes very high in the biofilm with multiple serotypes, so that the antibiotic resistance can easily be spread among the serotypes. Hence, co-colonization of multiple serotypes confers the development of supra-virulence and fitness in the pathogen for survival in the harsh environment of host [26].

We have further demonstrated the dominance of one serotype over the other in bacterial load when co-colonization is present. This difference in pneumococcal load among serotypes/serogroups in a co-colonization may suggest that there may be a competition among the serotypes for their growth due to limited nutrients and space. In mouse model, intra-species competition among pneumococci is demonstrated and found mediated by bacteriocin [27,28]. Epidemiological models also suggest the existence of competition among serotypes for initiation and persistence of colonization in children [16,17]. A study with mathematical modeling shows that direct (physical) competition and indirect (antibody mediated) competition do exit among the serotypes of pneumococcus in co-colonization [29]. We considered the 100 fold higher bacterial load, which we found in the dominant serotype, is due to direct competition as naturally acquired immune response due to colonization lasts for a short duration in unvaccinated young children. This is consistent with the finding of the mathematical modeling [29].

This study has limitations. Due to logistic problems, we were unable to bring all nasopharyngeal samples to Nagasaki from Vietnam for DNA extraction and nanofluidic real time PCR. First, we screened all the samples by culture, and only samples that grew alpha hemolytic colonies and Optochin sensitive isolates were brought to Nagasaki for molecular assays. It may have decreased the overall sensitivity of detection of pneumococcus and carriage rate. Minimum level of detection of the nanofluidic real time PCR was 30-300 copies per reaction; other limitations of the nanofluidic real time PCR have been described elsewhere [20].

Conclusions

This study shows a positive correlation of serotype/serogroup specific bacterial load with serotype/serogroup prevalence of pneumococcus in children. Higher bacterial load of a serotype in the nasopharynx may be an attributing factor for higher transmission of the serotype. The association of multiple serotypes of pneumococcus with ARI shows its link with increased pathogenicity, and dominance of one serotype over the other may infer the competition among serotypes when multiple serotypes are present in the nasopharynx.

Supporting Information

Table S1 Database of ARI and healthy children.

Table S2 Data dictionary file of database of ARI and healthy children.

Acknowledgments

We are grateful to children and their parents who participated in this study. We would like to thank the staffs from Khanh Hoa Health Service and the medical staff in Khanh Hoa General Hospital who helped to carry out this research. BGD is grateful to the Government of Japan, Ministry of Education, Culture, Sports, Science, and Technology for Monbukagakusho (MEXT) scholarship.

Author Contributions

Conceived and designed the experiments: LMY KA MY MS DAD. Performed the experiments: BGD MY HAN THV ATTN LMY. Analyzed the data: BGD MS KA MY LMY. Contributed reagents/materials/analysis tools: BGD HAN ATTN THV MS KA MY LMY. Wrote the paper: BGD KA MS LMY MY HAN THV ATTN DAD.

References

1. O'Brien KL, Wolfson LJ, Watt JP, Henkle E, Deloria-Knoll M, et al. (2009) Burden of disease caused by Streptococcus pneumoniae in children younger than 5 years: global estimates. Lancet 374: 893–902.
2. Simell B, Auranen K, Kayhty H, Goldblatt D, Dagan R, et al. (2012) The fundamental link between pneumococcal carriage and disease. Expert Rev Vaccines 11: 841–855.
3. Weinberger DM, Malley R, Lipsitch M (2011) Serotype replacement in disease after pneumococcal vaccination. Lancet 378: 1962–1973.
4. Huang SS, Hinrichsen VL, Stevenson AE, Rifas-Shiman SL, Kleinman K, et al. (2009) Continued impact of pneumococcal conjugate vaccine on carriage in young children. Pediatrics 124: e1–11.
5. Brueggemann AB, Peto TE, Crook DW, Butler JC, Kristinsson KG, et al. (2004) Temporal and geographic stability of the serogroup-specific invasive disease potential of Streptococcus pneumoniae in children. J Infect Dis 190: 1203–1211.
6. Abdullahi O, Karani A, Tigoi CC, Mugo D, Kungu S, et al. (2012) Rates of acquisition and clearance of pneumococcal serotypes in the nasopharynges of children in Kilifi District, Kenya. J Infect Dis 206: 1020–1029.
7. Tigoi CC, Gatakaa H, Karani A, Mugo D, Kungu S, et al. (2012) Rates of acquisition of pneumococcal colonization and transmission probabilities, by serotype, among newborn infants in Kilifi District, Kenya. Clin Infect Dis 55: 180–188.
8. Weinberger DM, Trzcinski K, Lu YJ, Bogaert D, Brandes A, et al. (2009) Pneumococcal capsular polysaccharide structure predicts serotype prevalence. PLoS Pathog 5: e1000476.
9. Hathaway LJ, Brugger SD, Morand B, Bangert M, Rotzetter JU, et al. (2012) Capsule type of Streptococcus pneumoniae determines growth phenotype. PLoS Pathog 8: e1002574.
10. Shak JR, Vidal JE, Klugman KP (2013) Influence of bacterial interactions on pneumococcal colonization of the nasopharynx. Trends Microbiol 21: 129–135.
11. Hare KM, Morris P, Smith-Vaughan H, Leach AJ (2008) Random colony selection versus colony morphology for detection of multiple pneumococcal serotypes in nasopharyngeal swabs. Pediatr Infect Dis J 27: 178–180.
12. Huebner RE, Dagan R, Porath N, Wasas AD, Klugman KP (2000) Lack of utility of serotyping multiple colonies for detection of simultaneous nasopharyngeal carriage of different pneumococcal serotypes. Pediatr Infect Dis J 19: 1017–1020.
13. Hansman D, Morris S, Gregory M, McDonald B (1985) Pneumococcal carriage amongst Australian aborigines in Alice Springs, Northern Territory. J Hyg (Lond) 95: 677–684.
14. Brugger SD, Hathaway LJ, Muhlemann K (2009) Detection of Streptococcus pneumoniae strain cocolonization in the nasopharynx. J Clin Microbiol 47: 1750–1756.
15. Ercibengoa M, Arostegi N, Marimon JM, Alonso M, Perez-Trallero E (2012) Dynamics of pneumococcal nasopharyngeal carriage in healthy children attending a day care center in northern Spain. Influence of detection techniques on the results. BMC Infect Dis 12: 69.
16. Lipsitch M, Abdullahi O, D'Amour A, Xie W, Weinberger DM, et al. (2012) Estimating rates of carriage acquisition and clearance and competitive ability for

pneumococcal serotypes in Kenya with a Markov transition model. Epidemiology 23: 510–519.
17. Auranen K, Mehtala J, Tanskanen A, S Kaltoft M (2010) Between-strain competition in acquisition and clearance of pneumococcal carriage–epidemiologic evidence from a longitudinal study of day-care children. Am J Epidemiol 171: 169–176.
18. Vu HT, Yoshida LM, Suzuki M, Nguyen HA, Nguyen CD, et al. (2011) Association between nasopharyngeal load of Streptococcus pneumoniae, viral coinfection, and radiologically confirmed pneumonia in Vietnamese children. Pediatr Infect Dis J 30: 11–18.
19. O'Brien KL, Nohynek H (2003) Report from a WHO working group: standard method for detecting upper respiratory carriage of Streptococcus pneumoniae. Pediatr Infect Dis J 22: 133–140.
20. Dhoubhadel BG, Yasunami M, Yoshida LM, Thi HA, Thi TH, et al. (2014) A novel high-throughput method for molecular serotyping and serotype-specific quantification of Streptococcus pneumoniae using a nanofluidic real-time PCR system. J Med Microbiol 63: 528–539.
21. Battig P, Hathaway LJ, Hofer S, Muhlemann K (2006) Serotype-specific invasiveness and colonization prevalence in Streptococcus pneumoniae correlate with the lag phase during in vitro growth. Microbes Infect 8: 2612–2617.
22. Azzari C, Resti M (2008) Reduction of carriage and transmission of Streptococcus pneumoniae: the beneficial "side effect" of pneumococcal conjugate vaccine. Clin Infect Dis 47: 997–999.
23. Brueggemann AB, Pai R, Crook DW, Beall B (2007) Vaccine escape recombinants emerge after pneumococcal vaccination in the United States. PLoS Pathog 3: e168.
24. Croucher NJ, Harris SR, Fraser C, Quail MA, Burton J, et al. (2011) Rapid pneumococcal evolution in response to clinical interventions. Science 331: 430–434.
25. Leung MH, Oriyo NM, Gillespie SH, Charalambous BM (2011) The adaptive potential during nasopharyngeal colonisation of Streptococcus pneumoniae. Infect Genet Evol 11: 1989–1995.
26. Marks LR, Reddinger RM, Hakansson AP (2012) High levels of genetic recombination during nasopharyngeal carriage and biofilm formation in Streptococcus pneumoniae. MBio 3.
27. Lipsitch M, Dykes JK, Johnson SE, Ades EW, King J, et al. (2000) Competition among Streptococcus pneumoniae for intranasal colonization in a mouse model. Vaccine 18: 2895–2901.
28. Dawid S, Roche AM, Weiser JN (2007) The blp bacteriocins of Streptococcus pneumoniae mediate intraspecies competition both in vitro and in vivo. Infect Immun 75: 443–451.
29. Zhang Y, Auranen K, Eichner M (2004) The influence of competition and vaccination on the coexistence of two pneumococcal serotypes. Epidemiology and Infection 132: 1073–1081.

A Biomarker Panel (Bioscore) Incorporating Monocytic Surface and Soluble TREM-1 Has High Discriminative Value for Ventilator-Associated Pneumonia

Vimal Grover[1,2,3], Panagiotis Pantelidis[2,4], Neil Soni[1,3], Masao Takata[3], Pallav L. Shah[5,6], Athol U. Wells[6], Don C. Henderson[2,4], Peter Kelleher[2,4], Suveer Singh[1,3,5]*

1 Magill Department of Anaesthesia, Critical Care and Pain, Chelsea and Westminster Hospital National Health Service Foundation Trust, London, United Kingdom, **2** Immunology Section, Department of Medicine, Imperial College, London, United Kingdom, **3** Department of Surgery and Cancer, Imperial College, London, United Kingdom, **4** Department of Immunology, Imperial College Healthcare National Health Service Trust, London, United Kingdom, **5** Department of Respiratory Medicine, Chelsea and Westminster Hospital National Health Service Foundation Trust, London, United Kingdom, **6** Department of Respiratory Medicine, Royal Brompton & Harefield Hospitals National Health Service Foundation Trust, London, United Kingdom

Abstract

Introduction: Ventilator-associated pneumonia (VAP) increases mortality in critical illness. However, clinical diagnostic uncertainty persists. We hypothesised that measuring cell-surface and soluble inflammatory markers, incorporating Triggering Receptor Expressed by Myeloid cells (TREM)-1, would improve diagnostic accuracy.

Methods: A single centre prospective observational study, set in a University Hospital medical-surgical intensive Care unit, recruited 91 patients into 3 groups: 27 patients with VAP, 33 ventilated controls without evidence of pulmonary sepsis (non-VAP), and 31 non-ventilated controls (NVC), without clinical infection, attending for bronchoscopy. Paired samples of Bronchiolo-alveolar lavage fluid (BALF) and blood from each subject were analysed for putative biomarkers of infection: Cellular (TREM-1, CD11b and CD62L) and soluble (IL-1β, IL-6, IL-8, sTREM-1, Procalcitonin). Expression of cellular markers on monocytes and neutrophils were measured by flow cytometry. Soluble inflammatory markers were determined by ELISA. A biomarker panel ('Bioscore'), was constructed, tested and validated, using Fisher's discriminant function analysis, to assess its value in distinguishing VAP from non VAP.

Results: The expression of TREM-1 on monocytes (mTREM-1) and neutrophils (nTREM-1) and concentrations of IL-1β, IL-8, and sTREM-1 in BALF were significantly higher in VAP compared with non-VAP and NVC ($p<0.001$). The BALF/blood mTREM-1 was significantly higher in VAP patients compared to non-VAP and NVC (0.8 v 0.4 v 0.3 $p<0.001$). A seven marker Bioscore (BALF/blood ratio mTREM-1 and mCD11b, BALF sTREM-1, IL-8 and IL-1β, and serum CRP and IL-6) correctly identified 88.9% of VAP cases and 100% of non-VAP cases.

Conclusion: A 7-marker bioscore, incorporating cellular and soluble TREM-1, accurately discriminates VAP from non-pulmonary infection.

Editor: Charles Dela Cruz, Yale University, United States of America

Funding: This work was supported by Chelsea and Westminster Health Charity (http://www.cwhc.org.uk/), Westminster Medical School Research Trust (JRC 09/10 SG006), and National Institute of Academic Anaesthesia, UK (http://www.niaa.org.uk/). The funders had no role in study design, data collection and analysis, decision to publish, or preparation of the manuscript.

Competing Interests: The authors have declared that no competing interests exist.

* Email: suveer.singh@imperial.ac.uk

Introduction

Ventilator-associated pneumonia (VAP) remains a common complication of critical illness, affecting over 10% of intubated patients, prolonging ICU stay, with an estimated attributable mortality of 13% [1–3]. This is despite the introduction of health improvement strategies such as Ventilator care bundles, which have apparently reduced the incidence [4,5], even though antibiotic prescriptions remain high for pulmonary sepsis in ICU [5]. Standardisation of diagnostic criteria for VAP is important for benchmarking, but no single best definition exists [6]. This in part has led to proposals for simplifying definitions into infective and non-infective ventilator associated complications [7].

Confirmatory diagnosis by microbiological culture is often too slow for clinical need, whilst even quantitative microbiological analysis is subject to the variations in the sampling site, or elusive despite other criteria being fulfilled [8]. Biomarkers may facilitate clinical confirmation and aid differentiation of pulmonary from non-pulmonary sepsis. This would allow earlier, targeted antibiotic intervention, direct clinicians' decision-making for 'antibiotic de-escalation' regimens and potentially reduce selective pressure for multi-resistant bacteria [9,10]. The role of inflammatory biomarkers including TREM-1 (Triggering Receptor Expressed on Myeloid Cells-1), IL-1, IL-6, IL-8, Procalcitonin (PCT) and more traditional indices, i.e. white cell count and CRP remains unclear. Only some show clinical diagnostic utility for VAP [11–14]. Differences in definitions of VAP patient populations, severity of disease, and assay techniques account for much of the conflicting data reported [15,16]. Furthermore, failure of many studies to consider the dynamic relationships between soluble and cell surface inflammatory proteins (e.g.TREM-1), differential expression of inflammatory markers by neutrophils and monocytes, and compartmentalization of inflammatory immune responses at the site of tissue infection in reference to blood, are likely contributory factors.

The aim of this study was to determine if, and which combination of paired blood and bronchoalveolar lavage fluid (BALF) inflammatory biomarkers (soluble and cell surface based, including TREM-1), could correctly classify patients with VAP from ventilated patients without evidence of pulmonary sepsis.

Materials and Methods

Study participants

Informed, witnessed and written assent was obtained from a relative or designated carer for all ventilated patients. Written consent was obtained from all day case bronchoscopy patients. Ethical permission was obtained from the local institutional board (Barking and Havering Local Research Ethics Committee, Ilford, Essex, UK), through the National Research Ethics Service (NRES) of the United Kingdom 08/H0702/61.

The study sample was selected from patients hospitalized between Feb 2009 and Aug 2011 in the Intensive Care unit, and Lady Kilmarnock bronchoscopy suite of the Chelsea and Westminster Hospital NHS Foundation Trust, London, United Kingdom. Adult patients (>18 years) were recruited into the following 3 groups; ventilator associated pneumonia, ventilated controls without evidence of pulmonary sepsis or with non-pulmonary sepsis (non-VAP), and non-ventilated non-infected controls (NVC).

In accordance with the 2005 guidelines of the American Thoracic Society/Infectious Diseases Society of America, the criteria for diagnosis of VAP were evidence of new infiltrates on chest radiographs after 48 hours of endotracheal intubation and presence of at least 2 of the following: fever (temperature >38°C or higher than basal temperature), abnormal white cell count (≥10 000/μL or <4000/μL), and purulent respiratory tract secretions [2]. As per recommendations, BALF samples were collected via directed bronchoscopy, semi-quantitatively reported (SQ) and cultured for microorganisms [17].

The clinical pulmonary infection score (CPIS) defined VAP and non-VAP [17,18]. Thus, VAP was predefined as CPIS >5 and positive BALF microbiology. Non-VAP was predefined as CPIS score <6 and negative microbiology. This was a modification of the original CPIS, by additionally incorporating SQ microbiological data. The patient cohorts comprised non-infected ventilated patients, or individuals with non-pulmonary infection (i.e. intra-abdominal, indwelling devices) confirmed on clinical, radiological and microbiological grounds. To control for the effects of mechanical ventilation on pulmonary inflammation, BALF and blood samples were obtained from a cohort of non-ventilated control patients (NVC) undergoing day case bronchoscopy for non-infective respiratory disorders (i.e., chronic obstructive pulmonary disease, COPD, interstitial lung disease, ILD, or solitary pulmonary nodules).

Comparison of CPIS with the European Hospitals in Europe Link for Infection Control through Surveillance programme (HELICS) criteria (PN4) revealed excellent concordance using the Cohen kappa statistic (0.95) [15,19]. Two patients with VAP would have been classified as non-VAP using HELICS and one patient with non-VAP could possibly have been placed into the VAP cohort. Initial chest radiographic interpretation was that of the clinical investigators, with all radiographs being independently confirmed by a radiologist.

Data on exclusion criteria, and description of procedures for obtaining informed consent and for sampling, processing of BALF and blood and group classification are provided in an online supplement.

Laboratory studies

Twenty two individual inflammatory markers were measured. In blood these consisted of six cell surface [3 monocytic and 3 neutrophilic (TREM-1, CD11b and CD62L)] and five soluble proteins sTREM-1, IL-6, PCT, CRP and the white cell count (WCC). In BALF, the same six cell surface markers were measured and five soluble proteins above the limit of detection for ELISA were sTREM-1, IL-1β, IL-6, IL-8 and PCT. Nine BALF/blood marker ratios were calculated.

Immunophenotypic analysis was performed on peripheral blood and BALF cell suspensions using 5-colour flow cytometry (Cytomics FC500 Beckman Coulter, Beckman-Coulter, Villepinte, France). Blood and BALF cells were isolated following standard centrifugation procedures, and washed in phosphate buffered saline/1% fetal calf serum (FCS). 100 μl aliquot cell suspensions were then stained with monoclonal antibodies for 30 minutes. Further details on monoclonal antibodies used, on instrumentation and software analysis are provided in an on line supplement. CD45 staining and side scatter properties were initially used to select CD14 and CD16 positive cells as markers of monocytes and neutrophils respectively. Isotype controls were used to delineate specific protein expression on the cell surface of inflammatory cells. Geometric mean fluorescent intensity (MFI) was used as an index of protein concentration expressed by a particular blood or BALF cell population. Details on measurement of cytokines and inflammatory mediators (sTREM-1, IL-1β, IL-6 and IL-8) and PCT are provided in an online supplement. Urea was determined by ELISA (Abcam, Cambridge, UK) and was used to correct for dilutional effects in BALF [20].

Statistical Analysis

Anthropometric data was reported as medians and inter-quartile ranges. Differences between the groups for individual biomarkers were determined using the Kruskal-Wallis test followed by the Mann-Whitney U test with Dunn's post-hoc correction for multiple analyses when there were any statistical differences between individual groups.

Fisher's discriminant function analysis (FDA) was used to determine the optimal combination of biomarkers that could discriminate between VAP and non-VAP patient groups. A variable was entered into the "model" if the significance level of its F-value was <0.05 and was removed if the significance level was ≥0.05. The model was then used to classify each of the 91 cases into a diagnostic group. In order to check that the result of the biomarker model was not skewed by the presence of outlier data the model was internally validated by means of the leave-one-out method, which involves omitting a single observation from the original sample, and then using the remaining observations to assign the omitted case either to the VAP or non-VAP patient group.

The model was cross-validated by repeat random sub-sampling - by repeatedly (10 times) randomly assigning original cases into a training cohort (60% of original cases) to obtain new classification function coefficients for the analytes derived from the original model. The new function coefficients obtained were applied to a test cohort that consisted of the remaining cases (40%), to confirm the reliability of the model [21–24]. Further statistical information is available in an online supplement. All analysis was conducted using the SPSS v19 software package (SPSS, Chicago, IL, USA) and GraphPad Prism software (California, USA). Independent statistical analysis was performed.

Results

Study participants

Ninety one patients were recruited consecutively. There were 27 VAP, 33 non-VAP and 31 NVC patients (Table 1). There were no statistically significant differences between the groups with respect to age, sex, history of cigarette smoking, presence of chest x-ray infiltrates and APACHE II score. Twenty eight-day mortality was 3 deaths in the VAP group, 4 in the non-VAP group (none in the NVC). The majority of patients in the VAP and non-VAP groups were receiving antibiotics at the time of sampling. Thirty percent of ventilated patients received steroids for sepsis. The distribution of steroids between VAP and non-VAP groups were not statistically significant. Nine VAP and 13 non-VAP patients were post-operative cases. Within the NVC group, 7 patients had lung cancer, 9 COPD, 2 pulmonary sarcoidosis, 1 lung fibrosis, 6 with benign lung nodules and 7 with normal findings.

The following organisms were isolated (patients): Serratia marcescens (2), Klebsiella spp (4), Pseudomonas spp (9), methicillin sensitive staphylococcal aureus, MSSA (4), methicillin resistant staphylococcal aureus, MRSA (3), Escherischia coli, (5), Acinetobacter baumanii (5), Stenotrophomonas (2) and Proteus mirabilis (2). Twenty eight organisms were isolated from VAP patients and the remaining eight bacteria were found in non-VAP patients (non-pulmonary infection).

The CRP was significantly elevated in VAP and non-VAP compared to NVC group ($p<0.001$). White cell count was significantly higher in VAP than NVC ($p<0.001$). Neither CRP nor WCC distinguished VAP from non-VAP.

Cellular and soluble inflammatory mediators in blood

In blood, there was no significant difference in the expression of cellular and soluble biomarkers between VAP and non-VAP (Table 2). However, the concentration of sTREM-1, IL-6, PCT and expression of CD62L on CD14 gated monocytes were significantly higher in VAP and non-VAP groups compared with NVC (Table 2). This suggests blood based biomarker activation resulting from ventilation, but that it is not discriminatory between VAP and non-VAP patients.

Cellular and soluble inflammatory mediators in BALF

By contrast, analysis of BALF showed significantly increased expression of cellular mTREM-1 and nTREM-1, and increased concentration of soluble IL-1β in VAP compared with non-VAP and NVC groups ($p<0.001$) (Table 2). Furthermore, whilst the increased expression of mTREM-1 from BALF in VAP was significant ($p<0.001$) (Figure 1a), this difference between VAP and the other two groups was greater when the compartmentalization ratio BALF/blood mTREM-1 was used (Figure 1b). This was not the case for BALF/Blood nTREM-1. The BALF/Blood ratios of CD11b on monocytes and sTREM-1 were also significantly higher

Table 1. Characteristics of patients recruited to study.

	VAP	Non-VAP	NVC
Number of patients	27	33	31
Age	68 (23–84)	62 (18–89)	59 (18–84)
Sex (% male/% female)	70/30	52/48	61/39
CPIS	7 (6–9)	3 (0–5)	N/A
Microbiology (% +ve)	100	12	0
APACHE II score	18 (5–45)	15 (2–24)	N/A
Smoking (% current/ex/none)	44/15/40	30/21/49	35/13/52
Antibiotics (% pre-BALF)	89	70	32
CXR (% with shadowing)	96	55	81
Steroids (%)	30	30	6
28-day mortality (%)	11	12	0
Post-surgical (%)	37	39	0
Burns injury (% of cases)	15	15	0
WCC ($x10^9/l$)	15 (4–24)	9 (3–27)	7 (3–18)*
CRP (mg/L)	84 (7–320)	102(2–341)†	6 (1–296)*

The median and range (lowest-highest) is shown for each group. APACHE II and CPIS are only applicable to the ventilated patients. Some variables are presented as percentages. Statistically significant differences between the groups were determined using the Mann-Whitney U test with post-hoc Dunn correction and are indicated as follows: VAP versus NVC ($p<0.001$)* and non-VAP versus NVC ($p<0.001$)†. CPIS = Clinical Pulmonary Infection Score. APACHE II = Acute Physiology and Chronic Health Evaluation II score. VAP = ventilator-associated pneumonia. NVC = non-ventilated control. Non-VAP = ventilated non-pulmonary infected control. CXR = Chest X-ray. WCC = White cell count. CRP = C-reactive protein.

Table 2. Expression of cell-surface and soluble proteins in study participants with VAP, non-VAP and NVC.

	VAP	Non-VAP	NVC
Blood			
mTREM-1	5.1 (3.2–8.6)	4.6 (3.1–6.1)	6.5 (4.3–10.9)
nTREM-1	4.7 (2.6–7.3)	3.8 (2.3–6.1)	4.5 (3.1–7.4)
mCD11b	47.2 (30.0–70.0)	43.3 (27.6–52.3)	39.2(21.7–51.8)
nCD11b	44.0 (33.4–91.9)	59.8 (43.4–82.9)	49.0 (38.0–81.0)
mCD62L	9.4 (7.3–15.1)	9.5 (7.4–13.2)	5.4 (3.9–9.4)*
nCD62L	9.6 (6.0–17.0)	8.3 (6.0–10.5)	8.6 (6.8–10.5)
sTREM-1 (μg/ml)	0.18 (0.01–0.03)	0.15 (0.08–0.30)	0.09 (0.06–0.15)[†,‡]
IL-1β (μg/ml)	N/A	N/A	N/A
IL-6 (μg/ml)	0.09 (0.03–0.21)	0.08 (0.03–0.17)	0.008 (0.005–0.02)[*]
IL-8 (μg/ml)	N/A	N/A	N/A
PCT (ng/ml)	1.3 (0.3–5.3)	2.9 (0.6–8.3)	N/A[*]
Corrected BALF			
mTREM-1	3.9 (2.5–5.4)	1.6 (1.1–2.3)	1.8 (1.2–2.9)[§]
nTREM-1	2.0 (1.7–3.3)	1.5 (1.2–2.2)**	1.7 (1.3–3.0)
mCD11b	25.2 (9.0–81.2)	18.6 (13.7–31.2)	21.0 (6.9–47.3)
nCD11b	47.0 (15.1–86.0)	32.9 (20.3–62.5)	24.0 (6.0–73.5)
mCD62L	1.2 (1.0–1.5)	1.1 (1.0–1.3)	1.2 (1.0–1.4)
nCD62L	1.4 (1.0–2.1)	1.1 (1.0–1.4)	1.2 (1.0–1.7)
sTREM-1 (μg/ml)	20.14 (9.45–43.94)	5.19 (2.83–10.96)[††]	7.61 (3.05–18.32)
IL-1β (μg/ml)	3.02 (1.47–8.59)	0.79 (0.36–1.51)	0.53 (0.19–2.79)[§]
IL-6 (μg/ml)	3.80 (1.32–17.71)	2.08 (1.23–5.75)	1.45 (0.52–2.52)[‡‡]
IL-8 (μg/ml)	48.60 (20.78–101.10)	12.16(5.71–17.3)[§§]	16.33 (3.12–67.15)
PCT (ng/ml)	16.8 (9.7–51.7)	12.5(6.8–27.4)	9.6(4.1–18.2)
Corrected BALF/blood ratio			
mTREM-1	0.8(0.5–1.0)	0.4(0.2–0.5)	0.3(0.2–0.4)[§]
nTREM-1	0.6(0.2–0.8)	0.4(0.3–0.8)	0.4(0.2–1.1)
mCD11b	0.53(0.4–2.3)	0.4(0.2–0.7)[§§]	0.5(0.2–1.3)
nCD11b	0.7(0.5–2.0)	0.5(0.2–0.9)	0.5(0.1–1.4)
mCD62L	0.2(0.1–0.5)	0.1(0.1–0.2)	0.2(0.1–0.3)
nCD62L	0.2(0.1–0.3)	0.2(0.1–0.2)	0.2(0.1–0.2)
sTREM-1	190(70–337)	30(11–85)[§§]	84(26–228)[ll]
IL-1β	N/A	N/A	N/A
IL-6	77(20–145)	43(41–230)	134(230–355)
IL-8	N/A	N/A	N/A
PCT	29(3–55)	4(2–23)	N/A

The median and interquartile range for each patient group is reported. Statistically significant differences between groups were determined using the Mann-Whitney U and post hoc Dunn correction as follows: VAP and non-VAP versus NVC ($p<0.001$)[*], VAP versus NVC ($p<0.001$)[†] and non-VAP versus NVC ($p<0.05$)[‡], VAP versus non-VAP and NVC ($p<0.001$)[§], VAP versus non-VAP ($p<0.01$)[**], VAP versus non-VAP ($p<0.001$)[††], VAP versus NVC ($p<0.01$)[‡‡], VAP versus non-VAP ($p<0.001$)[§§] and NVC> non-VAP ($p<0.01$)[ll]. The lower limits of detection for the sTREM-1, IL-1β, IL-6, IL-8 and PCT assays were 0.01 μg/ml, 0.001 μg/ml, 0.0007 μg/ml, 0.004 μg/ml and 0.05 ng/ml respectively. N/A indicates below assay detection limit. BALF levels were corrected for dilution occurring with bronchoscopy using urea analysis. BALF/blood ratios were only calculable if BALF and blood measurements were obtained. VAP = ventilator-associated pneumonia. Non-VAP = ventilated patients with no evidence of pulmonary infection. NVC = non-ventilated non-infected patients.

in VAP group compared to non-VAP, but not when compared to NVC (Table 2). The expression of cellular mTREM-1, nTREM-1, and CD11b was lower in BALF than blood (Table 2), although the reductions seen were notably less in patients with VAP, as compared with non-VAP and NVC groups, hence the higher BALF/blood ratio (Table 2). Other soluble markers IL-1β, IL-8 and sTREM-1 were significantly raised in the VAP compared with non-VAP groups. IL-6 was similar in VAP and non-VAP groups but higher than NVC (Figure 2). None of the individual markers in blood, BALF or BALF/blood ratios had sufficient accuracy in distinguishing VAP from non-VAP (data not shown).

Classification of individual cases within each study group using a biomarker panel

To determine whether a biomarker panel might have better discriminating ability than individual markers, and to separate the

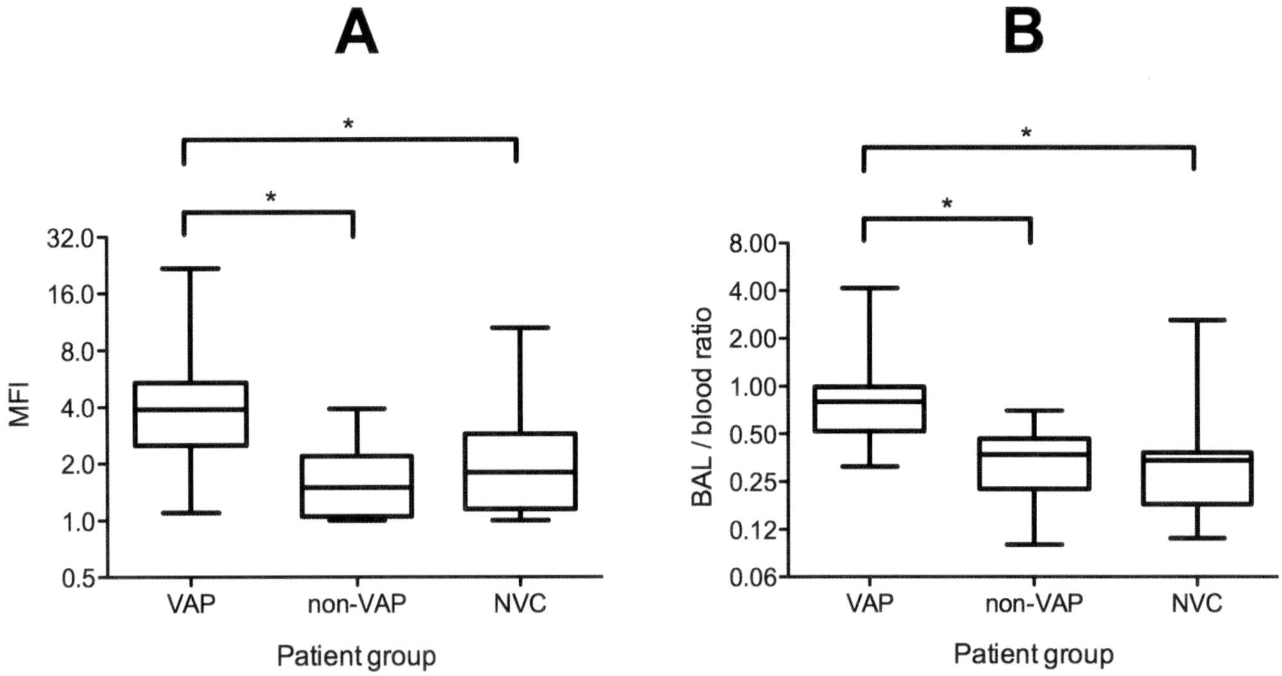

Figure 1. BALF levels and BALF/blood ratios of monocytic TREM-1. Box (interquartile) and whisker (range) plots showing expression of TREM-1 by CD14+ monocytes in BALF (Figure 1a) and the BALF/blood ratio of TREM-1 expression by monocytes in blood and BALF (Figure 1b) from patients with VAP, non-VAP (ventilated non-pulmonary infected control) and NVC (non-ventilated control). BALF levels were corrected for dilution occurring with bronchoscopy using urea measurement. Statistically significant differences between groups were determined using the Mann-Whitney U and post hoc Dunn correction as follows: monocyte TREM-1 levels for VAP versus non-VAP and NVC ($p<0.001$)* and BALF/blood monocytic TREM-1 ratio VAP versus non-VAP and NVC ($p<0.001$)*. MFI = mean fluorescence intensity.

effects of ventilation from infection, Fisher Discriminant Analysis (FDA) was performed to build a 'model' that could best predict to which group (VAP and non-VAP) a study participant belonged on the basis of the biological measurements alone. To build the model we used all the VAP and non-VAP cases in the study and the 22 different markers and their compartmentalized ratios. A seven marker Bioscore consisting of BALF/blood cell expression ratio for monocyte mTREM-1 and mCD11b, BALF levels of sTREM-1, IL-8 and IL-1β, blood levels of CRP and IL-6 was shown to discriminate between VAP and non-VAP patients.

The 7 marker-bioscore produced 100% correct classification of the non-VAP patients and 88.9% correct classification of VAP patients. The NVC group which was treated as an unknown was defined as non-VAP in 90.7% of the cases using this model. In order to control for the possibility that the findings of the biomarker panel might be skewed by results obtained from any particular patient, we performed a leave one out cross validation analysis which produced the same level of accuracy with the original model (100% for non-VAP, 88.9% for VAP).

In order to assess the robustness of the model further, individual cases were then randomly assigned into a training cohort (60% of original cases) to obtain new classification function coefficients for the 7 analytes and the remaining 40% were used as unknowns for classification. In this cross-validation model the average predictive accuracies for the patients in the testing cohort were 71.0% for VAP and 98.5% for non-VAP. The reduction in classification for VAP was largely driven by the model attributing a number of NVC as VAP and to the limited power of the testing cohort analysed.

Discussion

This study demonstrates that a combination of cell surface and soluble markers of inflammation, in particular TREM-1, sampled in blood and BALF simultaneously, can accurately discriminate VAP from ventilated patients without pulmonary sepsis. The use of a compartmentalization ratio, as a measure of site-specific immune response, results in a further improvement in diagnostic classification. These data have implications for the accurate diagnosis [25], antibiotic usage and management of VAP [26]. The results also address a potential weakness of previous studies which have measured only soluble mediators, often in one compartment. These may not fully account for the dynamic interaction between cell surface receptors and their soluble counterparts (e.g. mTREM-1 and sTREM-1 respectively), and site specific flux between the alveolar lung space and blood [27].

The findings suggest that monocytic surface receptor mTREM-1 and its neutrophilic counterpart nTREM-1 are compartmentalized within the lung, with increased expression in VAP. Although the expression of TREM-1 on pulmonary inflammatory cells has not to our knowledge previously been assessed in patients with VAP, the results are consistent with increased mTREM-1 reported in patients with community acquired pneumonia [28]. Soluble TREM-1 levels in BALF were significantly elevated and discriminatory in patients with VAP compared to non-VAP, in keeping with some, [12,14,29,30] but not all studies, [13,31,32]. The BALF/blood ratio of mTREM-1, mCD11b and sTREM-1 were significantly higher in patients with VAP compared to those without VAP suggesting site-specific utility. Pulmonary infection may be distinguished from abdominal infection by combining BALF sTREM-1 and blood Procalcitonin measurement, although with lesser discrimination than our use of combined cell surface/

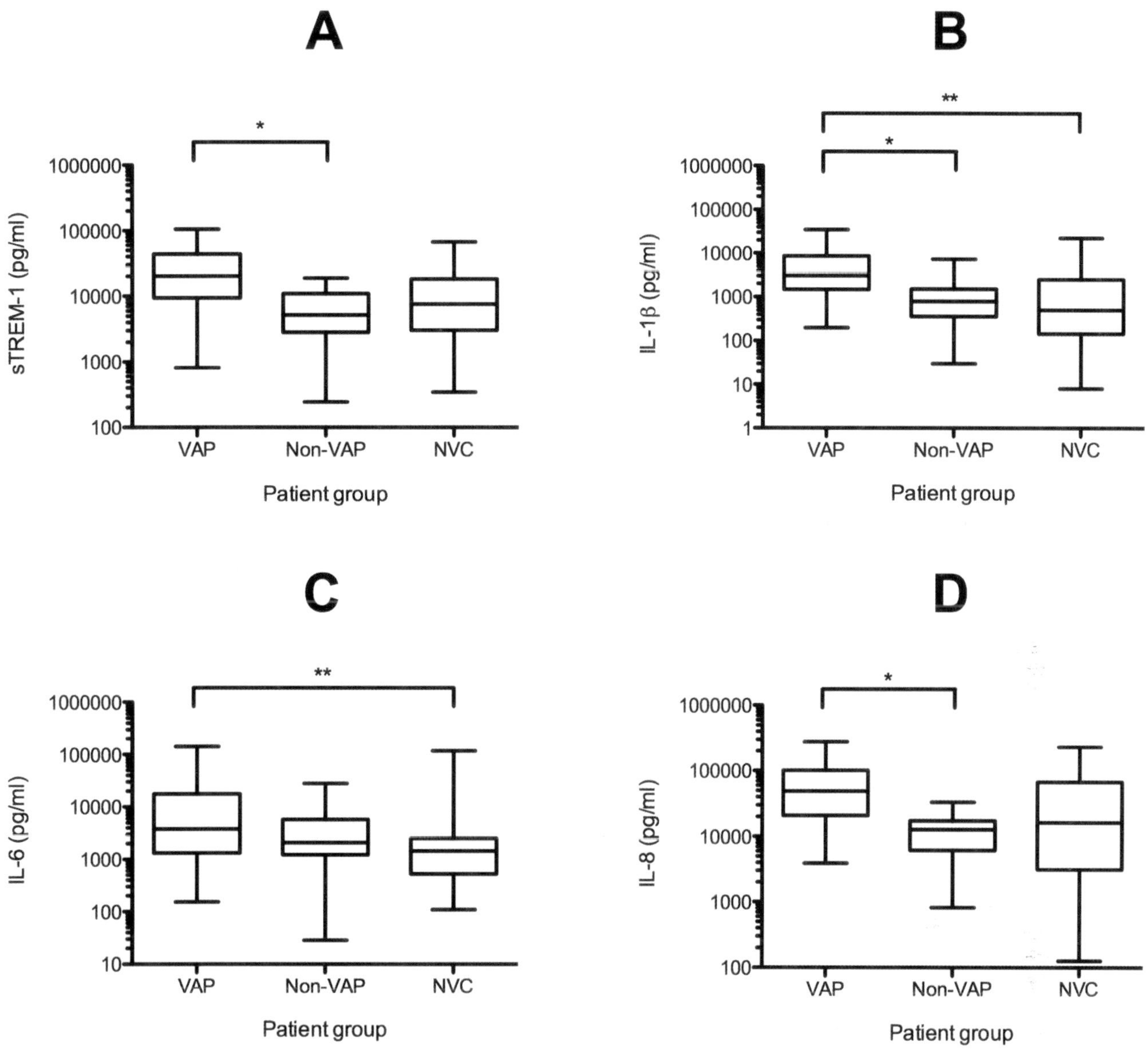

Figure 2. Soluble cytokine levels in BALF. Box (interquartile) and whisker (range) plots showing (a) sTREM-1, (b) IL-1β, (c) IL-6 and (d) IL-8 levels in BALF of patients with VAP, non-VAP (ventilated non-pulmonary infected control) and NVC (non-ventilated control). The BALF levels were corrected for dilution occurring with bronchoscopy using urea measurement. The concentration of BALF sTREM-1, IL-1β and IL-8 were significantly higher in VAP than non-VAP ($p<0.001$)*. BALF IL-1β and IL-6 were higher in the VAP compared with the NVC patient group ($p<0.001$)**.

soluble markers [12]. Ramirez et al reported the discriminative ability of site-sampled sTREM-1 for identifying pulmonary from abdominal infection in a critically ill cohort [33]. Thus, analysis of site-specific inflammatory markers may be useful in distinguishing infective sites, although measurement of cell surface markers over soluble proteins will not be influenced by dilutional variance from BALF.

The BALF/blood ratios of neutrophil-based nTREM-1 and nCD11b were not raised in VAP, unlike their monocytic counterparts. This difference is consistent with data from patients in septic shock, in whom blood mTREM-1 but not nTREM-1 levels increased compared with controls [34]. Expression of TREM-1 on neutrophils initially falls over minutes and then increases following in vitro LPS stimulation. In contrast TREM-1 levels on monocytes steadily increase over hours. It is possible that the recruitment timescale for VAP misses early neutrophilic changes [35]. Indeed, expression of TREM-1 by neutrophils may have passed its peak before time definitions of VAP allow measurement. Sampling individuals with suspected VAP at earlier time points may clarify differential kinetics of TREM-1 expression.

Surface TREM-1 may act as a link in the pathway from infective organism, to upregulation of the inflammatory cytokines. That said, it is unlikely to be specific for infection as opposed to inflammation. Experimentally, mTREM-1 activation in conjunction with lipopolysaccharide (LPS) increases IL-8 and IL-1β release, with amplification seen in septic shock, as in our study, [36,37]. Such changes in IL-8 and IL-1β are in accordance with Conway-Morris et al, who have demonstrated high area under the curve (AUC) for them in suspected VAP [13]. Others have found elevated BALF IL-1β and IL-6 levels in VAP, when using a lung to blood ratio like in this study [38]. The BALF/blood ratios of soluble cytokines were non-discriminatory in this study, perhaps due to significant compartmentalization by the time of sampling, producing very low blood levels.

The difference in expression of mTREM-1 in VAP from non-VAP was more notable in BALF than blood, although the MFI were lower in BALF (Table 2). This may be due to increased shedding of up-regulated BALF mTREM-1 within the lung, as evidenced by the significantly greater increase in soluble sTREM-1 compared with blood. A potential mechanism is suggested to involve the balance between bacterial induced metalloproteinase (MMP) mediated cleavage of TREM-1 from surface of monocytes and action of specific MMP inhibitors [39]. Moreover, neutrophil derived MMP production is seen to increase markedly in BALF as compared to plasma from patients with hospital acquired pneumonia, whereas the specific tissue inhibitors of MMP (TIMP) were increased in plasma compared to BALF [40].

The limitations of this study are addressed here. First, no gold standard for VAP diagnosis exists. We included patients, who based on the CPIS scoring system, plus semi-quantitative microbiological testing were highly likely to have the presence or absence of VAP in order to test putative biomarkers. CPIS has been criticized by some for its potentially low diagnostic accuracy based upon clinico-radiological criteria. However, all current definitions of VAP remain subject to limitations. We acknowledge that semi-quantitative microbiology is less specific than Quantitative, but as sensitive for identifying pulmonary infection [41]. However, even the use of quantitative microbiology from directed BALF will potentially miss an important group of VAP patients (defined by standard clinic-patho-radiological criteria), if not meeting the predefined cutoff values of colony forming units/ml (cfu/ml). The arbitrary 48 h requirement for mechanical ventilation in most definitions of VAP provides important standardization but will also miss some pulmonary sepsis in ventilated patients developing prior to that timepoint. In order to mitigate against these concerns, we redefined the VAP and non VAP patients by other well established validated international criteria. Thus, the diagnostic definitions used were highly concordant when the HELICS criteria for pneumonia were used [15]. Reassuringly, from a biological perspective, the raised BALF IL-1β and IL-8 levels in VAP from our study concur with a group utilizing different diagnostic methodology, implying the validity to such approaches [13]. Therefore, the type of diagnostic criteria, particularly quantitative microbiology, used were not a major influence on the bioscore's discriminability.

Second, this study did not encompass the whole range of infective aetiologies. For instance, no patients had mycoplasma, Legionella or proven respiratory viral pneumonias, and few had bilateral lung infiltrates. The management of viral pneumonias in particular, would benefit from early diagnostic biomarkers. Third, the absence of patients with ARDS does not allow us to comment on how the bioscore might perform in discriminating severe pulmonary inflammation from pulmonary infection. Fourth, and from a practical consideration, flow cytometry is a specialized technique. It requires samples with sufficient numbers of cells, which mandates adequate directed BALF samples, likely targeted bronchoscopy and makes serial biomarker analysis challenging. However, BALF samples are the current standard of care a microbiological diagnosis of VAP [16]. Fifth, a number of patients were receiving antibiotics and steroids at the time of sampling, with potential immunomodulatory activity. Given the prevalence of these key standard interventions in critically ill patients, we believe this pragmatic approach enhances the applicability of the findings. Sixth, the immune response to infecting pathogens in VAP, as in sepsis, is likely to involve neutrophils, monocytes and lymphocytes, [42]. As such we have not necessarily looked at all potentially relevant phagocytic or T cell markers. That said, the value of biomarker panels that include sTREM-1, PCT and CD64 on neutrophils has recently demonstrated the ability to predict sepsis in the setting of unselected critical illness, confirming the need to pursue such discriminatory panels in VAP, as in other disease states [42,43]. Finally, we acknowledge that these results require validation in an external cohort of patients with suspected VAP, to see whether the bioscore 7 panel retains its discriminatory accuracy. Moreover, such a study is needed to see how the biomarker components, particularly mTREM-1, sTREM-1, IL1 and IL8, will perform and whether the BALF/blood ratio offers improved accuracy.

In conclusion, a 7 biomarker panel comprising soluble and cell-surface inflammatory markers including TREM-1 in combination with BALF/blood ratio differentiates VAP from non-pulmonary infection with good diagnostic accuracy. Such an approach, that incorporates these practically relevant and easily measurable biomarkers, to confirm or refute suspected VAP, requires confirmation.

Supporting Information

Table S1 BALF bacterial growth in patient groups. The table shows the BALF microbiological results with patients of CPIS >6, CPIS <6 and CPIS = 6. CPIS = Clinical pulmonary infection score. VAP = Ventilator-associated pneumonia

Materials and Methods S1 Supporting information on study participants, biomarker measurement, biomarker panel construction and validation.

Acknowledgments

We would like to acknowledge the valuable assistance received by the Staff of the Intensive Care Unit, Operating Theatres, Bronchoscopy unit, and the Chelsea and Westminster Hospital ICU Patient's forum. We thank Dr Berge Azadian, clinical Microbiologist for his help comments. We thank Professor Athol Wells, internationally recognised in the respiratory field for his statistical knowledge and the use of complex data analysis, for providing independent statistical advice. He was not involved in study design, data collection or initial analysis.

Author Contributions

Conceived and designed the experiments: VG PP NS DCH PK SS. Performed the experiments: VG PLS SS. Analyzed the data: VG PP NS MT PLS AUW DCH PK SS. Contributed reagents/materials/analysis tools: VG PP NS MT PLS AUW DCH PK SS. Contributed to the writing of the manuscript: VG PP NS MT PLS AUW DH PK SS.

References

1. Alberti C, Brun-Buisson C, Burchardi H, Martin C, Goodman S, et al (2002) Epidemiology of sepsis and infection in ICU patients from an international multicentre cohort study. Int Care Med 28: 108–121.
2. American Thoracic Society and Infectious Diseases Society of America (2005) Guidelines for the management of adults with hospital-acquired, ventilator-associated, and healthcare-associated pneumonia. Am J Respir Crit Care Med 171: 388–416.
3. Melsen WG, Rovers MM, Groenwold RHH, Bergmans DCJJ, Camus C, et al (2013) Attributable mortality of ventilator-associated pneumonia: a meta-analysis of individual patient data from randomised prevention studies. Lancet Infect Dis 13: 665–71.

4. Bekaert M, Timsit JF, Vansteelandt S, Depuydt P, Vesin A, et al (2011) Attributable mortality of ventilator-associated pneumonia: a reappraisal using causal analysis. Am J Respir Crit Care Med 184: 1133–9.
5. Kollef MH, Hamilton CW, Ernst FR (2012) Economic impact of ventilator-associated pneumonia in a large matched cohort. Infect Control Hosp Epidemiol 33: 250–6.
6. Klompas M (2007) Does this patient have ventilator-associated pneumonia? JAMA 297: 1583–93.
7. Kollef MH (2012) Prevention of ventilator-associated pneumonia or ventilator-associated complications: a worthy, yet challenging, goal. Crit Care Med 40: 271–7.
8. Chastre J, Trouillet JL, Combes A, Luyt CE (2010) Diagnostic techniques and procedures for establishing the microbial etiology of ventilator-associated pneumonia for clinical trials: the pros for quantitative cultures. Clin Infect Dis 51 Suppl 1: S88–92.
9. Rea-Neto A, Youssef NC, Tuche F, Brunkhorst F, Ranieri VM, et al (2008) Diagnosis of ventilator-associated pneumonia: a systematic review of the literature. Crit Care 12: R56.
10. Lisboa T, Rello J (2008) Diagnosis of ventilator-associated pneumonia: is there a gold standard and a simple approach? Curr Opin Infect Dis 21: 174–8.
11. Gibot S, Cravoisy A, Levy B, Bene MC, Faure G, et al (2004) Soluble triggering receptor expressed on myeloid cells and the diagnosis of pneumonia. N Engl J Med 350: 451–8.
12. Gibot S, Cravoisy A, Dupays R, Barraud D, Nace L, et al (2007) Combined measurement of procalcitonin and soluble TREM-1 in the diagnosis of nosocomial sepsis. Scand J Infect Dis 39: 604–8.
13. Conway Morris A, Kefala K, Wilkinson TS, Moncayo-Nieto OL, Dhaliwal K, et al (2010) Diagnostic importance of pulmonary interleukin-1 beta and interleukin-8 in ventilator-associated pneumonia. Thorax 65: 201–7.
14. Anand NJ, Zuick S, Klesney-Tait J, Kollef MH (2009) Diagnostic implications of soluble triggering receptor expressed on myeloid cells-1 in BALF fluid of patients with pulmonary infiltrates in the ICU. Chest 135: 641–7.
15. Suetens C, Savey A, Labeeuw J, Morales I (2002) The ICU-HELICS programme: towards European surveillance of hospital-acquired infections in intensive care units. Euro Surveill 7: 127–8.
16. Conway Morris A, Kefala K, Simpson AJ, Wilkinson TS, Everingham K, et al (2009) Evaluation of the effect of diagnostic methodology on the reported incidence of ventilator-associated pneumonia. Thorax 64: 516–22.
17. Pugin J, Auckenthaler R, Mili N, Janssens JP, Lew PD, et al (1991) Diagnosis of ventilator-associated pneumonia by bacteriologic analysis of bronchoscopic and nonbronchoscopic "blind" bronchoalveolar lavage fluid. Am Rev Respir Dis 143: 1121–1129.
18. Luna CM, Blanzaco D, Niederman MS, Matarucco W, Baredes NC, et al (2003) Resolution of ventilator-associated pneumonia: prospective evaluation of the Clinical Pulmonary Infection Score as an early clinical predictor of outcome. Crit Care Med 31: 676–682.
19. Cohen J (1960) A coefficient of agreement for nominal scales. Educ Psychol Meas 20: 37–46.
20. Rennard SI, Basset G, Lecossier D, O'Donnell KM, Pinkston P, et al (1986) Estimation of volume of epithelial lining fluid recovered by lavage using urea as marker of dilution. J Appl Physiol 60: 532–8.
21. Beirne P, Pantelidis P, Charles P, Wells AU, Abraham DJ, et al (2009) Multiplex immune serum biomarker profiling in sarcoidosis and systemic sclerosis. Eur Resp J 34: 1376–82.
22. Picard R, Cook D (1984) Cross-Validation of Regression Models. J Am Stat Assoc 79 : 575–583.
23. Kohavi R (1995) A study of cross-validation and bootstrap for accuracy estimation and model selection. Proc of the Fourteenth Int Joint Conf on Art Intel 2: 1137–1143.
24. Efron B, Tibshirani R (1997) Improvements on cross-validation: The.632+ Bootstrap Method. J Am Stat Assoc 92: 548–560.
25. Chastre J, Fagon JY (2002) Ventilator-associated pneumonia. Am J Respir Crit Care Med 165: 867–903.
26. Leone M, Garcin F, Bouvenot J, Boyadjev I, Visintini P, et al (2007) Ventilator-associated pneumonia: breaking the vicious circle of antibiotic overuse. Crit Care Med 35: 379–385.
27. Gibot S, Massin F, Le Renard P, Bene MC, Faure GC, et al (2005) Surface and soluble triggering receptor expressed on myeloid cells-1: expression patterns in murine sepsis. Crit Care Med 33: 1787–93.
28. Richeldi L, Mariani M, Losi M, Maselli F, Corbetta L, et al (2004) Triggering receptor expressed on myeloid cells: role in the diagnosis of lung infections. Eur Respir J 24: 247–50.
29. Huh JW, Lim CM, Koh Y, Oh YM, Shim TS, et al (2008) Diagnostic utility of the soluble triggering receptor expressed on myeloid cells-1 in bronchoalveolar lavage fluid from patients with bilateral lung infiltrates. Crit Care 12: R6
30. Determann RM, Millo JL, Gibot S, Korevaar JC, Vroom MB, et al (2005) Serial changes in soluble triggering receptor expressed on myeloid cells in the lung during development of ventilator-associated pneumonia. Int Care Med 31: 1495–500.
31. Oudhuis GJ, Beuving J, Bergmans D, Stobberingh EE, ten Velde G, et al (2009) Soluble Triggering Receptor Expressed on Myeloid cells-1 in bronchoalveolar lavage fluid is not predictive for ventilator-associated pneumonia. Int Care Med 35: 1265–70.
32. Song Y, Lynch SV, Flanagan J, Zhuo H, Tom W, et al (2007) Increased plasminogen activator inhibitor-1 concentrations in bronchoalveolar lavage fluids are associated with increased mortality in a cohort of patients with Pseudomonas aeruginosa. Anesthesiology 106: 252–61.
33. Ramirez P, Kot P, Marti V, Gomez MD, Martinez R, et al (2011) Diagnostic implications of soluble triggering receptor expressed on myeloid cells-1 in patients with acute respiratory distress syndrome and abdominal diseases: a preliminary observational study. Crit Care 2011: R50.
34. Gibot S, Le Renard PE, Bollaert PE, Kolopp-Sarda MN, Bene MC, et al (2005) Surface triggering receptor expressed on myeloid cells 1 expression patterns in septic shock. Int Care Med 31: 594–7.
35. Knapp S, Gibot S, de Vos A, Versteeg HH, Colonna M, et al (2004) Cutting edge: expression patterns of surface and soluble triggering receptor expressed on myeloid cells-1 in human endotoxemia. J Immunol 173: 7131–4.
36. Bleharski JR, Kiessler V, Buonsanti C, Sieling PA, Stenger S, et al (2003) A role for triggering receptor expressed on myeloid cells-1 in host defense during the early-induced and adaptive phases of the immune response. J Immunol 170: 3812–8.
37. Bouchon A, Facchetti F, Weigand MA, Colonna M (2001) TREM-1 amplifies inflammation and is a crucial mediator of septic shock. Nature 410: 1103–7.
38. Millo JL, Schultz MJ, Williams C, Weverling GJ, Ringrose T et al (2004) Compartmentalisation of cytokines and cytokine inhibitors in ventilator-associated pneumonia. Int Care Med 30: 68–74.
39. Gomez-Pina V, Soares-Schanoski A, Rodriguez-Rojas A, Del Fresno C, Garcia F, et al (2007) Metalloproteinases shed TREM-1 ectodomain from lipopolysaccharide-stimulated human monocytes. J Immunol 179: 4065–73.
40. Hartog CM, Wermelt JA, Sommerfeld CO, Eichler W, Dalhoff K, et al (2003) Pulmonary matrix metalloproteinase excess in hospital-acquired pneumonia. Am J Respir Crit Care Med 167: 593–8.
41. Baselski V and Klutts JS (2013) Quantitative cultures of bronchoscopically obtained specimens should be performed for optimal management of Ventilator-Associated Pneumonia. J Clin Microbiol 51(3): 740–4.
42. Gibot S, Béné MC, Noel R, Massin F, Guy J, et al (2012) Combination biomarkers to diagnose sepsis in the critically ill patient. 186: 65–71.
43. Zethelius B, Berglund L, Sundstrom J, Ingelsson E, Basu S, et al (2008) Use of multiple biomarkers to improve the prediction of death from cardiovascular causes. N Engl J Med 358: 2107–2116.

Sheep Lung Segmental Delivery Strategy Demonstrates Adenovirus Priming of Local Lung Responses to Bacterial LPS and the Role of Elafin as a Response Modulator

Thomas I. Brown[1,2], David S. Collie[2,⁋,¶,*], Darren J. Shaw[2], Nina M. Rzechorzek[2], Jean-Michel Sallenave[1,⁋,¶,¤]

1 University of Edinburgh, Medical School, Edinburgh, Scotland, United Kingdom, 2 The Roslin Institute and R(D)SVS, The University of Edinburgh, Easter Bush Veterinary Centre, Roslin, Midlothian, United Kingdom

Abstract

Viral lung infections increase susceptibility to subsequent bacterial infection. We questioned whether local lung administration of recombinant adenoviral vectors in the sheep would alter the susceptibility of the lung to subsequent challenge with bacterial lipopolysaccharide (LPS). We further questioned whether local lung expression of elafin, a locally produced alarm anti-LPS/anti-bacterial molecule, would modulate the challenge response. We established that adenoviral vector treatment primed the lung for an enhanced response to bacterial LPS. Whereas this local effect appeared to be independent of the transgene used (Ad-o-elafin or Ad-GFP), Ad-o-elafin treated sheep demonstrated a more profound lymphopenia in response to local lung administration of LPS. The local influence of elafin in modulating the response to LPS was restricted to maintaining neutrophil myeloperoxidase activity, and levels of alveolar macrophage and neutrophil phagocytosis at higher levels post-LPS. Adenoviral vector-bacterial synergism exists in the ovine lung and elafin expression modulates such synergism both locally and systemically.

Editor: Jose Alejandro Chabalgoity, Facultad de Medicina, Uruguay

Funding: The authors acknowledge the Wellcome Trust (http://www.wellcome.ac.uk/) for funding this work (Clinical Research Training Award in Veterinary Medicine for T. Brown; 046712). The funders had no role in study design, data collection and analysis, decision to publish, or preparation of the manuscript.

Competing Interests: The authors have declared that no competing interests exist.

* Email: david.collie@ed.ac.uk

⁋ These authors contributed equally to this work.

¤ Current address: Inserm UMR1152, Physiopathologie et Epidémiologie des Maladies Respiratoires, Université Paris Diderot, Faculté de Médecine, site Bichat 16, Paris, France

¶ DSC and J-MS are joint senior authors on this work.

Introduction

Evidence from past flu pandemics indicates that secondary bacterial involvement frequently complicates primary viral lung infections and can extend to fatally compromise lung function [1,2]. Such viral-bacterial synergy is also observed in animals, particularly in domestic ruminants [3,4], and in pigs [5,6] where stress and viral respiratory infections commonly predispose towards secondary bacterial pneumonia. The specific nature of the mechanisms involved in enhancing the pathogenicity of what are often commensal bacteria is slowly being unravelled. Such mechanisms may include virus-induced epithelial damage exposing hidden bacterial binding sites [7,8], viruses altering alveolar macrophage [9–12] or polymorphonuclear [13,14] cell function, decreasing NK-cell activity [15] and/or increasing the production of either pro- or anti-inflammatory cytokines in a manner inappropriate to the clearance of the secondary bacterial infection.

Whilst lung-directed viral gene therapy offers the potential to treat or ameliorate a host of inflammatory, neoplastic and inherited lung diseases [16–19] the presence, nature and extent of any synergism that may exist between viruses and bacteria in the respiratory tract may impact on the safety of viral vectors in such a role. Whilst adenoviral vectors are commonly employed in clinical trials concern does exist that adverse effects may accompany their use [20–22]. Such effects may arise from the enhanced susceptibility to subsequent bacteria or LPS exposure [23]. Whilst this important phenomenon has been chiefly studied systemically, our own group has extended such studies to address whether potential exists for additive interactions between Ad-vectors and bacterial products at the local lung level. In this regard whilst we and others have shown no deleterious additive effect of Ad vectors in the context of bacterial and/or bacterial LPS instillation in murine lungs [24–27] the possible criticism, that extrapolating from such studies directly to man represents a tenuous assumption, drove us to consider the same issue in a large animal model system of arguably more potential relevance for pre-clinical validation of gene therapy protocols. We chose to evaluate these potential interactions and effects using the sheep as a model system. Our experience is that this system offers the advantage of studying local lung responses in relation to concomitant events elicited elsewhere in the lung and allows for the design of protocols wherein each animal serves as its own control [28–30]. In addition, the anatomy, physiology and immunological responsiveness of the respiratory system of sheep is more similar to humans than is that of rodents and the repertoire of Toll-like receptors (TLR) in sheep, which are pivotal in the initiation of the innate immune responses, show greater similarity to humans than do those of rodents [31]. Prior experience within our group has also demonstrated in mice that adenoviral expression of the anti-protease elafin is capable of augmenting lung innate immune responses to subsequent lipopolysaccharide (LPS)-mediated injury [25,26]. As mice do not normally carry a gene for elafin we considered the natural extension of such studies would be to explore the relevance of such observations in the sheep where elafin, in common with observations in people [32–36], behaves like a local acute phase reactant [36]. We and others have shown that this molecule is mainly produced at mucosal sites (including the lung) and have pleiotropic anti-microbial/immune-modulating properties in murine models of lung and intestinal inflammation (see Verrier et al (2012) [37] for a recent review).

We therefore used our previously characterised Ad-o-elafin vector [36] to address whether prior adenoviral mediated expression of ovine elafin would modulate subsequent innate immune responses to LPS.

Materials and Methods

All procedures were approved by the ethical review process of the University of Edinburgh and complied with the United Kingdom Animals (Scientific Procedures) Act 1986. The Ethical Review Committee of the University of Edinburgh reviewed and approved an application to the Home Office for a licence to carry out this research under the Act.

Adenoviral Constructs

A recombinant adenovirus encoding for the FLAG epitope tagged ovine elafin, (Trappin Ovine Molecule-1 (TOM-1)) cDNA (Ad-ovine elafin) was constructed as detailed elsewhere [36]. Ad expressing green fluorescent protein (Ad-GFP) was a kind gift from F. Graham and R. Marr, Department of Biology, McMaster University, Hamilton, Ontario, Canada. Both viruses were devoid of detectable LPS contamination (data not shown) and had very similar particles/plaque-forming unit (pfu) ratios (99 and 102, respectively).

ELISAs

A bovine tumor necrosis factor alpha (TNF-α) Screening Set (Endogen, Pierce Biotechnology, Inc., Rockford, IL, USA), used according to the manufacturer's instructions, established levels of TNF-α in bronchoalveolar lavage fluid (BALF) samples. A commercial ELISA kit for human pre-elafin/SKALP (Hycult Biotechnology b.v., AA Uden, The Netherlands) was used according to the manufacturer's instructions to determine elafin levels in BALF samples.

Production of Mannheimia haemolytica LPS

A 0.5 ml aliquot of M. haemolytica was inoculated into 50 ml of Nutrient Broth and incubated at 37°C overnight. 30 ml of this culture was then used to inoculate 3 litres of Nutrient Broth and incubated at 37°C for 18 hours in an orbital shaker at 100 rpm. The bacteria were then pelleted at 5000 g for 30 minutes and re-suspended in 50 ml of sterile distilled water. This suspension was then warmed to 68°C and an equal volume of 90% aqueous phenol at 68°C was added. The resultant mixture was maintained at 68°C for 10 minutes after which it was placed on ice to allow phase separation. After centrifugation at 5000 g for 30 minutes at 4°C, the upper aqueous phase was collected and dialysed for 36 hours against several changes of distilled water using Spectra/PorR dialysis tubing (3,500 molecular weight cut-off). The resultant solution was then lyophilized and diluted in sterile water to a final concentration of 150 µg/ml.

Animals

Sixteen commercially sourced crossbred sheep were used in this study. Animals were treated with anthelminthic prior to entry into the study. Freedom from unrelated pulmonary disease was subsequently confirmed at necropsy.

The sheep were anaesthetised and placed in a whole body plethysmograph as detailed elsewhere [29]. Briefly, each animal received 20 mg/kg body weight thiopentone sodium (Intraval sodium; Merial Animal Health Ltd., Harlow, Essex, UK) as a bolus after which the animals were intubated and maintained in a state of general anaesthesia by the use of 2–3% inhaled halothane in oxygen and nitrous oxide. The sheep were then placed in sternal recumbency in a plexiglass whole body negative pressure ventilator and ventilated via the endotracheal tube which was connected to the anaesthetic circuit via a junction in the wall of the plethysmograph. Extracorporeal pressure was varied via a bellows pump (Cuirass, Cape Road, Warwick, UK) allowing the maintenance of a sinusoidal tidal respiratory pattern. Tidal volume and end-tidal CO_2 were maintained at 10 ml/kg body weight and 4.5–5.5% respectively (CO_2 was measured using an Oxicap Monitor Model 4700, Ohmeda, Louisville).

Bronchoalveolar lavage

A flexible fibre-optic bronchoscope (5.3 mm OD)(Model FG-16X; Pentax U.K. Ltd.) was wedged in selected segmental bronchi. Two 20 ml aliquots of normal saline (0.9% NaCl solution) were used to collect BALF from selected lung segments. BALF samples were passed through sterile gauze into a sterile Falcon tube and immediately placed on ice until subsequent analysis.

BALF was spun at 400 g for seven minutes to separate out the cellular fraction. The resultant pellet was re-suspended in sterile phosphate-buffered saline (PBS) and the total cell number counted before subsequent preparation of cytospins for differential cytology. Supernatants were re-centrifuged at 1,000×g at 4°C for 20 min and stored at −70°C. Cells were counted using a Neubauer haemocytometer and values expressed per millilitre BALF. Cyto-centrifuge slides were prepared and stained using Diff Quick stain for differential counts on 500 cells. Cells were classified as neutrophils, macrophages, eosinophils, lymphocytes or mast cells according to standard morphological criteria.

Culture of BALF cells

Cells from BALF samples were plated out in 48 well tissue culture plates at 50,000 cells per well in RPMI containing 10% foetal calf serum (FCS), penicillin G (final concentration 100 U/ml), streptomycin sulphate (final concentration 100 µg/ml), L-glutamine (final concentration 2 µM) and amphotericin B (0.5%). After 6 hours non-adherent cells were washed off the wells and the adherent cells cultured for a further 7 days in fresh medium. Supernatants were then collected, spun at 13,000 rpm for 1 minute to remove cellular contamination, and stored at −30°C.

Optimisation of transfection efficiency in cultured alveolar macrophages

Adenovirus/calcium phosphate co-precipitates were formed by incubating, with gentle intermittent agitation, the specific amount of stock adenovirus solution (calculated to yield the requisite plaque-forming units (pfu)) with 1 ml of the freshly made calcium phosphate solution (2.14 µl 2.5 M $CaCl_2$ added per ml EMEM medium and vortexed well) at room temperature for 20 minutes before dilution to 5 ml with sterile PBS.

Cells from BALF samples were cultured in 24 well plates at a seeding density of 250,000 per well in RPMI containing 10% FCS, penicillin G (final concentration 100 U/ml), streptomycin sulphate (final concentration 100 ug/ml), L-glutamine (final concentration 2 uM) and amphotericin B (0.5%). After 6 hours non-adherent cells were washed off the wells and fresh medium added to each well.

Ad-GFP MOI (Multiplicity Of Infection = ratio of infectious virus particles to cells) 100 with or without calcium phosphate co-precipitation was applied to the cells for 20 minutes before removal and replacement of medium. 24 hours later the monolayers were photographed and infection efficiency assessed by visualisation of GFP using UV-microscopy.

Additionally, Ad-o-elafin was employed to transfect these cultures in a similar manner at MOIs of 100 and 200 both with and without co-precipitation. In this latter instance culture medium was collected after 4 days and elafin content assessed using Western blot analysis (see below).

Western blot analysis of cell culture supernatants

25 µl of supernatant along with known amounts of purified ovine elafin protein were reduced with 1% dithiothreitol and loaded on 4–12% gradient polyacrylamide gel using the Invitrogen NuPage gel system as recommended by the manufacturer. After running the gel proteins were transferred to Hybond ECL Nitrocellulose membrane (Amersham Pharmacia). Resultant membranes were blocked in 5% skimmed milk powder in TPBS (PBS and 0.1% Tween 20). Membranes were probed overnight at 4°C with Trab-2O monoclonal anti-elafin antibody (HyCult Biotechnology, Uden, the Netherlands) diluted 1 in 500–1000 in TPBS or anti-FLAG monoclonal antibody diluted 1 in 1000 in TPBS. Membranes were then washed in PBS-T before the secondary antibody was applied (Goat anti mouse IgG conjugated to HRP). This was followed by final washing, addition of Western LightningTM Chemiluminescent Reagent Plus (PerkinElmer Life Sciences, Inc.), and exposure to X-omat radiograph-quality film (Kodak).

Instillation of Adenovirus/calcium phosphate co-precipitates into the lung

A fibre-optic endoscope (5.3 mm OD) (Model FG-16X; Pentax U.K. Ltd.) was advanced and wedged in selected segmental bronchi. The adenovirus was diluted from stock solution into 5 ml sterile phosphate buffered saline (PBS) in order to achieve the required number of active particles (pfu). This 5 ml volume was then instilled into the segment, through a polyethylene catheter passed via the giving port of the endoscope. In order to direct each instillation towards the lung periphery the catheter (OD 1.6 mm) was advanced to the point of obstruction and its position retracted slightly before performing each instillation. Each instillation was performed in a carefully controlled manner in order to avoid flooding proximal to the tip of the endoscope and to facilitate dispersion of the instillate into the periphery of the subtended segment. Each instillation lasted approximately 30–60 seconds. At the end of the instillation air was allowed to enter the giving port of the endoscope to allow equilibration of pressures in the segment and the endoscope thereafter carefully withdrawn. No reflux of the adenovirus/PBS was observed.

Preliminary investigation of the use of adenoviral constructs in the sheep lung

Because calcium phosphate has been shown in other systems and mammals (mice, human) to improve Ad infections both in vitro and in vivo [38–40] two preliminary studies were conducted to firstly examine the benefits of this method with regards infection efficiency in the sheep (protocol 1) and secondly examine the duration of transgene expression following adenovirus-mediated gene delivery to the lung (protocol 2).

Protocol 1: One animal (MN (male neutered); Bodyweight (BW) 44 kg) was anaesthetised and instilled in one lung segment with 1×10^8 pfu Ad-GFP and in another lung segment with 1×10^8 pfu Ad-GFP co-precipitated with calcium phosphate. 48 hours after this infection the sheep was killed and cryosections were prepared from the two instilled segments and also a naive segment to allow visualisation of GFP-positive cells as described below.

48 hours after lung segmental instillation of Ad-GFP the animals were killed and the lungs removed and inflated for 2 hours with 4% paraformaldehyde at room temperature. The lungs were then rinsed twice with sterile PBS and inflated with 30% sucrose overnight at 4°C. Small representative portions of lung were carefully dissected and stored at 4°C in 30% sucrose. Small pieces of these portions were then mounted in optimal cutting temperature medium (OCT) and 10 µm sections cut and mounted on lysine- coated slides. The residual OCT was rinsed off with sterile PBS and then the slides were dipped in absolute alcohol to remove salts. The slides were subsequently dipped into 1 µg/ml DAPI (4',6-diamidino-2-phenylindole) in methanol for 2 seconds and then immediately dipped firstly into PBS and then into absolute ethanol before being air-dried. Cover slips were then affixed with DPX mounting fluid and GFP+ve cells counted by direct visualisation with UV-microscopy.

Protocol 2: Seven sheep (3 MN, 4F; BW 50 kg (median), range 32–58) were anaesthetised and each animal instilled with 1×10^8 pfu Ad-GFP with calcium phosphate (n = 7). After 3, 7 and 10 days these animals were anaesthetised and bronchoalveolar lavage fluid (BALF) collected from adenovirus instilled segments and also naïve segments in the contra-lateral lung to analyse alveolar macrophages for GFP expression.

Modulation of the local and systemic responses to bacterial LPS by the segmental administration of recombinant adenovirus

Three to four weeks prior to study commencement (Fig 1A), BALF was collected from eight female sheep (BW 35 kg (median), range 33–40) to confirm lung health status and provide baseline parameters with respect to the variables under study. Thereafter the sheep entered the experimental protocol as depicted in Fig 1 (B-D). The individual sheep were anaesthetised and each animal instilled with either 1×10^8 pfu Ad-GFP with calcium phosphate (n = 4) or 1×10^8 pfu Ad-o-elafin with calcium phosphate (n = 4). Virus was administered into one discrete lung segment of each animal. On day 10 after virus instillation M.haemolytica LPS (3 ml of a sterile solution in water at 150 µg/ml) was instilled into both a virus treated segment and a previously naïve segment in the contra-lateral lung. 6 hours after instillation of LPS the animals were re-anaesthetised and BALF recovered from both the LPS treated segments and also from a spatially distant 'new' naïve segment. The BALF samples were assessed for total and differential cell counts, phagocytosis assay, TNF-α and elafin content as detailed elsewhere.

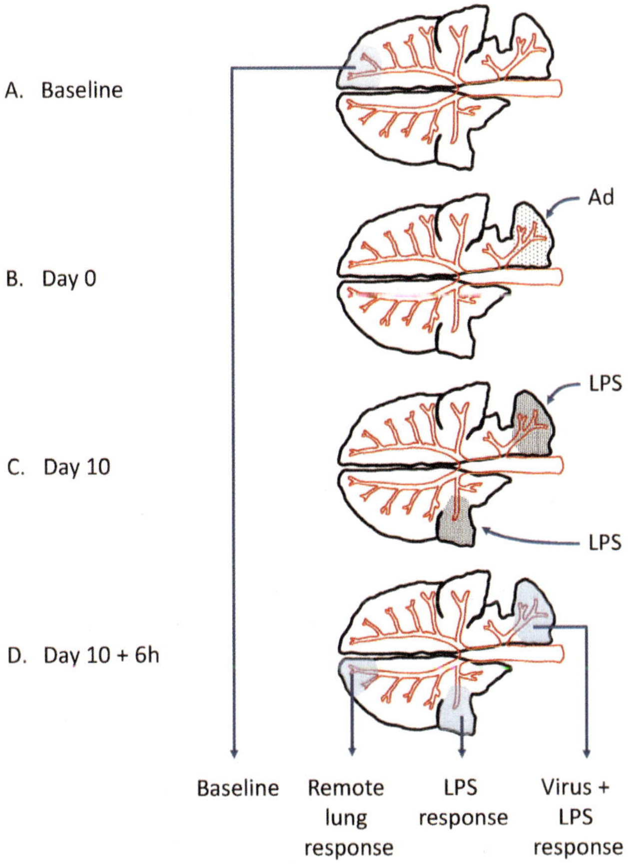

Figure 1. Experimental protocol for the examination of the effect of local up-regulation of ovine elafin on the response to bacterial LPS. A. Baseline sampling of BALF from a lung segment (3–4 weeks before the start of the experiment (day 0) B. Anaesthetised sheep were instilled on day 0 with either Ad-o-elafin-FLAG or Ad-GFP (as a control vector) co-precipitated with calcium phosphate in discrete lung segments. C. Ten days later, bacterial LPS was instilled into the same virus treated segments and also previously naïve segments (Pre-treatment blood samples were obtained immediately prior to anaesthetic induction on Day 10). D. 6 hours after LPS instillation, BALF was collected from these LPS treated segments and also a new 'remote lung' segment. The sample categories "Baseline", "Remote lung response", "LPS response" and "Virus + LPS response" correspond to the x-axes labels on the boxplots drawn in figure 6. In this design four samples of bronchoalveolar lavage fluid were derived, one sample obtained before any treatment was administered to the lung (Baseline), one sample derived from an area of the lung not subject to any direct treatment (Remote lung response) but obtained after treatments had been administered to other parts of the lung, and further samples from two areas of the lung, the first subject to direct treatment with LPS only (LPS response) and the second subject to treatment with LPS and adenoviral vector (Virus + LPS response).

Blood sampling

Jugular blood was collected by venepuncture into lithium heparin coated vacutainers for the subsequent analysis of total and differential cell counts by a haematology analyser (ABX Pentra 60; Horiba ABX, Montpelier, France).

Phagocytosis Assays

Opsonising E. coli. Four millilitres tetramethylrhodamine conjugated E. coli (E. coli (K-12 strain) BioParticlesR, Molecular Probes, Invitrogen, Paisley, UK) (1×10^7/ml) incubated with 400 ul heat inactivated serum at 37°C for 45 minutes, were spun at 800G for 15 minutes to form loose pellets. They were washed with RPMI, spun again twice and re-suspended in 4 ml serum-free RPMI to obtain a stock of approximately 10,000/µl which was kept on ice.

BALF Phagocytosis assay. 50,000 mobile cells were re-suspended into 100 µl RPMI to which 500,000 tetramethylrhodamine conjugated E. coli were added. Identical tubes were incubated on ice and at 37°C. After 20 and 30 minutes each tube was placed on ice and spun at 0°C for 5 minutes at 1300 rpm. Pellets were re-suspended in 500 µl of FACS Lyse solution, vigorously vortexed and incubated on ice for 10 minutes. Following a second spin, pellets were placed on ice and 100 µl trypan blue was added before a further spin and re-suspension in 300 µl RPMI for FACS analysis. Tubes incubated at 0°C served as controls for the test samples incubated at 37°C.

BALF Myeloperoxidase (MPO) Assay

BALF was spun at 13,000 rpm for 2 minutes and 50 µl added to a 96 well micro-titre assay plate. The MPO activity was determined using a tetramethylbenzidine substrate kit (ImmunoPure, Pierce, Rockford, IL). 100 µl tetramethylbenzidine substrate was added and the plate read by a plate reader at 405 nm with background of 560 nm. The reading was repeated after 10 minutes and the difference between the 2 readings gave a measure of MPO activity. MPO activity was related to the neutrophil count of the BALF sample and the data presented as a percentage change compared to pre-experimental data.

Statistical Analysis

Three to four weeks after initial baseline (Figure 1A) samples of BALF were obtained; three separate segments of the same lung were exposed to differing combinations of treatment regimes (no treatment, direct exposure to LPS, and direct exposure to virus). At a set interval after these treatments blood and BALF were again collected for analysis (Figure 1D). Blood samples were obtained prior to anaesthetic induction on Day 0 (baseline), Day 10 and on Day 10+6 hours).

Systemic Effect. A linear mixed-effect model, where sheep-specific responses were assumed a random effect, was used to analyse the influence of Ad-o-elafin and Ad-GFP and subsequent LPS instillation on blood parameters.

The time point (baseline, Day 10, Day 10+6 hours), treatment (Ad-o-elafin, Ad-GFP) and the interaction between the two were entered as fixed effects of interest. Lymphocyte data required log transformation prior to analysis in order to normalise the residuals. In all cases a $P<0.05$ was taken to indicate statistical significance.

Lung Effect. In addition to the obvious potential association between locally occurring phenomena arising as a direct consequence of locally administered treatments the potential also existed for such treatments to mediate influence on a whole-organ basis and this possibility was addressed through comparison with data obtained at baseline, prior to any treatments being given. As the data relating to the influence of Ad-o-elafin or Ad-GFP expression on LPS-induced local lung inflammation was nested in a hierarchical fashion the analysis was sub-divided into three components (Figure 1):

[i] Samples from un-instilled 'Remote lung' segments of the treated lung were compared to samples taken from segments at baseline;

[ii] Samples from un-instilled 'Remote lung' segments of the treated lung were compared to samples from lung segments that had been directly exposed to LPS;

[iii] Samples from treated lung segments that had been directly exposed to LPS were compared to samples from segments that had in addition previously been exposed to virus.

A generalised linear mixed-effect (GLME) model where the influence of sheep-specific responses was considered as a random effect was used as segments from the same sheep lung were being compared and the influence of two viruses being considered. For every component of the analysis, virus type, the particular analysis component and the interaction between the two were entered as fixed effects of interest. GLMEs with binomial errors were used for the proportion of AM, PMN and lymphocytes in BALF data, with standard GLMEs used for the other parameters. Total cell counts, AM phagocytosis, BALF Elafin, BALF MPO activity, and BALF TNF-α data required log transformation prior to analysis in order to normalise the residuals. In all cases a $P<0.05$ was taken to indicate statistical significance.

Results

Optimisation of transfection efficiency in cultured alveolar macrophages

The results of the *in vitro* experiments demonstrated that calcium phosphate up-regulates the infection efficiency of alveolar macrophages'. **Figures 2a and 2b** show the increased infection efficiency of alveolar macrophages by the incorporation of Ad-GFP in a calcium phosphate precipitate. The use of calcium phosphate increased both the number of macrophages infected and the intensity of fluorescence per infected cell. Similarly, **figure 2c** shows that the infection of alveolar macrophages with Ad-o-elafin-FLAG in conjunction with calcium phosphate increases the secretion of ovine elafin.

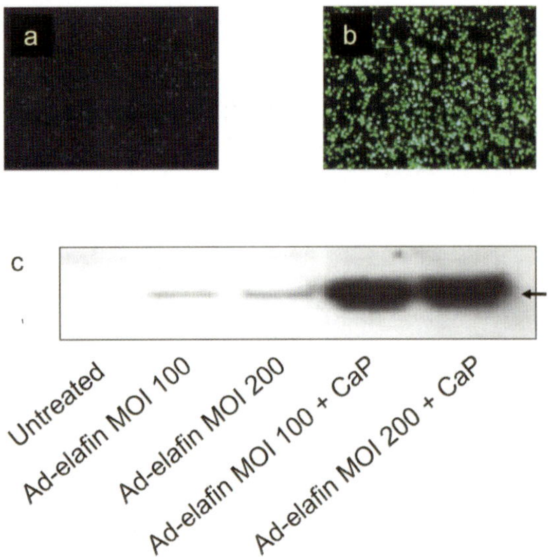

Figure 2. Incorporation of adenovirus into calcium phosphate precipitate increases the infection efficiency of alveolar macrophages in vitro. Ovine alveolar macrophages were cultured at a density of 250,000 per well in 48 well plates and were infected with Ad-GFP and Ad-o-elafin-FLAG at MOI 100 or 200 either pre-complexed with calcium phosphate or as virus alone. (a) – Ovine alveolar macrophages 24 hours after infection with Ad-GFP MOI 100 alone. (b) – Ovine alveolar macrophages 24 hours after infection withAd-GFP MOI 100/calcium phosphate co-precipitate. (c) – Western blot analysis of ovine alveolar macrophage supernatant using Trab-2O antibody 4 days after infection with Ad-o-elafin-FLAG at MOI 100 and 200 either with or without coprecipitation with calcium phosphate. Uninfected alveolar macrophage supernatant is included as a control.

Preliminary investigation of the use of adenoviral constructs in the sheep lung

In vivo instillation of Ad-GFP incorporated into a calcium phosphate precipitate (see protocol 1, Materials and Methods) led to the increased infection of both alveolar epithelial cells and alveolar macrophages, 48 hrs later, when compared to the instillation of Ad-GFP alone as seen in **figure 3a and 3b**.

This led us to use this calcium phosphate protocol for the kinetic experiment: GFP positive alveolar macrophages recovered from instilled segments 3, 7 and 10 days after Ad-GFP administration decreased in number with time as shown in **figure 4** (see protocol 2, Materials and methods). At no time point were any GFP+ve cells recovered from any naïve segments. Alveolar macrophages

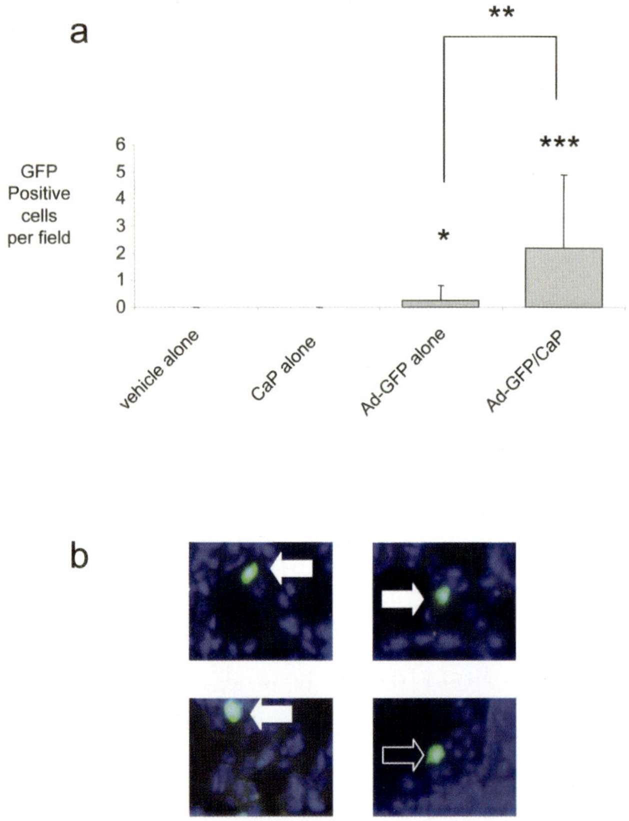

Figure 3. Incorporation of adenovirus into calcium phosphate precipitate increases the infection efficiency of alveolar macrophages and pulmonary respiratory epithelium in vivo. Cryo-sections were prepared from lung tissue 48 hours after instillation of vehicle, vehicle and calcium phosphate, 1×10^8 pfu Ad-GFP in PBS or 1×10^8 pfu Ad-GFP after pre-incubation with calcium phosphate. 24 random fields were counted at high power using UV light and the number of GFP+ve cells recorded. (a) – The number of GFP+ve cells is represented here as mean with error bars indicating standard deviation. *, ** and *** indicate $P<0.05$, $P<0.005$ and $P<0.0005$ respectively either comparing values to relevant control (i.e. vehicle alone or vehicle with calcium phosphate) or comparing virus treatment with and without calcium phosphate (indicated by a bar). Significance was calculated by non-paired T Test. (b) – Representative fields from the Ad-GFP/calcium phosphate segment showing infection of Type II epithelial cells (filled arrows) and an alveolar macrophage in an airway (open arrow). Counterstaining of nuclei is with DAPI.

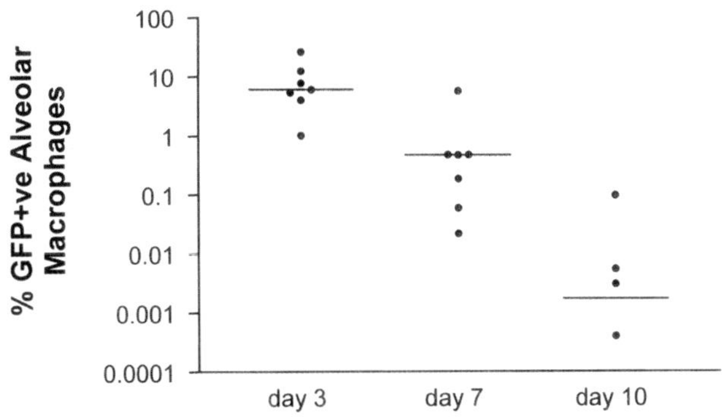

Figure 4. Transgene expression in alveolar macrophages is restricted to the segment infected with adenoviral vector. Alveolar macrophages were collected on day 3, 7 and 10 from sheep infected on day 0 with Ad-GFP/calcium phosphate from both segments infected with adenovirus and from naïve segments and assessed for GFP by UV microscopy after 24 hours in culture. Data is shown as scatter plots with the horizontal bars indicating the median. Macrophages from Ad-GFP infected segments on day 14 were negative for GFP. No GFP+ve macrophages were identified in BALF from any naïve segments at any time point (data not shown). NB Zero values are not shown due to the use of a log scale.

harvested at the same time points and sustained in culture for 7d indicate expression of Ad-o-elafin up to 10 days after instillation (data not shown).

Modulation of the local and systemic responses to bacterial LPS by the segmental administration of recombinant adenovirus

We, and others, have employed models whereby different treatments are applied to separate lung segments in order to study local lung responses. These models have hitherto proved valuable in the context of defining, at functional, cellular and immune levels, the local lung response to antigen challenge in both experimental animals and in man. Wherein responses can be considered local such an approach allows each animal to serve as its own control, thus reducing the extent of inter-animal variability associated with whole lung studies. Typically such studies have been interpreted through paired (within-subject) or un-paired comparisons between segments. The significant caveat to interpreting such studies arises when the possibility exists that a local treatment could exert an influence across the whole organ, or indeed systemically. In such circumstance, a simple comparison between treated and control segments may fail to demonstrate an effect, not because the treatment has no effect, but because the same influence extends to affect both areas of the lung in the same manner. The experimental design employed in this study (see Fig 1) whereby the viral vector-primed influence on a subsequent local lung response to LPS was the focus, carried this potential, and for this reason we obtained baseline samples and incorporated an overall 'remote lung response' effect as the first level of nesting in the analysis. In this way we were able to separate any potential whole-organ effects occurring as a consequence of locally instilled lung treatments from true local effects.

An interval of 10 days elapsed between treatment with the viral vectors and instillation of LPS. Our selection of this interval was influenced by observations in relation to natural and experimentally induced lung disease. Whilst shorter intervals have been employed in sheep to experimentally induce lung disease 5d after exposure to adenovirus [41], other experimental studies in ruminants indicate that viral-bacterial synergism occurs over at least 30-days [42] and naturally occurring outbreaks of pneumonic pasteurellosis in sheep usually occur 10–14 days after a stress [43].

Systemic effect. There were statistically significant differences in total white blood cells between the time points ($P = 0.011$, **Fig. 5a**). In sheep treated with Ad-o-elafin, relative to baseline total white blood cell counts, statistically significant reductions in total white blood cells occurred six hours after the administration of LPS (Day10 +6 hours, $P = 0.004$, **Fig. 5a**). Total white blood cell counts at this time point were also significantly lower than counts at the Day10 time point measured just before the addition of LPS ($P = 0.027$).

There was also a statistically significant interaction between time point and which virus (Ad-GFP or Ad-o-elafin) had been used ($P = 0.030$), with an observed reduction in total white blood cell counts in response to LPS at Day 10+6 hours compared to Day 10 in Ad-o-elafin treated sheep, but an increase in sheep treated with Ad-GFP (**Fig. 5a**).

There were also statistically significant differences in neutrophils between timepoints ($P = 0.008$, **Fig. 5b**), with increases in neutrophil numbers in response to LPS (Day 10+6 hours relative to Day 10) apparent for both Ad-o-elafin and Ad-GFP treated sheep ($P = 0.042$, 0.018, respectively, **Fig. 5b**). Day 10 neutrophil levels in Ad-o-elafin were also significantly lower than pre-treatment levels ($P = 0.047$, **Fig. 5b**).

Finally, statistically significant differences in lymphocyte numbers between time points occurred ($P < 0.001$, **Fig. 5c**), with pre-treatment levels higher than Day 10+6 hours in both Ad-o-elafin ($P < 0.001$) and Ad-GFP ($P = 0.036$) treated sheep (**Fig. 5c**). In addition, Day 10 levels in Ad-o-elafin were higher than Day 10+6 hours ($P < 0.001$). There was also a statistically significant interaction between time point and treatment ($P = 0.017$) with a larger decline in lymphocyte numbers in response to LPS (Day 10+6 hours relative to Day 10) being apparent for sheep treated with Ad-o-elafin than for Ad-GFP (**Fig. 5c**).

Lung Effect. The potential for the various treatments to have a 'global' or 'whole organ' effect and thereby influence the variables under study was assessed by comparing data from the control "Remote lung response" segments of the treated lungs to baseline data from separate segments obtained prior to any treatments being administered. A statistically significant increase in total cell counts ($P = 0.025$; **Fig. 6a** [i]) and MPO activity ($P = 0.040$; **Fig. 6h** [i]) and decrease in the proportion of BALF lymphocytes ($P = 0.026$; **Fig. 6f** [i]) occurred in Remote lung response segments relative to baseline. No other statistically significant differences in any other parameter occurred in Remote lung response segments relative to baseline as a consequence of treatment ($P > 0.070$). The nature of the virus used (Ad-o-elafin or Ad-GFP) had no statistically significant effect on any of the parameters, whether in relation to absolute values ($P > 0.131$), or the magnitude of response occurring as a consequence of lung treatment ($P > 0.069$).

Relative to remote lung response segments - exposing segments to LPS resulted in statistically significantly increased total cell counts ($P = 0.011$; **Fig. 6a** [ii]), BALF elafin ($P = 0.042$; **Fig. 6g** [ii]), and proportion of PMN ($P < 0.001$; **Fig. 6e** [ii]), but decreased AM phagocytosis ($P = 0.002$; **Fig. 6b** [ii]), BALF MPO activity ($P = 0.037$; **Fig. 6h** [ii]) and proportion of AM ($P < 0.001$; **Fig. 6d** [ii]).

Exposing segments to LPS did not significantly influence PMN phagocytosis, the proportion of lymphocytes or amount of TNF-α present in BALF ($P > 0.070$, **Figs. 6c, 6f and 6i** [ii]). The nature of the virus used (Ad-o-elafin or Ad-GFP) had no statistically significant effect on any of the parameters, whether in relation to

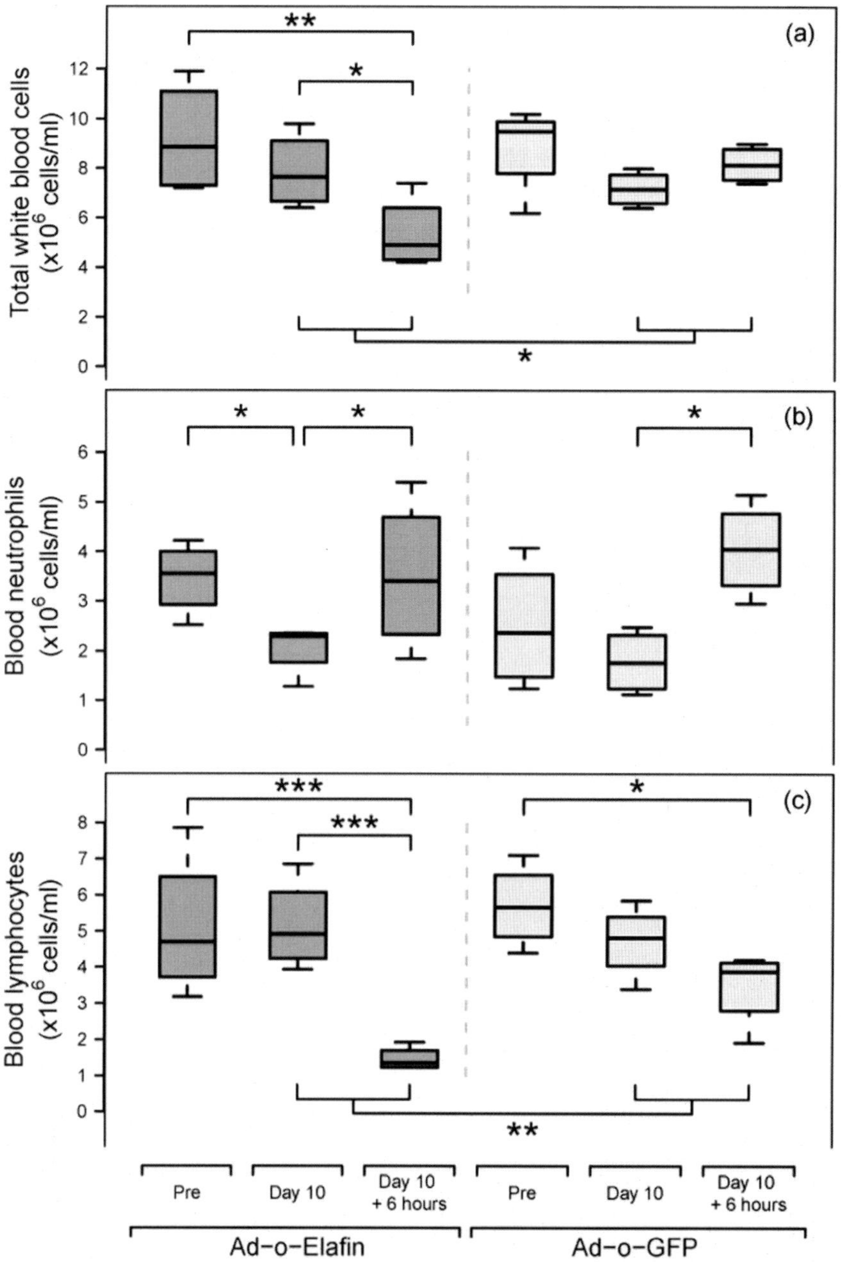

Figure 5. Systemic haematological responses to intrapulmonary adenoviral vector and LPS administration. Heparinised blood was collected by venepuncture at various time points throughout the experimental period (Pre-treatment (immediately prior to collection of baseline BALF samples), d10 and d10+6h). This blood was analysed for total white blood cell numbers, neutrophil numbers and lymphocyte numbers as indicated in a, b and c respectively. The boxplot tails reflect the range of data, the bottom and tops of the boxes the 25th and 75th percentiles respectively, and the thick horizontal line the median values. A linear mixed-effect model, where sheep-specific responses were assumed a random effect, was used to analyse the influence of Ad-o-elafin and Ad-GFP and subsequent LPS instillation on blood parameters. *, ** and *** represent $P<0.05$ and $P<0.01$ and $P<0.001$ respectively.

absolute values ($P>0.054$), or the magnitude of response occurring as a consequence of LPS treatment ($P>0.060$).

Exposing segments to virus statistically significantly altered the response of those segments to subsequent administration of LPS. This change took the form of increased total cell counts ($P<0.001$; **Fig. 6a** [iii]), BALF elafin ($P=0.004$; **Fig. 6g** [iii]), BALF TNF-α ($P<0.001$; **Fig. 6i** [iii]) and proportion of PMN ($P=0.004$; **Fig. 6e** [iii]), but decreased BALF MPO activity ($P=0.036$; **Fig. 6h** [iii]) and proportion of AM ($P=0.003$; **Fig. 6d** [iii]) as a consequence of LPS exposure. Prior exposure of segments to virus did not statistically significantly influence the extent of LPS-induced reduction in AM phagocytosis, nor influenced the observed lack of effect of LPS on PMN phagocytosis or the proportion of lymphocytes in BALF ($P>0.116$; **Figs. 6b, 6c and 6e** [iii]).

The nature of the virus used did appear to significantly impact on the response to LPS. The aforementioned virus-primed LPS-induced decrease in BALF MPO activity resulted in levels that

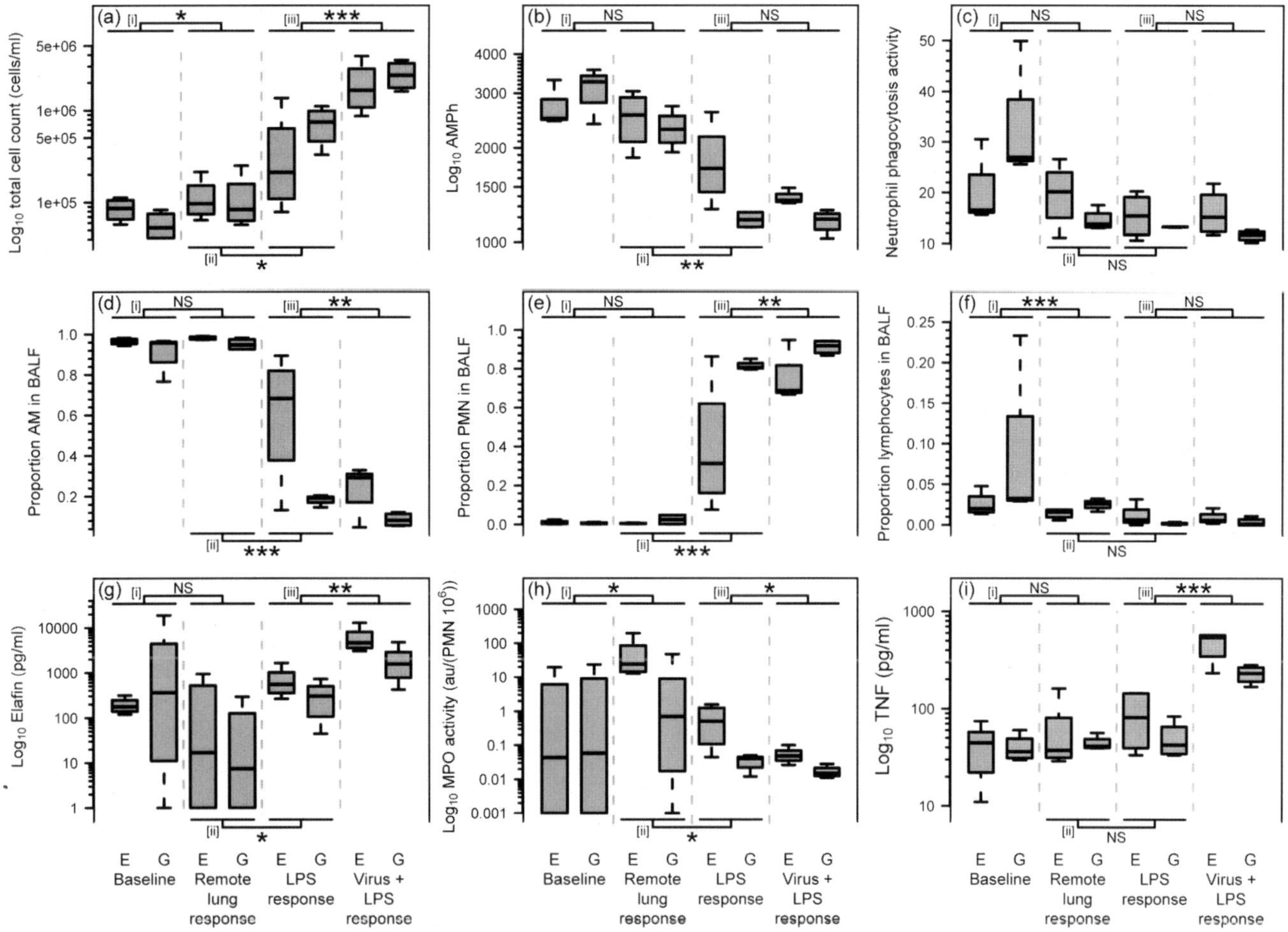

Figure 6. Local lung response to the instillation of adenoviral vectors and/or LPS. Boxplots depicting the (a) log10 Total cell counts (cells/ml); (b) Alveolar macrophage phagocytic activity (AMPh) (geometric mean fluorescence units); (c) neutrophil phagocytic activity activity (geometric mean fluorescence units); (d) proportion of AM in BALF; (e) proportion of PMN in BALF; (f) proportion of lymphocytes in BALF; (g) log10 Elafin (pg/ml); (h) log10 MPO activity (absorbance units (au)/PMN * 10^6); and (i) log10 TNF-α (pg/ml) data arising from analysis of BALF sampled from differentially treated lung segments of sheep exposed to either Ad-o-elafin (Virus E) or Ad-GFP (Virus G). The boxplot tails reflect the range of data, the bottom and tops of the boxes the 25th and 75th percentiles respectively, and the thick horizontal line the median values. The first pair of boxplots adjacent to the Y-axis reflect baseline data collected before lungs were exposed to treatment (Baseline). The next adjacent pair of boxplots depict data collected from non-treated control lung segments after other segments in the same lung had received different treatment regimes (Remote lung response). The third pair of boxplots reflect data collected from lung segments exposed to LPS six hours previously (LPS response). The last pair of boxplots reflect data collected from segments that had, in addition to LPS treatment six hours previously, been treated with adenoviral vectors ten days before, (Virus + LPS response). The results of statistical comparisons [i]-[iii] between these nested data sets are depicted by the interconnected horizontal lines above and below each separate graph (NS = no significant difference, *, ** & *** = $P<0.05$, 0.01 and 0.001 respectively). The bold font is simply used to emphasise the boxplot pairs across which the above statistical comparisons are directed. Whilst not explicitly annotated in this figure the virus-primed LPS-induced decrease in BALF MPO activity (6h) resulted in levels that were significantly greater for segments exposed to Ad-o-elafin ($P = 0.016$) when compared to segments treated with Ad-GFP, and levels of AM (6b) and PMN (6c) phagocytosis after LPS were significantly increased in segments exposed to Ad-o-elafin when compared to Ad-GFP ($P<0.023$).

were significantly greater for segments exposed to Ad-o-elafin ($P = 0.016$, **Fig. 6h**) when compared to segments treated with Ad-GFP.

In addition, whilst prior exposure of segments to virus did not appear to significantly influence the extent of LPS-induced reduction in AM phagocytosis nor influence the observed lack of effect of LPS on PMN phagocytosis, levels of AM and PMN phagocytosis after LPS were significantly increased in segments exposed to Ad-o-elafin when compared to Ad-GFP ($P<0.023$; **Figs. 6b, c**).

The nature of the virus used did not significantly impact on the post-LPS levels of any of the other parameters under study ($P> 0.053$), and neither were there any other statistically significant interaction demonstrable between virus type and the magnitude of the LPS-induced response ($P>0.100$).

Discussion

Whilst the concept of prior exposure to virus priming the innate immune response to subsequent bacterial products is widely acknowledged [5,6] this is less well established in the specific case of adenoviruses where the potential mechanisms involved in such priming are largely open to speculation. Regardless of any potential long-term influence, the short term effects of treatment with adenoviral vectors are likely to include the induction of inflammatory and immune responses. As well described [20,44,45], innate mechanisms initiate from recognition of pathogen-associated molecular patterns leading to signalling cascades and the expression of pro-inflammatory cytokines, type I interferons and activation of innate and adaptive immunity. Indeed, recent studies have shown that a critical aspect of the murine immune response to adenoviral vectors was the expression of adenoviral type I interferons with mechanisms of in vitro induction mediated by either TLR9 in plasmacytoid dendritic cells (DCs) or cytosolic detection of adenoviral DNA in non-plasmacytoid DCs [44]. Also, TLR-independent mechanisms of adenovirus recognition and type I interferon secretion have been described in splenic myeloid DCs, following in vivo systemic Ad administration [46]. Depending on the cell type, the signalling cascades include the induction of MAPK pathways, NFkB and ICAM-1 gene expression [20,44,45,47] as well as the SAPK/JNK pathway [46]. As many of the intracellular pathways are also used by key cytokines responding as part of the innate immune response the opportunity exists for interplay and interaction within cells responding to LPS and previous adenoviral exposure [48]. Indeed, recently, Fejer et al have shown that systemically- administered Ad vectors lead to LPS hypersensitivity via IFN-γ and epigenetic changes at the TNF-α promoter [46]. Whilst these observations merit further study with respect to identifying whether organ-specific mechanisms operate in murine systems we and others have previously shown that such Ad vector-evoked hypersensitivity may not operate in the context of lung bacterial infection or LPS administration [24–26,49]. To address this issue in an animal model more relevant to pre-clinical studies, we have chosen the sheep, a model amenable to a lung segmental approach to potentially differentiate between local and systemic effects.

Our data indicate that precipitating adenovirus with calcium phosphate is, as in other systems described in the literature, an effective method of optimising transfection efficiency in the sheep, particularly in alveolar macrophages, but also in alveolar epithelial cells (**Figs. 2 and 3**). That this optimisation strategy was not associated with any increase in inflammation or cytotoxicity over adenovirus alone was also confirmed (data not shown). We saw no evidence for infection of airway epithelial cells (**Fig. 3b**). This observation contrasts with those of Fasbender et al. [38] who demonstrated that the incorporation of Ad into a calcium phosphate precipitate markedly enhanced the efficiency of gene transfer to airway epithelia both in vitro and in vivo, in mice. Whether this contrast in targeting reflects delivery issues, or species-specific promoter tropisms remains unknown.

Adenoviral dose selection in this study was based on previous unpublished data (Brown, T.I. (2005) Anti-protease gene therapy in the lung. PhD thesis. University of Edinburgh) which indicated that at the dose used in this study (1×10^8 pfu Ad co-precipitated with calcium phosphate), only very local minor inflammation was elicited (PMNs <9% @ 48h) and was expected to resolve rapidly such that no long-term overt inflammatory sequelae would impact on the subsequent response to LPS in the treated segments ten days later. Clearly however, such a strategy will be insensitive to changes elicited at a molecular level and it would be naïve to assume that lack of influence at a phenotypic level would be a robust indicator of true 'lack of effect'.

Indeed, we establish here that previous exposure to an adenoviral vector per se potentiates the local lung inflammatory (TCC, PMN%, elafin & TNF-α levels) response to LPS (**Figs. 6a, 6e, 6g and 6i** [iii]). It should be noted, that although, the Trab-2O anti-elafin antibody does not discriminate endogenous from Ad-produced ovine elafin, we previously confirmed that lung Ad-instillation induces very little inflammation *per se* at the dose used in these experiments (data not shown). The increase in o-elafin production between the 'LPS response' and the 'Virus + LPS' arms of the experiment likely reflects the influence of LPS on the Ad-o-elafin construct and is in keeping with our reported findings (see ref 25 herein) that LPS up-regulates Ad-derived transgenes through up-regulating NF-kB (NF-kB responsive sequences are present in the MCMV promoter).

In addition, the decline in the MPO/PMN ratio occurring as a consequence of LPS treatment was more marked for segments previously treated with virus (**Fig. 6h** [iii]). Whilst seemingly at variance with the potentiated inflammatory response, it is conceivable that reduced MPO levels relative to PMN numbers may indicate the recruitment of immature neutrophil precursors into the lung, functionally altered cells, or the accumulation of degranulated but not yet apoptotic neutrophils.

Paralleling our observation, are the data showing that prior infection with RSV resulted in higher bacterial burden in the lungs of mice exposed a week later to Streptococcus pneumonia [13]. That this occurred in the face of a significantly greater influx of inflammatory cells was potentially explained by the finding that recruited neutrophils were functionally altered in containing less myeloperoxidase [13].

Whilst the nature of the virus (Ad-GFP or Ad-o-elafin) used did not significantly influence the PMN influx as a consequence of LPS treatment it would appear that a trend did exist for a greater influx in Ad-GFP treated sheep (**Fig. 6e** [ii]). Taken together with the previous observation it is conceivable that this again reflects a differential response with respect to neutrophil maturity. In that context, the specific influence of Ad-o-elafin in relation to BALF PMN MPO activity suggests that elafin is helping to maintain enzyme activity in these cells after exposure to LPS (**Fig. 6h** [ii]).

Similarly, elafin also had a protective effect in relation to alveolar macrophage phagocytic capacity that occurred as a consequence of LPS exposure (**Fig. 6b**). The influence of LPS in reducing the phagocytic capacity of alveolar macrophages was not dependent on whether the segment had previously been treated with virus. Whilst at variance with some reports suggesting that LPS either fails to influence macrophage function or improves it [50] our data is in agreement with the broader consensus that sepsis leads to impaired alveolar macrophage function [51].

Lymphopenia (two-fold reduction) and neutrophilia (four-fold increase) are commonly observed 6h after local lung instillation of E.coli LPS in sheep (DDSC data not published). Whilst it was anticipated that the low numbers of sheep involved in this study would preclude demonstration of any significant effect in this regard our data indicate a profound and significant five-fold reduction in circulating lymphocytes in only the elafin-treated animals. Indeed this reduction is the major influence behind the significant reduction in total white blood cell numbers occurring in response to local lung administration of LPS (**Fig. 5**). As blood lymphocyte numbers are maintained by recirculation through secondary lymphoid organs the possibility exists that local lung expression of elafin enhances the sequestration of lymphocytes in response to a local lung inflammation or recruits progenitors from the bone marrow and induces their differentiation and recruitment. These data, obtained in the sheep, potentially share a link with our own data obtained in mice, where we showed that over-expression of Ad-elafin in the lungs of mice had an adjuvant effect in a vaccination protocol [52].

The marginal though significant increase in the total cell number and reduced proportion of lymphocytes in BALF, and the increased MPO activity in remote lung segments relative to baseline (**Figs. 6a, 6f and 6h** [i]) indicate that systemic and/or whole organ effects have arisen as a consequence of the treatment regimes applied elsewhere in the lung. Certainly the aforementioned systemic lymphopenia parallels this observation and hints at the possibility that lymphocytes are being selectively sequestrated elsewhere. Whether, and to what extent, the observed remote lung response reflects systemic, whole organ, and/or spillover effects cannot be definitively established in this analysis. However, if spillover of LPS from treated to remote lung segments did occur then it would be reasonable to expect the nature of the remote lung response to be qualitatively similar to that seen in response to LPS instillation. This is not the case, as LPS instillation caused a significant decrease in BALF MPO activity, whereas the remote response was associated with a significant increase in this variable relative to baseline levels.

Taken together, in this sheep model, our results indicate that infection with an adenoviral vector appears to potentiate the inflammatory response to subsequent challenge with LPS.

Whilst the benefits of such augmentation in relation to handling subsequent bacterial infection are unknown in this model the suspicion is raised that adenoviral infection per se may have a negative influence in this regard through interfering with neutrophil function and phagocytic capacity. In contrast, Ad-o-elafin treated sheep restored neutrophil MPO activity and levels of AM and PMN phagocytosis at higher levels post LPS, compared to Ad-control treated animals. This newly described opsonic activity provides further evidence for the potential utility of elafin both as a local anti-LPS/antibacterial agent at mucosal surfaces and also as an influence in shaping adaptive immunity at a systemic level, by mobilising lymphocytes into the general circulation.

Lastly, our strategy of adopting a lung segmental approach to study design and the careful adoption of rigorous statistical method has demonstrated the feasibility of addressing relatively complex issues using a limited number of experimental animals. Such approaches, which are increasingly represented in the respiratory literature, clearly uphold the principles of reduction and refinement in research involving animals and indicate considerable potential for future strategic application.

Acknowledgments

We are grateful to Alison Baker, and Peter Tennant for technical assistance and to the animal care staff at Easter Bush Veterinary Centre for their assistance. The authors declare no conflict of interest.

Author Contributions

Conceived and designed the experiments: DSC TIB DS NMR J-MS. Performed the experiments: DSC TIB NMR. Contributed reagents/materials/analysis tools: DSC TIB DS NMR J-MS. Contributed to the writing of the manuscript: DSC TIB DS NMR J-MS.

References

1. Abrahams A, Hallows N, French H (1919) Influenzo-pneumococcal and influenzo-streptococcal septicemia: Epidemic influenzal "pneumonia of highly fatal type and its relation to "purulent bronchitis.". Lancet 1: 1–11.
2. Schwarzmann SW, Adler JL, Sullivan RJ, Jr., Marine WM (1971) Bacterial pneumonia during the Hong Kong influenza epidemic of 1968–1969. ArchInternMed 127: 1037–1041.
3. Brogden KA, Lehmkuhl HD, Cutlip RC (1998) Pasteurella haemolytica complicated respiratory infections in sheep and goats. VetRes 29: 233–254.
4. Hodgson PD, Aich P, Manuja A, Hokamp K, Roche FM, et al. (2005) Effect of stress on viral-bacterial synergy in bovine respiratory disease: novel mechanisms to regulate inflammation. Comparative and Functional Genomics 6: 244–250.
5. van GS, van RK, Pensaert M (2003) Interaction between porcine reproductive-respiratory syndrome virus and bacterial endotoxin in the lungs of pigs: potentiation of cytokine production and respiratory disease. JClinMicrobiol 41: 960–966.
6. Labarque G, van RK, van GS, Nauwynck H, Pensaert M (2002) Porcine reproductive-respiratory syndrome virus infection predisposes pigs for respiratory signs upon exposure to bacterial lipopolysaccharide. VetMicrobiol 88: 1–12.
7. Hakansson A, Kidd A, Wadell G, Sabharwal H, Svanborg C (1994) Adenovirus infection enhances in vitro adherence of Streptococcus pneumoniae. InfectImmun 62: 2707–2714.
8. Hers JF, Masurel N, Mulder J (1958) Bacteriology and histopathology of the respiratory tract and lungs in fatal Asian influenza. Lancet 2: 1141–1143.
9. Chang HW, Jeng CR, Lin TL, Liu JJ, Chiou MT, et al. (2006) Immunopathological effects of porcine circovirus type 2 (PCV2) on swine alveolar macrophages by in vitro inoculation. Veterinary Immunology and Immunopathology 110: 207–219.
10. Welsh MD, Adair BM, Foster JC (1995) Effect of BVD virus infection on alveolar macrophage functions. Veterinary Immunology and Immunopathology 46: 195–210.
11. Franke-Ullmann G, Pfortner C, Walter P, Steinmuller C, Lohmann-Matthes ML, et al. (1995) Alteration of pulmonary macrophage function by respiratory syncytial virus infection in vitro. Journal of Immunology 154: 268–280.
12. Nickerson CL, Jakab GJ (1990) Pulmonary antibacterial defenses during mild and severe influenza virus infection. InfectImmun 58: 2809–2814.
13. Stark JM, Stark MA, Colasurdo GN, LeVine AM (2006) Decreased bacterial clearance from the lungs of mice following primary respiratory syncytial virus infection. JMedVirol 78: 829–838.
14. Seki M, Higashiyama Y, Tomono K, Yanagihara K, Ohno H, et al. (2004) Acute infection with influenza virus enhances susceptibility to fatal pneumonia following Streptococcus pneumoniae infection in mice with chronic pulmonary colonization with Pseudomonas aeruginosa. ClinExpImmunol 137: 35–40.
15. Tripp RA, Moore D, Jones L, Sullender W, Winter J, et al. (1999) Respiratory syncytial virus G and/or SH protein alters Th1 cytokines, natural killer cells, and neutrophils responding to pulmonary infection in BALB/c mice. JVirol 73: 7099–7107.
16. Driskell RA, Engelhardt JF (2003) Current status of gene therapy for inherited lung diseases. AnnuRevPhysiol 65: 585–612.
17. Albelda SM, Wiewrodt R, Zuckerman JB (2000) Gene therapy for lung disease: hype or hope? AnnInternMed 132: 649–660.
18. Sallenave JM, Porteous DJ, Haslett C (1997) Gene therapy for lung inflammatory diseases: not so far away? Thorax 52: 742–744.
19. Curiel DT, Pilewski JM, Albelda SM (1996) Gene therapy approaches for inherited and acquired lung diseases. [Review] [211 refs]. American Journal of Respiratory Cell & Molecular Biology 14: 1–18.
20. Muruve DA (2004) The innate immune response to adenovirus vectors. HumGene Ther 15: 1157–1166.
21. Raper SE, Chirmule N, Lee FS, Wivel NA, Bagg A, et al. (2003) Fatal systemic inflammatory response syndrome in a ornithine transcarbamylase deficient patient following adenoviral gene transfer. MolGenetMetab 80: 148–158.
22. Shayakhmetov DM, Li ZY, Ni S, Lieber A (2005) Interference with the IL-1-signaling pathway improves the toxicity profile of systemically applied adenovirus vectors. Journal of Immunology 174: 7310–7319.
23. Fejer G, Szalay K, Gyory I, Fejes M, Kusz E, et al. (2005) Adenovirus infection dramatically augments lipopolysaccharide-induced TNF production and sensitizes to lethal shock. Journal of Immunology 175: 1498–1506.
24. Thorne PS, McCray PB, Howe TS, O'Neill MA (1999) Early-onset inflammatory responses in vivo to adenoviral vectors in the presence or absence of lipopolysaccharide-induced inflammation. American Journal of Respiratory Cell and Molecular Biology 20: 1155–1164.
25. Simpson AJ, Cunningham GA, Porteous DJ, Haslett C, Sallenave JM (2001) Regulation of adenovirus-mediated elafin transgene expression by bacterial lipopolysaccharide. HumGene Ther 12: 1395–1406.
26. Simpson AJ, Wallace WA, Marsden ME, Govan JR, Porteous DJ, et al. (2001) Adenoviral augmentation of elafin protects the lung against acute injury mediated by activated neutrophils and bacterial infection. Journal of Immunology 167: 1778–1786.
27. McMichael JW, Maxwell AI, Hayashi K, Taylor K, Wallace WA, et al. (2005) Antimicrobial activity of murine lung cells against Staphylococcus aureus is increased in vitro and in vivo after elafin gene transfer. InfectImmun 73: 3609–3617.
28. Collie DDS, McLean N, Sallenave JM, Baker A, Blundell R, et al. (2006) Local lung responses following endobronchial elastase and lipopolysaccharide instillation in the sheep. International Journal of COPD 1: 189–199.
29. Emerson M, Renwick L, Tate S, Rhind S, Milne E, et al. (2003) Transfection efficiency and toxicity following delivery of naked plasmid DNA and cationic lipid-DNA complexes to ovine lung segments. MolTher 8: 646–653.
30. Collie DD, Macaldowie CN, Pemberton AD, Woodall CJ, McLean N, et al. (2001) Local lung responses following local lung challenge with recombinant

lungworm antigen in systemically sensitized sheep. Clinical & Experimental Allergy 31: 1636–1647.

31. Nalubamba KS, Gossner AG, Dalziel RG, Hopkins J (2007) Differential expression of pattern recognition receptors in sheep tissues and leukocyte subsets. Veterinary Immunology and Immunopathology 118: 252–262.
32. Sallenave JM, Donnelly SC, Grant IS, Robertson C, Gauldie J, et al. (1999) Secretory leukocyte proteinase inhibitor is preferentially increased in patients with acute respiratory distress syndrome [see comments]. European Respiratory Journal 13: 1029–1036.
33. Tremblay GM, Sallenave JM, Israel-Assayag E, Cormier Y, Gauldie J (1996) Elafin/elastase-specific inhibitor in bronchoalveolar lavage of normal subjects and farmer's lung. AmJRespirCrit Care Med 154: 1092–1098.
34. van Bergen BH, Andriessen MP, Spruijt KI, van de Kerkhof PC, Schalkwijk J (1996) Expression of SKALP/elafin during wound healing in human skin. ArchDermatolRes 288: 458–462.
35. Wang Z, Beach D, Su L, Zhai R, Christiani DC (2008) A genome-wide expression analysis in blood identifies pre-elafin as a biomarker in ARDS. American Journal of Respiratory Cell and Molecular Biology 38: 724–732.
36. Brown TI, Mistry R, Collie DD, Tate S, Sallenave JM (2004) Trappin ovine molecule (TOM), the ovine ortholog of elafin, is an acute phase reactant in the lung. Physiol Genomics 19: 11–21.
37. Verrier T, Solhonne B, Sallenave JM, Garcia-Verdugo I (2012) The WAP protein Trappin-2/Elafin: a handyman in the regulation of inflammatory and immune responses. Int J Biochem Cell Biol 44: 1377–1380.
38. Fasbender A, Lee JH, Walters RW, Moninger TO, Zabner J, et al. (1998) Incorporation of adenovirus in calcium phosphate precipitates enhances gene transfer to airway epithelia in vitro and in vivo. Journal of Clinical Investigation 102: 184–193.
39. Walters R, Welsh M (1999) Mechanism by which calcium phosphate coprecipitation enhances adenovirus-mediated gene transfer. Gene Ther 6: 1845–1850.
40. Lee JH, Zabner J, Welsh MJ (1999) Delivery of an adenovirus vector in a calcium phosphate coprecipitate enhances the therapeutic index of gene transfer to airway epithelia. Human Gene Therapy 10: 603–613.
41. Lehmkuhl HD, Contreras JA, Cutlip RC, Brogden KA (1989) Clinical and microbiologic findings in lambs inoculated with Pasteurella haemolytica after infection with ovine adenovirus type 6. American Journal of Veterinary Research 50: 671–675.
42. Yates WD, Babiuk LA, Jericho KW (1983) Viral-bacterial pneumonia in calves: duration of the interaction between bovine herpesvirus 1 and Pasteurella haemolytica. CanJComp Med 47: 257–264.
43. Kopcha M (1998) Respiratory diseases of sheep and goats. In: Aiello SE, editor. The Merck Veterinary Manual: Merck & Co Inc, Whitehouse Station, NJ, USA. pp. 1107–1113.
44. Zhu J, Huang X, Yang Y (2007) Innate immune response to adenoviral vectors is mediated by both Toll-like receptor-dependent and -independent pathways. JVirol 81: 3170–3180.
45. Muruve DA, Cotter MJ, Zaiss AK, White LR, Liu Q, et al. (2004) Helper-dependent adenovirus vectors elicit intact innate but attenuated adaptive host immune responses in vivo. JVirol 78: 5966–5972.
46. Fejer G, Drechsel L, Liese J, Schleicher U, Ruzsics Z, et al. (2008) Key role of splenic myeloid DCs in the IFN-alphabeta response to adenoviruses in vivo. PLoSPathog 4: e1000208.
47. Tamanini A, Rolfini R, Nicolis E, Melotti P, Cabrini G (2003) MAP kinases and NF-kappaB collaborate to induce ICAM-1 gene expression in the early phase of adenovirus infection. Virology 307: 228–242.
48. Miller-Jensen K, Janes KA, Wong YL, Griffith LG, Lauffenburger DA (2006) Adenoviral vector saturates Akt pro-survival signaling and blocks insulin-mediated rescue of tumor necrosis-factor-induced apoptosis. JCell Sci 119: 3788–3798.
49. McMichael JW, Roghanian A, Jiang L, Ramage R, Sallenave JM (2005) The antimicrobial antiproteinase elafin binds to lipopolysaccharide and modulates macrophage responses. American Journal of Respiratory Cell and Molecular Biology 32: 443–452.
50. Frevert CW, Warner AE, Weller E, Brain JD (1998) The effect of endotoxin on in vivo rat alveolar macrophage phagocytosis. Experimental Lung Research 24: 745–758.
51. Frevert CW, Martin TR (2004) Sepsis and the lung host response. Semin Respir Crit Care Med 25: 85–93.
52. Roghanian A, Williams SE, Sheldrake TA, Brown TI, Oberheim K, et al. (2006) The antimicrobial/elastase inhibitor elafin regulates lung dendritic cells and adaptive immunity. American Journal of Respiratory Cell and Molecular Biology 34: 634–642.

Inhaled Lactonase Reduces *Pseudomonas aeruginosa* Quorum Sensing and Mortality in Rat Pneumonia

Sami Hraiech[1,2¶], Julien Hiblot[1¶], John Lafleur[3,4], Hubert Lepidi[1], Laurent Papazian[1,2], Jean-Marc Rolain[1], Didier Raoult[1], Mikael Elias[5], Mark W. Silby[3], Janek Bzdrenga[1], Fabienne Bregeon[1]*, Eric Chabriere[1]*

1 Unité de Recherche sur les Maladies Infectieuses et Tropicales Emergentes, UMR CNRS-IRD 6236, IFR48, Aix-Marseille Université, Marseille, France, **2** Réanimation - Détresses Respiratoires et Infections Sévères, APHM, CHU Nord, Marseille, France, **3** Department of Biology, University of Massachusetts Dartmouth, Dartmouth, Massachusetts, United States of America, **4** Department of Emergency Medicine, Alpert School of Medicine, Providence, Rhode Island, United States of America, **5** Weizmann Institute of Science, Biological Chemistry, Rehovot, Israel

Abstract

Rationale: The effectiveness of antibiotic molecules in treating *Pseudomonas aeruginosa* pneumonia is reduced as a result of the dissemination of bacterial resistance. The existence of bacterial communication systems, such as *quorum* sensing, has provided new opportunities of treatment. Lactonases efficiently quench acyl-homoserine lactone-based bacterial *quorum* sensing, implicating these enzymes as potential new anti-*Pseudomonas* drugs that might be evaluated in pneumonia.

Objectives: The aim of the present study was to evaluate the ability of a lactonase called *Sso*Pox-I to reduce the mortality of a rat *P. aeruginosa* pneumonia.

Methods: To assess *Sso*Pox-I-mediated quorum quenching, we first measured the activity of the virulence gene *lasB*, the synthesis of pyocianin, the proteolytic activity of a bacterial suspension and the formation of biofilm of a PAO1 strain grown in the presence of lactonase. In an acute lethal model of *P. aeruginosa* pneumonia in rats, we evaluated the effects of an early or deferred intra-tracheal treatment with *Sso*Pox-I on the mortality, lung bacterial count and lung damage.

Measurements and Primary Results: *Sso*Pox-I decreased PAO1 *lasB* virulence gene activity, pyocianin synthesis, proteolytic activity and biofilm formation. The early use of *Sso*Pox-I reduced the mortality of rats with acute pneumonia from 75% to 20%. Histological lung damage was significantly reduced but the lung bacterial count was not modified by the treatment. A delayed treatment was associated with a non-significant reduction of mortality.

Conclusion: These results demonstrate the protective effects of lactonase *Sso*Pox-I in *P. aeruginosa* pneumonia and open the way for a future therapeutic use.

Editor: Michael M. Meijler, Ben-Gurion University of the Negev, Israel

Funding: This study was funded by Aix Marseille University (AMU) and had no role in study design, data collection and analysis, decision to publish, or preparation of the manuscript.

Competing Interests: The authors have declared that no competing interests exist.

* Email: Fabienne.bregeon@ap-hm.fr (FB); Eric.chabriere@univ-amu.fr (EC)

¶ These authors contributed equally to this work.

Introduction

The dramatic increase of antibiotic resistance in bacterial isolates from intensive care unit (ICU) patients leads to an important reduction of therapeutic arsenal [1][2,3][4,5]. Alternative approaches to combat multidrug-resistant strains are under extensive research, especially using molecules that can reduce bacterial expression of virulence factors [1–3][6].

Expression of virulent phenotypes of numerous pathogenic bacteria is activated when the pathogen senses that a critical population density has been reached. This ability relates to the *quorum* sensing (QS) by which bacteria can sense messenger molecules thus virulence genes are activated [7]. This communication ability enables the bacteria to coordinate bacterial population behavior during the invasion of a host [8][9].

Acyl-Homoserine Lactones (AHLs) are QS molecule messengers used by a large number of Gram-negative bacteria, including *Pseudomonas aeruginosa* [10]. These bacteria are able to form biofilms whose maturation is regulated through QS [11]. Biofilms have been implicated in antibiotic resistance in chronic *P. aeruginosa* infections, primarily through the limitation of the diffusion of antibiotics into the bacterial colonies [12]. *P. aeruginosa* possesses two different AHL-based QS systems: the LasI/R and RhlI/R with their respective cognate 3-oxo-C12 AHLs and C4 AHLs messenger molecules [13].

The inhibition of bacterial virulence by targeting QS mechanism can be mediated by (i) the inhibition of the messenger production, (ii) inhibition of its detection, both known as QS inhibition/inhibitors [14,15][16], or (iii) the elimination of the messenger known as *quorum* quencher (QQ) [17,18] thus alteration of the *P. aeruginosa* QS system can attenuate its virulence. In pneumonia, the efficacy of QS modulation has been tested at the genomic level with reduction in lethality of infected animals [9]. Therapeutic management of animals with pneumonia has been tested with QS inhibitors such as furanones and patulin showing that these molecules can increase the clearance of bacteria in mice infected with *P. aeruginosa* [19,20][21]. Because some *in vitro* studies suggest toxicity of furanones and patulin [22][23], other QS inhibition options are under investigation [24] among which the use of lactonases or acylases enzymes [10][25]. Lactonases efficiently decrease the production of virulence factors and biofilm by *P. aeruginosa in vitro* [26][27], and may therefore represent an alternative and promising strategy for reducing bacterial virulence. The efficacy of lactonases to decrease bacterial virulence has been reported in several hosts [28,29][30]. In a recent *in vivo* study on mice with pneumonia [31], the use of a lactonase-producing *P. aeruginosa* mutant showed reduced lung injury and increased survival as compared to the wild strain. These encouraging results would suggest that the use of lactonases as a topic therapeutic agent could be effective in improving outcome in *P. aeruginosa* pneumonia.

The aim of our work was to test the efficacy of inhaled lactonase in improving survival of rats with acute *P. aeruginosa* pneumonia. To do this, we used an engineered variant of the hyperthermostable lactonase *Sso*Pox (first isolated from the extremophilic archaea *Sulfolobus solfataricus*) [32], *Sso*Pox-I, exhibiting a high stability and an improved ability to hydrolyze 3-oxo-C12 AHLs. We first tested *in vitro* the ability of our molecule to reduce, in a *P.aeruginosa* PAO1 strain, the virulence gene *lasB* activity, the pyocianin synthesis, the proteolytic activity and the biofilm formation. Thus, we evaluated the effect of *Sso*Pox-I when delivered early or late intra-tracheally to animals with lungs infected with *P. aeruginosa*.

Material and Methods

Protein production & purification

The plasmid encoding *Sso*Pox-I protein was commercially obtained (GeneArt, Invitrogen; Germany). *Sso*Pox-I protein was synthesized in *E. coli* strain BL21(DE_3)-pGro7/GroEL (TaKaRa) in ZYP medium [33] containing 100 μg/ml ampicillin and 34 μg/ml chloramphenicol as previously described [22]. The proteins were purified as previously described [34]. Briefly, the culture was incubated at 70°C for 30 minutes, followed by differential ammonium sulfate precipitation, dialysis and exclusion size chromatography. The proteins were quantified using a nanospectrophotometer (Nanodrop, ThermoFisher Scientific, France) and the protein molar extinction coefficient was determined using the protein primary sequence in PROT-PARAM (ExPASy tool software) [35]. The protein yield was approximately 10 mg/L for *Sso*Pox-I, and the identity and purity of the purified protein was assessed through sodium dodecyl sulfate polyacrylamide gel electrophoresis (SDS-PAGE) and mass spectrometry (Plateforme Timone, Marseille, France). The enzymes were stored and used in phosphate-buffered saline (PBS) (Biomerieux; France).

In vitro experiments

P. aeruginosa culture. *P. aeruginosa* (strain PA01 ATCC 15692) was grown at 37°C in Luria-Bertani (LB) medium (BD, France) with shaking (200 rpm). When required, 1.5% bacto agar was added to solidify the LB.

For *in vivo* experiments [36], aliquots containing *P. aeruginosa* PAO1 strain were thawed and cultured on COS (Biomerieux, France) (Columbia with 5% Sheep blood) agar plates. Ten fresh PAO1 colonies were sampled and cultured at 37°C in tryptic soy broth (TSB, Biomerieux, France) with continuous shaking until the $OD_{600\ nm} = 1$. Serial dilutions were subsequently performed to adjust the bacterial amount, and the precise concentrations were confirmed after plating serial dilutions on the appropriate culture medium and counting the resulting colonies.

LasB reporter system. A 50-μl aliquot from an 18-hour culture of *P. aeruginosa* PAO1 carrying P*lasB-luxCDABE* (QS reporter) was added to the wells of a 96-well plate. A ten-fold dilution series from 50 μg to 0.05 μg of *Sso*Pox-I was added to the wells containing the *P. aeruginosa* reporter strain. LB was added to each well to generate a final volume of 100 μl. The plates were incubated at 37°C for 90 minutes, with shaking every 10 minutes, and subsequently analyzed using a Varioskan Flash multimode plate reader. The luminescence was measured every 10 minutes to determine the QS reporter activity.

Quantification of pyocianin synthesis. Quantification of pyocyanin was performed as previously described [37]. Briefly, *P. aeruginosa* PAO1 strain was grown in 1 mL of Glycerol-alanine (GA) minimum medium (10 $mL.L^{-1}$ glycerol, 6 $g.L^{-1}$ L-alanine, 2 $g.L^{-1}$ $MgSO_4$, 0.1 $g.L^{-1}$ K_2HPO_4, 0.018 $g.L^{-1}$ $FeSO_4$) with and without 14 μM of filtered (0.2 μm pore) *Sso*Pox-I enzyme during 24 h at 37°C and 450 rpm shaking in 48-well plate (Greiner Bio-One, Germany). Cells were centrifuged 15 min at 12.000 *g* and the supernatant was filtered (0.2 μm pore). Extraction of pyocyanin was performed on 500 μL of supernatant using 0.5× volume of chloroform and absorbance was subsequently measured at 690 nm. Blank assay was realized using 500 μL of culture medium with and without 14 μM of filtered (0.2 μm pore) *Sso*Pox-I enzyme.

Proteolytic activity. Measurement of the proteolytic activity was made using azocasein enzymatic assay as previously described [38]. Briefly, *P. aeruginosa* PAO1 strain was grown in 200 μL of LB medium with and without 14 μM of filtered (0.2 μm) *Sso*Pox-I enzyme during 24 h at 37°C and 450 rpm shaking in 96-well plate. The *Sso*Pox-I enzyme stock solution being in PBS buffer, control cultures were supplemented with equivalent PBS quantity. Cells were centrifuged 15 min at 12.000 *g*. The reaction was performed in 0.3 M TrisHCl buffer (pH 7.5) with 50 μL of azocasein (Sigma, St. Louis, USA) (30 $mg.mL^{-1}$ dissolved in water) and with 50 μL of culture's supernatant for a final volume of 1.5 mL. The reaction was incubated at 37°C for 1 h and subsequently stopped by addition of 250 μL of 20% (w/v) trichloroacetic acid (TCA). The blank assay was realized using 50 μL of culture medium with and without 14 μM of filtered (0.2 μm pore) *Sso*Pox-I enzyme. After centrifugation at 12.000 *g* for 10 min, optical density was measured at 366 nm. The proteolytic activity was defined as the increase in absorbance at 366 $nm.h^{-1}$ per number of cells (OD_{600}).

Biofilm formation assays. Liquid cultures of *P. aeruginosa* PAO1 were grown for 18 hours, and subsequently diluted 1:50 in 10% TSB. To examine biofilm susceptibility to *Sso*Pox-I, 100 μl aliquots were dispensed onto Calgary Biofilm Device 96-well plates (MBEC Assay for Physiology & Genetics, Innovotech Inc., Edmonton, Alberta, Canada). A three-fold dilution series from 50 μg to 0.5 μg of *Sso*Pox-I was added to the wells containing *P. aeruginosa*. The plates were incubated for 4 hours with rocking at 120 Hz at 37°C, and subsequently, the MBEC device with adherent *P. aeruginosa* biofilms was placed on a fresh 96-well plate containing 100 µl of 1% crystal violet dye in each well for 15 minutes. The MBEC device was subsequently washed three times with 100 µl of water to remove excess dye and allowed to dry. Crystal violet stain was solubilized from the biofilms after placing the MBEC device on a 96-well plate with 100 µl of 100% ethanol in each well. The solubilized crystal violet dye was measured at 600 nm using a Varioskan Flash multimode plate reader (Thermo). The optical density at 600 nm was also used to assess *P. aeruginosa* PAO1 planktonic growth on the original 96-well plate to determine the effect of *Sso*Pox-I on *P. aeruginosa* planktonic growth.

In vivo experiments

Ethics statement. The experiments and protocols were performed in accordance with the European law and the French version of this law details the statutory requirements for the live animal experiments (articles R214-87 to R215-10 of Code Rural, law #76–629 from July 10th, 1976/law #2001-464 from May 29th, 2001 (published in JORF on May 31st, 2001)). Consistent with these laws, the experiments were performed under the direct control of the researcher authorized through the Préfecture-des-Bouches-du-Rhone Administration (authorization number: 13–437). The animal experiments were performed in accordance with 'Animal Research: Reporting In Vivo Experiments' (ARRIVE Guidelines http://www.nc3rs.org.uk) and the guidelines of the Guide for the Care and Use of Laboratory Animals. All animal experiments were authorized through the National Animal Ethics Committee («Comité National de Réflexion Ethique sur l'Expérimentation Animale (Comité d'éthique de Marseille)»). The experiments were performed in the Faculté de Pharmacie-Aix-Marseille University.

The animals were euthanized with an intra-peritoneal injection of a lethal dose of thiopental (Panpharma, France).

General procedures. Adult Sprague-Dawley male pathogen-free rats, weighing 250 to 300 g, were obtained from SAS Janvier (Le-Genest-St-Isle, France) and housed in individual plastic cages (4 animals per cage) in a ventilated pressurized cabinet (A-BOX 160, Noroit, Rezé, France) with free access to water and standard diet food. The rats were anesthetized with 5% Sévoflurane (Abbott, Rungis, France) in 100% oxygen (anesthetizing box, Harvard Apparatus, Les Ulis, France). The trachea was exposed, and they were intubated using a 16-gauge catheter for drug and/or bacterial administration. The awakened rats were housed under the same conditions and weighed daily. At the end of each experiment, the rats were euthanized with an intra-peritoneal injection of a lethal dose of thiopental (Panpharma, France).

Rat tolerance of inhaled *Sso*Pox-I. The tolerance to intra-tracheal treatment with *Sso*Pox-I was examined in a preliminary study on 3 groups of animals (n = 3 per group) receiving 250 µl of *Sso*Pox-I at a concentration of 0.1, 1 or 10 mg/ml and compared with 5 control animals receiving 250 µl of PBS. After the treatment, signs of bad tolerance of the molecule were investigated *i.e.* shortness of breathing, prostration and atony or weight loss above 10% from baseline. Spontaneous mortality was also recorded. One animal from each group was sacrificed after 6, 24 and 48 hours. The remaining animals were sacrificed after 48 hours. Subsequently, the lungs were removed, macroscopically examined, and preserved in formaldehyde for histological assessment of lung damage.

Rat respiratory infection model and *Sso*Pox-I treatment. Three groups of 20 animals were infected through intra-tracheal inoculation with 250 µl of a PBS solution containing 10^8 CFU/ml of *P. aeruginosa* PAO1.

Among the 3 groups of infected rats, one group received immediately after infection 250 µl of PBS (non-treated group: NT), while another group was treated with 250 µl of *Sso*Pox-I at a concentration of 1 mg/ml (immediate treatment group: IT). The last group received 250 µl of 1 mg/ml *Sso*Pox-I at 3 hours after infection (deferred treatment group: DT). *Sso*Pox-I and additional PBS were delivered intra-tracheally using the same anesthetic procedure as used for the infection.

Lung processing and blood or spleen samples. After infection, the animals were observed for 2 days, and spontaneous mortality was examined. Animals' conditions and clinical status were checked every 2 hours. Humane endpoints were used during the survival study. If animals had one of the following signs, they were anesthetized and euthanized with an intra-peritoneal injection of a lethal dose of thiopental (Panpharma, France) to avoid suffering:

- Major dyspnea with noisy breathing and head or neck movements associated with breathing
- Prostration and atony
- Weight loss>20% of initial body weight.

The remaining rats were euthanized after 48 hours. Subsequently, the lungs were removed aseptically. The right lung was homogenized in PBS for bacterial culture, and the left lung was preserved for histological analysis. The blood and spleen were sampled and cultured on agar plates to assess systemic diffusion of the bacteria.

Histological severity score (HSS). Sections (3 mm thick) were obtained from the upper, mid and lower parts of the lungs, including the entire circumference. The sections were stained with hematoxylin and eosin. A pathologist blinded to the group identity (H. L.) examined the samples. The HSS was calculated based on the number of bronchopneumonia lesions (0, no lesions; 1, 30 lesions/lung; 2, ≥30 lesions/lung; 3, confluent lesions of bronchopneumonia), as previously reported [39,40].

Statistics

The number of studied animals (20 animals per group) was calculated based on a mortality reduction from 80% in the NT group infected with PAO1 to an expected mortality rate of 50% in the treated groups, with 90% statistical power and a two-sided alpha value of 0.05. The data were expressed as the means ± standard deviation (SD) or median [inter-quartile range, IQR] according to the distribution of the data. Student's *t*-test or the Mann-Whitney rank-sum test were used for inter-group comparisons. Kaplan-Meier analysis was performed to evaluate 48-h mortality. Intergroup differences were evaluated using the log rank test. The data analysis was performed with SPSS for Windows (Chicago, IL), version 12.0. A value of $p \leq 0.05$ was considered statistically significant.

Results

Protein production & purification

See Fig. S1 in supplementary material.

In vitro experiments

We monitored the *lasB* activity in a *P. aeruginosa* PAO1 strain carrying the P*lasB-luxCDABE* plasmid. We showed that the addition of *Sso*Pox-I significantly reduced the levels of *lasB* activity (**Fig. 1A**). Moreover, this inhibition exhibited a dose-dependent profile with a half inhibition concentration ($[C_{1/2}]$) of the enzyme of approximately 0.5 µg/ml (**Fig. 1A**).

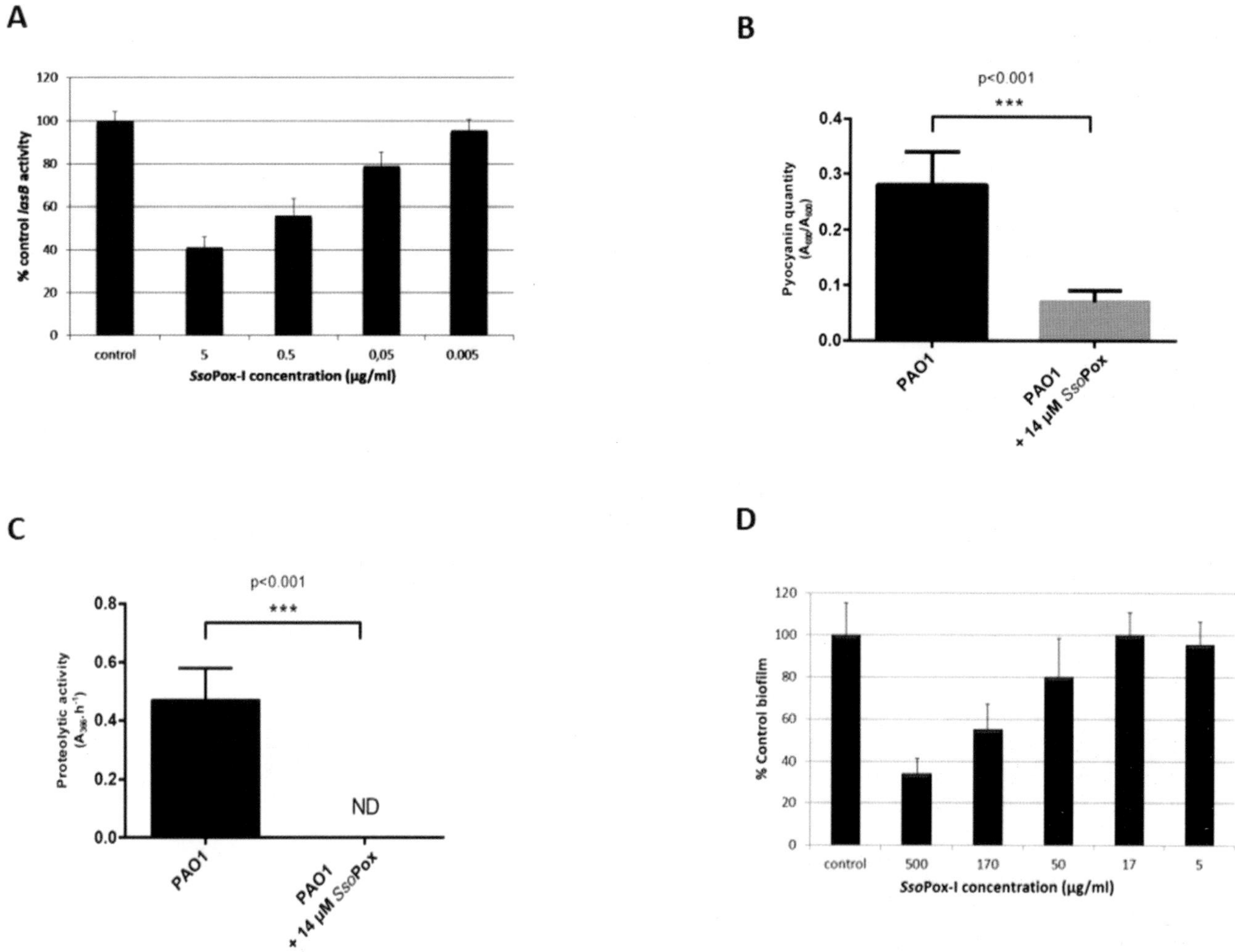

Figure 1. Effects of *Sso*Pox-I on PAO1 virulence factors expression and biofilm formation. 1A: *lasB* activity. The chart shows the *lasB* activity in treated cultures, expressed as the percentage of that in untreated controls (no *Sso*Pox-I), and these data represent the average of three independent experiments, each with three technical replicates. The error bars represent 95% confidence intervals. Student's t test $p<0.05$ for *Sso*Pox-I. T tests were used for the comparison of baseline with the highest dose of enzyme. **1B: pyocianin synthesis.** Pyocyanin quantification of *P. aeruginosa* PAO1 strain after 24 h growth in GA medium was assessed in presence (black) or absence (gray) of 14 µM of *Sso*Pox-I lactonase. Pyocyanin quantity was followed at A_{690} as per number of cells (A_{600}). **1C: proteolytic activity.** Proteolytic activity of *P. aeruginosa* PAO1 strain after 24 h growth in LB medium was assessed in presence (black) or absence (grey) of 14 µM of *Sso*Pox-I lactonase. Proteolytic activity was measured by the azocasein assay ($A_{366}.h^{-1}$) as per number of cells (A_{600}). ND stands for non-detected activity. **1D: biofilm formation.** Biofilms were grown in an MBEC device as described in the methods section. The dose-dependent inhibition of *P. aeruginosa* biofilm formation through *Sso*Pox-I was observed and analyzed using Student's t test $p=0.05$ for *Sso*Pox-I.

Pyocyanin secretion was affected by the presence of *Sso*Pox-I and presented a 4 fold drop in quantity as compared to the control **(Fig. 1B)**.

Cultures of PAO1 made in presence of 14 µM *Sso*Pox-I showed after 24 h a clear drop of protease activity followed using azocasein assay. Protease activity in presence of *Sso*Pox-I was beyond detection limit **(Fig. 1C)**.

The biofilm assay showed that *Sso*Pox-I reduced biofilm formation in a dose-dependent manner with a $[C_{1/2}]\sim170$ µg/ml (**Fig. 1D**).

Interestingly, *Sso*Pox-I did not significantly affect the rate of *P. aeruginosa* growth. Indeed, even at the highest enzyme dose (5 mg/ml), the optical density of the cell culture did not significantly differ from that of the control experiment with no treatment (**Fig. S2**).

In vivo experiments

Rat tolerance to inhaled *Sso*Pox-I. The effects of *Sso*Pox-I treatment on rat tissues were investigated. On the 9 rats that received *Sso*Pox-I into the trachea, none exhibited any sign of bad tolerance including in the group that received the highest dose. The weight curve of treated rats was not different to control animals and no animal loosed weight. There was no spontaneous mortality after 48-hours observation in the treated group as well as in the control group. After sacrifice, the lungs were harvested and the macroscopic examination showed no signs of injury. Histological assessment showed that there was no sign of lung damage 6, 24 or 48 hours after the treatment including in the group receiving the highest dose of *Sso*Pox-I.

Rat respiratory infection model and *Sso*Pox-I treatment. The influence of *Sso*Pox-I on pulmonary *P. aeruginosa* infection was monitored in 3 groups of 20 rats. The spontaneous mortality rate was 75% (15/20) in the non-treated group (NT). When the rats were treated with *Sso*Pox-I (1 mg/ml) immediately after infection (IT), the mortality rate was significantly reduced to 20% (4/20) ($p = 0.0001$ vs. NT). The protective effect of lactonase on mortality was less significant in the deferred treatment (DT) group, where the treatment was administered at 3 hours after the infection (mortality rate of 50% (10/20) (p = ns vs. NT) (**Fig. 2**). However, in the DT group, the mean delay of mortality was significantly longer than that in the control group (respectively 26±9.5 vs. 17±9.2 hours; p = 0.04).

In addition to death, other parameters were monitored during the infection, including the weight of the animals. We observed that the loss of body weight, measured from the day of infection until the day of death, was significantly less important in the IT group than in the NT group (11.3±12 g vs. 20.4±9.3 g respectively; $p = 0.01$). The DT group lost 25.6±1.82 g of body weight (p = ns vs. NT group).

Notably, consistent with the increased survival rate observed in the IT group, we also observed that compared with the NT group, the damage to the lungs of the animals in the IT group was less significant (**Fig. 3**), as revealed by a significantly lower HSS (HSS IT group vs. NT group: 1.27±0.6 *vs.* 2.64±0.4; $p = 0.005$). In the DT group, the mean HSS was not significantly different from that in the NT group.

Moreover, we also investigated the potential effects of lactonase treatment on the lung bacterial count, associated with the increased survival observed in the IT group. We observed that the lung bacterial count did not significantly differ between the 3 groups (CFU/g of lung in median [inter-quartile range]: 3.3×10^5 [$5.6\times10^3-1.3\times10^6$] in the NT group; 1.3×10^5 [$9.2\times10^3-10^6$] in the IT group; and 10^5 [$8.4\times10^4-7.8\times10^5$] in the DT group) (**Fig. 4**).

Finally, there was no difference concerning the number of animals with positive blood or spleen culture at the time of death between the 3 groups (n/tot (%): 8/20 (40%) in the NT group; 7/20 (35%) in the IT group; 10/20 (50%) in the DT group; p = NS).

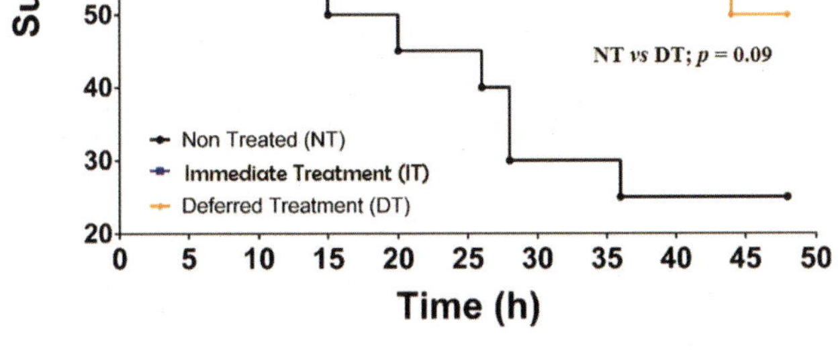

Figure 2. Forty-eight-hour survival curves for the 3 groups of animals after infection. The animals were infected with 10^8 CFU/ml (2.5×10^7 CFU/rat) of *P. aeruginosa* PAO1 in the following treatment groups: non-treated (NT), immediate-treatment (IT) or deferred treatment (DT) who received treatment with *Sso*Pox-I at 3 hours after infection.

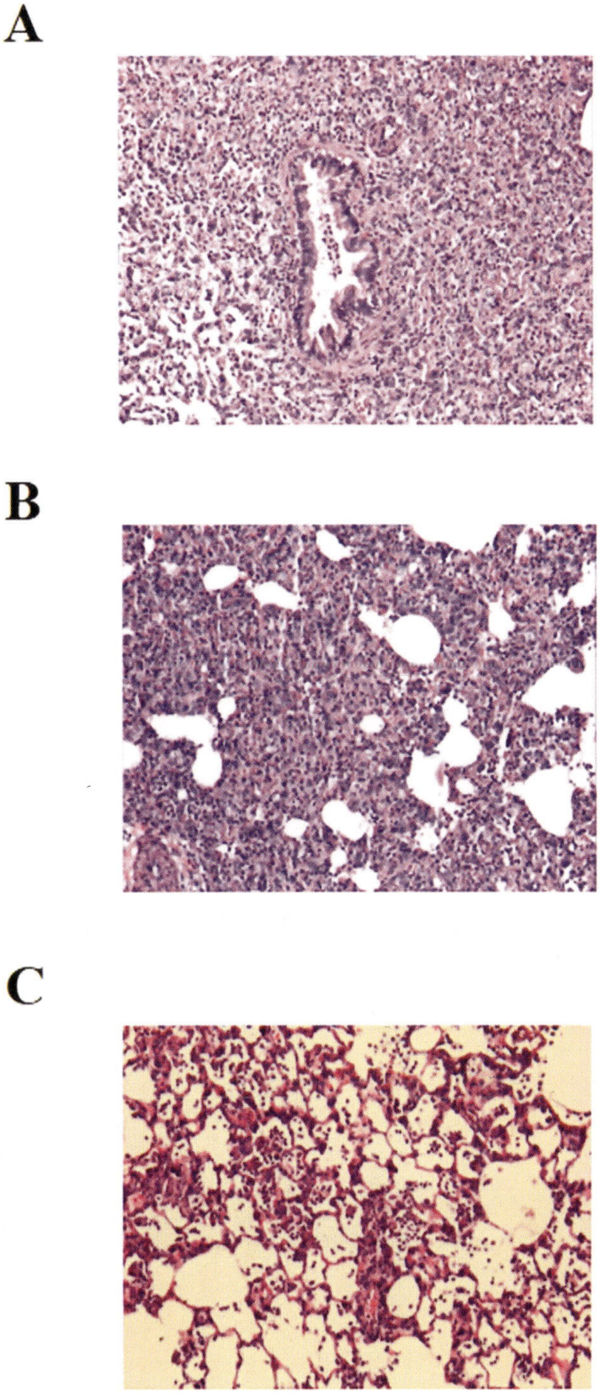

Figure 3. Lung histological examination after infection. Pathological mapping of the lungs of non-treated (NT) (**A**), deferred-treatment (DT) (**B**) and immediate-treatment (IT) (**C**) groups. Photomicrographs of the pathological Giemsa staining of the lung sections (100X). Mean histological severity score (HSS) was 2.64±0.4 (mean ± SD) for the NT group, 1.27±0.6 for the IT group (p = 0.005 *vs.* NT) and 2.32±0.4 for the DT group (p = NS *vs.* NT).

Discussion and Conclusions

In the present study, we used both *in vitro* and *in vivo* experiments to show that the lactonase *Sso*Pox-I was able to decrease the activity of *lasB* virulence gene, the synthesis of

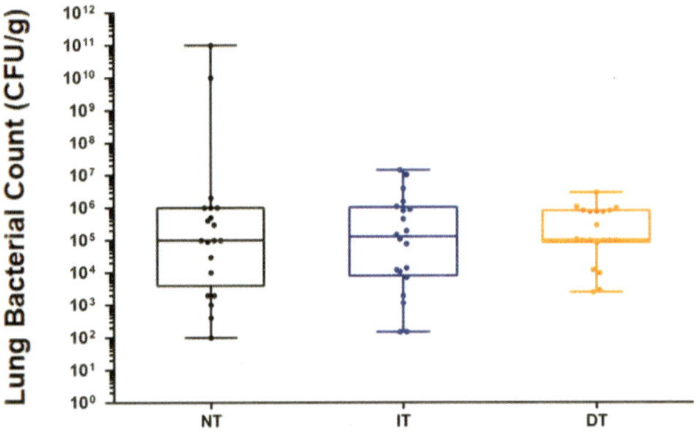

Figure 4. Lung bacterial count after infection. The lung bacterial count was adjusted according to the lung weight. The box plots limits represent the 25th and 75th percentiles, and the bars represent the 5th and 95th percentiles. The median is represented as a horizontal line. NT= non-treated group; IT= immediate treatment group; DT= deferred treatment group.

pyocianin, the proteolytic activity and the biofilm formation of the *P. aeruginosa* PAO1 strain. In addition, the treatment with *Sso*Pox-I was associated with an important improve in survival in a rat model of highly lethal acute pneumonia.

Originally, this work focuses on the lactonase *SsoPox*-I QQ activity with a design trying to approach clinical settings by giving the enzyme as a therapeutic drug. Similarly, QS inhibitor molecules such as furanones have been shown to increase the bacterial clearance in animal models of *P. aeruginosa* pneumonia but data on reduction of mortality are lacking [16] [19,20]. In one study in mice using indirect demonstration of QQ effects of lactonases in animal models of pneumonia [31], Migiyama *et al.* showed a decrease in mortality and lung damage when animals were infected with a lactonase-producing *P. aeruginosa* strain. The main difference between Migiyama's study and ours is that we used a wild strain of *P. aeruginosa* for infections and we treated the animals with a synthetic lactonase given after infection as a therapeutic drug.

The catalytic efficiency and quenching activity of the QS lactonase *Sso*Pox-I against 3-oxo-C12 AHLs has been previously improved through protein engineering [32]. While the QS activity of the wild-type enzyme has been previously demonstrated *in vitro* [26], the efficiency of this enzyme *in vivo* has not been explored. *Sso*Pox-I inhibits the *lasB* gene activity, a classical virulence factor [41], at concentrations as low as 0.5 μg/ml. *Sso*Pox-I is also able to decrease the pyocianin synthesis as well as the proteolytic activity of a *P.aeruginosa* PAO1 strain. Moreover, the effect of *Sso*Pox-I on *P. aeruginosa* goes beyond the inhibition of virulence-associated genes. Indeed, *Sso*Pox-I also inhibited biofilm formation, albeit at much higher concentrations (170 μg/ml). This discrepancy in the active dose of the enzyme might reflect the distinct regulation of biofilm formation and maturation [12] [42]. Indeed, multiple quorum sensing-regulated genes are modulated without affecting lasRI, rhlRI or the production of N-acyl-L-homoserine lactones. In particular, the transcriptional regulator MvfR may contribute more to biofilm formation of *P. aeruginosa*. This could explain why in our experiments *Sso*Pox-I seemed to have a better efficacy on *lasB* gene down regulation than on decrease in biofilm formation [43,44].

We further investigated the potential consequences of the observed *in vitro* effects. For this, we used an acute lethal model of *P. aeruginosa* pneumonia. Our model was consistent with previous ones showing a high and early lethality within the 24–48 first hours [45–47]. On histological analysis, the lungs of untreated animals exhibited important and confluent lesions of broncho-pneumonia arguing for the correlation between death and severity of pneumonia. In addition, nearly one half of the animals had bacteremia which probably contributed to the high mortality rate. In this model, *Sso*Pox-I significantly decreased the mortality rate from 75% in the non-treated group to 20% in the group treated immediately after infection. This observation is consistent with the dramatic reduction in the lung damage observed in the treated group. The results are also consistent with previous studies showing that infections with QS-deleted strains of *P. aeruginosa* were less severe in several infection models [48][49].

*Sso*Pox-I did not significantly reduce lung lesions and rat mortality when administrated at 3 hours after the onset of infection. This ineffectiveness might be due to the use of a highly lethal model of infection (death in 48 hours). The preventive action of *Sso*Pox-I might be higher than its curative effect as previously observed for QSI [22]. QS is indeed under a positive retro-control regulation [50]: when the bacterial *quorum* is reached, the inhibition of QS is more difficult because of the self-stimulating properties of bacteria.

In our study, the innovative molecule *Sso*Pox-I was administered intra-tracheally within the 3 first hours of infection. This design was chosen to approach clinical preventive therapeutic methods used in patients at risk for *P. aeruginosa* infections, such as ICU patients. However, our model did not totally mimic clinical settings primarily because of the high amount of bacteria given in one inoculation.

No difference in the lung bacterial burden was observed between the control group and the 2 treated groups regardless the time of administration of the molecule. While surprising, these results are consistent with our *in vitro* findings on bacterial cultures in which lactonase adjunction to the media did not influence *P. aeruginosa* growth. These results agree with those of Migiyama *et al.* [31] who showed similar bacterial count with animals infected with wild-type *P. aeruginosa* and their lactonase-producing mutant strain. It remains however unknown whether the improved survival could be due to a less invasive activity of the microorganism towards the lung parenchyma and/ or to change in the host-pathogen interaction regardless the bacterial load.

In summary, *Sso*Pox-I presents several properties that could increase the therapeutic arsenal, particularly in the field of nosocomial pneumonia. In contrast to antibiotics, *quorum*-quenching strategies do not impose drastic selection pressure on bacterial survival. Therefore, treatments with lactonases such as *Sso*Pox-I might not or only slightly, promote the emergence of resistance [7][51]. Interestingly, due to their ability to reduce biofilm formation, lactonases could restore susceptibility to antibiotics in drug-resistant strains as previously observed with tobramycin in animal models [52]. Because of its mechanisms of action involving a modulation of the QS, azythromycin has been recently shown in a randomized controlled trial to reduce the incidence of ventilator-acquired pneumonia in pseudomonas colonized patients [53] showing the growing interest of QS inhibitors in clinics.

To conclude, our results open the way to further investigations assessing *Sso*Pox-I as a possible tool in antimicrobial strategy.

Supporting Information

Figure S1 SDS-PAGE of *Sso*Pox-I. Twenty-five μg of *Sso*Pox-I (left band) were deposited next to a Molecular weight Marker (MwM, right panel) (Mulicolor broad range protein ladder, Euromedex).

Figure S2 The growth of *P. aeruginosa* in the presence of *Sso*Pox-I. A small decrease in *P. aeruginosa* growth was observed at the highest concentration of *Sso*Pox-I; however, this effect was not significant (Student's t test p = 0.67). The chart shows percentage of controls (no *Sso*Pox I) and represents the data obtained from four independent experiments, each performed with three technical replicates. The error bars represent 95% confidence intervals.

Checklist S1 Arrive guidelines.

Acknowledgments

We acknowledge Dr JM Brunel and Mr Janek Bzdrenga for their contribution to this work.

Author Contributions

Conceived and designed the experiments: SH JH FB EC LP MS ME JL. Performed the experiments: SH JH FB MS ME JL HL. Analyzed the data: SH JH FB EC MS ME JL. Contributed reagents/materials/analysis tools: LP JMR DR. Wrote the paper: SH JH FB EC MS ME JL HL.

References

1. Stanton TB (2013) A call for antibiotic alternatives research. Trends Microbiol 21: 111-113. S0966-842X(12)00199-0 [pii];10.1016/j.tim.2012.11.002 [doi].
2. Garcia-Quintanilla M, Pulido MR, Lopez-Rojas R, Pachon J, McConnell MJ (2013) Emerging therapies for multidrug resistant Acinetobacter baumannii. Trends Microbiol 21: 157–163. S0966-842X(12)00225-9 [pii];10.1016/j.tim.2012.12.002 [doi].
3. Breidenstein EB, Fuente-Nunez C, Hancock RE (2011) Pseudomonas aeruginosa: all roads lead to resistance. Trends Microbiol 19: 419–426. S0966-842X(11)00086-2 [pii];10.1016/j.tim.2011.04.005 [doi].
4. Agodi A, Barchitta M, Cipresso R, Giaquinta L, Romeo MA, et al.(2007) Pseudomonas aeruginosa carriage, colonization, and infection in ICU patients. Intensive Care Med 33: 1155–1161. 10.1007/s00134-007-0671-6 [doi].
5. Adair CG, Gorman SP, Feron BM, Byers LM, Jones DS, et al. (1999) Implications of endotracheal tube biofilm for ventilator-associated pneumonia. Intensive Care Med 25: 1072–1076. 90251072.134 [pii].
6. Hoiby N, Bjarnsholt T, Givskov M, Molin S, Ciofu O (2010) Antibiotic resistance of bacterial biofilms. Int J Antimicrob Agents 35: 322–332. S0924-8579(10)00009-9 [pii];10.1016/j.ijantimicag.2009.12.011 [doi].
7. Schuster M, Sexton DJ, Diggle SP, Greenberg EP (2013) Acyl-homoserine lactone quorum sensing: from evolution to application. Annu Rev Microbiol 67: 43–63. 10.1146/annurev-micro-092412-155635 [doi].
8. Wagner VE, Frelinger JG, Barth RK, Iglewski BH (2006) Quorum sensing: dynamic response of Pseudomonas aeruginosa to external signals. Trends Microbiol 14: 55–58. S0966-842X(05)00333-1 [pii];10.1016/j.tim.2005.12.002 [doi].
9. Lesprit P, Faurisson F, Join-Lambert O, Roudot-Thoraval F, Foglino M, et al. (2003) Role of the quorum-sensing system in experimental pneumonia due to Pseudomonas aeruginosa in rats. Am J Respir Crit Care Med 167: 1478–1482. 10.1164/rccm.200207-736BC [doi];200207-736BC [pii].
10. Grabiner MA, Fu Z, Wu T, Barry KC, Schwarzer C, et al. (2014) Pseudomonas aeruginosa Quorum-Sensing Molecule Homoserine Lactone Modulates Inflammatory Signaling through PERK and eI-F2alpha. J Immunol. jimmunol.1303437 [pii];10.4049/jimmunol.1303437 [doi].
11. Parsek MR, Greenberg EP (2005) Sociomicrobiology: the connections between quorum sensing and biofilms. Trends Microbiol 13: 27–33. S0966-842X(04)00261-6 [pii];10.1016/j.tim.2004.11.007 [doi].
12. Costerton JW, Stewart PS, Greenberg EP (1999) Bacterial biofilms: a common cause of persistent infections. Science 284: 1318–1322.
13. Williams P, Camara M (2009) Quorum sensing and environmental adaptation in Pseudomonas aeruginosa: a tale of regulatory networks and multifunctional signal molecules. Curr Opin Microbiol 12: 182–191. S1369-5274(09)00008-3 [pii];10.1016/j.mib.2009.01.005 [doi].
14. Galloway WR, Hodgkinson JT, Bowden S, Welch M, Spring DR (2012) Applications of small molecule activators and inhibitors of quorum sensing in Gram-negative bacteria. Trends Microbiol 20: 449–458. S0966-842X(12)00113-8 [pii];10.1016/j.tim.2012.06.003 [doi].
15. Kalia VC (2013) Quorum sensing inhibitors: an overview. Biotechnol Adv 31: 224–245. S0734-9750(12)00185-1 [pii];10.1016/j.biotechadv.2012.10.004 [doi].
16. Rasmussen TB, Givskov M (2006) Quorum-sensing inhibitors as anti-pathogenic drugs. Int J Med Microbiol 296: 149–161. S1438-4221(06)00078-6 [pii];10.1016/j.ijmm.2006.02.005 [doi].
17. Dong YH, Wang LH, Xu JL, Zhang HB, Zhang XF, et al. (2001) Quenching quorum-sensing-dependent bacterial infection by an N-acyl homoserine lactonase. Nature 411: 813–817. 10.1038/35081101 [doi].
18. Amara N, Krom BP, Kaufmann GF, Meijler MM (2011) Macromolecular inhibition of quorum sensing: enzymes, antibodies, and beyond. Chem Rev 111: 195–208. 10.1021/cr100101c [doi].
19. Hentzer M, Wu H, Andersen JB, Riedel K, Rasmussen TB, et al. (2003) Attenuation of Pseudomonas aeruginosa virulence by quorum sensing inhibitors. EMBO J 22: 3803–3815. 10.1093/emboj/cdg366 [doi].
20. Rasmussen TB, Skindersoe ME, Bjarnsholt T, Phipps RK, Christensen KB, et al. (2005) Identity and effects of quorum-sensing inhibitors produced by Penicillium species. Microbiology 151: 1325–1340. 151/5/1325 [pii];10.1099/mic.0.27715-0 [doi].
21. Jakobsen TH, van GM, Phipps RK, Shanmugham MS, Christensen LD, et al. (2012) Ajoene, a sulfur-rich molecule from garlic, inhibits genes controlled by quorum sensing. Antimicrob Agents Chemother 56: 2314–2325. AAC.05919-11 [pii];10.1128/AAC.05919-11 [doi].
22. O'Loughlin CT, Miller LC, Siryaporn A, Drescher K, Semmelhack MF, et al. (2013) A quorum-sensing inhibitor blocks Pseudomonas aeruginosa virulence and biofilm formation. Proc Natl Acad Sci U S A 110: 17981–17986. 1316981110 [pii];10.1073/pnas.1316981110 [doi].
23. Baveja JK, Willcox MD, Hume EB, Kumar N, Odell R, et al. (2004) Furanones as potential anti-bacterial coatings on biomaterials. Biomaterials 25: 5003–5012. 10.1016/j.biomaterials.2004.02.051 [doi];S0142961204002005 [pii].
24. Bjarnsholt T, Tolker-Nielsen T, Hoiby N, Givskov M (2010) Interference of Pseudomonas aeruginosa signalling and biofilm formation for infection control. Expert Rev Mol Med 12: e11. S1462399410001420 [pii];10.1017/S1462399410001420 [doi].
25. Uroz S, Oger PM, Chapelle E, Adeline MT, Faure D, et al. (2008) A Rhodococcus qsdA-encoded enzyme defines a novel class of large-spectrum quorum-quenching lactonases. Appl Environ Microbiol 74: 1357–1366. AEM.02014-07 [pii];10.1128/AEM.02014-07 [doi].
26. Ng FS, Wright DM, Seah SY (2011) Characterization of a phosphotriesterase-like lactonase from Sulfolobus solfataricus and its immobilization for disruption of quorum sensing. Appl Environ Microbiol 77: 1181–1186. AEM.01642-10 [pii];10.1128/AEM.01642-10 [doi].
27. Pei R, Lamas-Samanamud GR (2014) Inhibition of biofilm formation by T7 bacteriophages producing quorum quenching enzymes. Appl Environ Microbiol. AEM.01434-14 [pii];10.1128/AEM.01434-14 [doi].
28. Dong YH, Xu JL, Li XZ, Zhang LH (2000) AiiA, an enzyme that inactivates the acylhomoserine lactone quorum-sensing signal and attenuates the virulence of Erwinia carotovora. Proc Natl Acad Sci U S A 97: 3526–3531. 10.1073/pnas.060023897 [doi];060023897 [pii].
29. Stoltz DA, Ozer EA, Taft PJ, Barry M, Liu L, et al. (2008) Drosophila are protected from Pseudomonas aeruginosa lethality by transgenic expression of paraoxonase-1. J Clin Invest 118: 3123–3131. 10.1172/JCI35147 [doi].
30. Papaioannou E, Wahjudi M, Nadal-Jimenez P, Koch G, Setroikromo R, et al. (2009) Quorum-quenching acylase reduces the virulence of Pseudomonas aeruginosa in a Caenorhabditis elegans infection model. Antimicrob Agents Chemother 53: 4891–4897. AAC.00380-09 [pii];10.1128/AAC.00380-09 [doi].
31. Migiyama Y, Kaneko Y, Yanagihara K, Morohoshi T, Morinaga Y, et al. (2013) Efficacy of AiiM, an N-acylhomoserine lactonase, against Pseudomonas aeruginosa in a mouse model of acute pneumonia. Antimicrob Agents Chemother 57: 3653–3658. AAC.00456-13 [pii];10.1128/AAC.00456-13 [doi].
32. Hiblot J, Gotthard G, Elias M, Chabriere E (2013) Differential active site loop conformations mediate promiscuous activities in the lactonase SsoPox. PLoS One 8: e75272. 10.1371/journal.pone.0075272 [doi];PONE-D-13-20233 [pii].
33. Studier FW (2005) Protein production by auto-induction in high density shaking cultures. Protein Expr Purif 41: 207–234.
34. Hiblot J, Gotthard G, Chabriere E, Elias M (2012) Characterisation of the organophosphate hydrolase catalytic activity of SsoPox. Sci Rep 2: 779. 10.1038/srep00779 [doi].
35. Wilkins MR, Gasteiger E, Bairoch A, Sanchez JC, Williams KL, et al. (1999) Protein identification and analysis tools in the ExPASy server. Methods Mol Biol 112: 531–552.
36. Hraiech S, Roch A, Lepidi H, Atieh T, Audoly G, et al. (2013) Impaired virulence and fitness of a colistin-resistant clinical isolate of Acinetobacter baumannii in a rat model of pneumonia. Antimicrob Agents Chemother 57: 5120–5121. AAC.00700-13 [pii];10.1128/AAC.00700-13 [doi].
37. Price-Whelan A, Dietrich LE, Newman DK (2007) Pyocyanin alters redox homeostasis and carbon flux through central metabolic pathways in Pseudomonas aeruginosa PA14. J Bacteriol 189: 6372–6381. JB.00505-07 [pii];10.1128/JB.00505-07 [doi].

38. Nicodeme M, Grill JP, Humbert G, Gaillard JL (2005) Extracellular protease activity of different Pseudomonas strains: dependence of proteolytic activity on culture conditions. J Appl Microbiol 99: 641–648. JAM2634 [pii];10.1111/j.1365-2672.2005.02634.x [doi].
39. Marquette CH, Wermert D, Wallet F, Copin MC, Tonnel AB (1999) Characterization of an animal model of ventilator-acquired pneumonia. Chest 115: 200–209.
40. Hraiech S, Bregeon F, Brunel JM, Rolain JM, Lepidi H, et al. (2012) Antibacterial efficacy of inhaled squalamine in a rat model of chronic Pseudomonas aeruginosa pneumonia. J Antimicrob Chemother 67: 2452–2458. dks230 [pii];10.1093/jac/dks230 [doi].
41. Wagner VE, Gillis RJ, Iglewski BH (2004) Transcriptome analysis of quorum-sensing regulation and virulence factor expression in Pseudomonas aeruginosa. Vaccine 22 Suppl 1: S15–S20. S0264-410X(04)00613-9 [pii];10.1016/j.vaccine.2004.08.011 [doi].
42. Dickschat JS (2010) Quorum sensing and bacterial biofilms. Nat Prod Rep 27: 343–369. 10.1039/b804469b [doi].
43. Deziel E, Gopalan S, Tampakaki AP, Lepine F, Padfield KE, et al. (2005) The contribution of MvfR to Pseudomonas aeruginosa pathogenesis and quorum sensing circuitry regulation: multiple quorum sensing-regulated genes are modulated without affecting lasRI, rhlRI or the production of N-acyl-L-homoserine lactones. Mol Microbiol 55: 998–1014. MMI4448 [pii];10.1111/j.1365-2958.2004.04448.x [doi].
44. Ilangovan A, Fletcher M, Rampioni G, Pustelny C, Rumbaugh K, et al. (2013) Structural basis for native agonist and synthetic inhibitor recognition by the Pseudomonas aeruginosa quorum sensing regulator PqsR (MvfR). PLoS Pathog 9: e1003508. 10.1371/journal.ppat.1003508 [doi];PPATHOGENS-D-12-03063 [pii].
45. Bakker-Woudenberg IA, ten Kate MT, Guo L, Working P, Mouton JW (2002) Ciprofloxacin in polyethylene glycol-coated liposomes: efficacy in rat models of acute or chronic Pseudomonas aeruginosa infection. Antimicrob Agents Chemother 46: 2575–2581.
46. Rezaiguia S, Garat C, Delclaux C, Meignan M, Fleury J, et al. (1997) Acute bacterial pneumonia in rats increases alveolar epithelial fluid clearance by a tumor necrosis factor-alpha-dependent mechanism. J Clin Invest 99: 325–335. 10.1172/JCI119161 [doi].
47. Wen J, Li CM, Gu L, Yin SJ, Li W, et al. (2014) Aging reduces the expression of lung CINC and MCP-1 mRNA in a P. aeruginosa rat model of infection. Inflammation 37: 933–941. 10.1007/s10753-014-9813-5 [doi].
48. Pearson JP, Feldman M, Iglewski BH, Prince A (2000) Pseudomonas aeruginosa cell-to-cell signaling is required for virulence in a model of acute pulmonary infection. Infect Immun 68: 4331–4334.
49. Smith RS, Harris SG, Phipps R, Iglewski B (2002) The Pseudomonas aeruginosa quorum-sensing molecule N-(3-oxododecanoyl)homoserine lactone contributes to virulence and induces inflammation in vivo. J Bacteriol 184: 1132–1139.
50. Seed PC, Passador L, Iglewski BH (1995) Activation of the Pseudomonas aeruginosa lasI gene by LasR and the Pseudomonas autoinducer PAI: an autoinduction regulatory hierarchy. J Bacteriol 177: 654–659.
51. Rutherford ST, Bassler BL (2012) Bacterial quorum sensing: its role in virulence and possibilities for its control. Cold Spring Harb Perspect Med 2. 2/11/a012427 [pii];10.1101/cshperspect.a012427 [doi].
52. Christensen LD, van GM, Jakobsen TH, Alhede M, Hougen HP, et al. (2012) Synergistic antibacterial efficacy of early combination treatment with tobramycin and quorum-sensing inhibitors against Pseudomonas aeruginosa in an intraperitoneal foreign-body infection mouse model. J Antimicrob Chemother 67: 1198–1206. dks002 [pii];10.1093/jac/dks002 [doi].
53. van DC, Kohler T, Brunner-Ferber F, Francois B, Carlet J, et al. (2012) Azithromycin to prevent Pseudomonas aeruginosa ventilator-associated pneumonia by inhibition of quorum sensing: a randomized controlled trial. Intensive Care Med 38: 1118–1125. 10.1007/s00134-012-2559-3 [doi].

22

Polymerase Discordance in Novel Swine Influenza H3N2v Constellations Is Tolerated in Swine but Not Human Respiratory Epithelial Cells

Joshua D. Powell[1], Daniel Dlugolenski[1], Tamas Nagy[2], Jon Gabbard[1], Christopher Lee[1], Stephen M. Tompkins[1], Ralph A. Tripp[1]*

1 Department of Infectious Diseases, Animal Health Research Center, University of Georgia, Athens, Georgia, United States of America, **2** Department of Pathology, College of Veterinary Medicine, University of Georgia, Athens, Georgia, United States of America

Abstract

Swine-origin H3N2v, a variant of H3N2 influenza virus, is a concern for novel reassortment with circulating pandemic H1N1 influenza virus (H1N1pdm09) in swine because this can lead to the emergence of a novel pandemic virus. In this study, the reassortment prevalence of H3N2v with H1N1pdm09 was determined in swine cells. Reassortants evaluated showed that the H1N1pdm09 polymerase (PA) segment occurred within swine H3N2 with ~80% frequency. The swine H3N2-human H1N1pdm09 PA reassortant (swH3N2-huPA) showed enhanced replication in swine cells, and was the dominant gene constellation. Ferrets infected with swH3N2-huPA had increased lung pathogenicity compared to parent viruses; however, swH3N2-huPA replication in normal human bronchoepithelial cells was attenuated - a feature linked to expression of IFN-β and IFN-λ genes in human but not swine cells. These findings indicate that emergence of novel H3N2v influenza constellations require more than changes in the viral polymerase complex to overcome barriers to cross-species transmission. Additionally, these findings reveal that while the ferret model is highly informative for influenza studies, slight differences in pathogenicity may not necessarily be indicative of human outcomes after infection.

Editor: Toru Takimoto, University of Rochester Medical Center, United States of America

Funding: The studies were funded through a contract with the Center of Excellence for Influenza Research and Surveillance (CEIRS; HHSN266200700006C). The funders had no role in study design, data collection and analysis, decision to publish, or preparation of the manuscript.

Competing Interests: The authors have declared that no competing interests exist.

* Email: ratripp@uga.edu

Introduction

Influenza pandemics occur when an animal influenza virus to which humans have no or limited immunity acquires the ability through genetic reassortment or mutation to cause sustained human-to-human transmission leading to community-wide outbreaks. Influenza A viruses (IAV) have the capacity to exchange viral RNA segments when a host cell is co-infected with two IAV strains. IAV reassortment in swine is of global concern as swine support replication and reassortment of human, avian and swine IAV [1–3]. The term "mixing vessel" is often associated with IAV in pigs [4,5] and is embodied by the widely circulating "triple reassortant of internal genes" (TRIG) constellation. The TRIG cassette comprises avian-origin PB2 and PA, human H3N2-origin PB1, and swine-origin M, NP and NS genes [6]. Initially identified in swine in 1998 [7], the TRIG-cassette is hypothesized to have a competitive advantage over other swine influenza virus (SIV) gene constellations [8], and it is thought that this feature helps maintain continued circulation in both H1 and H3 SIV lineages.

In 2009, five of six TRIG genes (with M gene from classical swine) emerged in the form of the human H1N1 pandemic (pdm09) [9]. Presently, pdm09 remains the dominant H1N1 circulating strain in humans emphasizing the need for continued pdm09 studies [10]. During the 2009 human pandemic, via reverse zoonosis, pdm09 was reintroduced back into swine [11] where 10 reassortant H3N2 SIV genotypes harboring one to six pdm09 genes were identified circulating in North American swine herds [12,13]. Numerous SIV surveillance case-reports have also identified pdm09 genes within swine H1N1 and H1N2 subtypes on multiple continents [14–18]. The actual number of SIV constellations containing pdm09 segments is likely much higher, as globally swine surveillance is inconsistent and limited [19]. Given these concerns, determining which of the 256 possible reassortant combinations are compatible during co-infection between pdm09 and circulating endemic SIV strains is highly warranted, but remains largely uncharacterized.

While human infections with H1N1 and H3N2 SIV have been sporadically reported from 1990–2010 [20–22], commonly referred to as "variant" infections, in July 2011 the first H3N2 variant (H3N2v) containing a human-derived pdm09 segment (rH3N2p) was identified in humans [23]. There were 320 confirmed cases of H3N2v documented over this period, where many of these cases were linked to direct contact with swine [24]. It was estimated that that total number of H3N2v related infections exceeded 2000 cases [25].

Whole-genome sequencing of 14 human H3N2v infections has identified the pdm09 M gene consistently occurring within swine H3N2-TRIG viruses [26]. The pdm09 M gene is linked to increased transmissibility [27] [28]; therefore, this segment within H3N2v may represent a critical determinant for swine-to-human transmission. To address the reassortment potential of pdm09 and swine H3N2-TRIG viruses to combine as an H3N2v constellation, and generate infectious (compatible) or non-infectious (incompatible) pdm09-based reassortants, swine cells from a porcine kidney epithelial cell line (PK-1) and a primary normal swine bronchoepithelial cell line isolated from euthanized pigs [29,30] were co-infected with the pdm09 strain (A/California/04/09) and a recently characterized H3N2-TRIG virus (A/Sw/PA/62170-1/2010). This swine H3N2-TRIG isolate was selected as it has established virulence and contact transmissibility in pigs [31]. Furthermore, the HA gene is of cluster-IV lineage, similar to H3N2v human cases [8], and over 99% identical to an isolate found in a human swine farmer in Ontario, Canada in 2005 [22], given its potential for human infection.

In this study, examination of 750 influenza virus isolates from plaques in NSBE cells or PK-1 swine cells co-infected with pdm09 and swine H3N2 viruses showed reassortment for the 6 IAV segments tested (NA, HA, NS, M, PA, and PB1). Later, NP and PB2 IAV segments were deduced for a subset of reassortants. Interestingly, the polymerase acidic (PA) segment of pdm09 occurred within seven genes of H3N2-TRIG (swH3N2-huPA), and this feature was shown to have both a reassortment and replication advantage in the swine cell lines which is consistent with its known functions in the RNA polymerase complex having both endonuclease and cap binding function [32,33]. A second protein encoded within the PA segment, PA-X, is synthesized as a ribosomal frame-shift, and has been shown to modulate virulence and host innate responses and suppress host protein synthesis [34,35]. Given the critical functions of the PA gene, and the continued circulation of pdm09 PA viruses in both swine and humans [36], it was important to determine if the PA gene represents a barrier to viral fitness in swH3N2-huPA reassortants, and determine if differences in replication could be linked to differences in the antiviral host response comprising type I and III interferons (IFNs). Interestingly, replication of one reassortant virus harboring both PA and PB1 pdm09 polymerase genes (swH3N2-huPA-PB1) was attenuated in swine cells and human cells, suggesting that PA-PB1 is a feature that may govern attenuation at the innate cell level in swine and human epithelial cells. Ferrets infected with swH3N2-huPA isolates had increased lung pathogenicity compared to parent viruses confirming the role of the pdm09 PA, and these isolates induced high expression of IFN-β and IFN-λ genes in human but not swine cells. These findings provide evidence that genetic reassortment resulting from co-infection of swine with endemic SIV and human IAV strains may result in novel reassortant viruses with varied degrees of pathogenicity attributed to in part by the the polymerase complex.

Materials and Methods

Ethics statement

All ferret experiments were performed in accordance to the national guidelines provided by the "The Guide for Care and Use of Laboratory Animals" and The University of Georgia Institutional Animal Care and Use Committee (IACUC). The animal use protocol A2012 06-025-Y2-A2 was approved by the University of Georgia IACUC.

Viruses

The H3N2 swine isolate A/Sw/PA/62170-1/2010 [swH3N2] was acquired from the National Veterinary Services Laboratory (NVSL). Pathogenesis, transmission and genetic sequence characterization for this swH3N2 in pigs has been previously established [31]. The human H1N1 virus, A/California/04/2009 (pdm09), was provided by the Center for Disease Control and Prevention (Atlanta, GA) and has been previously characterized [37].

Cells

Viruses were propagated in Madin-Darby Canine Kidney (MDCK; ATTC #CCL-34) cells. The PK-1 cell line was acquired from ATCC (#CL-101). The isolation, culturing and differentiation of primary NSBE has been described previously [30]. NSBE cells were verified by University of Georgia Veterinary Medical Diagnostic Laboratory (VMDL) as PCR-negative for influenza, circovirus and porcine reproductive respiratory syndrome virus before use. Primary normal human bronchoepithelial (NHBE) cells were purchased (Lonza CC-2540). Both NSBE and NHBE cells were cultured at air-liquid-interface.

Co-infection and plaque isolation

Co-infection of swine cells was performed at MOI = 3 in infection media (DMEM, 1 mM L-glutamine, 0.5 μg/mL trypsin). The cell supernatant was collected at 18 h post-infection (hpi) and the PFU/mL determined by plaque assay as previously described [38]. PK-1 and NSBE cell supernatants were added to confluent MDCK cells in 15-cm^2 tissue culture dishes for 1 h in DMEM, washed 2X PBS, and overlaid with infection media supplemented with 0.225% sodium bicarbonate and 2% agarose. Serial dilutions were optimized to ensure adequate spacing between virus plaques (<100 plaques). Plaques isolated from agar were amplified in 48-well plates using the NSBE cells or PK-1 cells for 48 h before RNA extraction and multiplex qPCR analysis. Additionally, select reassortants were propagated in MDCK cells in the presence of 1 μg/ml trypsin to generate viral stocks for downstream experiments. After propagation in MDCK, the PCR Ct values for viral stocks were verified to confirm that there was no mixed infection.

qPCR multiplex

Supernatants from virus-infected PK-1 and NSBE cells cultured in 48-well plates of were RNA purified using an RNeasy Mini-kit (Qiagen). 500 ng of RNA was used for cDNA synthesis with a Verso cDNA kit (Thermo Scientific) using random hexamer primers according to manufacturer's instructions. cDNA reactions were diluted 10-fold and used as template for qPCR analysis. Multiplex qPCR primer/probe sequences and their location within genome segments of SwH32-PA [TaxID: 938271] and huH1N1-CA [TaxID: 641501] are noted in Fig. S1. After primers were initially verified for specificity by using SYBR GreenER Supermix PCR (Life Technologies), Quencher probes Iowa Black FQ-Cy5 and ZEN-double-quenched probes specific for 6-FAM and HEX, (Integrated DNA Technologies) were implemented in a 3-plex reaction using a Quanti-Tech Multiplex PCR kit (Qiagen). cDNA from each corresponding plaque was analyzed in 4 separate reactions specific for either swine or human HA-NA-NS1 and swine or human PB2-PA-M. Ct values for swH3N2 and huH1N1 positive controls isolated as described above and the schematic for qPCR analysis is shown in Fig. S2, confirming the specificity of the 2×3-plex six gene assay. The remaining two influenza genes, PB1 and NP for select reassortants were deduced by SYBR GreenER supermix PCR (Life Technologies) (Fig. S1,bottom). All qPCR reactions were carried out in an Agilent Mx3005P qPCR instrument with an initial 5 min denaturation, and 40 cycles of denaturation at 95°C, 15 sec of annealing at 57°C, 15 sec, and 15 sec of extension at 72°C.

Co-infection studies

Supernatants (1 µL) from the 24-well virus isolates at the corresponding MOI were used to co-infect PK-1 cells or NSBE cells for 48 h. For each respective passage, the cells were washed 2X in PBS, and the infections proceeded for an additional 48 h. This was repeated for all subsequent passages. At passage 8, a multiplex qPCR was used to determine the six influenza gene segments. The additional two genes, PB1 and NP, were determined by SYBR GreenER Supermix qPCR (Life Technologies).

Viral kinetics

Virus stocks of selected reassortants were analyzed in PK-1 cells, MDCK cells, undifferentiated normal swine bronchoepithelial cells, fully differentiated normal swine bronchoepithelial (dNSBE) cells, and fully-differentiated normal human bronchoepithelial (dNHBE) as described [30,39] at an MOI = 0.01 for 24, 48, 56 and 72 hpi. All viral titers were determined by the 50% tissue culture infectious dose ($TCID_{50}$) assay [40]. Peak titers were confirmed by plaque assay using 1.2% Avicel, and by $TCID_{50}$ assay. The dNHBE and dNSBE cell infections were performed using DMEM without exogenous trypsin at an MOI = 0.01, the cells washed 3X in PBS, and infections allowed to progress at the air-liquid interface. Apical titers were determined by gently washing cells 2×500 µL PBS. Basolateral titers were directly deduced from primary growth media.

Plaque morphology and size

Ten-fold serial dilutions of supernatant from virally infected cells was overlaid with 2% agarose in 1X overlay media for 4 days and stained with crystal violet [41]. Selected plaques, totaling 10–20 plaques/well from 2–3 representative wells, were scanned using a standard flatbed Hewlett Packard Inkjet scanner. Relative plaque diameters were measured using Photoshop 5.0 software.

qPCR gene expression in dNHBE and dNSBE cells

Taqman qPCR primer probes for determining the innate signaling response were purchased from Life Technologies and used per the manufacturer suggestion. RNA extraction and cDNA synthesis reagents were performed as described above for qPCR multiplex. 500 ng of total RNA was used in cDNA synthesis and diluted to a final concentration of 2.5 ng for each qPCR reaction. Primer-probes were commercially prepared from Life Technologies are as previously noted [30].

Ferret studies

Outbred 0.8–1.0 kg juvenile female ferrets (Triple F Farms, Sayre, PA), were tested and determined to seronegative by hemagglutination inhibition assay to influenza virus. Only seronegative ferrets were used for the studies. Prior to infection, a subcutaneous implantable temperature transponder (BioMedic Data Systems, Seaford, DE) was used to monitor body temperature. Ferrets were anesthetized with isoflurane and intranasally inoculated with 0.2 ml of virus (0.1 ml per nostril) at 10^6 PFU/ml totaling 2×10^5 PFU. Weights and temperatures were monitored every other day for 8 days pi, and at day 15 pi prior to euthanasia. Nasal washes were obtained from ferrets on days 2, 4, 6, and 8 days pi. Ferrets were anesthetized with ketamine (30 mg/kg), and nasal washes isolated as described previously [37]. Both $TCID_{50}$ and plaque assays (PFU/ml) were used to confirm viral load in nasal washes. Five ferrets (n = 5) were used for each experiment.

Histopathological examination of ferret tissues

In addition to ferret nasal wash studies, three ferrets per virus were used to determine histopathology at day 3 pi (2×10^5 PFU) with swH3N2, pdm09 or swH3N2-huPA virus, and two ferrets were mock-infected with PBS. At day 3 pi, ferrets were euthanized and the head and lungs fixed in 10% buffered formalin for histological examination. Bone was decalcified for 14 days prior to nasal turbinate analysis. Both hematoxylin and eosin (H&E) staining and immunohistochemical (IHC) analysis was performed as previously reported [37]. Briefly, lung and nasal turbinates were embedded in paraffin wax, sectioned 4–5 µm thick, and placed on glass slides. Tissues were examined by IHC and using H&E staining to detect lesions consistent with viral infection. For IHC, primary mouse anti-NP influenza mouse monoclonal antibody (ATCC; *H16-L10-4R5*) was used at 5 µg/ml.

Immunofluorescence co-localization analysis

Co-localization studies in dNSBE and dNSBE cell studies were performed as previously described [39]. Briefly, cells were stained for α2,6 or α2,3 sialic acids, permeabilized, and stained with anti-NP influenza antibody [ATCC; *H16-L10-4R5*] and AlexaFluor 488 (Molecular Probes). Images were obtained with a Zeiss LSM 710 confocal microscope.

Statistical analysis

Statistical analysis was performed using GraphPad Prism 5 software. One-way ANOVA analysis was performed using GraphPad Prism software with $p<0.05$ as indicated by an asterisk (*).

Results

Swine H3N2-TRIG viruses containing the pdm09 PA gene have a reassortant advantage

A 6-gene multiplex qPCR assay for segments PA, PB2, M, NS, NA and HA was utilized to delineate the parent segment for selected plaques. In total, 363 of 408 PK-1 cell plaques, and 323 of 351 NSBE cell plaques were distinguished as to the origin of the parent viral segment (Fig 1). While a majority of plaques were not reassortants for the six genes analyzed, 45 of 323 NSBE cell plaques (14%; Fig. 1, left), and 121 of 363 PK-1 cell plaques (33%; Fig. 1, right) were reassortants. qPCR multiplex profiling confirmed the PA segment of pdm09 was the most frequent reassortant gene which was identified in 93 of 121 PK-1 cell reassortants, in 39 of 45 NSBE cell reassortants, and was the primary gene detected in the swine H3N2 HA/NA backbone. The top six reassortant constellations identified from plaques is summarized in Figure 1. Interestingly, only five PK-1 cell-derived reassortants were identified that contained HA or NA genes of pdm09 origin. While reassortment frequency was lower in NSBE cells compared to PK-1 cells, a higher degree of diversity in genotypes was derived from NSBE cells implying fundamental differences in co-infection outcomes for swine cells of kidney origin (PK-1 cells) compared to those isolated as primary lung respiratory epithelial cells. Nonetheless, both swine cell lines revealed preferential pdm09 PA gene incorporation within the swine H3N2 backbone. Of note, due to the high nucleotide similarity of NP and PB1 for parent strains, determining the parental viruses in a high-throughput screening approach was not viable using quencher probes. However, subsequent SYBR green qPCR primers were designed to target a more unique region of PB1

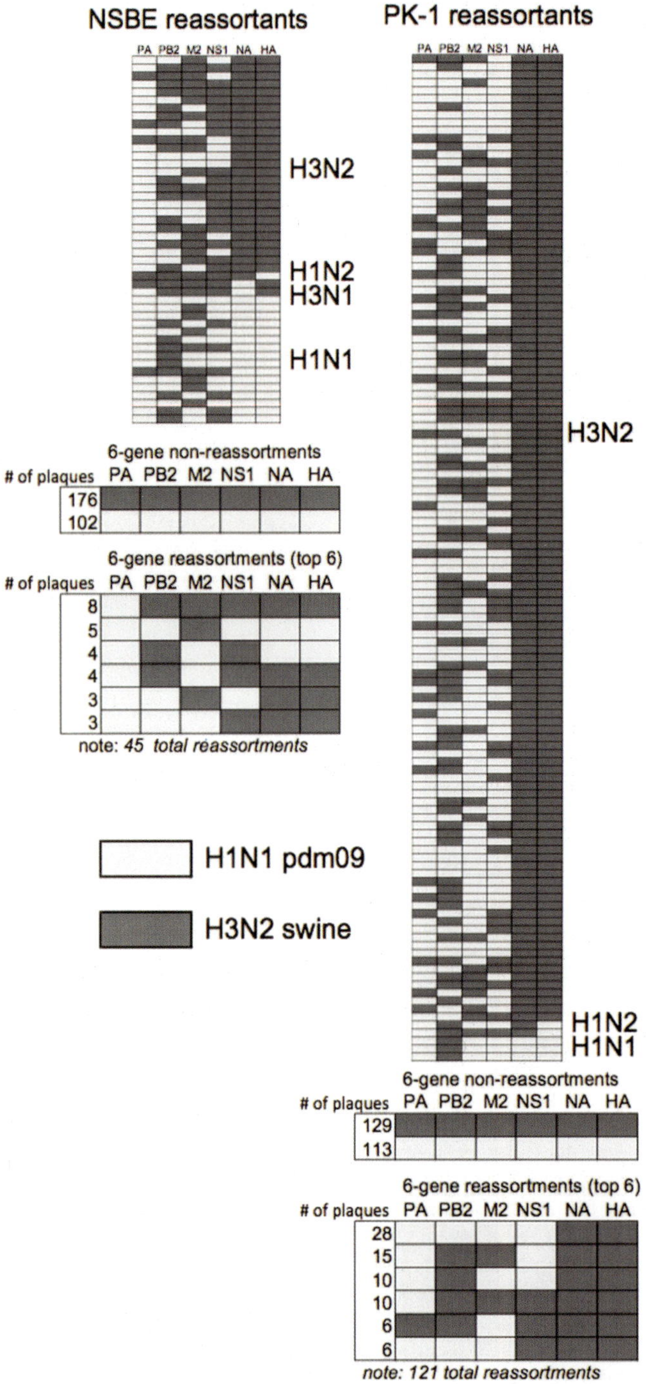

Figure 1. Reassortment outcomes following human H1N1 pdm09 and swine H3N2 co-infection. Segments originating from pdm09 origin (light colored) and swH3N2 (dark-colored) are shown after co-infection in NSBE cells (left) and PK-1 cells. Primer and probes specific to parental strains pdm09 and swH3N2 gene segments were used and from left to right in the matrix correspond to PA, PB2, M, NS, NA and HA. All reassortant plaques identified are categorized by HA and NA backbone type. In total, 121 reassortants for PK-1 cells and 45 reassortants for NSBE cells were evaluated. The number of virus plaques showing 6-gene non-reassortment and the top 6 reassortant types are summarized below profile matrix.

and NP (Fig. S1) which was specific, thus both qPCR approaches were used to determine all eight gene segments for reassortants reported.

pdm09 PA gene reassortment

To determine if a dominant reassortant genotype occurred after co-infection with pdm09 and swH3N2 viruses in swine cells, a multiplex qPCR approach (Fig. 1) was combined with SYBR green qPCR for NP and PB1 that enabled all viral segments to be determined. An equivalent starting MOI = 1:1, or 10-fold bias (MOI = 1.0:0.1 or 1.0:0.1) for pdm09 and swH3N2 was used to infect PK-1 cells (Fig. 2A) and primary NSBE cells (Fig. 2B). Although in limited cases a dominant genotype for a given gene segment could not be definitively identified by qPCR, and were

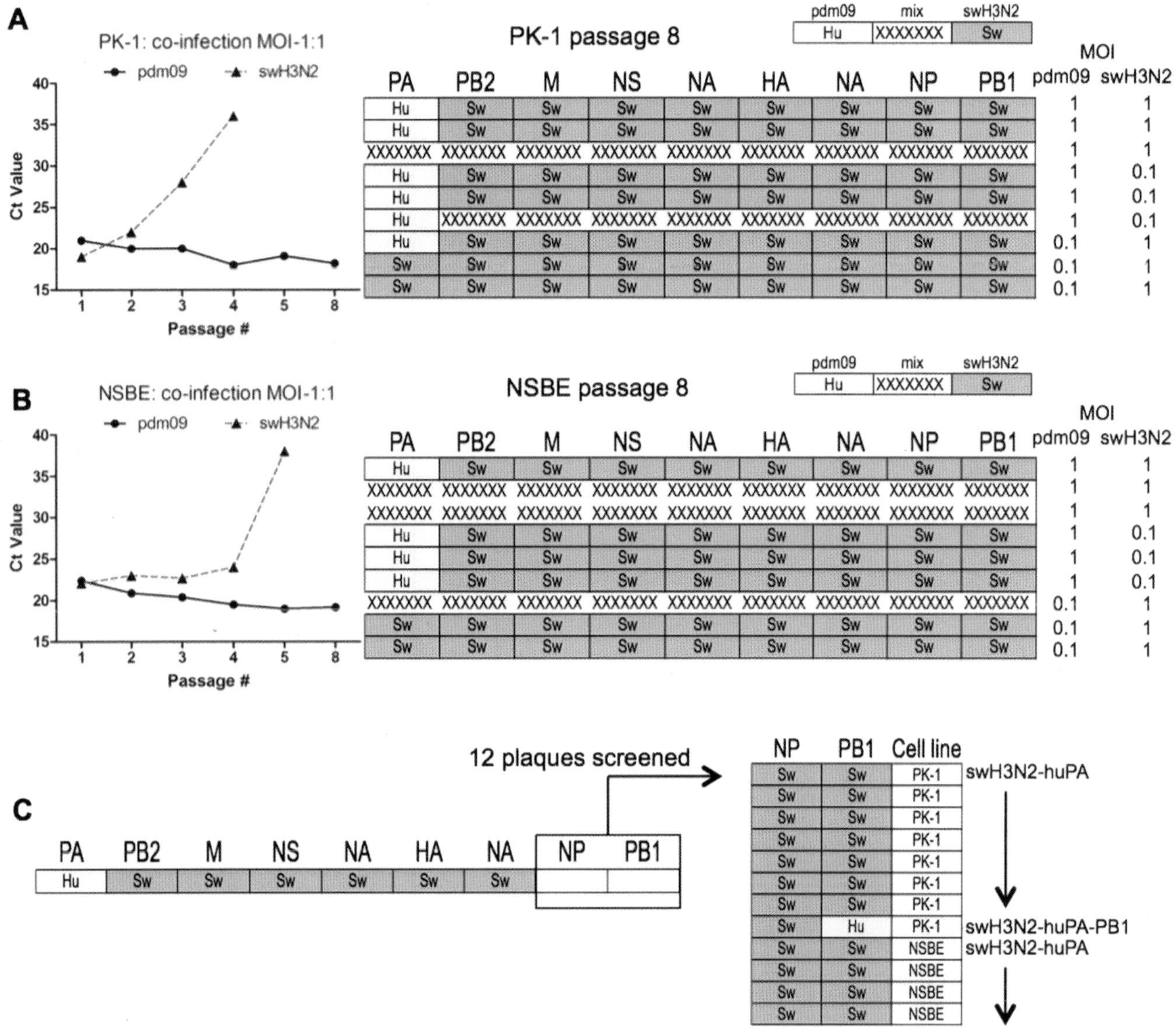

Figure 2. Reassortment findings after eight serial passages. Co-infection was performed in (A) PK-1 cells and (B) NSBE cells. While pdm09 and swH3N2 parent viruses were evident the only reassortant constellation identified was the PA segment of human pdm09 (light colored, "Hu") within seven gene segments from swH3N2 (dark colored, "Sw"). Mixed gene segments with Ct values <8 are depicted as hash marks. Serial passaging was done in triplicate with a starting MOI of either 1.0 or 0.1 for each virus as indicated. To the left of (A) PK-1 cells and (B) NSBE cells is the kinetics of PA acquisition and loss for a MOI = 1:1. Depicted is the first replicate shown from matrix. (C) 12 plaques with PA gene of pdm09 and 5 segments of swH3N2 from reassortant studies (Fig. 1) were subjected to qPCR do delineate the final two segments, NP and PB1. Depicted on right, 11 of 12 reassortants were determined to be swH3N2-huPA, and 1 of 12 reassortants to be swH3N2-huPA-PB1.

identified as multiple viral isolates are denoted as "mixed" in Fig. 2 (X-dashed), there was a high propensity for human "hu" pdm09 PA incorporation within swine "sw" H3N2 backbone (Fig. 2B). Subsequently, viral RNA from the supernatant of MOI = 1:1 cultures was probed to determine pdm09 PA gene acquisition and swH3N2 PA gene loss for all eight serial passages. It was confirmed that pdm09 PA was acquired between passages 3–5 (Fig. 2, left). Of note, cDNA from 12 plaques isolated (Fig. 1) having a gene constellation from swH3N2 and pdm09 PA were also screened for incorporation of the other polymerase genes and NP (Fig. 2C). Consistent with passaging studies (Fig. 2A, B), only one-of-twelve isolates had additional pdm09 polymerase segments corresponding to the PB1 of pdm09 virus (Fig. 2C). Of note, neither PB1 nor PB2 genes from pdm09 were present in swH3N2 after passaging Collectively; these results indicate that the PA gene of pdm09 provides a reassortment advantage without the preferential need of pdm09 segments PB1 and PB2. Given these findings, swH3N2-huPA, the single swH3N2-huPA-PB1 reassortant (Fig. 2C) and the parent viruses, swH3N2 and pdm09, were further studied.

The pdm09 PA gene facilitates replication in swine cells

Reassortment profiles (Fig. 1) and replication trends (Fig. 2A, B) infer that the swH3N2-huPA gene constellation improves viral fitness and replication. Thus, the replication kinetics of swH3N2-huPA compared to its parent strains was determined for the three virus isolates. In addition, the swH3N2-huPA-PB1 isolate (Fig. 2C) was also evaluated. As anticipated, all three swH3N2-huPA

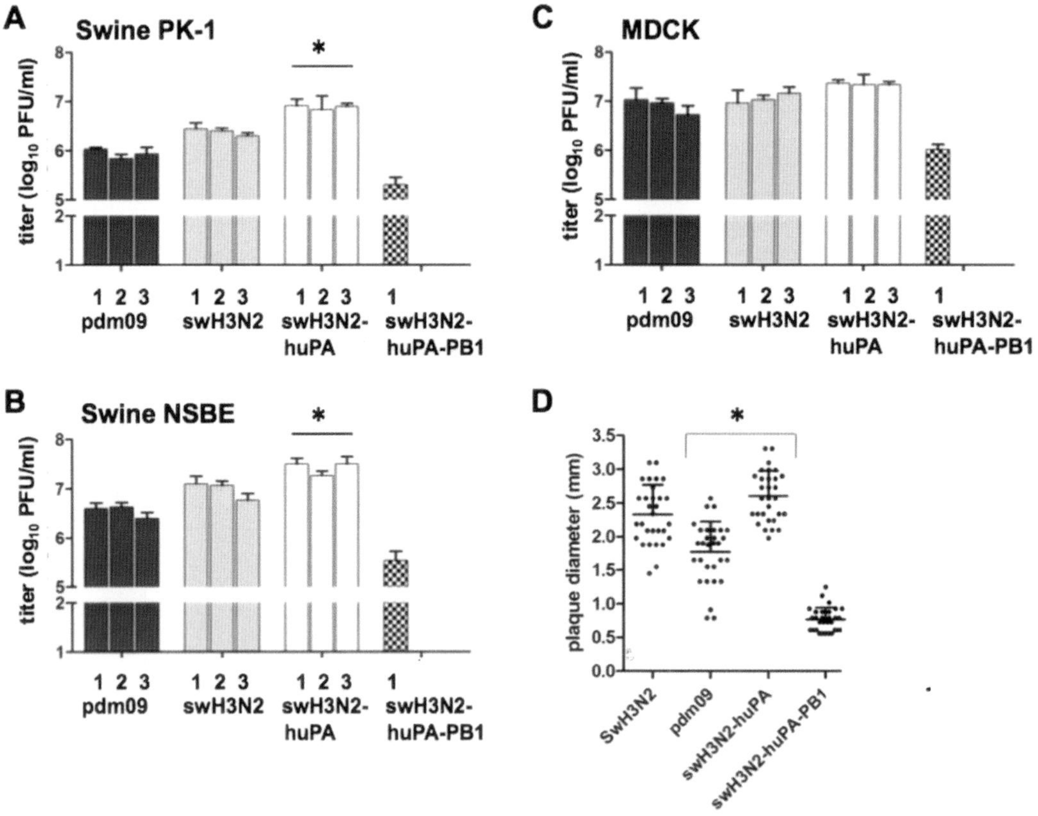

Figure 3. Peak virus titers from plaque isolates with pdm09, swH3N2, swH3N2-huPA, and swH3N2-huPA-PB1 gene constellations. The cell lines used are: (A) PK-1 cells, (B) NSBE cells, and (C) MDCK cells. Significant ($p < 0.05$) differences in viral titer for swH3N2-huPA and both parental strains is indicated by an asterisk (*). Of note, only one swH3N2 reassortant with huPA-PB1 genes was identified (Fig. 2C). All infections used a MOI = 0.01. (D) Plaque diameter were measured 96 h pi in 2% agarose overlay solution. Cumulative plaque total measured from 2–3 separate six-well plates with 10–20 total plaques dilutions per well. * denotes significant difference between pdm09 and swH3N2-huPA.

isolates exhibited higher peak virus titers in PK-1 cells (Fig. 3A) and undifferentiated NSBE cells (Fig. 3B) compared to parent strains. In MDCK cells, although not significant, higher peak virus titers trended for swH3N2-huPA compared to the parent strains (Fig. 3C). The swH3N2-huPA-PB1 reassortant was appreciably attenuated in all three cell lines (Fig. 3A, B, C), a feature that may explain the limited detection of this constellation after passaging (Fig. 2C). Agarose plaque assays used to determine plaque morphology revealed that the acquisition of the pdm09 PA gene for swH3N2-huPA resulted in plaque morphology similar to the swH3N2 virus. This finding was more pronounced when the agarose concentration was increased to 2%, a feature that allows for larger plaque size and was revealed for swH3N2-huPA compared to swH3N2 viruses (Fig. 3D). These findings suggest there is enhanced replicative fitness for swH3N2-huPA virus compared to swH3N2-huPA-PB1 virus, or the parental strains. Notably, a swH3N2-huPB2 constellation was not detected in the initial screen (Fig. 1), subsequently 22 virus plaques which had 6 gene segments of swH3N2 (Fig. 1) were screened for pdm09 PB1 and NP within swH3N2, but neither pdm09 PB1, PB2 or NP was detected within the seven remaining swH3N2 segments.

swH3N2-huPA reassortants have increased pathogenicity in a ferret model

Based on the findings showing increased replicative fitness for swH3N2-huPA virus (Fig. 3), and the reassortment profiles and genotyping (Fig. 1 and 2), the ferret model was used to assess the pathogenicity of the swH3N2-huPA virus (Fig. 4). Nasal inoculation of ferrets with pdm09, swH3N2 or swH3N2-huPA viruses revealed increased nasal wash virus titers for swH3N2-huPA at day 2 pi, and considerably increased virus titers at day 4 pi compared to parent virus titers (Fig. 4A). Morbidity was assessed by the percent body weight change during the course of infection. At day 4 pi, although not significant ($p > 0.05$), there was a trend toward increased body weight loss in ferrets infected with swH3N2-huPA (Fig. 4B). Notably, at day 4 pi, there was a thick nasal discharge in 4 of 5 ferrets infected with swH3N2-huPA, but only 2 of 5 swH3N2-infected ferrets, and 1 of 5 pdm09-infected ferrets displayed substantial nasal discharge. At day 6 pi, clinical symptoms of infection had dissipated in all ferrets cohort. Hematoxylin and Eosin (H&E) pathology studies were performed at day 3 pi in ferrets infected with pdm09, swH3N2 or swH3N2-huPA viruses (Fig. 4C). The findings revealed increased rhinitis and inflammation of the mucous membrane in nasal turbinates of swH3N2-huPA infected ferrets compared to ferrets infected with parent viruses, as well as elevated levels of infiltrating cells (Fig. 4C, asterisk), and thinning of the epithelial cell lining. At day 3 pi, 2 of 3 swH3N2-huPA infected ferrets had detectable influenza NP antigen by IHC, and pulmonary cell infiltration as assessed by H&E staining (Fig. 4D vs. 4E). In contrast, very few NP-positive cells were detected in the lungs ferrets infected with swH3N2 virus (1 of 3 ferrets), or ferrets infected with pdm09 virus (1 of 3 ferrets) at day 3 pi. The pathology findings (Fig. 4C, D, E) and the enhanced nasal virus shedding observed at day 2 and 4 pi

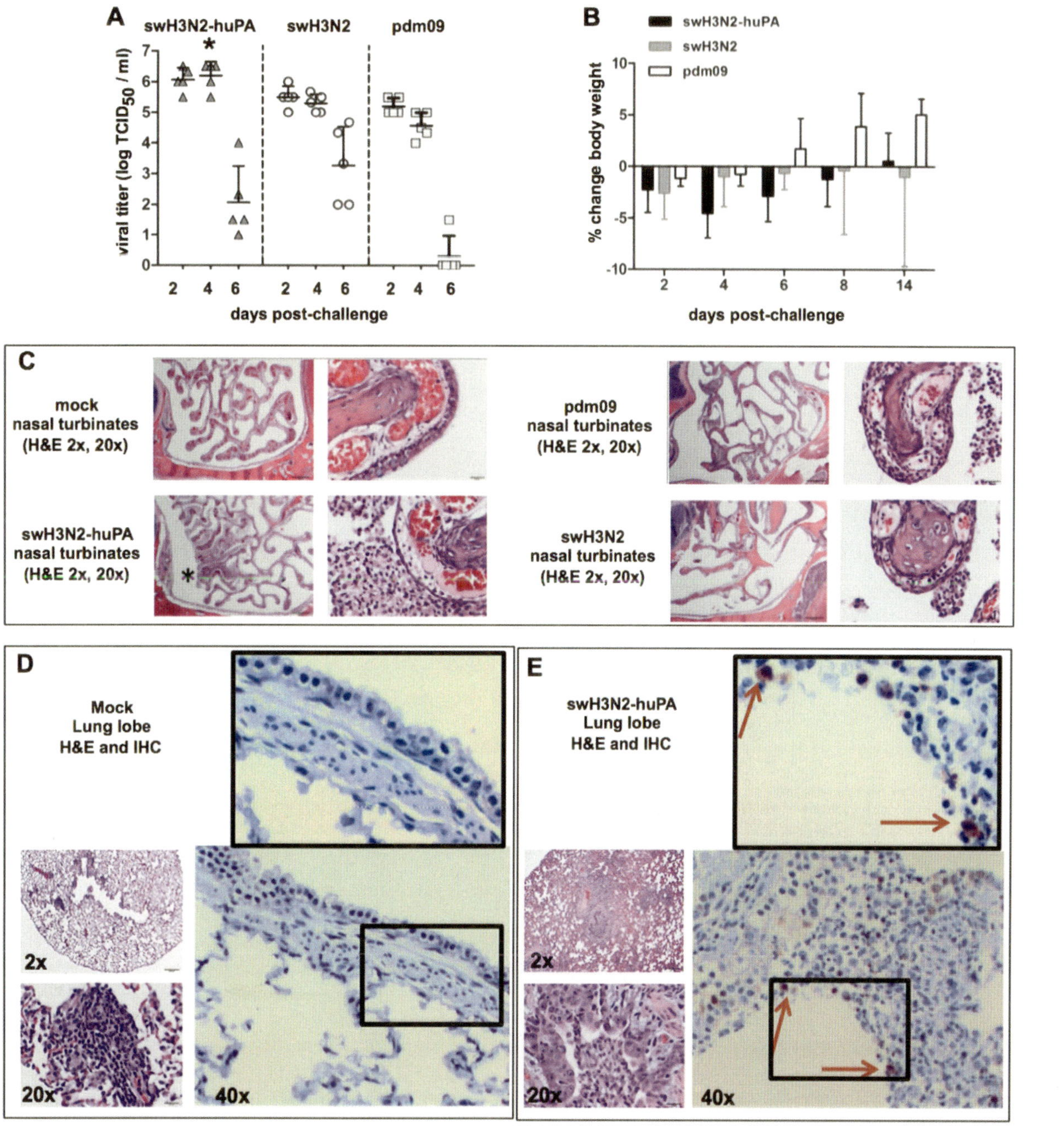

Figure 4. swH3N2-huPA infection is linked to increased nasal virus titers and pathology at early time points post-infection in ferrets (A). Virus titers from nasal washes indicate an increased viral load for swH3N2 at day 2 and 4 pi. An asterisk (*) denotes a significant ($p<0.05$) difference between swH3N2-huPA and both parental strains at day 4 pi. (B) Percent change in body weight over the course of infection as a measure of morbidity at day 4 pi following swH3N2-huPA infection. (C). Representative H&E images from nasal turbinates at 3 days pi. 2× magnification (left) and 20× magnification for mock, swH3N2-huPA and parent viruses. Asterisks show the region of magnification for swH3N2-huPA, and highlight the increased rhinitis in nasal turbinates and accompanying cell infiltration. Representative lung images following mock (D) and swH3N2-huPA (E) infection at day 3 pi showing H&E at 2X and 20X (left) and IHC stains at 40X. Arrows denote NP-positive cells with magnification of boxed area for viewing clarity. All ferrets excluding mock animals were infected with 2×10^5 PFU.

(Fig. 4A), suggest that pdm09 PA gene reassortants cause increased pathogenesis in a ferret model.

swH3N2-huPA viruses replicate efficiently in differentiated swine respiratory epithelial cells

A majority of influenza pathogenesis studies are performed in the ferret model. Although these studies provide insight, the findings do not fully reflect the range of disease associated in humans infected with influenza virus. In contrast, primary normal bronchial epithelial cells from humans or swine can provide a surrogate model of lung disease to help elucidate some of the mechanisms of disease pathogenesis in the airways [30,39,42]. Primary normal swine bronchoepithelial cells and primary normal human bronchoepithelial cells cultured at air-liquid interface polarize and form a three dimensional cell architecture comparable to typical lung architecture [30,39,42]. During differentia-

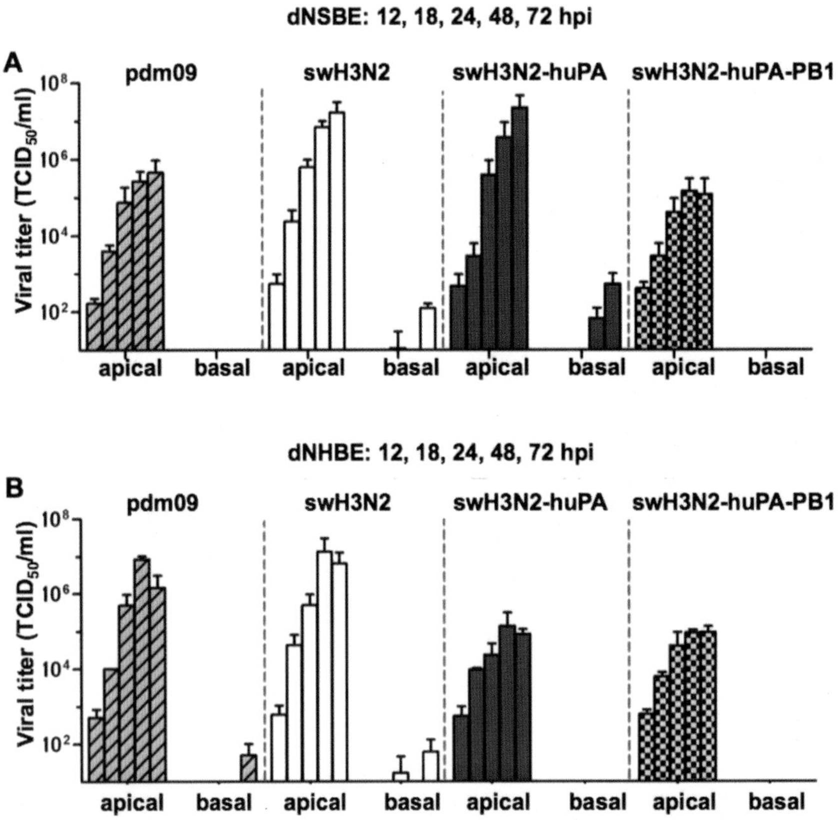

Figure 5. Kinetics of parent and reassortant virus replication in dNSBE and dNHBE cells. Replication kinetics in (A) swine dNSBE cells and (B) dNHBE cells at air-liquid interface. Viruses were infected on the apical side (left) and assessed for the ability to migrate through both the mucus layer and the polarized multi-layer epithelial architecture to the basolateral side [4].

tion of NSBE (dNSBE) and NHBE cells (dNHBE), these cells form tight junctions and are capable of secreting mucus. dNHBE and dNSBE cells express sialic acid (sias) receptor α2–6, and lower levels of α2–3 sias [39,43,44]. To determine if differences in Type I or III IFNs by dNSBE and dNHBE cells responding to IAV infection were a barrier restricting cross-species infection, and/or reassortment, comparative studies were performed. The results showed that H3N2-huPA-PB1 replication was attenuated in both cell lines, and swH3N2-huPA was attenuated in dNHBE cells but not dNSBE cells (Fig. 5A vs. Fig. 5B). These findings indicated innate antiviral host response differences between swine and human epithelial cells.

The kinetics of swH3N2, pdm09, swH3N2-huPA and swH3N2-huPA-PB1 replication in dNSBE cells (Fig. 5A) were consistent with that in PK-1 cells and undifferentiated NSBE cells (Fig. 3A, B). This was evident for swH3N2-huPA by the level of virus isolated from apical washes, and by detection in the basolateral media. These findings support the concept of enhanced replication fitness for swH3N2-huPA compared to the parent strains in dNSBE cells. Interestingly, when the viruses were assessed for replication in dNHBE cells, there was an approximate 2-log attenuation of replication for the reassortant viruses compared to parental strains (Fig. 5B), and no virus was isolated from the basolateral media. These findings show that neither pdm09 PA alone, or in combination with pdm09 PB1 in a swine H3N2 context enhances replicative fitness in human dNHBE cells.

Given the differences in virus replication in dNSBE cells compared to dNHBE cells some of the features linked to virus tropism were investigated. The level of α2–3 and α2–6 sias expression on dNHBE and dNSBE cells was determined (Fig. 6). Immunofluorescence co-localization studies of α2–3 sias (Fig. 6A) and α2–6 sias (Fig. 6B) on dNHBE cells following swH3N2-huPA infection showed no substantial difference in expression among the sias as indicated by the level of sias co-localization (yellow; Fig. 6). As expected from earlier related studies [39], swH3N2-huPA virus infection co-localized with α2–6 sias (Fig. 6B, C), but was not exclusively reliant on α2–6 expression for infection based on influenza NP staining and α2–3 and α2–6 sias staining of dNHBE and dNSBE cells. Consistent with the replication kinetics (Fig. 5), levels of influenza NP (green staining) appeared less abundant at 24 h pi for reassortants compared to parental viruses post-infection (MOI = 0.01) of dNHBE cells (Fig. 6A, B). Attenuation of virus replication was also confirmed at 48 h pi in dNHBE cells (representative images in Fig. S3), indicating that viral attenuation (Fig. 5) may relate to NP abundance as determined by immunofluorescence (Fig. 6B, S3). Higher resolution (60X) images for swH3N2-huPA infection of dNHBE or dNSBE cells showed similar tropism based on immunofluorescence and co-staining of α2–3 and α2–6 sias despite the scant cells infected (Fig. 6C). Of note, >10% of dNSBE cells were positive for α2–3 sias (Fig.6C, right), while <5% of NHBE cells expressed α2–3 sias (Fig. 6C, left). Interestingly α2–3 sias staining for both dNSBE and dNHBE cells showed patchy expression (Fig. 6C). These findings indicate that the differences between swH3N2-huPA and parent virus replication in normal fully differentiated swine or human bronchoepithelial cells is not based on differences in cell tropism linked to α2–3 and α2–6 sias expression.

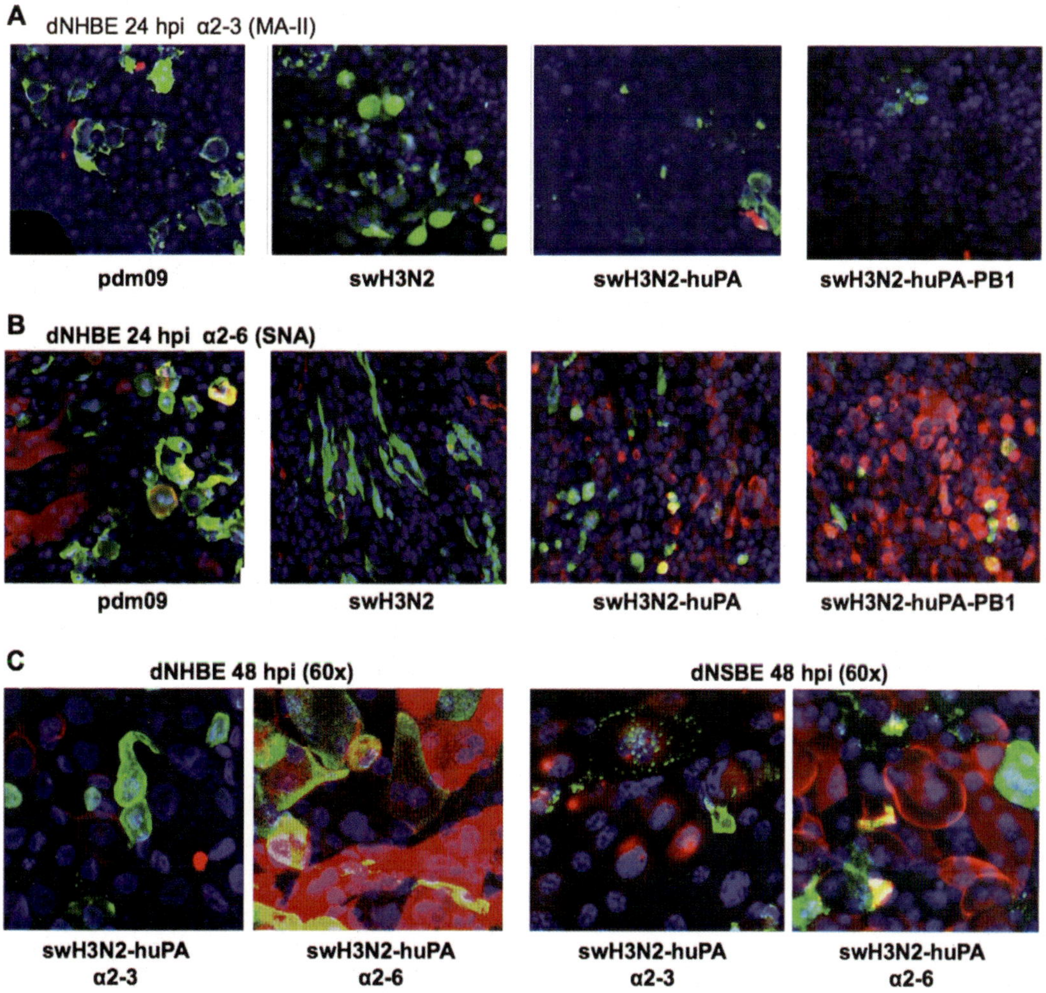

Figure 6. Immunofluorescence co-localization studies of virus and sialic acid expression on dNHBE cells. To determine co-localization of virus with sialic acid expression, cells were examined for either (A) α2–3 sialic acid by MAA-II lectin stain (red) or (B) α2–6 SNA lectin stain (red). DAPI was used for nuclear staining (blue). Yellow indicates co-localization of the NP with sialic acids. (C) 60× magnification of swH3N2-huPA reassortant showed similar localization profiles as other viruses in dNHBE cells (left) and dNSBE cells [4] revealing minimal to no localization (yellow) in α2–3 stained cells versus more noticeable NP co-localization with α2–6 sialic acid.

As differences in α2–3 and α2–6 sias expression did not solely account for differences in swH3N2-huPA or parent virus replication in dNHBE and dNSBE cells (Fig. 6), differences in the expression of interferon (IFN) IFN-α and IFN-β was explored (Fig. 7). Both type I interferon and type III IFN-λ genes (IL-28 and IL-29) are antiviral and can modulate virus replication [45]. qPCR analysis showed that infection of dNSBE with the parental viruses does not appreciably induce IFN-α (Fig. 7A), IFN-β (Fig. 7B) or IFN-λ IL-29 (Fig. 7C) expression at early time points of infection which is in agreement with previously qPCR findings in dNSBE cells infected with avian, swine and human IAV strains [30]. However, IL28, the only other detectable type III interferon in swine [46], was highly up-regulated at the transcript level in NSBE, a novel and yet unreported finding regarding IAV infection in swine (Fig. 7D).

Comparison of type I and III IFN expression in dNSBE and dNHBE cells following infection with reassortant and parent viruses showed modest IFN-α induction (Fig. 7A) at 48 h and 72 h pi for reassortant viruses in human but not swine cells. Notable are the findings in dNSBE following swH3N2-huPA-PB1 infection, and to a lesser extent, the findings following swH3N2-huPA infection which showed increased IFN-β (Fig. 7B), IFN-λ (Fig. 7C) and IL-28 (Fig. 7D) expression at earlier time-points. Cytokine expression that occurs earlier (8 h to 48 h pi) compared to later time-points (72 h pi) likely has a greater impact on viral replication (Fig. 5). Reassortant virus replication was attenuated in human dNHBE, a finding consistent with the antiviral IFN profiles. IFN-stimulated genes (ISGs) ISG15, Mx1 and OAS1 were explored (Fig. 8) as these genes also function to regulate virus replication [47]. As predicted from the IFN expression results (Fig. 7), parental and reassortant viruses induced high ISG expression in dNSBE cells at 24 h pi (Fig. 8A) and 72 h pi (Fig. 8B). Interestingly, in dNSBE cells, expression of all three antiviral effectors were substantially higher compared to in dNHBE cells at 24 h pi, and the trend contrasted at 72 hpi indicating that there are kinetic differences in the antiviral response between human and swine respiratory epithelium. By 72 h pi, dNHBE cells exhibited pronounced up-regulation of IFN genes, while IFN expression levels in dNSBEs appeared unaltered between the 24 h and 72 h time-points (Fig. 8A vs. 8B). These anti-viral differences may account for virus replication differences between swine and human cell types.

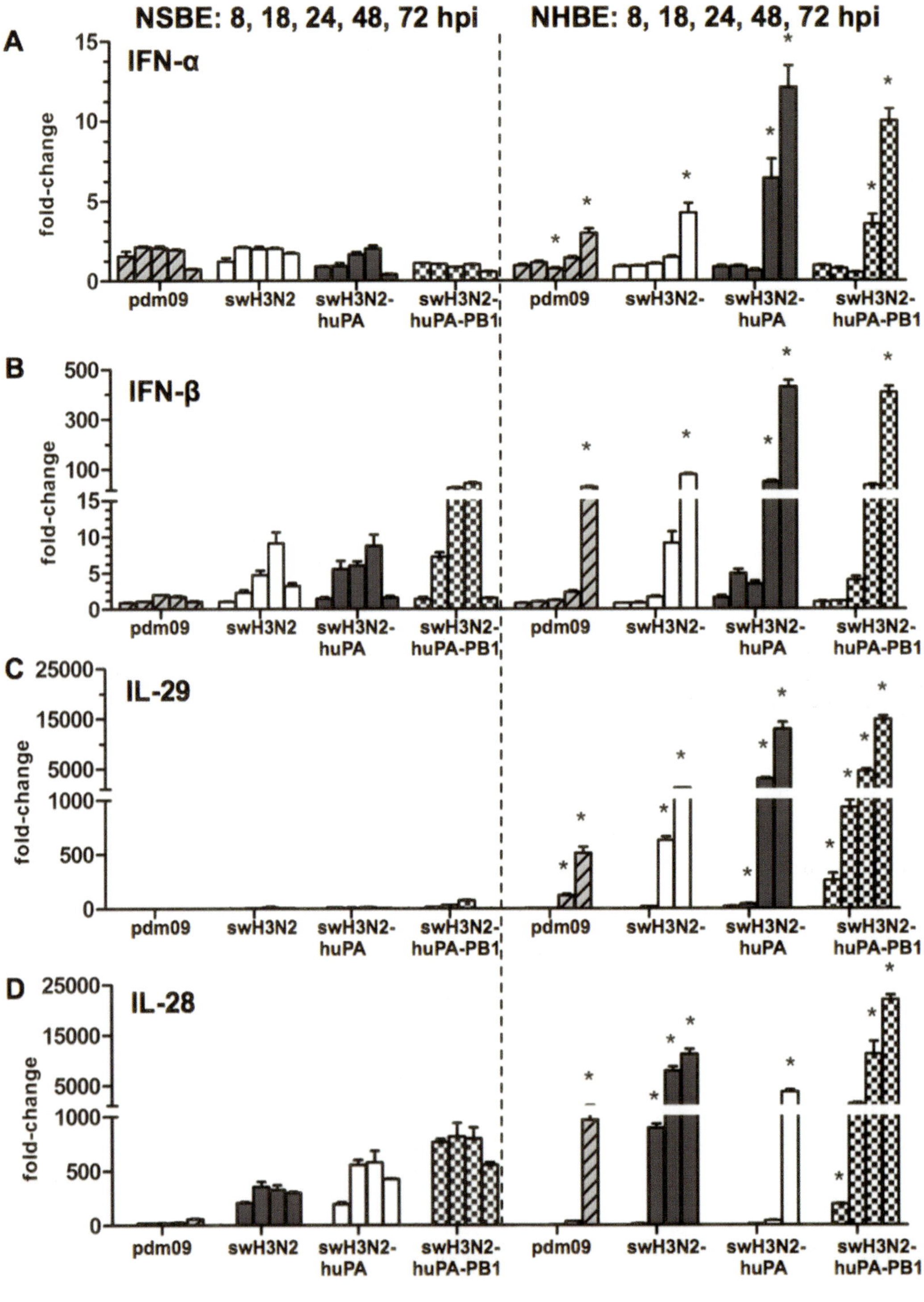

Figure 7. qPCR analysis of the type I and III IFN response in dNSBE and dNHBE cells. The qPCR fold-changes at 8 h, 18 h, 24 h, 48 h, and 72 h pi are shown for virus-infected dNSBE (left) and NHBE cells [4]. Shown is type I interferons (A) IFN-α (B) IFN-β and type III interferons (C) IL-29 (D) IL-28. Time-points that were significant (* = $p<0.05$) by one-way ANOVA comparing swine and human gene expression are indicated. Fold-changes and standard deviations were calculated from Ct values run in quadruplicate relative mock and the housekeeping gene HPRT1.

Discussion

Identification of reassortment trends between endemic circulating SIVs and seasonal human strains of IAV can provide a framework for identifying potential factors involved in pathogenicity and novel gene constellations that enable zoonosis. The emergence of new influenza A viruses with pandemic potential requires crossing species barriers for transmission to humans. There is evidence that this process is mediated by particular viral genes and their reassortment, in particular, the viral polymerase complex (PA, PB1, PB2). In this study, the ability of polymerase genes to allow reassortant viruses to cross-species barriers was

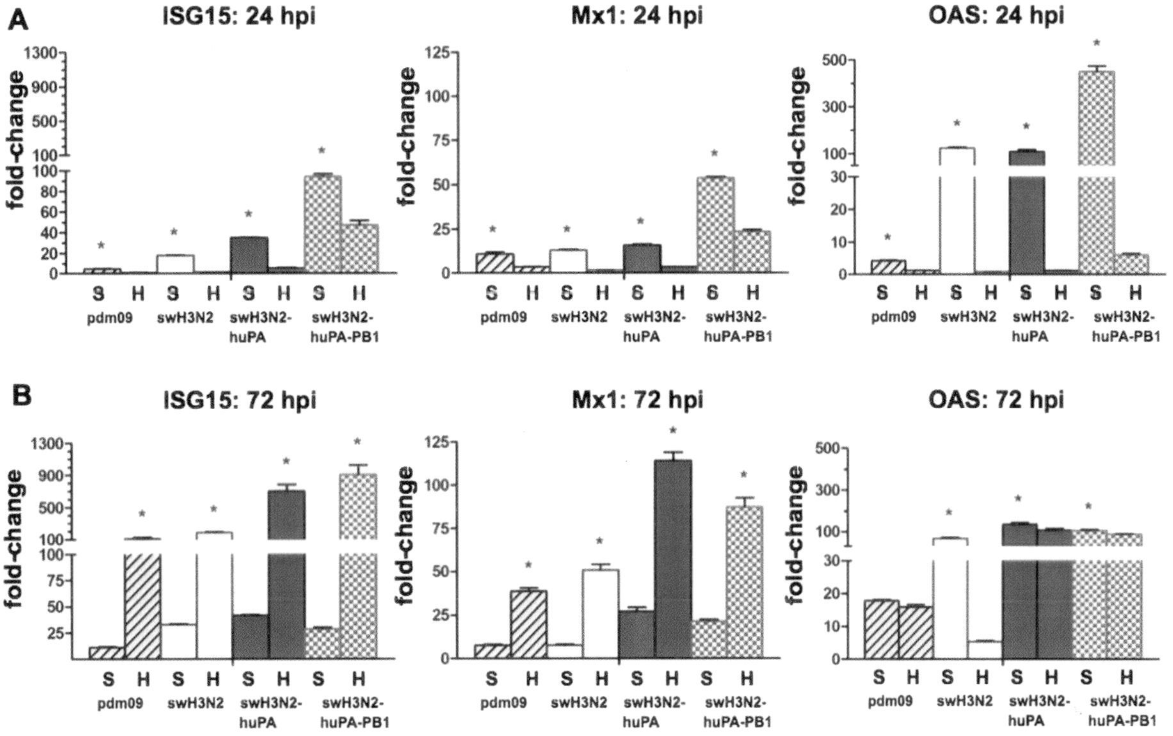

Figure 8. qPCR analysis of IFN-stimulated genes (ISGs). Expression of ISG15 (left), MX1 (middle) and OAS1 [4] was determined at (A) 24 h and (B) 72 h pi where "S" denotes swine dNSBE and "H" denotes human dNHBE cells. Fold-changes and standard deviations were calculated from Ct values run in quadruplicate relative mock and the housekeeping gene HPRT1. Time points that were significant between NSBE and NHBE cells are noted (* = $p<0.05$).

examined in normal fully-differentiated swine and human bronchoepithelial cells because the origin of most pandemic strains appears to originate in swine, which are considered 'mixing vessels'. Our results show that human-origin PA has a preferential reassortment advantage within a swine influenza virus polymerase complex, but is restricted in human but to a lesser degree in swine respiratory epithelial cells.

To identify features that contribute to viral attenuation, virulence, and novel reassortment of polymerase gene constellations, the reassortment prevalence for six gene segments was analyzed initially in PK-1 cells and subsequently in NSBE cells. The analysis revealed 33% reassortment prevalence in PK-1 cells, and 14% prevalence in NSBE cells. The true number of reassortants is possibly higher as the qPCR assay was limited to six genes, omitting PB1 and NP in the initial multiplex screen. Despite this limitation, the methods used to screen have an advantage over a reverse-genetics system as they allow comparative profiling of the reassortment prevalence after co-infection with parental strains (pdm09 and swH3N2), and is consistent with the natural reassortment of H3N2v in swine. Based on the reassortment profiles, PA, PB1, PB2 and NP from pdm09 contribute to viral fitness, whereas displacement of any of these four genes by a swine H3N2 segment counterpart is not well tolerated. In support are the findings here showing not one reassortant virus being detected having a huH1N1-swPA constellation compared to the common swH3N2-huPA constellation.

The swH3N2-huPA constellation was closely evaluated as PA is essential for polymerase function, and because of the limited knowledge regarding whether the reassortment of PA subunits with different viral origins affects species tropism. Studies examining the PA gene of pdm09 within a swine H3N2 architecture were also pursued based on previous studies reporting that the pdm09 PA within seven genes of highly pathogenic avian influenza (HPAI) H5N1 enabled respiratory droplet transmission in a guinea pig model and enhanced polymerase activity in humans cells [48]. Recent studies have shown that pdm09 PA can also lessen species-specific host restriction within an avian viral polymerase complex in 293T cells to expand tropism [49].

While the PA segment encodes PA-X, an immune modulator, there was no evidence of excess type I or III IFN responses to pdm09 or swH3N2 relative to swH3N2-huPA or swH3N2-huPA-PB1 response in dNHBE cells. These results suggest that pdm09 PA, and/or differences in the NS1 gene, a regulator of the host IFN response, are not exclusively responsible for attenuation of swH3N2-huPA replication and the high levels of IFN gene expression observed. Sequencing of all parent viruses and reassortants did not reveal any genetic mutations to PA and NS segments. It should be noted that the IAV polymerase complex can inhibit activation of the IFNβ promoter independent of NS1 function [50]. It is conceivable that an all-inclusive polymerase cassette of PA, PB1 and PB2 from swH3N2, or pdm09 may be needed to optimally replicate in dNHBE cells without triggering a robust IFN response. pdm09-PA and swH3N2-PB1 and -PB2 polymerase constellations in swH3N2-huPA may conceivably be tolerated to a greater extent in dNSBE cells but not dNHBE cells. Alternatively, acquisition of PB1 in the form of swH3N2-huPA-PB1 may not be tolerated in both swine dNSBE and human dNHBE cells.

In summary, IAV polymerase segments appear to contribute to both reassortment and viral fitness by promoting adaption to cross-species barriers of replication. Changes that affect the host range affect pandemic potential. Based on the findings from this study and others [48], it is clear that pdm09 PA reduces the barrier to species-specific host restriction particularly for the swine pdm09 PA reassortant (swH3N2-huPA). Potential differences in expression of α2–3 or α2–6 sias did not account for the attenuated replication phenotype of swH3N2-huPA or parent virus replication in dNHBE and dNSBE cells. Reassortant or parental virus infection of dNHBE cells was characterized by a pronounced type I and III IFN and ISG antiviral response, while attenuation of virus replication was not evident in the swine-derived dNSBE cells. These findings indicate that differences in the type I and III IFN response dictates in large part cross-species barriers to infection of reassortant viruses. Additionally, the discrepancy between increased lung pathology in ferrets infected with swH3N2-huPA, but apparent attenuation of replication in human cells, is intriguing and suggests additional studies are needed to determine which of these two systems may be translationally more informative. Nonetheless, the studies reported here provide a framework for understanding pandemic potential and host cell features that affect influenza virus reassortment in humans and swine.

Supporting Information

Figure S1 Primer and probe sequences used in multiplex qPCR and SYBR green qPCR to determine parent viral segments during reassortment studies. Noted in primer sequence is the following: IAbRQsp: Iowa Black Quencher short wavelength emission; IABFQ: Iowa Black far wavelength emission; ZEN: Zen Quencher; Probe: denotes same probe used for both virus gene segments due to high sequence similarity within amplified region, SYBR: SYBR Green qPCR assay used to discern PB1 and NP gene segments of select assortments.

Figure S2 qPCR multiplex for determining A/Sw/PA/62170-1/2010 [taxid: 938271] and A/California/04/2009 [taxid: 641501] genome segments. A). Plaques were analyzed in one of two 3-plex qPCR assays for each virus to deduce reassortment trends for 6 of the 8 genome segments. qPCR multi-plex dCT values, shown in bold font reveal specificity for 3-plex qPCR assay. See Fig. S1 for specified primer-probe sequences.

Figure S3 Immunofluorescence analysis of swH3N2-huPA and pdm09 viruses at 48h pi in dNHBE cells. These studies show attenuation of viral spread in dNHBE cells following a starting MOI = 0.01. Blue: DAPI, Green: Influenza NP, Red: α2–6 sialic acid, and merged panels, shown at (A) 20× and (B) 40× magnified view.

Acknowledgments

We thank Geraldine Saavedra for sequencing, and Bianca Stewart for assistance in RNA extraction and qPCR analysis. Swine H3N2 virus was kindly provided by Dr. Sabrina Swenson at the National Veterinary Services Laboratory.

Author Contributions

Conceived and designed the experiments: JP DD RAT SMT. Performed the experiments: JP DD JG CL TN. Analyzed the data: JP DD SMT RAT. Contributed reagents/materials/analysis tools: JP DD SMT RAT. Wrote the paper: JP DD SMT RAT.

References

1. Crisci E, Mussa T, Fraile L, Montoya M (2013) Review: influenza virus in pigs. Mol Immunol 55: 200–211.
2. Krueger WS, Gray GC (2013) Swine influenza virus infections in man. Curr Top Microbiol Immunol 370: 201–225.
3. Ma W, Lager KM, Vincent AL, Janke BH, Gramer MR, et al. (2009) The role of swine in the generation of novel influenza viruses. Zoonoses Public Health 56: 326–337.
4. Shu LL, Lin YP, Wright SM, Shortridge KF, Webster RG (1994) Evidence for interspecies transmission and reassortment of influenza A viruses in pigs in southern China. Virology 202: 825–833.
5. Kida H, Ito T, Yasuda J, Shimizu Y, Itakura C, et al. (1994) Potential for transmission of avian influenza viruses to pigs. J Gen Virol 75 (Pt 9): 2183–2188.
6. Ma W, Lager KM, Lekcharoensuk P, Ulery ES, Janke BH, et al. (2010) Viral reassortment and transmission after co-infection of pigs with classical H1N1 and triple-reassortant H3N2 swine influenza viruses. J Gen Virol 91: 2314–2321.
7. Zhou NN, Senne DA, Landgraf JS, Swenson SL, Erickson G, et al. (1999) Genetic reassortment of avian, swine, and human influenza A viruses in American pigs. Journal of virology 73: 8851–8856.
8. Ma W, Lager KM, Lekcharoensuk P, Ulery ES, Janke BH, et al. (2010) Viral reassortment and transmission after co-infection of pigs with classical H1N1 and triple-reassortant H3N2 swine influenza viruses. The Journal of general virology 91: 2314–2321.
9. Smith GJ, Vijaykrishna D, Bahl J, Lycett SJ, Worobey M, et al. (2009) Origins and evolutionary genomics of the 2009 swine-origin H1N1 influenza A epidemic. Nature 459: 1122–1125.
10. CDC (2013) Update: influenza activity - United States, September 29-December 7, 2013. MMWR Morb Mortal Wkly Rep 62: 1032–1036.
11. Howden KJ, Brockhoff EJ, Caya FD, McLeod LJ, Lavoie M, et al. (2009) An investigation into human pandemic influenza virus (H1N1) 2009 on an Alberta swine farm. The Canadian veterinary journal La revue veterinaire canadienne 50: 1153–1161.
12. Nelson MI, Vincent AL, Kitikoon P, Holmes EC, Gramer MR (2012) Evolution of novel reassortant A/H3N2 influenza viruses in North American swine and humans, 2009–2011. Journal of virology 86: 8872–8878.
13. Kitikoon P, Nelson MI, Killian ML, Anderson TK, Koster L, et al. (2013) Genotype patterns of contemporary reassorted H3N2 virus in US swine. The Journal of general virology 94: 1236–1241.
14. Ali A, Khatri M, Wang L, Saif YM, Lee CW (2012) Identification of swine H1N2/pandemic H1N1 reassortant influenza virus in pigs, United States. Veterinary microbiology 158: 60–68.
15. Charoenvisal N, Keawcharoen J, Sreta D, Chaiyawong S, Nonthabenjawan N, et al. (2013) Genetic characterization of Thai swine influenza viruses after the introduction of pandemic H1N1 2009. Virus genes.
16. Vijaykrishna D, Poon LL, Zhu HC, Ma SK, Li OT, et al. (2010) Reassortment of pandemic H1N1/2009 influenza A virus in swine. Science 328: 1529.
17. Matsuu A, Uchida Y, Takemae N, Mawatari T, Yoneyama SK, et al. (2012) Genetic characterization of swine influenza viruses isolated in Japan between 2009 and 2012. Microbiology and immunology 56: 792–803.
18. Harder TC, Grosse Beilage E, Lange E, Meiners C, Dohring S, et al. (2013) Expanded co-circulation of stable subtypes, emerging lineages and new sporadic reassortants of porcine influenza viruses in swine populations in Northwest Germany. Journal of virology.
19. Detmer S, Gramer M, Goyal S, Torremorell M, Torrison J (2013) Diagnostics and surveillance for Swine influenza. Curr Top Microbiol Immunol 370: 85–112.
20. Shu B, Garten R, Emery S, Balish A, Cooper L, et al. (2012) Genetic analysis and antigenic characterization of swine origin influenza viruses isolated from humans in the United States, 1990–2010. Virology 422: 151–160.
21. Cox CM, Neises D, Garten RJ, Bryant B, Hesse RA, et al. (2011) Swine influenza virus A (H3N2) infection in human, Kansas, USA, 2009. Emerging infectious diseases 17: 1143–1144.
22. Olsen CW, Karasin AI, Carman S, Li Y, Bastien N, et al. (2006) Triple reassortant H3N2 influenza A viruses, Canada, 2005. Emerging infectious diseases 12: 1132–1135.
23. CDC (2011) Swine-origin influenza A (H3N2) virus infection in two children–Indiana and Pennsylvania, July-August 2011. MMWR Morbidity and mortality weekly report 60: 1213–1215.
24. Jhung MA, Epperson S, Biggerstaff M, Allen D, Balish A, et al. (2013) Outbreak of variant influenza A(H3N2) virus in the United States. Clin Infect Dis 57: 1703–1712.
25. Biggerstaff M, Reed C, Epperson S, Jhung MA, Gambhir M, et al. (2013) Estimates of the Number of Human Infections With Influenza A(H3N2) Variant Virus, United States, August 2011–April 2012. Clinical infectious diseases: an official publication of the Infectious Diseases Society of America 57 Suppl 1: S12–15.
26. Kitikoon P, Nelson MI, Killian ML, Anderson TK, Koster L, et al. (2013) Genotype patterns of contemporary reassorted H3N2 virus in US swine. J Gen Virol 94: 1236–1241.
27. Campbell PJ, Danzy S, Kyriakis CS, Deymier MJ, Lowen AC, et al. (2014) The M segment of the 2009 pandemic influenza virus confers increased NA activity,

filamentous morphology and efficient contact transmissibility to A/Puerto Rico/8/1934-based reassortant viruses. J Virol.
28. Chou YY, Albrecht RA, Pica N, Lowen AC, Richt JA, et al. (2011) The M segment of the 2009 new pandemic H1N1 influenza virus is critical for its high transmission efficiency in the guinea pig model. J Virol 85: 11235–11241.
29. Garten RJ, Davis CT, Russell CA, Shu B, Lindstrom S, et al. (2009) Antigenic and genetic characteristics of swine-origin 2009 A(H1N1) influenza viruses circulating in humans. Science 325: 197–201.
30. Hauser MJ, Dlugolenski D, Culhane MR, Wentworth DE, Tompkins SM, et al. (2013) Antiviral responses by Swine primary bronchoepithelial cells are limited compared to human bronchoepithelial cells following influenza virus infection. PloS one 8: e70251.
31. Kitikoon P, Vincent AL, Gauger PC, Schlink SN, Bayles DO, et al. (2012) Pathogenicity and transmission in pigs of the novel A(H3N2)v influenza virus isolated from humans and characterization of swine H3N2 viruses isolated in 2010–2011. Journal of virology 86: 6804–6814.
32. Dias A, Bouvier D, Crepin T, McCarthy AA, Hart DJ, et al. (2009) The cap-snatching endonuclease of influenza virus polymerase resides in the PA subunit. Nature 458: 914–918.
33. Yuan P, Bartlam M, Lou Z, Chen S, Zhou J, et al. (2009) Crystal structure of an avian influenza polymerase PA(N) reveals an endonuclease active site. Nature 458: 909–913.
34. Jagger BW, Wise HM, Kash JC, Walters KA, Wills NM, et al. (2012) An overlapping protein-coding region in influenza A virus segment 3 modulates the host response. Science 337: 199–204.
35. Desmet EA, Bussey KA, Stone R, Takimoto T (2013) Identification of the N-terminal domain of the influenza virus PA responsible for the suppression of host protein synthesis. J Virol 87: 3108–3118.
36. Manz B, Schwemmle M, Brunotte L (2013) Adaptation of avian influenza A virus polymerase in mammals to overcome the host species barrier. J Virol 87: 7200–7209.
37. Smith JH, Nagy T, Driskell E, Brooks P, Tompkins SM, et al. (2011) Comparative pathology in ferrets infected with H1N1 influenza A viruses isolated from different hosts. Journal of virology 85: 7572–7581.
38. Matrosovich M, Matrosovich T, Garten W, Klenk HD (2006) New low-viscosity overlay medium for viral plaque assays. Virology journal 3: 63.
39. Oshansky CM, Pickens JA, Bradley KC, Jones LP, Saavedra-Ebner GM, et al. (2011) Avian influenza viruses infect primary human bronchial epithelial cells unconstrained by sialic acid alpha2,3 residues. PloS one 6: e21183.
40. Potter CW, Oxford JS (1979) Determinants of immunity to influenza infection in man. British medical bulletin 35: 69–75.
41. Smith JH, Nagy T, Driskell E, Brooks P, Tompkins SM, et al. (2011) Comparative pathology in ferrets infected with H1N1 influenza A viruses isolated from different hosts. J Virol 85: 7572–7581.
42. Villenave R, Thavagnanam S, Sarlang S, Parker J, Douglas I, et al. (2012) In vitro modeling of respiratory syncytial virus infection of pediatric bronchial epithelium, the primary target of infection in vivo. Proc Natl Acad Sci U S A 109: 5040–5045.
43. Kogure T, Suzuki T, Takahashi T, Miyamoto D, Hidari KI, et al. (2006) Human trachea primary epithelial cells express both sialyl(alpha2–3)Gal receptor for human parainfluenza virus type 1 and avian influenza viruses, and sialyl(alpha2–6)Gal receptor for human influenza viruses. Glycoconj J 23: 101–106.
44. Chan RW, Yuen KM, Yu WC, Ho CC, Nicholls JM, et al. (2010) Influenza H5N1 and H1N1 virus replication and innate immune responses in bronchial epithelial cells are influenced by the state of differentiation. PloS one 5: e8713.
45. Durbin RK, Kotenko SV, Durbin JE (2013) Interferon induction and function at the mucosal surface. Immunol Rev 255: 25–39.
46. Sang Y, Rowland RR, Blecha F (2010) Molecular characterization and antiviral analyses of porcine type III interferons. J Interferon Cytokine Res 30: 801–807.
47. Sadler AJ, Williams BR (2008) Interferon-inducible antiviral effectors. Nat Rev Immunol 8: 559–568.
48. Zhang Y, Zhang Q, Kong H, Jiang Y, Gao Y, et al. (2013) H5N1 hybrid viruses bearing 2009/H1N1 virus genes transmit in guinea pigs by respiratory droplet. Science 340: 1459–1463.
49. Bussey KA, Desmet EA, Mattiacio JL, Hamilton A, Bradel-Tretheway B, et al. (2011) PA residues in the 2009 H1N1 pandemic influenza virus enhance avian influenza virus polymerase activity in mammalian cells. J Virol 85: 7020–7028.
50. Iwai A, Shiozaki T, Kawai T, Akira S, Kawaoka Y, et al. (2010) Influenza A virus polymerase inhibits type I interferon induction by binding to interferon beta promoter stimulator 1. J Biol Chem 285: 32064–32074.

Permissions

All chapters in this book were first published in PLOS ONE, by The Public Library of Science; hereby published with permission under the Creative Commons Attribution License or equivalent. Every chapter published in this book has been scrutinized by our experts. Their significance has been extensively debated. The topics covered herein carry significant findings which will fuel the growth of the discipline. They may even be implemented as practical applications or may be referred to as a beginning point for another development.

The contributors of this book come from diverse backgrounds, making this book a truly international effort. This book will bring forth new frontiers with its revolutionizing research information and detailed analysis of the nascent developments around the world.

We would like to thank all the contributing authors for lending their expertise to make the book truly unique. They have played a crucial role in the development of this book. Without their invaluable contributions this book wouldn't have been possible. They have made vital efforts to compile up to date information on the varied aspects of this subject to make this book a valuable addition to the collection of many professionals and students.

This book was conceptualized with the vision of imparting up-to-date information and advanced data in this field. To ensure the same, a matchless editorial board was set up. Every individual on the board went through rigorous rounds of assessment to prove their worth. After which they invested a large part of their time researching and compiling the most relevant data for our readers.

The editorial board has been involved in producing this book since its inception. They have spent rigorous hours researching and exploring the diverse topics which have resulted in the successful publishing of this book. They have passed on their knowledge of decades through this book. To expedite this challenging task, the publisher supported the team at every step. A small team of assistant editors was also appointed to further simplify the editing procedure and attain best results for the readers.

Apart from the editorial board, the designing team has also invested a significant amount of their time in understanding the subject and creating the most relevant covers. They scrutinized every image to scout for the most suitable representation of the subject and create an appropriate cover for the book.

The publishing team has been an ardent support to the editorial, designing and production team. Their endless efforts to recruit the best for this project, has resulted in the accomplishment of this book. They are a veteran in the field of academics and their pool of knowledge is as vast as their experience in printing. Their expertise and guidance has proved useful at every step. Their uncompromising quality standards have made this book an exceptional effort. Their encouragement from time to time has been an inspiration for everyone.

The publisher and the editorial board hope that this book will prove to be a valuable piece of knowledge for researchers, students, practitioners and scholars across the globe.

List of Contributors

B. David Persson and Aron B. Jaffe
Developmental and Molecular Pathways, Novartis Institutes for BioMedical Research, Cambridge, Massachusetts, United States of America

Rachel Fearns
Department of Microbiology, Boston University School of Medicine, Boston, Massachusetts, United States of America

Henry Danahay
Respiratory Disease Area, Novartis Institutes for BioMedical Research, Horsham, United Kingdom

Youhui Si, Jianguo Li, Yuqiang Niu, Xiuying Liu, Lili Ren, Li Guo, Min Cheng, Hongli Zhou, Jianwei Wang, Qi Jin and Wei Yang
Ministry of Health Key Laboratory of Systems Biology of Pathogens, Institute of Pathogen Biology, Chinese Academy of Medical Sciences and Peking Union Medical College, Beijing, China

Daan de Gouw, Marien I. de Jonge, Peter W. M. Hermans, Aldert Zomer, Alinda Berends and Dimitri A. Diavatopoulos
Laboratory of Pediatric Infectious Diseases, Department of Pediatrics, Radboud University Medical Centre, Nijmegen, The Netherlands
Laboratory of Medical Immunology, Department of Laboratory Medicine, Radboud University Medical Centre, Nijmegen, The Netherlands

Frits R. Mooi
Laboratory of Pediatric Infectious Diseases, Department of Pediatrics, Radboud University Medical Centre, Nijmegen, The Netherlands
Laboratory of Medical Immunology, Department of Laboratory Medicine, Radboud University Medical Centre, Nijmegen, The Netherlands
Netherlands Centre for Infectious Disease Control, National Institute for Public Health and the Environment (RIVM), Bilthoven, The Netherlands

Hans J. C. T. Wessels
Nijmegen Centre for Mitochondrial Disorders, Department of Laboratory Medicine, Radboud Proteomics Centre, Radboud University Medical Centre, Nijmegen, The Netherlands

Guy A. Berbers
Netherlands Centre for Infectious Disease Control, National Institute for Public Health and the Environment (RIVM), Bilthoven, The Netherlands

Catherine Pratt
Public Health England, Centre for Emergency Preparedness and Response, Porton Down, Salisbury, United Kingdom

Benjawan Khuntirat, In-Kyu Yoon, Robert V. Gibbons and Darunee Buddhari
Department of Virology, Armed Forces Research Institute of Medical Sciences, Bangkok, Thailand

Malinee Chittaganpitch, Krongkaew Supawat and Pathom Sawanpanyalert
National Institute of Health, Ministry of Public Health, Nonthaburi, Thailand

Whitney S. Krueger, Gary L. Heil, John A. Friary and Gregory C. Gray
College of Public Health and Health Professions and Emerging Pathogens Institute, University of Florida, Gainesville, Florida, United States of America

Patrick J. Blair
Naval Medical Research Center - Asia, Singapore, Singapore

Shannon D. Putnam
Naval Health Research Center, San Diego, California, United States of America

Sven Brandau, Kirsten Bruderek and Stephan Lang
Department of Otorhinolaryngology, University Hospital Essen, Essen, Germany

Mark Jakob and Friedrich Bootz
Department of Otorhinolaryngology, University Hospital Bonn, Bonn, Germany

Bernd Giebel and Stefan Radtke
Institute of Transfusion Medicine, University Hospital Essen, Essen, Germany

Katharina Mauel, Marcus Jäger and Stefanie B. Flohé
Surgical Research, Department of Trauma Surgery, University Hospital Essen, Essen, Germany

Gideon W. Blumstein, Arya Parsa, Anthony K. Park, Beverly L. P. McDowell, Melissa Arroyo-Mendoza, Marie Girguis, Jill P. Adler-Moore, Jon Olson and Nancy E. Buckley
Department of Biological Sciences, California State Polytechnic University, Pomona, California, United States of America

Jean-Michel Sallenave
University of Edinburgh, Medical School, Edinburgh, Scotland, United Kingdom

Thomas I. Brown
University of Edinburgh, Medical School, Edinburgh, Scotland, United Kingdom
The Roslin Institute and R(D)SVS, The University of Edinburgh, Easter Bush Veterinary Centre, Roslin, Midlothian, United Kingdom

David S. Collie, Darren J. Shaw and Nina M. Rzechorzek
The Roslin Institute and R(D)SVS, The University of Edinburgh, Easter Bush Veterinary Centre, Roslin, Midlothian, United Kingdom

Yohannes Adama Melaku, Berhe Weldearegawi Sahle, Fisaha Haile Tesfay, Afework Mulugeta Bezabih, Alemseged Aregay and Semaw Ferede Abera
Department of Public Health, College of Health Sciences, Mekelle University, Mekelle, Ethiopia

Loko Abreha
School of Medicine, College of Health Sciences, Mekelle University, Mekelle, Ethiopia

Gordon Alexander Zello
College of Pharmacy and Nutrition, University of Saskatchewan, Saskatoon, Canada

Lai-Giea Seng, Janet Daly, Kin-Chow Chang and Suresh V. Kuchipudi
School of Veterinary Medicine and Science, University of Nottingham, Sutton Bonington Campus, Leicestershire, United Kingdom

Sven Schmiedl and Petra Thürmann
Department of Clinical Pharmacology, School of Medicine, Faculty of Health, Witten/Herdecke University, Witten, Germany
Philipp Klee-Institute for Clinical Pharmacology, HELIOS Clinic Wuppertal, Wuppertal, Germany

Rainald Fischer
Pneumologische Praxis München-Pasing, Munich, Germany

Luisa Ibáñez
Fundació Institut Catalàde Farmacologia, Hospital Universitari Vall d'Hebron, Barcelona, Spain
Departament de Farmacologia, Terapèutica i Toxicologia, Universitat Autònoma de Barcelona, Barcelona, Spain

Joan Fortuny
Novartis Farmaceutica S.A., Barcelona, Spain

Olaf H. Klungel
Utrecht Institute for Pharmaceutical Sciences, Division Pharmacoepidemiology and Clinical Pharmacology, Utrecht University, Utrecht, the Netherlands

Robert Reynolds
Epidemiology, Pfizer, New York, New York, United States of America

Roman Gerlach and Martin Tauscher
National Association of Statutory Health Insurance Physicians of Bavaria, Munich, Germany

Joerg Hasford and Marietta Rottenkolber
Institute for Medical Information Sciences, Biometry, and Epidemiology, Ludwig-Maximilians-Universitaet, Munich, Germany

Stefan Schilling
Department for Internal Medicine, Staedtische Kliniken Moenchengladbach, Moenchengladbach, Germany

Francesco Maria Fusco, Vincenzo Puro and Giuseppe Ippolito
Department for Infectious Diseases, National Institute for Infectious Diseases "Lazarro Spallanzani", Rome, Italy

Giuseppina De Iaco
Department for Internal Medicine, Azienda Ospedaliero, Universitaria Ospedali Riuniti delle Marche, Torrette, Italy

Barbara Bannister
Department for Infectious Diseases, The Royal Free Hospital, London, United Kingdom

Helena C. Maltezou
Department for Interventions in Health-Care Facilities, Hellenic Center for Disease Control and Prevention, Athens, Greece

Gail Carson
Department of Rare and Imported Pathogens, Health Protection Agency, Porton, United Kingdom

Rene Gottschalk
Department for Infectious Diseases, Port Health Authorities, Frankfurt am Main, Germany

Hans-Reinhard Brodt
Department for Infectious Diseases, Goethe University Frankfurt, Frankfurt am Main, Germany

Philippe Brouqui
Department for Infectious Diseases and Tropical Medicine, Marseilles University, Marseille, France

Paul Schnitzler
Department of Infectious Diseases, Virology, University of Heidelberg, Heidelberg, Germany

Julia Tabatabai
Department of Infectious Diseases, Virology, University of Heidelberg, Heidelberg, Germany
London School of Hygiene and Tropical Medicine, London, United Kingdom

Christiane Prifert
Institute of Virology and Immunobiology, University of Würzburg, Würzburg, Germany

Jürgen Grulich-Henn
Department of Pediatrics, University of Heidelberg, Heidelberg, Germany

Johannes Pfeil
Department of Pediatrics, University of Heidelberg, Heidelberg, Germany
German Centre for Infectious Diseases (DZIF), Heidelberg, Germany

Juan Wang, Karin Engvall, Greta Smedje and Dan Norbäck
Department of Medical Sciences, Uppsala University and University Hospital, Uppsala, Sweden

John Lusingu, Allvan Butichi, Paminus Lushino and Martha Lemnge
Korogwe Research Laboratory, National Institute for Medical Research, Tanga, Tanzania

Coline Mahende
Korogwe Research Laboratory, National Institute for Medical Research, Tanga, Tanzania
Department of Medical Entomology and Parasitology, School of Public Health, Muhimbili University of Health and Allied Sciences, Dar es Salaam, Tanzania

Billy Ngasala and Zul Premji
Department of Medical Entomology and Parasitology, School of Public Health, Muhimbili University of Health and Allied Sciences, Dar es Salaam, Tanzania

Julien Hiblot, Hubert Lepidi, Jean-Marc Rolain, Didier Raoult, Janek Bzdrenga, Fabienne Bregeon and Eric Chabriere
Unité de Recherche sur les Maladies Infectieuses et Tropicales Emergentes, UMR CNRS-IRD 6236, IFR48, Aix-Marseille Université, Marseille, France

Sami Hraiech and Laurent Papazian
Unité de Recherche sur les Maladies Infectieuses et Tropicales Emergentes, UMR CNRS-IRD 6236, IFR48, Aix-Marseille Université, Marseille, France
Réanimation - Détresses Respiratoires et Infections Sévères, APHM, CHU Nord, Marseille, France

Mark W. Silby
Department of Biology, University of Massachusetts Dartmouth, Dartmouth, Massachusetts, United States of America

John Lafleur
Department of Biology, University of Massachusetts Dartmouth, Dartmouth, Massachusetts, United States of America
Department of Emergency Medicine, Alpert School of Medicine, Providence, Rhode Island, United States of America

Mikael Elias
Weizmann Institute of Science, Biological Chemistry, Rehovot, Israel

Susan J. Pizzutto
Menzies School of Health Research, Charles Darwin University, Brinkin, Northern Territory, Australia

Stephanie T. Yerkovich
Menzies School of Health Research, Charles Darwin University, Brinkin, Northern Territory, Australia
Queensland Lung Transplant Service, The Prince Charles Hospital, Chermside, Queensland, Australia
School of Medicine, The University of Queensland, St Lucia, Queensland, Australia

Anne B. Chang
Menzies School of Health Research, Charles Darwin University, Brinkin, Northern Territory, Australia
The Department of Respiratory Medicine, Royal Children's Hospital, Herston, Queensland, Australia
Queensland Children's Medical Research Institute, Royal Children's Hospital, Herston, Queensland, Australia

John W. Upham
School of Medicine, The University of Queensland, St Lucia, Queensland, Australia
Department of Respiratory Medicine, Princess Alexandra Hospital, Wooloongabba, Queensland, Australia

Belinda J. Hales and Wayne R. Thomas
Telethon Kids Institute, The University of Western Australia, Crawley, Western Australia, Australia

Aurélie Francart, Sophie Lamoral and Michael Kalai
National Reference Centre of Rabies, Viral Diseases, Scientific Institute of Public Health (WIV-ISP), Brussels, Belgium

Sanne Terryn and Steven Van Gucht
National Reference Centre of Rabies, Viral Diseases, Scientific Institute of Public Health (WIV-ISP), Brussels, Belgium
Laboratory of Virology, Department of Virology, Parasitology and Immunology, Faculty of Veterinary Medicine, Ghent University, Merelbeke, Belgium

Anna Hultberg, Heidi Rommelaere, Angela Wittelsberger, Filip Callewaert, Thomas Stohr, Kris Meerschaert, Ingrid Ottevaere, Catelijne Stortelers and Peter Vanlandschoot
Ablynx NV, Gent, Belgium

Marinus C. Lamers
Max Planck Institute of Immunobiology and Epigenetics, Freiburg, Germany

Sebastian Scheer
Max Planck Institute of Immunobiology and Epigenetics, Freiburg, Germany
International Max Planck Research School of Molecular and Cellular Biology, Freiburg, Germany
University of Freiburg, Freiburg, Germany

Christine Krempl
Institute of Virology and Immunology, University of Wuerzburg, Wuerzburg, Germany

Carsten Kallfass and Peter Staeheli
Institute for Virology, Department of Medical Microbiology and Hygiene, University Medical Center Freiburg, Freiburg, Germany

Stefanie Frey and Thilo Jakob
Allergy Research Group, Department of Dermatology, University Medical Center Freiburg, Freiburg, Germany

Gabriel Mouahid
Univ. Perpignan Via Domitia, Ecologie et Evolution des Interactions, UMR 5244, F-66860, Perpignan, France

Hélène Moné
CNRS, Ecologie et Evolution des Interactions, UMR 5244, F-66860, Perpignan, France

Annette Schmitt-Gräff
Institute of Pathology, University of Freiburg, Freiburg, Germany

Pallav L. Shah
Department of Respiratory Medicine, Chelsea and Westminster Hospital National Health Service Foundation Trust, London, United Kingdom
Department of Respiratory Medicine, Royal Brompton and Harefield Hospitals National Health Service Foundation Trust, London, United Kingdom

Athol U. Wells
Department of Respiratory Medicine, Royal Brompton and Harefield Hospitals National Health Service Foundation Trust, London, United Kingdom

Deborah H. Strickland, Vanessa Fear, Mathew E. Wikstrom and Alexander N. Larcombe
Telethon Institute for Child Health Research and Centre for Child Health Research, University of Western Australia, Perth, W.A., Australia

Seth Shenton and Philip A. Stumbles
Telethon Institute for Child Health Research and Centre for Child Health Research, University of Western Australia, Perth, W.A., Australia
School of Veterinary and Life Sciences, Murdoch University, Perth, W.A., Australia

Graeme Zosky
Telethon Institute for Child Health Research and Centre for Child Health Research, University of Western Australia, Perth, W.A., Australia
School of Medicine, University of Tasmania, Hobart, Tasmania, Australia

Patrick G. Holt
Telethon Institute for Child Health Research and Centre for Child Health Research, University of Western Australia, Perth, W.A., Australia
Queensland Children's Medical Research Institute, University of Queensland, Brisbane, Qld., Australia

Christophe von Garnier
Telethon Institute for Child Health Research and Centre for Child Health Research, University of Western Australia, Perth, W.A., Australia
Pulmonary Medicine, Bern University Hospital and Department of Clinical Research, Berne University, Berne, Switzerland

Cassandra Berry
School of Veterinary and Life Sciences, Murdoch University, Perth, W.A., Australia

Yíngyún Caì, Shuǐqìng Yú, Elena N. Postnikova, Steven Mazur, John G. Bernbaum, Robin Burk, Téngfēi Zhāng, Laura Bollinger, Lisa E. Hensley, Peter B. Jahrling and Jens H. Kuhn
Integrated Research Facility at Fort Detrick, National Institute of Allergy and Infectious Diseases, National Institutes of Health, Fort Detrick, Frederick, Maryland, United States of America

Sheli R. Radoshitzky
United States Army Medical Research Institute of Infectious Diseases, Fort Detrick, Frederick, Maryland, United States of America

Marcel A. Müller
Institute of Virology, University of Bonn Medical Centre, Bonn, Germany

Ingo Jordan
Pro Bio Gen AG, Berlin, Germany

Daniel J. Smith and David W. Reid
Department of Thoracic Medicine, The Prince Charles Hospital, Brisbane, Queensland, Australia
School of Medicine, University of Queensland, Brisbane, Queensland, Australia
Infection and Inflammation Laboratory, QIMR Berghofer Medical Research Institute, Brisbane, Queensland, Australia

Scott C. Bell
Department of Thoracic Medicine, The Prince Charles Hospital, Brisbane, Queensland, Australia
School of Medicine, University of Queensland, Brisbane, Queensland, Australia
Queensland Children's Medical Research Institute, Royal Children's Hospital, Brisbane, Queensland, Australia

Geoffrey R. Hill
Bone Marrow Transplant Laboratory, QIMR Berghofer Medical Research Institute, Brisbane, Queensland, Australia

Anne E. Mayer and Griffith D. Parks
Department of Microbiology and Immunology, Wake Forest School of Medicine, Winston-Salem, NC 27101, United States of America

Shamir Jacobino and Jeanette H. W. Leusen
Laboratory of Translational Immunology, Immunotherapy group, UMC Utrecht, Utrecht, The Netherlands

Gerco den Hartog
Laboratory of Translational Immunology, Immunotherapy group, UMC Utrecht, Utrecht, The Netherlands
Cell Biology and Immunology, Wageningen University, Wageningen, The Netherlands

Louis Bont
Laboratory of Translational Immunology, Immunotherapy group, UMC Utrecht, Utrecht, The Netherlands
Department of Pediatrics, UMC Utrecht, Utrecht, The Netherlands

R. J. Joost van Neerven
Cell Biology and Immunology, Wageningen University, Wageningen, The Netherlands
Friesland Campina, Amersfoort, The Netherlands

Linda Cox
Bioceros, Utrecht, The Netherlands

Laurien H. Ulfman
FrieslandCampina, Amersfoort, The Netherlands

Mei-Ling Cheng
Department of Biomedical Sciences, College of Medicine, Chang Gung University, Tao-Yuan, Taiwan
Healthy Aging Research Center, Chang Gung University, Tao-Yuan, Taiwan
Metabolomics Core Laboratory, Chang Gung University, Tao-Yuan, Taiwan

Hung-Yao Ho
Healthy Aging Research Center, Chang Gung University, Tao-Yuan, Taiwan
Department of Medical Biotechnology and Laboratory Science, College of Medicine, Chang Gung University, Tao-Yuan, Taiwan
Office of Research and Development, Chang Gung Memorial Hospital, Tao-Yuan, Taiwan

Shiue-Fen Weng and Chih-Hao Kuo
Department of Medical Biotechnology and Laboratory Science, College of Medicine, Chang Gung University, Tao-Yuan, Taiwan

Michio Yasunami and Motoi Suzuki
Department of Clinical Medicine, Institute of Tropical Medicine, Nagasaki University, Nagasaki, Japan

Bhim Gopal Dhoubhadel and Koya Ariyoshi
Department of Clinical Medicine, Institute of Tropical Medicine, Nagasaki University, Nagasaki, Japan
Graduate School of Biomedical Sciences, Nagasaki University, Nagasaki, Japan

Duc Anh Dang, Hien Anh Thi Nguyen and Thu Huong Vu
Department of Bacteriology, National Institute of Hygiene and Epidemiology, Hanoi, Vietnam

Ai Thi Thuy Nguyen
Department of Microbiology, Khanh Hoa General Hospital, NhaTrang, Vietnam

Lay-Myint Yoshida
Department of Pediatric Infectious Diseases, Institute of Tropical Medicine, Nagasaki University, Nagasaki, Japan

Vimal Grover
Magill Department of Anaesthesia, Critical Care and Pain, Chelsea and Westminster Hospital National Health Service Foundation Trust, London, United Kingdom
Immunology Section, Department of Medicine, Imperial College, London, United Kingdom
Department of Surgery and Cancer, Imperial College, London, United Kingdom

Neil Soni
Magill Department of Anaesthesia, Critical Care and Pain, Chelsea and Westminster Hospital National Health Service Foundation Trust, London, United Kingdom
Department of Surgery and Cancer, Imperial College, London, United Kingdom

Suveer Singh
Magill Department of Anaesthesia, Critical Care and Pain, Chelsea and Westminster Hospital National Health Service Foundation Trust, London, United Kingdom
Department of Surgery and Cancer, Imperial College, London, United Kingdom
Department of Respiratory Medicine, Chelsea and Westminster Hospital National Health Service Foundation Trust, London, United Kingdom

Panagiotis Pantelidis, Don C. Henderson and Peter Kelleher
Immunology Section, Department of Medicine, Imperial College, London, United Kingdom
Department of Immunology, Imperial College Healthcare National Health Service Trust, London, United Kingdom

Masao Takata
Department of Surgery and Cancer, Imperial College, London, United Kingdom
Department of Immunology, Imperial College Healthcare National Health Service Trust, London, United Kingdom

Joshua D. Powell, Daniel Dlugolenski, Jon Gabbard, Christopher Lee, Stephen M. Tompkins and Ralph A. Tripp
Department of Infectious Diseases, Animal Health Research Center, University of Georgia, Athens, Georgia, United States of America

Tamas Nagy
Department of Pathology, College of Veterinary Medicine, University of Georgia, Athens, Georgia, United States of America

Index